FIFTH EDITION

Critical Care
Handbook of the
Massachusetts
General Hospital

FIFTH EDITION

Critical Care Handbook of the Massachusetts General Hospital

Senior Editor
Luca M. Bigatello, MD

Associate Editors
Hasan B. Alam, MD
Rae M. Allain, MD
Edward A. Bittner, MD, PhD
Dean R. Hess, PhD, RRT
Richard M. Pino, MD, PhD
Ulrich Schmidt, MD, PhD

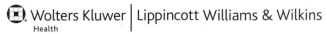 Wolters Kluwer | Lippincott Williams & Wilkins
Health

Philadelphia • Baltimore • New York • London
Buenos Aires • Hong Kong • Sydney • Tokyo

Acquisitions Editor: Frances DeStefano
Product Manager: Nicole Dernoski
Production Manager: Bridgett Dougherty
Senior Manufacturing Manager: Benjamin Rivera
Marketing Manager: Angela Panetta
Design Coordinator: Terry Mallon
Production Service: Aptara, Inc.

© 2010 by LIPPINCOTT WILLIAMS & WILKINS, a WOLTERS KLUWER business
530 Walnut Street
Philadelphia, PA 19106 USA
LWW.com

Printed in China

Library of Congress Cataloging-in-Publication Data

Critical care handbook of the Massachusetts General Hospital / senior editor,
Luca M. Bigatello ; associate editors, Hasan Alam . . . [et al.]. — 5th ed.
    p. ; cm.
  Includes bibliographical references and index.
  ISBN 978-0-7817-9566-1 (alk. paper)
  1. Critical care medicine—Handbooks, manuals, etc. I. Bigatello, Luca M. II.
Massachusetts General Hospital.
  [DNLM: 1. Critical Care—Handbooks. 2. Postoperative Complications—Handbooks.
WX 39 C934 2009]
  RC86.8C76 2009
  616.02′809744—dc22
                                                                        2009033023

To purchase additional copies of this book, call our customer service department at (800)
638-3030 or fax orders to (301) 223-2320. International customers should call (301) 223-2300.

Visit Lippincott Williams & Wilkins on the Internet: at LWW.com. Lippincott Williams &
Wilkins customer service representatives are available from 8:30 am to 6 pm, EST.

                                                            10 9 8 7 6 5 4 3 2 1

To Our Patients

PREFACE

The *Critical Care Handbook of the Massachusetts General Hospital* is a pragmatic review of the basis of adult critical care, designed for all trainees and practitioners who are interested in working in an intensive care unit (ICU). Although our practice over many years has consisted primarily of surgical patients, we always ensured that learning, teaching, and clinical plans of care be developed with a multidisciplinary approach. For this reason, this *Handbook* is authored by intensivists from anesthesia, surgery, and medicine, as well as critical care nurses, respiratory therapists, and pharmacists. Over the years, the glue that has kept this diverse faculty together has been *physiology*, because the body works the same way in patients admitted to a surgical, medical, or neurological ICU. The principles of physiology applied to critical care are illustrated in the chapters that open the *Handbook*, including hemodynamic and respiratory monitoring, acid—base, principles of mechanical ventilation, and the bases of antimicrobial therapy and nutritional support. However, as the practice of critical care evolves, we now have *evidence* from a number of well-designed trials to guide our therapeutic choices, so the *Handbook* emphasizes the evidence that exists behind our recommendations. Further progress in patient outcomes has been achieved by implementing *safety* in the ICU, where the fast pace and invasive procedures may at times hurt our patients. We have added chapters on prophylaxis of nosocomial complications, on the safe transport of critically ill patients, and on what intensivists offer outside the ICU.

As the *Handbook* has evolved over the years, its authors and its contents have changed, but part of the older information has been conserved, sometimes even verbatim. Here, we acknowledge all the authors of the past editions, many of whom have moved on to successful professional careers, and hopefully still cherish the chapters they wrote during their busy times of residency and fellowship.

Finally, as I leave this famed institution after nearly 20 years, I thank the innumerous individuals who have made our Ellison 4 Surgical ICU (and her various previous incarnations) an extraordinary place to work. First, I thank our patients and their families, who, through their suffering, have taught us about their illness, allowing us to save some of those who followed. Then, I thank our incredible staff—the nurses, doctors, respiratory therapists, unit assistants, students, and anyone of the thousands who over the years have worked in this unit, not as spectators but as protagonists of this dream.

Luca M. Bigatello

CONTRIBUTORS

Hasan B. Alam, MD
Program Director, Fellowship in Surgical Critical Care
Department of Surgery
Massachusetts General Hospital
Associate Professor of Surgery
Harvard Medical School
Boston, Massachusetts

Rae M. Allain, MD
Director, Vascular Anesthesia
Department of Anesthesia and Critical Care
Massachusetts General Hospital
Assistant Professor of Anesthesia
Harvard University
Boston, Massachusetts

Kathrin Allen, MD
Clinical Fellow in Critical Care
Department of Anesthesia and Critical Care
Massachusetts General Hospital
Harvard Medical School
Boston, Massachusetts

Theodore A. Alston, MD, PhD
Associate Anesthetist
Department of Anesthesia and Critical Care
Massachusetts General Hospital
Assistant Professor of Anesthesia
Harvard Medical School
Boston, Massachusetts

Houman Amirfarzan, MD
Resident in Anesthesiology
Anesthesia Department
Tufts New England Medical Center
Boston, Massachusetts

Emily A. Apsell, MD
Resident in Anesthesiology
Department of Anesthesia and Critical Care
Massachusetts General Hospital
Clinical Fellow in Anesthesiology
Harvard Medical School
Boston, Massachusetts

Aranya Bagchi, MD
Resident in Anesthesiology
Department of Anesthesia and Critical Care
Massachusetts General Hospital
Clinical Fellow in Anesthesia
Harvard Medical School
Boston, Massachusetts

Karsten Bartels, MD
Resident in Anesthesiology
Department of Anesthesia and Critical Care
Massachusetts General Hospital
Clinical Fellow in Anesthesia
Harvard Medical School
Boston, Massachusetts

William J. Benedetto, MD
Assistant in Anesthesia
Massachusetts General Hospital
Instructor in Anesthesia
Harvard Medical School
Boston, Massachusetts

Lorenzo Berra, MD
Resident in Anesthesiology and Beecher Research Scholar
Department of Anesthesia and Critical Care
Massachusetts General Hospital
Harvard Medical School
Boston, Massachusetts

Luca M. Bigatello, MD
Chief, Anesthesia and Critical Care Service
Veterans Administration Boston Healthcare System
Associate Vice Chairman
Massachusetts General Hospital
Associate Professor of Anesthesia
Harvard Medical School
Boston, Massachusetts

Edward A. Bittner, MD, PhD
Program Director, Anesthesia-Critical Care Fellowship
Department of Anesthesia and Critical Care
Massachusetts General Hospital
Instructor in Anesthesia
Harvard Medical School
Boston, Massachusetts

Ross Blank, MD
Clinical Lecturer
Division of Critical Care
Department of Anesthesiology
University of Michigan Health System
Ann Arbor, Michigan

Jonathan D. Bloom, MD
Resident in Anesthesiology
Department of Anesthesia and Critical Care
Massachusetts General Hospital
Clinical Fellow in Anesthesia
Harvard Medical School
Boston, Massachusetts

Sharon E. Brackett, RN, BS
Staff Nurse, Surgical ICU
Massachusetts General Hospital
Boston, Massachusetts

Jonathan E. Charnin, MD
Assistant in Anesthesia
Department of Anesthesia and Critical care
Massachusetts General Hospital
Instructor in Anesthesia
Harvard Medical School
Boston, Massachusetts

Sherry Chou
Staff Physician
Department of Neurology
Brigham and Women's Hospital
Instructor
Harvard Medical School
Boston, Massachusetts

Claudia Crimi
Research Fellow
Department of Anesthesia and Critical Care
Massachusetts General Hospital
Harvard Medical School
Boston, Massachusetts

Ettore Crimi, MD
Resident in Anesthesiology
Department of Anesthesia and Critical Care
Massachusetts General Hospital
Harvard Medical School
Boston, Massachusetts

Marc A. de Moya, MD, FACS
Director of Surgical Core Clerkship
Department of Surgery
Massachusetts General Hospital
Assistant Professor of Surgery
Harvard Medical School
Boston, Massachusetts

Alan DiBiasio, RPh
Senior Attending Pharmacist
Department of Pharmacy
Massachusetts General Hospital
Boston, Massachusetts

Anahat Dhillon, MD
Staff Anesthesiologist
Department of Anesthesiology
Ronald Regan Medical Center
Assistant Professor
University of California Los Angeles
Los Angeles, California

Michael G. Fitzsimons, MD
Operations Director, Cardiac Anesthesia
Department of Anesthesia and Critical Care
Massachusetts General Hospital
Assistant Professor of Anesthesia
Harvard Medical School
Boston, Massachusetts

Jonathan Frederick Fox, MD
Clinical Fellow in Critical Care
Department of Anesthesia and Critical Care
Harvard Medical School
Massachusetts General Hospital
Boston, Massachusetts

Eugene Y. Fukudome, MD
Clinical Fellow in Surgery
Department of Surgery
Harvard Medical School
Massachusetts General Hospital
Boston, Massachusetts

Henning A. Gaissert, MD
Associate Visiting Surgeon
Division of Thoracic Surgery
Massachusetts General Hospital
Associate Professor of Surgery
Harvard Medical School
Boston, Massachusetts

Cosmin Gauran, MD
Staff Anesthesiologist
Department of Anesthesia and Critical Care
Massachusetts General Hospital
Instructor in Anesthesia
Harvard Medical School
Boston, Massachusetts

Edward E. George, MD, PhD
Medical Director
Post Anesthesia Care Units
Massachusetts General Hospital
Assistant Professor of Anesthesia
Harvard Medical School
Boston, Massachusetts

Fiona K. Gibbons, MD
Assistant in Medicine
Pulmonary and Critical Care Unit
Massachusetts General Hospital
Instructor in Medicine
Harvard Medical School
Boston, Massachusetts

Jeremy W. Goldfarb, MD
Resident in Anesthesiology
Department of Anesthesia and Critical Care
Harvard Medical School
Massachusetts General Hospital
Boston, Massachusetts

Robert L. Goulet, MS, RRT
Senior Respiratory Therapist
Respiratory Care Services
Massachusetts General Hospital
Boston, Massachusetts

David M. Greer, MD, MA
Assistant in Neurology
Department of Neurology
Massachusetts General Hospital
Assistant Professor of Neurology
Harvard Medical School
Boston, Massachusetts

Robin K. Guillory, MD
Assistant Professor of Anesthesiology
Department of Anesthesiology
Washington University in St. Louis School of Medicine
St. Louis, Missouri

Robert Hallisey, MS, RPh
Director, Clinical Systems
Department of Pharmacy
Massachusetts General Hospital
Assistant Professor of Clinical Pharmacy
Massachusetts College of Pharmacy and Health Sciences
Boston, Massachusetts

Bishr Haydar, MD
Resident in Anesthesiology
Department of Anesthesia and Critical Care
Massachusetts General Hospital
Boston, Massachusetts

Judith Hellman
Department of Anesthesia and Perioperative Care
Associate Professor
University of California, San Francisco
San Francisco, California

Dean R. Hess, PhD, RRT
Assistant Director
Respiratory Care Services
Associate Professor of Anesthesia
Harvard Medical School
Boston, Massachusetts

Daniel W. Johnson, MD
Clinical Fellow in Critical Care
Department of Anesthesia and Critical Care
Massachusetts General Hospital
Harvard Medical School
Boston, Massachusetts

Kathryn Davis Kalafatas, RPh
Senior Attending Pharmacist
Department of Pharmacy
Massachusetts General Hospital
Boston, Massachusetts

Erik B. Kistler, MD, PhD
Assistant Professor
Department of Anesthesia
University of California, San Diego
San Diego, California

Corry "Jeb" Kucik, MD
Clinical Fellow in Critical Care
Department of Anesthesia and Critical Care
Massachusetts General Hospital
Instructor in Anesthesia
Harvard Medical School
Boston, Massachusetts

Jean Kwo, MD
Director, Pre-Admission Testing Clinic
Department of Anesthesia and Critical Care
Massachusetts General Hospital
Assistant Professor in Anesthesia
Harvard Medical School
Boston, Massachusetts

Laura H. Leduc, MD
Resident in Anesthesiology
Department of Anesthesia and Critical Care
Harvard Medical School
Massachusetts General Hospital
Boston, Massachusetts

Nicolas Melo
Resident in Surgery
Department of Surgery
Harvard Medical School
Massachusetts General Hospital
Boston, Massachusetts

Beverly J. Newhouse, MD
Instructor in Anesthesia and Critical Care
Department of Anesthesia and Critical Care
Massachusetts General Hospital
Clinical Instructor in Anesthesiology
Harvard Medical School
Boston, Massachusetts

Ara Nozari, MD, PhD
Instructor in Anesthesia
Department of Anesthesia and Critical Care
Massachusetts General Hospital
Instructor in Anesthesia
Harvard Medical School
Boston, Massachusetts

Amy Ortman, MD
Chief Resident
Department of Anesthesia and Critical Care
Massachusetts General Hospital
Instructor in Anesthesia
Harvard Medical School
Boston, Massachusetts

Robert L. Owens, MD
Clinical and Research Fellow
Pulmonary and Critical Care Unit
Massachusetts General Hospital
Instructor in Anesthesiology
Harvard Medical School
Boston, Massachusetts

Richard M. Pino, MD, PhD
Associate Anesthetist
Department of Anesthesia and Critical Care
Massachusetts General Hospital
Associate Professor
Harvard Medical School
Boston, Massachusetts

Steven J. Russell, MD, PhD
Assistant in Medicine
Department of Medicine, Endocrine Division
Massachusetts General Hospital
Instructor of Medicine
Harvard Medical School
Boston, Massachusetts

Elizabeth A. Sailhamer, MD, MMSc
Resident in General Surgery
Department of Surgery
Massachusetts General Hospital
Harvard Medical School
Boston, Massachusetts

Ulrich Schmidt, MD, PhD
Director, Surgical Intensive Care Unit
Department of Anesthesia and Critical Care
Massachusetts General Hospital
Asistant Professor of Anesthesia
Harvard Medical School
Boston, Massachusetts

Lee H. Schwamm, MD, FAHA
Vice-Chairman
Department of Neurology
Massachusetts General Hospital
Associate Professor
Harvard Medical School
Boston, Massachusetts

Todd A. Seigel, MD
Clinical Associate
Department of Anesthesia and Critical Care
Massachusetts General Hospital Assistant
Professor in Emergency Medicine
Brown University
Providence, Rhode Island

Robert L. Sheridan, MD
Chief, Burn Surgery Service
Shriner's Hospitals for Children—Boston
Associate Professor of Surgery
Harvard Medical School
Boston, Massachusetts

Kevin N. Sheth, MD
Assistant Professor
Departments of Neurology
University of Maryland School of Medicine
Baltimore, Maryland

Jagmeet Singh
Cardiac Arrhythmia Service
Massachusetts General Hospital
Assistant Professor
Harvard University
Boston, Massachusetts

David J.R. Steele, MD
Assistant Physician
Department of Medicine
Massachusetts General Hospital
Assistant Professor
Harvard Medical School
Boston, Massachusetts

H. Thomas Stelfox, MD, PhD
Departments of Critical Care Medicine
Medicine and Community Health Sciences
Foothills Medical Centre
Asistant Professor
University of Alberta
Calgary, Alberta

Dorothea Strozyk, MD
Vascular Neurology and Critical Care Fellow
Department of Neurology
Massachusetts General Hospital
Clinical and Research Fellow
Harvard Medical School
Boston, Massachusetts

B. Taylor Thompson, MD
Chief, Medical Intensive Care Unit
Pulmonary and Critical Care Unit
Massachusetts General Hospital
Associate Professor of Medicine
Harvard Medical School
Boston, Massachusetts

Arthur J. Tokarczyc, MD
Assistant Anesthesiologist
Department of Anesthesiology
North Shore University Health System
Clinical Instructor
University of Chicago
Chicago, Illinois

Jeffrey S. Ustin, MD, MS
Fellow
Trauma, Emergency Surgery, Surgical Critical Care
Massachusetts General Hospital
Instructor in Surgery
Harvard Medical School
Boston, Massachusetts

Jason A. Wertheim, MD, PhD
Resident in Surgery
Department of Surgery
Harvard Medical School
Massachusetts General Hospital
Boston, Massachusetts

Susan R. Wilcox, MD
Clinical Fellow in Critical Care
Department of Anesthesia and Critical Care
Massachusetts General Hospital
Harvard Medical School
Boston, Massachusetts

CONTENTS

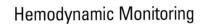

Hemodynamic Monitoring

Erik Kistler and Luca Bigatello

I. **The goal of hemodynamic monitoring** is to be able to measure or infer hemodynamic parameters necessary to maintain adequate organ perfusion. In critically ill patients, hypoperfusion of vital organs may lead to multiple-system organ dysfunction and death. The aim of this chapter is to guide the clinician through the interpretation of hemodynamic data based on the application of basic circulatory physiology.

   A. **Cardiovascular performance and tissue perfusion.** Organ perfusion is grossly determined by the difference between arterial and venous pressures divided by its resistance to flow:

$$\text{Flow} = \frac{(P_{\text{arterial}} - P_{\text{venous}})}{\text{Resistance}}$$

   In the absence of a method for measuring blood flow to individual organs, measurement of the systemic arterial pressure is used as a surrogate for estimating organ perfusion, assuming constant venous pressure and constant resistance.

   1. The **mean arterial pressure (MAP)** value provides the closest measure of perfusion pressure. A MAP of greater than **65 mm Hg** is a reasonable target for most patients. At times (e.g., chronic hypertension, acute tubular necrosis, or central nervous system ischemia), higher levels are necessary.

   2. Under normal circumstances, organ blood flow is maintained within normal range by **autoregulation**, which provides constant blood flow through constriction or dilation of the afferent vessels during changes in arterial blood pressure. However, pathologic conditions such as chronic hypertension, trauma, and sepsis impair autoregulation significantly, and flow may become directly dependent on perfusion pressure (**Fig. 1-1**).

II. **Pressure-based hemodynamic monitoring**

   A. **Main determinants of hypotension.** Hypotension is the most common reason for instituting invasive hemodynamic monitoring in critically ill surgical patients. A simple approach to the physiologic determinants of hypotension is shown in **Fig 1-2**. Hypotension is due to either **low cardiac output** or **low vascular tone**. A low cardiac output ([**CO**] = **stroke volume × heart rate**)

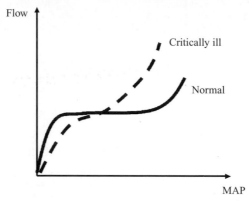

FIGURE 1-1 Autoregulation provides constant blood flow in healthy individuals over a wide range of blood pressure, but it may be impaired in critically ill patients, and flow may become dependent on perfusion pressure. MAP, mean arterial pressure.

can be due to a primary decrease in heart rate (HR) or to a decrease in **stroke volume**. A decrease in stroke volume can be due to a decrease in **venous return** (volume depletion or, less frequently, obstruction to heart filling) or to **ventricular dysfunction**. Commonly, several of these mechanisms may coexist in critically ill patients. As the complexity of a patient's presentation increases, it may become increasingly difficult to discern which mechanism is responsible for the circulatory failure. Hence, invasive hemodynamic monitoring can provide information to help understand and treat hemodynamic instability.

B. **Arterial blood pressure measurement**
1. **Noninvasive blood pressure** measurement involves temporarily occluding an artery by a pressurized cuff. Various techniques can be used, including manual auscultation of Korotkoff's sounds and automated auscultation systems. Most automated devices measure blood pressure

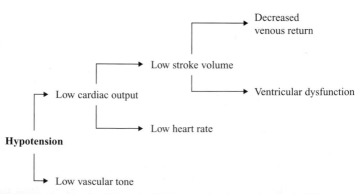

FIGURE 1-2 Algorithm describing a physiologic approach to hypotension (Section IIA).

by **oscillometry**. The **MAP** correlates well with the lowest pressure at which maximum oscillations occur. The systolic and diastolic pressures are determined by proprietary algorithms, but generally correlate with the initial rise and final fall of oscillations about the maximum. Blood pressure cuffs should cover about two-thirds of the upper arm or thigh; that is, the width of the cuff should be 20% more than the diameter of the limb; cuffs that are too narrow may produce falsely high measurements and cuffs that are too wide may produce falsely low values. Cycle times less than 2 minutes apart should be avoided to minimize the risk of compromised perfusion or resultant nerve damage.

2. **Intra-arterial blood pressure monitoring** is the gold standard of arterial blood pressure measurement. When correctly positioned and calibrated, the catheter–transducer monitor system provides a highly accurate measurement of systemic blood pressure. **Indications** include **hemodynamic instability**, instances where **rigorous control of blood pressure** is mandatory (e.g., leaking aortic aneurysm, traumatic injury of the aorta, central nervous system ischemia), and the need for **frequent arterial blood sampling**.

3. **Sites, techniques**, and **complications**. The **radial artery** at the wrist is the preferred site for an indwelling arterial catheter. The hand usually has good collateral blood supply through the ulnar artery, and the wrist is an easy area for access and maintenance of the catheter. Acceptable alternative sites in adults include the femoral, axillary, brachial, and *dorsalis pedis* arteries. The choice of sites depends on individual habits and on the patient's underlying medical condition. For example, the femoral artery may be considered in the septic hypotensive patient because the radial artery pressure may underestimate central pressure and lead to excessive vasopressor administration. **Vascular complications** of clinical significance are rare but can be devastating. Fastidious attention to the adequacy of distal perfusion is of great importance. All sites are at risk for ischemic complications because of their small caliber (radial and *dorsalis pedis* arteries), lack of adequate collateral circulation (brachial and axillary arteries), or the frequent presence of atherosclerotic vascular disease (femoral and *dorsalis pedis* arteries). **Infectious complications** are rare, probably due to the high blood flow rate through and around the catheter. However, they do occur, and arterial catheters should be treated like any indwelling device; that is, using sterile technique and frequently inspecting the site for signs of inflammation and infection.

4. **Function of the catheter–transducer monitor system**. The accuracy of intra-arterial blood pressure measurement depends on the proper setup and function of the catheter–transducer monitor system.

   a. **Reference level.** The level at which the arterial transducer should be referenced is not strictly codified—it should be at the level of interest. For example, in neurosurgical patients, it may be at the height of the external meatus of the ear to reference the blood pressure to the intracranial circulation. In the majority of critically ill patients, the object of blood pressure monitoring is overall tissue perfusion, and the arterial pressure transducer is set at the level of the heart.

   b. **Calibration.** Clinicians should be familiar with the principles of calibration of a blood pressure monitoring system to be able to troubleshoot catheter malfunction.

      (1) **Static calibration.** Given the high precision of the current monitors and disposable transducers, the calibration routine is often limited

to **zeroing** the transducer. The transducer is opened to air and the recorded pressure (the atmospheric pressure) is used by convention as the 0 mm Hg reference value. A second step of the static calibration, the **high calibration**, entails the application of a higher level of pressure (e.g., 200 mm Hg) to ensure accurate recordings over a clinically relevant pressure range, and is performed automatically by most current monitors.

(2) **Dynamic calibration.** There are two components of a dynamic calibration of an oscillating system: damping and resonance. **Damping** indicates the tendency of an oscillating system to return to its resting state. With increased damping, the pressure waveform appears flattened. Factors that increase damping include loose connections, kinks, and large air bubbles. The ideal damping coefficient is 0.707 (with 1 corresponding to no oscillations [critically damped]). Properly set up, modern transducers have minimal damping. **Resonance** indicates the property of a system to vibrate (resonate) when excited by a certain force. When the systolic pressure "hits" the elastic arterial wall, this vibrates and, just like a musical fork, generates an infinite series of sine waves of increasing frequency and decreasing amplitude. The lowest frequency of the sine waves (**fundamental frequency**) is the HR, and the subsequent sine wave frequencies (**harmonics**) are its multiples. If the system resonates at a frequency lower than the 8th to the 10th harmonics (decreased resonant frequency), the pressure trace will appear "whipped" or "flinging," that is, with a higher systolic pressure and a more pronounced dicrotic notch. Excessive tubing length, multiple stopcocks, large-bore catheters, and inadequate debubbling of the system predispose to a decrease in its resonant frequency. The resonant frequency of a system can be tested with a **flush test,** by applying a pressure burst to the transducer by flushing the system. Displayed on a strip chart recorder, the resonant frequency of the system can be calculated by measuring the distance between two subsequent peaks of the trace (**Fig. 1-3**).

(3) **Arterial blood pressure waveform on the monitor.** In contrast to central venous pressure (CVP), the arterial blood pressure is only minimally affected by changes in intrathoracic pressure relative to its absolute value. Therefore, the numeric values displayed on the monitor screen, which reflect an average over time (a few seconds) of each beat, are reasonably accurate for clinical purposes. Arterial pressure traces differ from individual to individual and from site to site (**Fig. 1-4**). For example, a pressure waveform recorded at the root of the aorta looks rounded, with a dicrotic notch located at the beginning of the descending portion of the curve. As arterial pressure is recorded more distally, the trace is progressively more peaked, and the dicrotic notch migrates away from the peak. Note, however, that the MAP does not vary widely as one measures more distally, except in situations of stenotic or compromised flow.

C. **Central pressures: significance, indications.** A central venous catheter can be used to determine the **CVP** in the systemic circulation. A pulmonary artery (**PA**) catheter can be used to determine, in addition to the CVP, the pulmonary artery pressure (**PAP**), the pulmonary artery occlusion pressure (**PAOP**), and the cardiac output (**CO**). The measurement of central vascular pressures is affected by a number of variables, including the proper setup of the monitoring system, the patient's position, the circulating volume status,

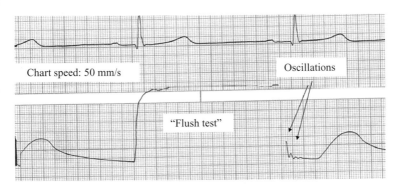

FIGURE 1-3 Flush test. The catheter–transducer system is pressurized by opening the flush ("square-wave sign") and then letting go of it. As the pressure rapidly returns to the patient's arterial pressure, the system "resonates." The resonance frequency is calculated by dividing the strip chart speed by the distance between two successive oscillations generated by the flush test. In this case, the distance is 2–3 mm, which holds a resonance frequency of 20 Hz. This is a common frequency of properly set up transducers, which will accurately reproduce most arterial traces at heart rates up to 120 beats/min.

interactions between systemic and pulmonary circulations, and the dynamic changes in the respiratory system over the breathing cycle. Not surprisingly, the accurate interpretation of central vascular pressures can be difficult, and a number of studies have challenged their clinical usefulness. The following sections are designed to provide basic physiological principles that will enhance the accuracy of central vascular pressures measurement in ICU patients.

We tend to measure an intravascular pressure in order to estimate a circulating volume. In general, we assume that

CVP ≅ Right ventricular end-diastolic volume (RVEDV)

PAOP ≅ Left ventricular end-diastolic volume (LVEDV)

However, variables in addition to the intravascular volume status of the systemic and pulmonary circulations can affect the measurement of central pressures.

1. **Interpretation—physiology of central pressures.** There are four main physiologic conditions that may alter the foregoing relationships:

   a. **Abnormal compliance of a cardiac chamber.** The relationship between pressure and volume (*compliance*) of a cardiac chamber at end diastole is not linear and is affected by pathologic conditions. For example, in a patient with **concentric left ventricle (LV) hypertrophy** secondary to chronic hypertension or aortic stenosis, the left ventricular compliance is decreased, and the measured pressure (PAOP) tends to overestimate the respective volume (LVEDV).

   b. **Increased intrathoracic pressure.** The measured vascular pressures are intended to be **transmural pressures** (pressure inside the vessel minus the pressure outside); that is, the pressure that actually distends the blood vessel and cardiac chamber. However, the pressure that we measure with a central catheter is the **intravascular pressure**, which is affected both by the volume of blood in the vessel and any other pressure applied to the outside of the vessel, such as the

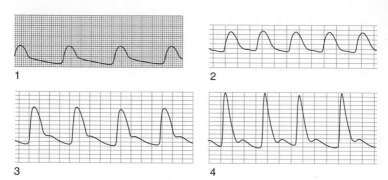

FIGURE 1-4 Arterial blood pressure traces from different patients, all obtained with properly calibrated transducers. The first three traces are from radial artery catheters, the fourth trace is from a dorsalis pedis catheter.

intrathoracic pressure. Common causes of increased intrathoracic pressure in critically ill patients include positive-pressure ventilation, applied positive end-expiratory pressure (PEEP), intrinsic PEEP (see **Chapter 2**), and possibly, increased abdominal pressure. The effect of intrathoracic pressure changes on the measured vascular pressures (CVP, PAOP) is minimal at end-expiration, when it approaches atmospheric pressure. For this reason, central **pressures are read at end-expiration**. However, the alveolar pressure can be increased at end-expiration by **PEEP** or **intrinsic PEEP**. One can estimate the fraction of alveolar pressure that is transmitted to the pleural space based on the compliance of the lung and chest wall. Normally, these two values are nearly equal, and approximately half of the alveolar pressure is transmitted across the lung to the pleural space. Remembering to convert the units of measurement (centimeters of water for airway pressure, millimeters of mercury for vascular pressure), we find that 10 cm H_2O of PEEP will increase a CVP/PAOP by approximately 3 mm Hg (5 cm $H_2O \times 0.74$). When the compliance of the lung is significantly decreased (e.g., in acute respiratory distress syndrome), a smaller fraction of pressure is transmitted. When the compliance of the lung is increased (e.g., in chronic obstructive pulmonary disease) or the compliance of the chest wall is decreased (e.g., in abdominal distension), a larger fraction of the applied pressure is transmitted. We do not recommend discontinuing the applied PEEP to improve the accuracy of central pressure readings: *first*, PEEP discontinuation may cause lung derecruitment and hypoxemia; *second*, the pressure exerted on the blood vessel is real and has hemodynamic effects; hence, by discontinuing PEEP we create a situation that may be less relevant to the current patient's physiology.

c. **Severe stenotic valvular lesions** of the atrioventricular valves (tricuspid and mitral stenoses) limit the ability to estimate the pressure in the respective ventricles. In these valvular lesions, the pressure in the atria can be significantly higher than the pressure in the ventricles, which, with progression of the lesion, tend to be underfilled. Therefore, pressure readings will overestimate ventricular volumes.

   d. **Ventricular interdependence.** When the right ventricle **(RV) is dilated** from volume and pressure overload (e.g., from pulmonary hypertension, primary RV failure), the interventricular septum moves leftward and impinges onto the LV, decreasing its compliance. In these cases, an elevated PAOP is in part determined by the overload of the RV and may overestimate filling of the LV.
   e. Despite the aforementioned sources of inaccuracy, measurement of central pressures with or without CO measurement is widely used to diagnose the causes of hypotension and guide therapy. Clearly, the hemodynamic values have to be put in the patient's context and interpreted in the light of relevant clinical variables, and trends may be more important than absolute numbers in the interpretation of the data.

2. **Monitoring with a CVP catheter.** Standard central venous catheters permit monitoring the CVP without the capability of measuring the CO.
   a. **Indications** for central venous cannulation include:
      (1) Measurement of right heart filling pressures and of central venous oxygen saturation (see **Section II. C. 6** and **Chapters 6** and **30**) as a guide to intravascular volume estimates and volume resuscitation.
      (2) Access for administration of drugs or parenteral nutrition into the central circulation.
      (3) Intravenous access in patients with difficult peripheral access.
   b. **Sites of cannulation.** Techniques of central venous catheter insertion have been described extensively, and we refer to the *Clinical Anesthesia Procedures of the Massachusetts General Hospital, 7th Edition,* **Chapter 10,** for review and illustrations. The most common sites of cannulation are the internal jugular and the subclavian veins. The tip of the catheter should be positioned at the junction of the superior vena cava and the right atrium. It is controversial whether central pressure can be accurately measured through a femoral vein access, and we do not recommend it. The **ideal site of cannulation** varies with the characteristics of the patient and the indication for central vein cannulation. For example, the subclavian site should not be chosen in a coagulopathic patient, and the femoral vein may be ideal in an emergency because of ease of cannulation. **Table 1-1** summarizes the advantages and disadvantages of the most commonly used sites for central vein access.
   c. **Complications** of CVP catheter insertion and use include dysrhythmias, **pneumothorax,** pericardial tamponade, hydrothorax, air embolism, **arterial puncture** and **injury,** and **infection.** Transient **dysrhythmias** (premature atrial and ventricular contractions [PACs, PVCs]) may occur while threading the guide wire but should resolve after retrieving it from the right atrium. Occasionally, the tip of the catheter may either be placed or migrate into the right atrium or ventricle, causing recurrent arrhythmias. Subclavian vein cannulation should be avoided in patients at increased risk for bleeding because the subclavian artery cannot be effectively compressed if accidentally punctured. **Catheter-related bloodstream infections** are associated with increased mortality and significant costs and are avoidable. Recommendations for the prevention of this important nosocomial complication are described in **Chapter 13.**
   d. **Waveform readings.** The zero reference point for venous pressures is at the fourth intercostal space on the midaxillary line, which corresponds to the position of the right and left atria when the patient is supine. The

TABLE 1-1 Risks and Benefits of Different Central Line Access Approaches

Cannulation Site	Infection Risk	Bleeding Risk	Thrombotic Risk	Pneumothorax Risk	Patient Comfort	Comments
Internal jugular	++	+	++	++	++	Fewest immediate complications, compressible, low pneumothorax risk
Subclavian	+	+++	+	+++	+++	Higher risk of pneumothorax, difficult area to compress in case of bleeding, low infection rate
Femoral	+++	+	+++	−	+	Easiest to place in an emergency, higher infection rate
External jugular	−	+	+	+	++	Essentially a peripheral venous line
PICC	+	−	++	+	+++	Good for long-term venous access, limited number of ports, low flow rate

+, low risk (or comfort); ++, higher risk (or comfort); +++, highest risk (or most comfortable); −, not applicable; PICC, peripherally inserted central catheter.

transducer is maintained at the same level with respect to the patient during sequential measurements. It should be noted that **changes in position may significantly affect the CVP,** even with correct leveling of the transducer. The CVP, like all central vascular pressures, is read at end-expiration, when the pleural pressure is close to 0. A normal CVP is on the order of 2 to 6 mm Hg. The CVP tracing contains three positive deflections, the **a-, c-, and v-waves (Fig. 1-5).** These correspond respectively to atrial contraction (seen after the P wave on ECG), bulging of the tricuspid valve during isovolumic ventricular contraction, and right atrial filling against a closed tricuspid valve. The x-descent is thought to be caused by the downward displacement of the atrium during ventricular systole and the y-descent by tricuspid valve opening during diastole. a-waves are absent in atrial fibrillation, while large a-waves **(cannon a-waves)** may occur when the atrium contracts against a closed valve, such as during atrioventricular dissociation. **Abnormally large v-**waves can be associated with tricuspid regurgitation; they begin immediately after the QRS complex and often incorporate the c-wave. Large v-waves are also observed during right ventricular failure and ischemia, constrictive pericarditis, or cardiac tamponade, due to the volume and/or pressure overload associated with these conditions.

e. **Interpretation.** Considering the number of variables that influence the measurement of the CVP in addition to the volume status of the systemic circulation, it is not surprising that it is frequently difficult to interpret CVP values. When the CVP is available as part of a monitoring system that can measure the CO, such as a PA catheter (see **Section II.C.3**) or a transthoracic thermodilution monitor, its

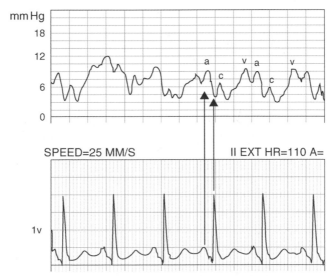

FIGURE 1-5 The central venous pressure trace contains three positive deflections, which correspond to atrial contraction, (a) ventricular contraction in systole, (c) and right atrial filling (v) (see Section II.C). HR, heart rate. Shown here in relationship with the ECG tracing.

value is significantly increased. When no measure of CO is available, changes in MAP can be used as a surrogate of CO in response to a volume challenge.

3. Monitoring with a **PA catheter** permits measurement of CVP, PAP, PAOP, and CO.

  a. **Indications.** The main indication for the placement of a PA catheter is the presence of **hemodynamic instability** (hypotension) of unclear physiologic etiology. Other indications include sampling of **mixed venous oxygen saturation (SvO$_2$)** and **pacing capability.**

  b. **Insertion.** The internal jugular vein is used most commonly because of easy access from the head of the patient and the lower incidence of pneumothorax. **Figure 1-6** shows the characteristic pressure waveforms seen as the pulmonary catheter is advanced through the successive structures of the heart. The PA catheter is first inserted to a depth of 20 cm, where the monitor should confirm a CVP waveform. The balloon is inflated with 1 to 1.5 mL of air, and the catheter is advanced until a right ventricular pressure waveform is seen. This should occur at a depth of approximately 30 to 35 cm. PVCs and, less often, bursts of ventricular tachycardia can occur at this time; the

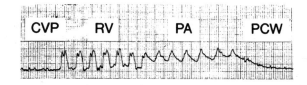

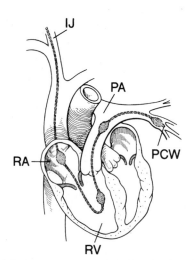

FIGURE 1-6 Characteristic pressure waves seen during insertion of a pulmonary artery catheter. CVP, central venous pressure; IJ, internal jugular; PA, pulmonary artery; PCW, pulmonary capillary wedge; RA, right atrium; RV, right ventricle.

catheter should be advanced rapidly out of the RV into the PA, where the dysrhythmias generally cease. The catheter is then advanced slowly until a PAOP trace is obtained (generally at a depth of 50–55 cm). The PA trace should reappear with deflation of the balloon. If it does not, the catheter is withdrawn until the PA tracing reappears. **A high degree of caution** must be applied to **the transition from a PA to a PAOP** trace; sometimes, the change is not quite apparent, and the catheter may be advanced when it is already in the occlusion position, causing disastrous complications (PA rupture, see below). Such a situation may occur particularly in the presence of a large *v*-wave on the PAOP trace (mitral regurgitation, congestive heart failure) which may be confused with a persistent PAP trace. Occasionally, the PA catheter may have to be placed under direct fluoroscopic guidance. Indications include the presence of a recently placed (generally 6 weeks) permanent pacemaker, the need for selective PA placement (e.g., following a right pneumonectomy), and the presence of significant structural abnormalities, such as severe right ventricular dilatation, and large intracardiac shunts.

c. **Complications** in addition to those relevant to central venous cannulation include:

(1) **PVCs, ventricular tachycardia,** and **right bundle-branch block (RBBB).** Most arrhythmias occur during placement (see prior discussion) and are transient. However, in the presence of a left bundle-branch block, the onset of an RBBB will cause **complete heart block;** the catheter may not be able to float out of the RV and the block may persist. Clinical judgment must be used prior to inserting a PA catheter in a patient with a left bundle-branch block. Appropriate measures include setting up pacing capability, transcutaneous or transvenous, and aborting the procedure.

(2) **PA rupture** is rare but has a high mortality. Factors predisposing to PA rupture include severe pulmonary hypertension, the presence of a suture line, and possibly, anticoagulation. The fundamental measure for avoiding PA rupture is using appropriate technique. Balloon inflation should be slow, and stopped immediately when a PAOP tracing is obtained; the balloon should never be kept inflated for an extended period of time. The PAP trace should be monitored at all times to rule out the migration into the occluded position. Although somewhat counterintuitive, there is no evidence that the number of occlusions performed correlates with the incidence of rupture. Instead, one may argue that by not performing sufficient occlusions over time, the clinician is deprived of important information needed to guide optimal patient therapy. Hence, we tend to perform occlusion pressures as frequently as we record all other hemodynamic parameters.

(3) **Pulmonary infarction** is another rare complication related mainly to poor technique. Although less devastating than a PA rupture, infarction is a serious complication and can be avoided using proper technique.

(4) PA catheters may occasionally form a **knot.** Fluoroscopic guidance may be needed to untangle and remove the catheter.

(5) **Balloon rupture.** At no time should the balloon be filled with more than 1.5 mL of air.

4. **Thermodilution CO** is determined by injecting a fixed volume of cold (room temperature or lower) solution into the CVP port. The cold tracer mixes

with the blood as it passes through the right heart, and the temperature of the mixture is measured as it passes a thermistor near the tip of the PAC. The computation of the CO uses a formula (*Stewart-Hamilton* equation) that must properly account for the volume and temperature of the injectate, the thermodynamic properties of blood, injectate solution and catheter used, and the integral of the temperature–time curve. Determining the CO allows diagnosis of a low-tone state, a low CO, or both. Concurrent measurement of HR will help to determine whether this is related to the HR or ventricular performance. Instead of the CO, the **cardiac index** may be calculated by dividing CO by the body surface area (BSA). At the extremes of body sizes, using the CI may allow easier comparison between patients.

a. **Accuracy and reliability.** Serial measurements (generally three) are recommended for each CO determination. Even then, the CO measurement can vary by as much as 10% without a change in the clinical condition of the patient. CO can vary over the **respiratory** cycle, depending on the mode of ventilation and baseline levels of venous return and cardiac performance. Accordingly, the timing of injection affects the measurement of a thermodilution CO measurement. If a consistent trend is desired, it is probably best to inject at a constant point in the respiratory cycle, usually at end-expiration. Note that this is not necessary for transthoracic CO determinations. If an average over the respiratory cycle is desired, it is usual to take the mean of three measurements obtained at random times throughout the respiratory cycle.

b. **Low-output states** can affect the accuracy of the CO measurement, especially when room-temperature indicator solutions are injected. Iced injectate gives more accurate measurements because of the larger temperature gradient.

c. **Tricuspid regurgitation** may produce both erroneously high and erroneously low readings. When the cold indicator fluid is recycled back and forth across the tricuspid valve, the thermodilution curve is prolonged (which may lead to a low reading) and has a low amplitude (which may lead to a high reading).

d. **Intracardiac shunts** can also produce erroneous measurements (tend to be increased) because they create a difference between right and left ventricular outputs.

5. **PA pressure and PA occlusion pressure**

a. **Measurement.** For an accurate measurement of PAOP, one should be able to detect a proper atrial pressure trace, similar to "*a-c-v*" trace described for the CVP in **Section II.C.2.d.**

b. **Values.** The PAP is considered normal between 15 and 20 mm Hg systolic pressure and 5 to 12 mm Hg diastolic pressure. The PAOP is intended to estimate the left atrial pressure, which in turn should correlate with the left ventricular end-diastolic pressure, an estimate of left ventricular end-diastolic volume (LVEDV). Because of the interposed lung, this estimate is delayed and dampened. **The *a*- and *c*-waves** typically are not very large. Consequently, the mean pressure (that is, midway between the *a*- and *c-waves*) at end-expiration is taken to reflect the left atrial pressure. A normal PAOP is between 5 and 12 mm Hg. As highlighted in the discussion of central pressure measurements, volume is only one parameter that influences the PAOP measurements; other variables (e.g., cardiac compliance, intrathoracic pressure, and ventricular interdependence) have to be kept in mind when interpreting the measured values (**Section II.C.1**).

6. **Mixed venous oxygen saturation.** The oxygen saturation in the PA (**SvO$_2$**) can be monitored continuously with an oximetric PA catheter, or it can be measured *in vitro* with a blood sample obtained from the distal port of the catheter. SvO$_2$ rises with increases of perfusion above requirements and falls with increasing oxygen extraction ratio as perfusion becomes inadequate. Thus, a low SvO$_2$ may indicate either a decreased rate of oxygen delivery (anemia, low CO) or an increased rate of oxygen consumption (see also **Chapter 6**). SvO$_2$ can be estimated (central SvO$_2$ or **ScvO$_2$**) in the absence of a PAC by measurements obtained from a CVP. ScvO$_2$ tends to overestimate SvO$_2$ because blood from the SVC tends to have a higher PO$_2$ than blood from the IVC; however, in pathologic states such as sepsis with decreased oxygen extraction, this relationship may be reversed.

7. **PA catheters** with **pacing ports** provide specially positioned ports to pass temporary pacing wires, usually one port for atrial pacing and one port for ventricular pacing. Without pacing wires in place, these ports can also be used for drug infusions.

D. **Controversy on PA catheters.** With the introduction of flow-directed balloon-tipped catheters in 1970, the PA catheter became accessible to many physicians and was soon adopted as a tool for guiding cardiovascular therapy in perioperative and critical care medicine. The effect of this technology on patient-centered outcomes was not initially tested in randomized trials. Since the mid-1990s, several large outcome studies assessing the benefit of PA catheters have been conducted and have not shown clear evidence of such benefit. Although these results are not sufficiently convincing to discourage the use of invasive hemodynamic monitoring, they underscore the importance of using appropriate indications for invasive monitoring and of correctly interpreting the data obtained.

1. The assumption, explicit or otherwise, is that monitoring devices should be able to improve outcomes. Monitoring devices provide information, which can used to direct patient care. They are not, however, a clinical intervention that can cure patients per se.

2. Clearly, not all patients may benefit from the insertion of a PA catheter. Patients should be selected based on specific questions to be answered, such as an uncertain cardiac status, the adequacy of the CO, the choice of a vasoactive substance, difficulty in titrating fluid volume, and so on.

3. In some patients there may, in fact, be little correlation between PA catheter measurements and fluid status.

III. **Alternatives to pressure monitoring.** Numerous noninvasive or less invasive monitors have been developed as alternatives to PA and CVP catheters. They use a multitude of different algorithms, typically based on arterial waveform analysis and CO determinations, and have different strengths and weaknesses. Some of the commercially available methods of hemodynamic monitoring include:

A. **Respiratory-induced systolic blood pressure variation (SBPV)** takes into account the change in the height of the arterial waveform that occurs with inspiration during positive pressure ventilation (**Fig. 1-7**).

1. The magnitude of this change is inversely correlated to the **circulating volume status** and directly correlated to the degree of **change in intrathoracic pressure** caused by the positive pressure breath. Hence, a

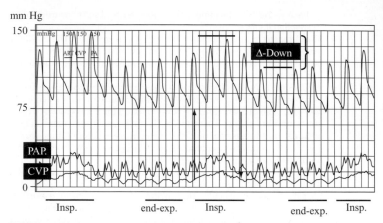

FIGURE 1-7 Respiratory-induced BP variation. PAP and CVP show a rise in pressure during inspiration. CVP, central venous pressure; end-exp, end-expiration; Insp., inspiration; PAP, pulmonary artery pressure. From Magder S. Clinical usefulness of respiratory variations in arterial pressure. *Am J Respir Crit Care Med* 2004;169:151–155, with permission.

pronounced SBPV (often defined as >15%–20% variation during the respiratory cycle) may be due to hypovolemia, a high intrathoracic pressure change, or a combination of both. Regardless, the subsequent administration of fluid volume will reduce such BPV and will tend to increase systemic blood pressure and CO. Hence, the BPV has been defined as an index of **fluid responsiveness**, that is, not of absolute hypovolemia, but of hypovolemia *relative* to specific intrathoracic pressure changes.

2. The concept of measuring fluid responsiveness rather than absolute volume status is new and may be of great importance in the management of critically ill patients. Measurements similar to the SBPV include the **pulse pressure variation** and the **stroke volume variation**. They are all based on the analysis of the arterial pressure trace during mechanical ventilation, which can also be used to extrapolate the beat-to-beat stroke volume (**pulse contour analysis**).

3. The proper interpretation of any measurement of respiratory-induced variations in hemodynamics requires that the patient be **fully ventilated** without spontaneous efforts and that the mechanics of lung and chest wall be in a steady state.

B. TTE indicator-dilution allows measurement of CO without performing a right heart catheterization. Different commercially available monitors may use cold saline solution or other indicators. They use a manual determination of the CO to calibrate additional, continuous CO measurements obtained from the pulse contour analysis.

1. A common advantage of all these devices is their less invasive nature than the PA catheter.

2. One particular monitor provides volumetric indices calculated from the thermodilution curve—the **global end-diastolic volume** and the **extravascular lung water index**. Both these parameters are potentially useful clinically, particularly in situations where pressure-based monitoring has clear limitations (see **Section II.C.1**). However, these indices are calculated using complicated proprietary algorithms that include a number of assumptions, whose validity is difficult to confirm in the clinical setting.

C. **Ultrasound** may be used to assess the contractile properties of both the ventricles, their degree of filling, the function of the cardiac valves, and whether there is a hemodynamically significant pericardial effusion. Measurement devices fall into two general categories: standard echocardiography and Doppler techniques. Most commercially available Doppler techniques use a transesophageal (TEE) approach. Ultrasound applications to ICU practice are reviewed in **Chapter 3**.

1. **Echocardiography** can be used to calculate systolic and diastolic volumes in one, two, or three dimensions as well as aortic outflow, enabling CO determinations. Accuracy increases as the number of dimensions measured increases; limitations include the need for a skilled operator and single time-point measurements. The TEE approach typically has better resolution than a TTE view, which is often limited by body habitus, bandages, and so on. TEE is limited to intubated or sedated patients and there is risk for ulceration and bleeding with extended placement.

2. **Doppler techniques.** TEE Doppler uses a continuous wave mode aligned with the descending thoracic aorta to determine directly stroke volume and CO of the passing blood using the Doppler principle. Small sensors are available which can be left in place for extended periods of time. Drawbacks include the need for optimal placement and the tendency of probes to migrate or move after placement.

D. **Impedance cardiography** uses changes in electrical impedance across the chest over the cardiac cycle to determine stroke volume and thus CO. Advances in phased-array and signal processing technologies have improved impedance cardiography, largely overcoming artifact due to electrode placement, HR and rhythm disturbances, and differences in body habitus. Extravascular fluid accumulation may still contribute to uncertainty in error, however.

E. **The Fick principle** calculates CO using the assumption that the rate of oxygen consumption is equal to the CO times the difference in oxygen content from the arterial side to the venous side. The Fick principle can be applied as such, by administering a precisely known fraction of oxygen, for example, through a canopy, and is also used commercially in a modified fashion, by measuring CO_2 rather than oxygen, using an intermittent partial rebreathing circuit (see **Chapter 2, Fig. 2-6**).

F. **End-organ perfusion monitors** are still in their infancy. Since end-organ perfusion is arguably the goal of patient monitoring, development of these devices is of considerable interest. Some of the issues to be resolved are as follows: (a) In which organs should tissue perfusion be measured? (b) How is adequate organ perfusion measured? (c) How should measurement be standardized? (d) What does end-organ perfusion mean for other (nonmeasured) organs or even the organism as a whole? Monitors that exist today include those that measure bilateral cerebral oxygenation, microcirculatory flow in surface tissues (i.e., loose skin under the eye) using **orthogonal polarization spectral imaging,** and distal muscle perfusion using **near-infrared spectral monitoring (NIRS)**. NIRS is particularly appealing because of its ease of use and relatively low cost. However, the precision of the currently available probes needs to improve in order to confer to this technique a clinically significant value as a guide to resuscitation.

Selected References

Dunn PF, Alston T, Baker K, Davison JK, eds. *Clinical anesthesia procedures of the Massachusetts General Hospital.* 7th ed. Baltimore: Lippincott Williams & Wilkins, 2007.

Guyton AC. Venous return. In: Dow P, Hamilton WF, eds. *Handbook of physiology. Section 2, Vol. 2: Circulation.* Washington, DC: American Physiological Society, 1963:1099–1133.

Harvey S, Harrison DA, Singer M, et al; PAC-Man study collaboration. Assessment of the clinical effectiveness of pulmonary artery catheters in management of patients in intensive care (PAC-Man): a randomised controlled trial. *Lancet* 2005;366:472–477.

Isakow W, Schuster D. Extravascular lung water measurement and hemodynamic monitoring in the critically ill: bedside alternatives to the pulmonary artery catheter. *Am J Physiol Lung Cell Mol Physiol* 2006;291:1118–1131.

Jacobson E, Chorn R, O'Connor M. The role of the vasculature in regulating venous return and cardiac output: historical and graphical approach. *Can J Anaesth* 1997;44:849–867.

Kleinman B, Powell S, Kumar P, et al. The fast flush test measures the dynamic response of the entire blood pressure monitoring system. *Anesthesiology* 1992;77:1215–1220.

Magder S. Clinical usefulness of respiratory variations in arterial pressure. *Am J Respir Crit Care Med* 2004;169:151–155.

Magder S. Central venous pressure: a useful but not simple measurement. *Crit Care Med* 2006;34:2224–2227.

O'Quin R, Marini JJ. Pulmonary artery occlusion pressure: clinical physiology, measurement, and interpretation. *Am Rev Respir Dis* 1983;128:319–326.

Pinsky M. Pulmonary artery occlusion pressure. *Intensive Care Med* 2003;29:19–22.

Richard C, Warszawski J, Anguel N, et al. Early use of the pulmonary artery catheter and outcomes in patients with shock and acute respiratory distress syndrome: a randomized controlled trial. *JAMA* 2003;290:2713–2720.

Sharkey SW. Beyond the wedge: clinical physiology and the Swan-Ganz catheter. *Am J Med* 1987;83:111–122.

Slogoff S, Keats AS, Arlund C. On the safety of radial artery cannulation. *Anesthesiology* 1983;59:42–47.

Soller BR, Yang Y, Soyemi OO, et al. Noninvasively determined muscle oxygen saturation is an early indicator of central hypovolemia in humans. *J Appl Physiol* 2008;104:475–481.

Teboul JL, Pinsky MR, Mercat A, et al. Estimating cardiac filling pressure in mechanically ventilated patients with hyperinflation. *Crit Care Med* 2000;28:3631–3636.

Wheeler AP, Bernard GR, Thompson BT, et al; National Heart, Lung, and Blood Institute ARDS Clinical Trials Network. Pulmonary artery vs. central venous catheter to guide treatment of acute lung injury. *N Engl J Med* 2006;354:2213–2224.

2

Respiratory Monitoring

Ettore Crimi and Dean Hess

I. **Monitoring** is a continuous, or nearly continuous, evaluation of the physiologic function of a patient in real time to guide management decisions, including when to make therapeutic interventions and assessment of those interventions.

   A. Monitoring is often performed to assure patient **safety.** For example, pulse oximetry is used to detect hypoxemia, and airway pressure is monitored to detect a mechanical ventilator disconnection. Although monitoring has improved patient safety, its impact on patient outcome in the ICU is less clear.

   B. Invasive and noninvasive monitoring is commonly used in the ICU **to assess patient response** to clinical interventions. Titration of the inspired oxygen fraction (Fio_2) is commonly guided by pulse oximetry, the level of pressure support is guided by respiratory rate and tidal volume, and the inspiratory-to-expiratory ratio (I:E ratio) is guided by measurement of intrinsic positive end-expiratory pressure (auto-PEEP).

II. **Gas exchange**

   A. **Arterial blood gases and pH.** Arterial blood gas analysis is often considered the gold standard for assessment of pulmonary gas exchange.

   1. **Arterial partial pressure of oxygen (Pao_2).** The normal arterial Pao_2 is 90 to 100 mm Hg breathing room air at sea level.

   2. **Decreased Pao_2 (hypoxemia)** occurs with pulmonary diseases resulting in shunt ($\dot{Q}_S/\dot{Q}_T$), ventilation–perfusion ($\dot{V}/\dot{Q}$) mismatch, hypoventilation, and diffusion defect. A low mixed venous Po_2 (e.g., decreased cardiac output) will magnify the effect of shunt on Pao_2. The Pao_2 is also decreased with decreased inspired oxygen (e.g., at high altitude).

   3. **Increased Pao_2 (hyperoxemia)** may occur when breathing supplemental oxygen. The Pao_2 also increases with hyperventilation.

   4. **Effect of Fio_2.** The Pao_2 should always be interpreted in relation to the level of supplemental oxygen. For example, a Pao_2 of 95 mm Hg breathing 100% oxygen is quite different from a Pao_2 of 95 mm Hg breathing air (21% oxygen).

   5. **Arterial partial pressure of CO_2 ($Paco_2$).** The $Paco_2$ reflects the balance between carbon dioxide production ($\dot{V}co_2$) and alveolar ventilation ($\dot{V}_A$):

$$Paco_2 = \dot{V}co_2/\dot{V}_A$$

   a. $Paco_2$ varies directly with carbon dioxide production and inversely with alveolar ventilation.

   b. $Paco_2$ is determined by **alveolar ventilation,** *not* minute ventilation per se.

   c. Minute ventilation affects $Paco_2$ only to the extent that it affects the alveolar ventilation.

   6. **Arterial pH** is determined by bicarbonate (HCO_3^-) concentration and $Paco_2$, as predicted by the **Henderson-Hasselbalch equation:**

$$pH = 6.1 + \log [HCO_3^-/(0.03 \times Paco_2)]$$

7. Blood gas errors

  a. Care must be taken to avoid sample contamination with air, as the Po_2 and Pco_2 of room air are approximately 160 mm Hg (at sea level) and approximately 0 mm Hg, respectively. Care should also be taken to avoid contamination of the sample with saline or venous blood.

  b. A specimen stored in a plastic syringe at room temperature should be analyzed within 30 minutes.

  c. Leukocyte larceny (spurious hypoxemia, pseudohypoxemia). The Pao_2 in samples drawn from subjects with very high leukocyte counts can decrease rapidly. Immediate chilling and analysis is necessary.

8. Blood gases and pH are measured at 37°C. Using empiric equations, the blood gas analyzer can adjust the measured values to the patient's body temperature. This issue is becoming increasingly important with the use of induced hypothermia after cardiac arrest and with focal cerebral ischemia.

  a. With **alpha-stat** management, $Paco_2$ is maintained at 40 mm Hg when measured at 37°C.

  b. With **pH-stat** management, $Paco_2$ is corrected to the patient's actual body temperature.

  c. Because of increased gas solubility during hypothermia, the alpha-stat strategy results in relative hyperventilation. The pH-stat approach results in improved cerebral blood flow and neurologic outcomes.

B. Venous blood gases reflect Pco_2 and Po_2 at the tissue level.

  1. There is a large difference between Pao_2 and **venous Po_2 (Pvo_2)**. Moreover, Pvo_2 is affected by oxygen delivery and oxygen consumption, whereas Pao_2 is affected by lung function. Thus, Pvo_2 should not be used as a surrogate for Pao_2.

  2. Normally, **venous pH** is slightly lower than arterial pH, and **venous Pco_2 ($Pvco_2$)** is slightly higher than $Paco_2$. However, the difference between arterial and venous pH and Pco_2 is increased by hemodynamic instability. During cardiac arrest, for example, it has been shown that $Pvco_2$ can be very high even when $Paco_2$ is low.

  3. When venous blood gases are used to assess acid–base balance, **mixed venous** or central venous samples are preferable to peripheral venous samples.

  4. Mixed venous oxygen level provides a global indication of the level of tissue oxygenation. Normal mixed venous Po_2 is 35 to 45 mm Hg and normal mixed venous So_2 is 65% to 75%. Factors affecting mixed venous oxygen level can be illustrated by the following equation, which is a rearrangement of the **Fick equation:**

$$S\bar{v}o_2 = Sao_2 - \dot{V}o_2/\dot{Q} \times Hb \times 1.34$$

C. CO-oximetry. Spectrophotometric analysis of arterial blood is used to measure levels of oxyhemoglobin (oxygen saturation of hemoglobin), carboxyhemoglobin (carbon monoxide saturation of hemoglobin), and methemoglobin (amount of hemoglobin in the oxidized ferric form rather than the reduced ferrous form).

  1. Oxyhemoglobin (Hbo_2) measured by CO-oximetry is the gold standard for determination of oxygen saturation and is superior to other means of determining oxygen saturation, such as that calculated empirically by a blood gas analyzer or that measured by pulse oximetry. Normal Hbo_2 is approximately 97%.

  2. Carboxyhemoglobin (HbCO) levels should be performed whenever carbon monoxide inhalation is suspected. Endogenous carboxyhemoglobin levels are 1% to 2% and can be elevated in cigarette smokers and in those living in polluted environments. Because carboxyhemoglobin does not transport oxygen, the HbO_2 is effectively reduced by the $Hbco$ level.

3. **Methemoglobin.** The iron in the hemoglobin molecule can be oxidized to the ferric form in the presence of a number of oxidizing agents, the most notable being nitrates. Because methemoglobin (Hbmet) does not transport oxygen, the HbO_2 is effectively reduced by the Hbmet level.

D. **Point-of-care blood gas monitoring** is performed near the site of patient care. Point-of-care analyzers are available to measure blood gases, pH, electrolytes, glucose, lactate, urea nitrogen, hematocrit, and clotting studies (activated clotting time [ACT], prothrombin time [PT], and partial thromboplastin time [PTT]).

1. **Advantages.** Point-of-care analyzers are small and portable (some are handheld), they use very small blood volumes (several drops), and they provide rapid reporting of results (a few minutes). They are relatively easy to use (e.g., self-calibrating) and typically incorporate a disposable cartridge that contains the appropriate biosensors.

2. **Disadvantages.** The cost benefit of these devices is unclear. Furthermore, appropriate quality control is necessary for compliance with the Clinical Laboratory Improvement Amendments or Joint Commission requirements.

E. **Pulse oximetry**

1. **Principles of operation.** The commonly used pulse oximeter passes two wavelengths of light (e.g., 660 and 940 nm) from light-emitting diodes through a pulsating vascular bed to a photodetector. A variety of probes are available in disposable or reusable designs and include digital probes (finger or toe), ear probes, and nasal probes.

2. **Accuracy.** Pulse oximeters use empiric calibration curves developed from studies of healthy volunteers. The accuracy of pulse oximetry is $\pm 4\%$ at saturations of greater than 80% (and less at lower saturations). The implications of this accuracy relate to the oxyhemoglobin dissociation curve (**Fig. 2-1**). If the pulse oximeter displays an oxygen saturation

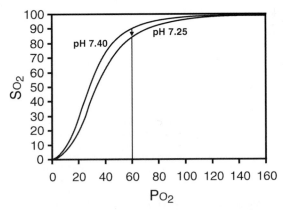

FIGURE 2-1 Oxyhemoglobin dissociation curve. Note that small changes in oxygen saturation relate to large changes in partial pressure of oxygen (Po_2) when the saturation is greater than 90%. Also note that the saturation can change without a change in Po_2 if there is a shift of the oxyhemoglobin dissociation curve.

(SpO_2) of 95%, the true saturation could be as low as 90% or as high as 100%. This range of SpO_2 translates to a PaO_2 range from as low as about 60 mmHg to greater than 150 mmHg.

3. Multiple wavelength pulse oximeters measure and report $HbCO$, $Hbmet$, and hemoglobin concentration in addition to SpO_2.

4. **Limitations** of pulse oximetry should be recognized and understood by everyone who uses pulse oximetry data.

   a. **Saturation versus PO_2.** Because of the shape of the oxyhemoglobin dissociation curve, pulse oximetry is a poor indicator of hyperoxemia. It is also an insensitive indicator of hypoventilation. If the patient is breathing supplemental oxygen, significant hypoventilation can occur without HbO_2 desaturation.

   b. **Ventilation versus oxygenation.** Pulse oximetry provides little, if any, clinical information related to $PaCO_2$ and acid–base balance.

   c. **Differences between devices and probes.** Calibration curves vary from manufacturer to manufacturer. The output of the light-emitting diodes of pulse oximeters varies from probe to probe. For these reasons, the same pulse oximeter and probe should be used for each SpO_2 determination for a patient.

   d. **The penumbra effect** occurs when the pulse oximeter probe does not fit correctly and light is shunted from the light-emitting diodes directly to the photodetector.

   e. **Dyshemoglobinemia.** Traditional pulse oximeters use only two wavelengths of light and therefore evaluate only two forms of hemoglobin: oxyhemoglobin and deoxyhemoglobin. **Carboxyhemoglobinemia** and **methemoglobinemia** result in significant inaccuracy of pulse oximetry. Carboxyhemoglobinemia produces an SpO_2 greater than the true oxygen saturation and methemoglobinemia causes the SpO_2 to move toward 85%. Multiple wavelength pulse oximeters address these issues by measuring $HbCO$ and $metHb$. Fetal hemoglobin does not affect the accuracy of pulse oximetry.

   f. **Endogenous and exogenous dyes and pigments** such as intravascular dyes (particularly methylene blue) affect the accuracy of pulse oximetry. Nail polish can also affect the accuracy of pulse oximetry; although this may be less problematic in newer generations of pulse oximeter, it is nonetheless prudent to remove nail polish before application of the pulse oximetry probe. Hyperbilirubinemia does not affect the accuracy of pulse oximetry.

   g. **Skin pigmentation.** The accuracy and performance of pulse oximetry may be affected by deeply pigmented skin.

   h. **Perfusion.** Pulse oximetry becomes unreliable during conditions of low flow such as low cardiac output or severe peripheral vasoconstriction. An ear probe may be more reliable than a digital probe under these conditions. A dampened plethysmographic waveform suggests poor signal quality. Newer technology uses signal processing software that improves the reliability of pulse oximetry with poor perfusion.

   i. **Anemia.** Although pulse oximetry is generally reliable over a wide range of hematocrit, it becomes less accurate under conditions of severe anemia.

   j. **Motion** of the oximeter probe can produce artifact and inaccurate pulse oximetry readings. Newer-generation oximeters incorporate noise-canceling algorithms to lessen the effect of motion on signal interpretation. Newer technology uses signal processing software that improves the reliability of pulse oximetry with motion of the probe.

k. **High-intensity ambient light,** which can affect pulse oximeter performance, can be corrected by shielding the probe.

l. **Abnormal pulses.** Venous pulsations and a large dicrotic notch can affect the accuracy of pulse oximetry.

5. **Respiratory variation in the plethysmographic waveform.** Photoplethysmography of peripheral perfusion is displayed by some pulse oximeters. The beat-to-beat plethysmogram displayed on the pulse oximeter reflects beat-to-beat changes in local blood volume. The cyclic changes in blood pressure and plethysmographic waveform can be caused by changes in intrathoracic pressure relative to the intravascular volume (pulsus paradoxus).

a. Perfusion index (PI) is a measurement displayed on many pulse oximeters. It is the ratio of the pulsatile blood flow to the nonpulsatile and thus represents a noninvasive measure of peripheral perfusion.

b. Plethysmographic variability index (PVI) is a measure of the dynamic changes in the PI that occur during the respiratory cycle. The lower the number, the lesser the variability.

c. PVI may be increased in patients with severe airflow obstruction and in patients who are hypovolemic.

6. **Guidelines for use.** Although pulse oximetry improves the detection of desaturation, there is little evidence that its use improves patient outcome. In spite of this, pulse oximetry has become a standard of care in the ICU (particularly for mechanically ventilated patients). Pulse oximetry is useful for titrating supplemental oxygen in mechanically ventilated patients. An SpO_2 of greater than or equal to 92% reliably predicts a PaO_2 of greater than or equal to 60 mm Hg in white patients (SpO_2 ≥95% in black patients). SpO_2 should be periodically confirmed by blood gas analysis. Assessment of the plethysmographic waveform may be useful to monitor response to therapy in patients with severe airflow obstruction and those who are being volume resuscitated although individual variability in waveform amplitude can represent a limitation (**Fig. 2-2**).

F. **Capnometry** is the measurement of CO_2 at the airway and **capnography** is the display of a CO_2 waveform called the **capnogram** (**Fig. 2-3**). The PCO_2 measured at end-exhalation is called the **end-tidal PCO_2** ($PetCO_2$).

1. **Principles of operation.** Quantitative capnometers measure CO_2 using the principles of infrared spectroscopy, Raman spectroscopy, or mass spectroscopy. Nonquantitative capnometers indicate CO_2 by a color change of an indicator material. Mainstream capnometers place the measurement chamber directly on the airway, whereas sidestream capnometers aspirate gas through tubing to a measurement chamber in the capnometer.

2. The **$PetCO_2$** represents alveolar PCO_2; it is determined by the rate at which CO_2 is added to the alveolus and the rate at which CO_2 is cleared from the alveolus. Thus, the $PetCO_2$ is a function of the ($\dot{V}/\dot{Q}$): with a normal ($\dot{V}/\dot{Q}$), the $PetCO_2$ approximates the $PaCO_2$. With a high ($\dot{V}/\dot{Q}$) (deadspace effect), the $PetCO_2$ is lower than the $PaCO_2$. With a low ($\dot{V}/\dot{Q}$) (shunt effect), the $PetCO_2$ approximates the mixed-venous PCO_2. The $PetCO_2$ can be as low as the inspired PCO_2 (zero) or as high as the mixed venous PCO_2. Changes in $PetCO_2$ can be due to changes in CO_2 production, CO_2 delivery to the lungs, or changes in alveolar ventilation.

3. **Abnormal capnogram.** The shape of the capnogram can be abnormal with obstructive lung diseases (**Fig. 2-4**).

4. **Limitations.** There is considerable intra- and interpatient variability in the relationship between $PaCO_2$ and $PetCO_2$. The P(a-et)CO_2 is often too

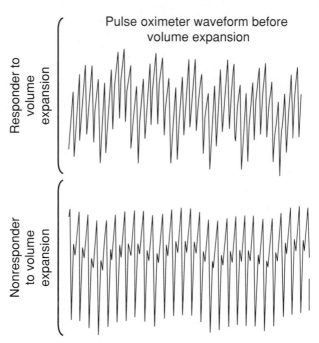

FIGURE 2-2 Pulse oximeter waveform from a patient who responded to volume expansion and from another who did not respond to volume expansion. From Cannesson M, Desebbe O, Rosamel P, et al. Pleth variability index to monitor the respiratory variations in the pulse oximeter plethysmographic waveform amplitude and predict fluid responsiveness in the operating theatre. *Br J Anaesth* 2008;101:200–206.

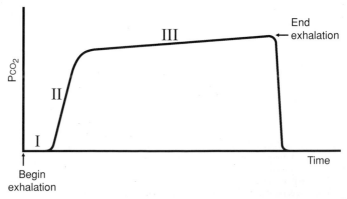

FIGURE 2-3 Normal capnogram. Phase I, anatomic dead space; phase II, transition from dead space to alveolar gas; phase III, alveolar plateau.

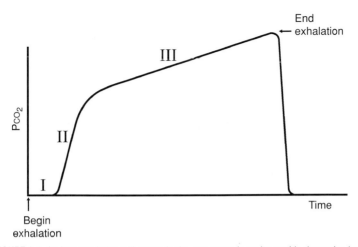

FIGURE 2-4 An increased phase III occurs in the capnogram in patients with obstructive lung disease.

variable in critically ill patients to allow precise prediction of $Paco_2$ from $Petco_2$.

5. **Guidelines for clinical use.** The utility of $Petco_2$ to predict $Paco_2$ is limited in the ICU. Capnometry is useful for detecting esophageal intubation. $Petco_2$ monitoring to confirm tracheal intubation is generally regarded as a standard of care. Low-cost disposable devices are commercially available that produce a color change in the presence of exhaled CO_2.

6. **Volume-based capnometry** displays exhaled CO_2 as a function of exhaled tidal volume (**Fig. 2-5**). Note that the area under the volume-based

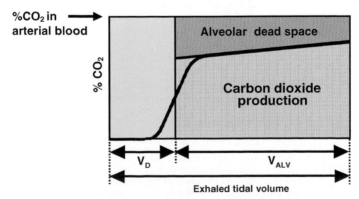

FIGURE 2-5 The volume-based capnogram. Note that the area under the curve represents carbon dioxide elimination, which equals carbon dioxide production during steady-state conditions.

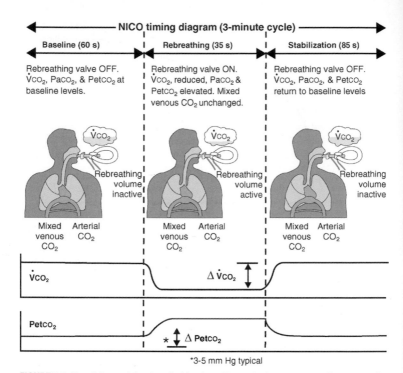

FIGURE 2-6 Use of the partial carbon dioxide rebreathing method to measure cardiac output using capnometry. Assuming that changes in pulmonary capillary carbon dioxide content (Cc'_{CO_2}) are proportional to changes in end-tidal CO_2 ($P_{et}CO_2$), we can use the following equation to calculate pulmonary capillary blood flow (PCBF): $PCBF = \Delta \dot{V}_{CO_2}/(S \times \Delta P_{et}CO_2)$, where $\Delta \dot{V}_{CO_2}$ is the change in CO_2 output and S is the slope of the CO_2 dissociation curve. Cardiac output is determined from PCBF and pulmonary shunt: $\dot{Q} = PCBF/(1 - \dot{Q}s/\dot{Q}t)$. Noninvasive estimation of pulmonary shunt ($\dot{Q}s/\dot{Q}t$) is adapted from Nunn's isoshunt plots, which are a series of continuous curves for the relationship between partial pressure of oxygen (P_aO_2) and inspired oxygen (F_iO_2) for different levels of shunt. P_aO_2 is estimated using a pulse oximeter. P_aCO_2, arterial partial pressure of CO_2. (NICO timing diagram courtesy of Novametrix, Wallingford, CT.)

capnogram is the volume of CO_2 exhaled. Assuming steady-state conditions, this represents **carbon dioxide production** ($\dot{V}_{CO_2}$). Because ($\dot{V}_{CO_2}$) is determined by metabolic rate, this can be used to estimate **resting energy expenditure** (REE):

$$REE = \dot{V}_{CO_2}(L/min) \times 5.52 \text{ kcal/L} \times 1{,}440 \text{ min/d}$$

Normal ($\dot{V}_{CO_2}$) is approximately 200 mL/min (2.6 mL/kg/min).

7. Using volume-based capnometry and a partial-rebreathing circuit allows measurement of **pulmonary capillary blood flow** using a modification of the Fick equation (**Fig. 2-6**). With corrections for intrapulmonary shunt, this allows noninvasive estimation of cardiac output. Studies of the accuracy of this method in critically ill patients have been mixed, and further validation in this patient population is needed.

G. **Transcutaneous blood gas monitoring. Transcutaneous Po_2 ($Ptco_2$) and transcutaneous Pco_2 ($Ptcco_2$)** have been used in the neonatal ICU, but with limited acceptance in the care of adults.

1. **Principle of operation.** The $Ptco_2$ electrode uses a polarographic principle and the $Ptcco_2$ uses a Severinghaus electrode. To produce a $Ptco_2$ similar to Pao_2, the electrode is heated. The increase in Po_2 caused by heating roughly balances the decrease in Po_2 caused by skin oxygen consumption and diffusion of oxygen across the skin. The $Ptcco_2$ is consistently greater than $Paco_2$ and for this reason manufacturers incorporate a correction factor so that the displayed $Ptcco_2$ approximates $Paco_2$.

2. **Limitations.** A number of factors limit the usefulness of transcutaneous monitoring in adults. The heated electrode can cause skin burns, and its position must be changed frequently to prevent burns. $Ptco_2$ and $Ptcco_2$ are unreliable for 15 to 20 minutes after the electrode is placed. Compromised hemodynamics causes underestimation of Pao_2 and overestimation of $Paco_2$. Additional information regarding metabolic status (e.g., pH, bicarbonate) is not provided.

3. A **combined pulse oximeter and transcutaneous Pco_2 monitor** is available for monitoring of adult patients in the ICU.
   a. The sensor clips onto the earlobe and warms the skin to $42°C$.
   b. The sensor is removed and calibrated every 8 hours; the membrane needs to be changed every 28 days.

III. **Lung function**
   A. **Indices of oxygenation**
      1. **Shunt fraction** is the gold standard index of oxygenation. It is calculated from the **shunt equation:**

$$\dot{Q}_S/\dot{Q}_T = (Cc'o_2 - Cao_2)/(Cc'o_2 - C\overline{v}o_2)$$

where $Cc'o_2$ is the pulmonary capillary oxygen content, Cao_2 is the arterial oxygen content, and $C\overline{v}o_2$ is the mixed venous oxygen content. Oxygen content is calculated from

$$Co_2 = (1.34 \times Hb \times Hbo_2) + (0.003 \times Pao_2)$$

To calculate $Cc'o_2$, we assume the pulmonary capillary Po_2 is equal to the alveolar Po_2 and the pulmonary capillary hemoglobin is 100% saturated with oxygen. If measured when the patient is breathing 100% oxygen, the $\dot{Q}_S/\dot{Q}_T$ represents shunt (i.e., blood that flows from the right heart to the left heart without passing functional alveoli). If measured at Fio_2 less than 1.0, the $\dot{Q}_S/\dot{Q}_T$ represents shunt and $\dot{V}/\dot{Q}$ mismatch.

2. Pao_2, $P(A-a)o_2$, Pao_2/PAo_2. The alveolar Po_2 (PAo_2) is calculated from the alveolar gas equation:

$$PAo_2 = (Fio_2 \times EBP) - [Paco_2 \times (Fio_2 + (1 - Fio_2)/R)]$$

where EBP is the effective barometric pressure (barometric pressure minus water vapor pressure) and R is the respiratory quotient. For calculation of PAo_2, an R of 0.8 is commonly used. For Fio_2 greater than or equal to 0.6, the effect of R on the alveolar gas equation becomes

$$PAo_2 = (Fio_2 \times EBP) - (Paco_2)$$

For Fio_2 less than 0.6, the alveolar gas equation becomes

$$PAo_2 = (Fio_2 \times EBP) - (1.2 \times Paco_2)$$

An increased difference between $P_{A_{O_2}}$ and Pa_{O_2}, the **P(A-a)o$_2$ gradient**, can be due to shunt, $\dot{V}/\dot{Q}$ mismatch, or diffusion defect. The $P(A-a)o_2$ is normally equal to or less than 10 mmHg breathing room air and equal to or less than 50 mmHg breathing 100% oxygen. The ratio of the Pa_{O_2} to $P_{A_{O_2}}$ (**Pao$_2$/Pao$_2$**) can also be calculated as an index of lung function and is normally greater than 0.75 at any Fi_{O_2}.

3. **Pao$_2$/Fio$_2$** is the easiest of the indices of oxygenation to calculate. The acute respiratory distress syndrome (ARDS) is associated with Pa_{O_2}/Fi_{O_2} less than 200, and acute lung injury (ALI) is associated with Pa_{O_2}/Fi_{O_2} less than 300.

4. The **oxygenation index (OI)** is calculated from the Fi_{O_2}, mean airway pressure ($\overline{P}aw$), and Pa_{O_2}:

$$OI = \frac{(Fi_{O_2} \times \overline{P}aw \times 100)}{Pa_{O_2}}$$

The OI is commonly calculated for critically ill neonates, but it is seldom used in the care of critically ill adults.

B. **Indices of ventilation**

1. **Dead space** (V_D/V_T) is calculated from the **Bohr equation**, which measures the ratio of dead space to total ventilation:

$$\frac{V_D}{V_T} = \frac{(Pa_{CO_2} - P\overline{E}_{CO_2})}{Pa_{CO_2}}$$

where $P\overline{E}_{CO_2}$ is the mixed exhaled P_{CO_2}. To determine $P\overline{E}_{CO_2}$, exhaled gas is collected in a bag from the expiratory port of the ventilator and its CO_2 concentration is measured with a blood gas analyzer or capnometer. Alternatively, $P\overline{E}_{CO_2}$ can be determined using volumetric capnometry:

$$P\overline{E}_{CO_2} = \frac{(\dot{V}_{CO_2} \times Pb)}{\dot{V}_E}$$

where Pb is barometric pressure. The normal V_D/V_T is 0.3 to 0.4.

IV. **Lung mechanics**

A. **Plateau pressure** (Pplat) is the peak alveolar pressure during mechanical ventilation.

1. **Measurement.** Pplat is measured by applying an end-inspiratory breath-hold for 0.5 to 2.0 seconds. During the breath-hold, pressure equilibrates throughout the system so that the pressure measured at the proximal airway approximates the peak alveolar pressure (**Fig. 2-7**). For valid measurement of Pplat, the patient must be relaxed and breathing in synchrony with the ventilator.

2. **An increased Pplat** indicates a greater risk of alveolar overdistention during mechanical ventilation. Many authorities recommend that Pplat be maintained at less than or equal to 30 cmH$_2$O in patients with acute respiratory failure. This assumes that chest wall compliance is normal. Higher plateau pressures may be necessary if chest wall compliance is decreased (e.g., abdominal distension).

B. **Auto-PEEP**

1. **Measurement.** Auto-PEEP is measured by applying an end-expiratory pause for 0.5 to 2.0 seconds (**Fig. 2-8**). The pressure measured at the end of this maneuver that is in excess of the PEEP set on the ventilator represents the amount of auto-PEEP. For a valid measurement, the patient must be relaxed and breathing in synchrony with the ventilator—active

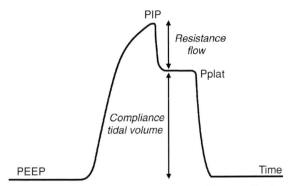

FIGURE 2-7 Peak alveolar pressure (Pplat) is determined by applying an end-inspiratory breath-hold. The peak inspiratory pressure (PIP)–Pplat difference is determined by resistance and end-inspiratory flow, and the Pplat–positive end-expiratory pressure (PEEP) difference is determined by compliance and tidal volume.

breathing will invalidate the measurement. Measurement of auto-PEEP during active breathing requires the use of an esophageal balloon.

2. **Clinical implications.** Auto-PEEP is determined by the ventilator settings (tidal volume and expiratory time) and lung function (airways resistance and lung compliance). The level of auto-PEEP can be decreased by reducing the minute ventilation with a decrease in either tidal volume or respiratory rate (permissive hypercapnia). Increasing the expiratory time may also decrease the level of auto-PEEP. This can be achieved by changing the I:E ratio (i.e., shortening the inspiratory time) or decreasing the respiratory rate; decreasing the rate more effectively increases the expiratory time than changing the I:E. The level of auto-PEEP can also be reduced by decreasing airways resistance (i.e., secretion clearance or bronchodilator administration).

3. **Occlusion pressure ($P_{0.1}$)** is the negative airway pressure generated 100 ms after the onset of inhalation against an occluded airway.

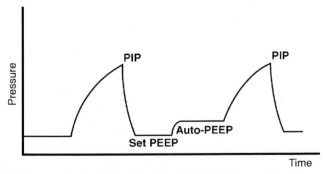

FIGURE 2-8 Auto–positive end-expiratory pressure (auto-PEEP) is measured by applying an end-expiratory breath-hold. An increase in pressure above the level of PEEP set indicates the presence of auto-PEEP. PIP, peak inspiratory pressure.

  a. $P_{0.1}$ is an index of ventilatory drive. It can be measured manually and/or automatically on some ventilators.
  b. Normal $P_{0.1}$ is 3 to 4 cm H_2O.
  c. A $P_{0.1}$ greater than 6 cm H_2O has been associated with weaning failure.
  4. Maximum inspiratory pressure (Pi_{max} or MIP), the most negative pressure generated during a maximal inspiratory effort against an occluded airway
  a. Pi_{max} is an index of the strength of the inspiratory muscles.
  b. The off-ventilator manual measurement technique uses a one-way valve allowing exhalation, but not inhalation, and an occlusion for approximately 15 to 20 seconds provided no arrhythmias or desaturation occur. Some ventilators perform this measurement electronically, by occluding both inspiratory and expiratory valves.
  c. Normal Pi_{max} is < -100 cm H_2O (varies with sex and age).
  d. Although $Pi_{max} > -30$ cm H_2O has been associated with weaning failure, its predictive value is poor.
  5. Maximum expiratory pressure (Pe_{max} or MEP), the most positive pressure generated during a maximal inspiratory effort against an occluded airway
  a. Pe_{max} is an index of the strength of the expiratory muscles.
C. Esophageal pressure
  1. Measurement. Esophageal pressure is measured from a thin-walled balloon, which contains a small volume of air (<1 mL) placed into the lower esophagus. The measurement and display of esophageal pressure are facilitated by commercially available systems.
  2. Esophageal pressure changes reflect changes in pleural pressure, but the absolute esophageal pressure does not reflect absolute pleural pressure.
  a. Changes in esophageal pressure can be used to assess respiratory effort and work of breathing during spontaneous breathing and patient-triggered modes of ventilation, to assess chest wall compliance during full ventilatory support, and to assess auto-PEEP during spontaneous breathing and patient-triggered modes of ventilation.
  b. If exhalation is passive, the change in esophageal (i.e., pleural) pressure required to reverse flow at the proximal airway (i.e., trigger the ventilator) reflects the amount of auto-PEEP. Negative esophageal pressure changes that produce no flow at the airway indicate failed trigger efforts—in other words, the patient's inspiratory efforts are insufficient to overcome the level of auto-PEEP and trigger the ventilator (**Fig. 2-9**). Clinically, this is recognized as a patient respiratory rate (observed by inspecting chest wall movement) that is greater than the trigger rate on the ventilator.
  c. The increase in esophageal pressure ($\Delta Peso$) during passive inflation of the lungs can be used to calculate chest wall compliance (Ccw): Ccw = $V_T / \Delta Peso$.
  d. Changes in esophageal pressure, relative to changes in alveolar pressure, can be used to calculate transpulmonary pressure (lung stress). This may allow more precise setting of tidal volume (and Pplat) in patients with reduced chest wall compliance. In this case, transpulmonary pressure (difference between Pplat and Peso) is targeted at <27 cm H_2O.
  e. Although esophageal pressure has been used to target the appropriate setting for PEEP, its clinical application is debated. The concept is that patients with a higher Peso require more PEEP to counterbalance the alveolar collapsing effect of the higher pleural pressure.
  f. An alternative to esophageal pressure to assess changes in pleural pressure is respiratory variation in the central venous pressure.

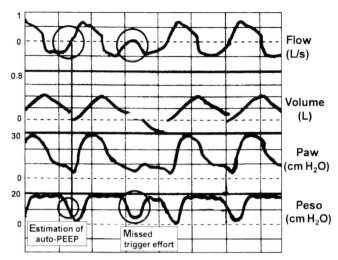

FIGURE 2-9 Use of esophageal pressure to determine auto–positive end-expiratory pressure (auto-PEEP). The change in esophageal pressure required to trigger the ventilator is the level of auto-PEEP. Also note the presence of missed trigger efforts in which the inspiratory effort of the patient is not sufficient to overcome the amount of auto-PEEP. Paw, mean airway pressure; Peso, esophageal pressure.

D. Gastric pressure
1. Gastric pressure is measured by a balloon-tipped catheter similar to that used to measure esophageal pressure. It reflects changes in intra-abdominal pressure. An alternative for measuring gastric pressure is measuring **bladder pressure**.
2. **Clinical implications.** During a spontaneous inspiratory effort, gastric pressure normally increases because of contraction of the diaphragm. A decrease in gastric pressure with spontaneous inspiratory effort is consistent with diaphragmatic paralysis (**Fig. 2-10**). A high baseline gastric pressure reflects elevated intra-abdominal pressure, which may affect chest wall compliance and lung function.

E. Compliance (the inverse of elastance) is the change in volume (usually tidal volume) divided by the change in pressure required to produce that volume.
1. Respiratory system, chest wall, and lung compliance
   a. **Respiratory system compliance** is most commonly calculated in the ICU:

$$C = \frac{\Delta V}{\Delta P} = \frac{\text{tidal volume}}{(\text{Pplat} - \text{PEEP})}$$

   Respiratory system compliance is normally 100 mL/cm H_2O and is reduced to 50 to 100 mL/cm H_2O in mechanically ventilated patients, likely due to the supine or semirecumbent position and microatelectasis. It is determined by the compliance of the chest wall and the lungs. This measurement is often called *static compliance*, meaning that the measurement was performed in conditions of no flow or, more likely, a very low flow (quasistatic conditions) achieved by the end-inspiratory pause.

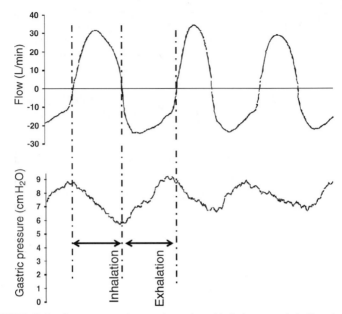

FIGURE 2-10 Gastric pressure measurement in a patient with diaphragm paralysis. Note that the gastric pressure decreases during the inspiratory phase.

    b. **Chest wall compliance** is calculated from changes in esophageal pressure (pleural pressure) during passive inflation. Chest wall compliance is normally 200 mL/cm H_2O and can be decreased because of abdominal distension, chest wall edema, chest wall burns, and thoracic deformities (e.g., kyphoscoliosis). It is also decreased with an increase in muscle tone (e.g., a patient who is bucking the ventilator) and increased with flail chest and paralysis.

    c. **Lung compliance** is calculated from changes in transpulmonary pressure. **Transpulmonary pressure** is the difference between alveolar pressure (Pplat) and pleural pressure (esophageal). Normal lung compliance is 100 mL/cm H_2O. Lung compliance is decreased with pulmonary edema (cardiogenic or noncardiogenic), pneumothorax, consolidation, atelectasis, pulmonary fibrosis, pneumonectomy, and mainstream intubation and is increased with emphysema.

2. **Clinical implications.** When compliance is decreased, a larger transpulmonary pressure is required to deliver a given tidal volume into the lungs. Thus, a decreased compliance will result in a higher Pplat and peak inspiratory pressure (PIP). To avoid dangerous levels of airway pressure, lower tidal volumes are used to ventilate the lungs of patients with decreased compliance. Decreased lung compliance also increases the work of breathing, decreasing the likelihood of successful weaning from the ventilator.

F. **Mean airway pressure** ($\overline{P}aw$) is the average pressure applied to the lungs over the entire ventilatory cycle.

1. Most current generation microprocessor ventilators display $\overline{P}aw$ from integration of the airway pressure waveform.

2. Typical $\overline{P}aw$ for passively ventilated patients are 5 to 10 cm H_2O (normal), 10 to 20 cm H_2O (airflow obstruction), and 15 to 30 cm H_2O (ALI/ARDS).
3. Factors affecting $\overline{P}aw$ are PIP (an increase in PIP increases $\overline{P}aw$), PEEP (increasing PEEP increases $\overline{P}aw$), I:E ratio (the longer the inspiratory time, the higher the $\overline{P}aw$), inspiratory pressure waveform (a rectangular inspiratory pressure waveform produces higher $\overline{P}aw$ than a triangular inspiratory pressure waveform).

G. Airways resistance is determined by the driving pressure and the flow.
1. **Inspiratory airways resistance** can be estimated during volume ventilation from the PIP–Pplat difference and the end-inspiratory flow:

$$R_I = \frac{(PIP - Pplat)}{\dot{V}_I}$$

where $\dot{V}_I$ is the end-inspiratory flow. A simple way to make this measurement is to set the ventilator for a constant inspiratory flow of 60 L/min (1 L/s). Using this approach, we have that the inspiratory airways resistance is the PIP–Pplat difference.
2. Expiratory resistance can be estimated from the time constant (τ) of the lung (**Fig. 2-11**):

$$R_E = \tau/C$$

3. **Common causes** of increased airways resistance are bronchospasm and secretions. Resistance is also increased with a small–inner-diameter endotracheal tube. For intubated and mechanically ventilated patients, airways resistance should be less than 10 cm $H_2O/L/s$ at a flow of 1 L/s. Expiratory airways resistance is typically greater than inspiratory airways resistance.

H. Work of breathing
1. **The Campbell diagram** (**Fig. 2-12**) is used to determine the work of breathing. The Campbell diagram includes the effects of chest wall compliance, lung compliance, and airway resistance on the work of breathing. Work of breathing is increased with decreased chest wall compliance, decreased lung compliance, or increased airways resistance.

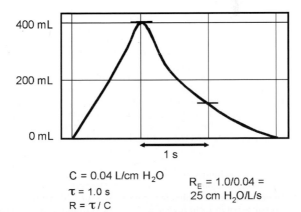

FIGURE 2-11 Use of the tidal volume waveform to measure time constant (τ) and calculate expiratory airways resistance.

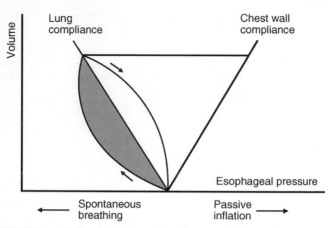

FIGURE 2-12 Campbell diagram. The chest wall compliance curve is determined by plotting volume as a function of esophageal pressure during positive-pressure breathing with the chest wall relaxed. The lung compliance curve is determined from the point of zero flow at end-exhalation to the point of zero flow at end-inhalation during spontaneous breathing. Because of airways resistance, the esophageal pressure is more negative than predicted from the lung compliance curve. The areas indicated on the curve represent elastic work of breathing and resistive work of breathing. Note that a decreased chest wall compliance will shift that compliance curve to the right, thus increasing the elastic work of breathing. A decrease in lung compliance shifts that curve to the left, also increasing the work of breathing. An increased airways resistance causes a more negative esophageal pressure during spontaneous breathing, increasing the resistive work of breathing.

    2. Clinical implications. Work of breathing requires special equipment and an esophageal balloon to quantify, and for that reason it is not frequently measured. Moreover, it is not clear that measuring work of breathing improves patient outcome. It may be useful for quantifying patient effort during mechanical ventilation, but this can often be achieved by simply observing the respiratory variation on a central venous pressure tracing. Large inspiratory efforts produce large negative deflections of the central venous pressure trace during inspiratory efforts. Increasing the level of ventilatory assistance should reduce these negative deflections.

I. The **static pressure–volume curve** measures the pressure–volume relationship of the respiratory system.

    1. Measurement. The manual method with a supersyringe is relatively simple but requires disconnecting the patient from the ventilator to perform the maneuver. Alternatively, a pressure–volume curve can be performed automatically in selected ventilators without disconnecting the patient from the ventilator. The multiple occlusion method performs repeated end-inspiratory breath occlusions at different lung volumes, and the constant flow technique measures the change in airway opening pressure with a constant slow flow ($\leq$10 L/min). The best technique is unknown.

    2. Lower and upper inflection points can be determined from the pressure–volume curve (**Fig. 2-13**). Some authors have suggested that the level of PEEP should be set above the lower inflection point to avoid alveolar collapse and Pplat should be set below the upper

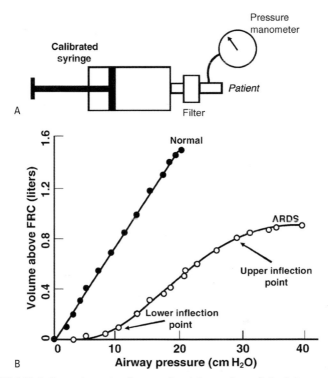

FIGURE 2-13 A. Supersyringe set-up for measuring static compliance. **B.** Inspiratory pressure–volume curve for a patient with normal lung function and for a patient with acute respiratory distress syndrome (ARDS). FRC, functional residual capacity.

inflection point to avoid alveolar overdistention. However, the clinical benefits of this approach are not clear, and setting the ventilator using the pressure–volume curve is not currently recommended because there are important limitations to the clinical use of pressure–volume curves. Accurate measurements require heavy sedation (and often paralysis); it is unclear whether the inflation or deflation curve should be assessed; it can be difficult to precisely determine the inflection points; the respiratory system pressure–volume curve can be affected by both the lungs and the chest wall; and the pressure–volume curve models the lungs as a single compartment.

J. **Ventilator graphics,** typically scalar graphs of pressure, flow, and volume, can be displayed by many microprocessor-based ventilators. Flow-volume and pressure–volume graphics can also be displayed but these are less useful. Dynamic pressure–volume loops typically reflect how the ventilator delivers flow and are of limited usefulness for detecting lower and upper inflection points.

  1. Airway pressure graphics
    a. An airway pressure waveform that varies from breath to breath indicates the presence of dyssynchrony (**Fig. 2-14**).

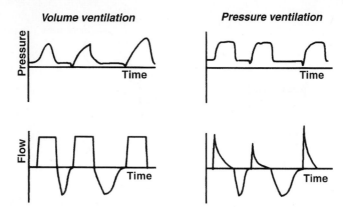

FIGURE 2-14 Patient–ventilator dyssynchrony. During volume-controlled ventilation, the pressure waveform varies from breath to breath. During pressure-controlled ventilation, the flow waveform varies from breath to breath.

    b. The stress index is the coefficient b of a power equation (airway pressure $= a \times$ inspiratory time^b + c), fitted on the airway opening pressure segment corresponding to the period of constant-flow inflation during constant flow, volume-controlled ventilation. For stress index values of less than 1, the airway pressure curve presents a downward concavity, suggesting a decrease in elastance during constant-flow inflation. For stress index values higher than 1, the curve presents an upward concavity, suggesting a increase in elastance. For a stress index value equal to 1, the curve is straight, suggesting the absence of tidal variations in elastance (**Fig. 2-15**).

  2. The airway flow waveform

    a. Expiratory flow does not return to a zero baseline in the presence of auto-PEEP (**Fig. 2-16**). Although the flow waveform is useful for detecting auto-PEEP, it does not quantitatively indicate the amount of auto-PEEP.

  3. The volume waveform

    a. The difference between the inspiratory and expiratory tidal volumes indicates the volume of a leak (e.g., bronchopleural fistula) (**Fig. 2-17**).

K. Functional residual capacity (FRC) is the lung volume at the end of a normal exhalation.

  1. FRC is decreased in patients with ALI and it is increased in patients with obstructive lung disease.

  2. Some modern ventilators are able to measure FRC using a nitrogen washout procedure. The FRC procedure takes two measurements of approximately 20 breaths each. When an FRC measurement is started, the system first measures a baseline N_2 concentration. A constant Fio_2 is needed to accurately establish a baseline N_2 concentration for the nitrogen washout process. Once the baseline N_2 concentration is found, Fio_2 is changed by 10%. Because the only gases that are present are O_2, CO_2, and N_2, it is possible to determine the N_2 concentration indirectly by measurement of O_2 and CO_2. FRC can be calculated from the washout of N_2 during the step change in Fio_2.

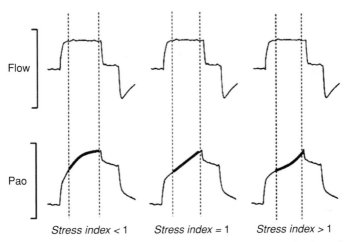

FIGURE 2-15 The pressure–time curve and the stress index. Note that the patient is ventilated with constant flow volume ventilaton. The pressure versus time curves are of stress indice <1 (alveolar recruitment), = 1, and > 1 (alveolar over-distention). (From Grasso S, Stripoli T, DeMicheleM, et al. ARDSnet ventilatory protocol and alveolar hyperinflation: role of positive end-expiratorypressure. *Am J Respir Crit Care Med* 2007;176(8):761–767).

L. **Electrical impedance tomography (EIT)** is an imaging technique in which the conductivity is inferred from surface electrical measurements. EIT adhesive electrodes are applied to the skin and an electric current, typically a few milliamperes of alternating current at a frequency of 10 to 100 kHz, is applied across two or more electrodes. The resulting electrical potentials are measured, and the process repeated for numerous different configurations of applied current. The lungs become less conductive as the alveoli

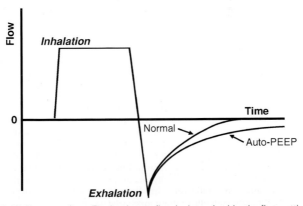

FIGURE 2-16 Flow waveform. The inspiratory flow is determined by the flow setting on the ventilator. Expiratory flow should return to zero. If the expiratory flow does not return to zero, auto–positive end-expiratory pressure is present. Auto-PEEP, auto–positive end-expiratory pressure.

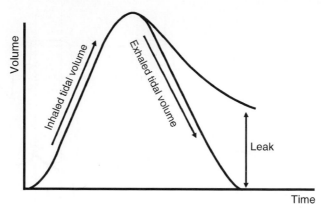

FIGURE 2-17 Volume waveform. If the exhaled volume does not equal the inhaled volume, a leak is present in the system.

become filled with air and more conductive if alveoli become airless (collapsed, edematous, or consolidated).

M. Ventilator function

1. **Alarms** are numerous on mechanical ventilators. The most important is the disconnect alarm.

    a. A loss of airway pressure **(low-pressure alarm)** indicates a ventilator disconnect or a gross leak in the system. A **high-pressure alarm** indicates the presence of an elevated airway pressure. The high-pressure alarm also serves to cycle the ventilator to the expiratory phase to avoid injury due to overpressurization of the lungs. Appropriate setting of the high-pressure alarm is particularly important during volume ventilation. Common causes of a high-pressure alarm are obstruction of the ventilator circuit or the patient's airways (e.g., kinked ventilator circuit, kinked endotracheal tube, secretions, bronchospasm), a sudden decrease in lung compliance (pneumothorax, mainstream intubation, congestive heart failure), or patient–ventilator dyssynchrony ("bucking the ventilator").

    b. **Exhaled tidal volume** should be monitored during volume-controlled ventilation to detect a leak. During pressure-controlled ventilation, the tidal volume should be monitored to detect changes in respiratory system compliance, resistance, auto-PEEP, or patient breathing efforts.

    c. **Fio$_2$.** Although the blenders in mechanical ventilators are reliable, it is prudent to monitor Fio$_2$ in mechanically ventilated patients.

    d. **Apnea.** With spontaneous breathing modes, such as pressure support, there is risk of hypoventilation due to loss of respiratory drive. Current-generation ventilators initiate backup ventilatory support if the patient does not breathe during a preset period of time.

2. **Inspired gas conditioning.** Because the upper airway is bypassed, the inspired gas is warmed and humidified during mechanical ventilation. This has been traditionally accomplished using an active heated humidifier. Recently, there has been increased use of passive humidifiers (artificial noses) during mechanical ventilation.

    a. **Airway temperature** is typically monitored during mechanical ventilation when active humidifiers are used. High temperatures should be monitored to avoid airway burns and low temperatures should be monitored to avoid delivery of inadequately humidified gas.

3. **Humidity** is not measured by current mechanical ventilators. The adequacy of delivered humidity can be assessed by observing the ventilator circuit near the patient for the presence of condensation. If the inspiratory circuit near the patient is dry, the delivered humidity is inadequate and steps should be taken to increase the level of humidification to avoid occlusion of the artificial airway with secretions. If an artificial nose is used, adequate humidification of the inspired gas is indicated by condensation within the proximal end of the endotracheal tube.

Selected References

Albaiceta GM, Blanch L, Lucangelo U. Static pressure-volume curves of the respiratory system: were they just a passing fad? *Curr Opin Crit Care* 2008;14:80–86.

Banner MJ, Jaeger MJ, Kirby RR. Components of the work of breathing and implications for monitoring ventilator-dependent patients. *Crit Care Med* 1994;22:515–523.

Batchelder PB, Raley DM. Maximizing the laboratory setting for testing devices and understanding statistical output in pulse oximetry. *Anesth Analg* 2007;105(6 Suppl):S85–S94.

Bendjelid K. The pulse oximetry plethysmographic curve revisited. *Curr Opin Crit Care* 2008;14:348–353.

Bendjelid K, Schütz N, Stotz M, et al. Transcutaneous PCO_2 monitoring in critically ill adults: clinical evaluation of a new sensor. *Crit Care Med* 2005;33:2203–2206.

Blanch L, Bernabé F, Lucangelo U. Measurement of air trapping, intrinsic positive end-expiratory pressure, and dynamic hyperinflation in mechanically ventilated patients. *Respir Care* 2005;50:110–124.

Cannesson M, Desebbe O, Rosamel P, et al. Pleth variability index to monitor the respiratory variations in the pulse oximeter plethysmographic waveform amplitude and predict fluid responsiveness in the operating theatre. *Br J Anaesth* 2008;101:200–206.

Cheifetz IM, Myers TR. Should every mechanically ventilated patient be monitored with capnography from intubation to extubation? *Respir Care* 2007;52:423–442.

Dhand R. Ventilator graphics and respiratory mechanics in the patient with obstructive lung disease. *Respir Care* 2005;50:246–261.

Fernández-Pérez ER, Hubmayr RD. Interpretation of airway pressure waveforms. *Intensive Care Med* 2006;32:658–659.

Gehring H, Nornberger C, Matz H, et al. The effects of motion artifact and low perfusion on the performance of a new generation of pulse oximeters in volunteers undergoing hypoxemia. *Respir Care* 2002;47:48–60.

Georgopoulos D, Prinianakis G, Kondili E. Bedside waveforms interpretation as a tool to identify patient-ventilator asynchronies. *Intensive Care Med* 2006;32:34–47.

Grasso S, Stripoli T, DeMicheleM, et al. ARDSnet ventilatory protocol and alveolar hyperinflation: role of positive end-expiratorypressure. *Am J Respir Crit Care Med* 2007;176(8): 761–767.

Hess D. Detection and monitoring of hypoxemia and oxygen therapy. *Respir Care* 2000; 45:65–80.

Hess DR, Bigatello LM. The chest wall in acute lung injury/acute respiratory distress syndrome. *Curr Opin Crit Care* 2008;14:94–102.

Hess DR, Medoff MD, Fessler MB. Pulmonary mechanics and graphics during positive pressure ventilation. *Int Anesthesiol Clin* 1999;37(3):15–34.

Jubran A. Advances in respiratory monitoring during mechanical ventilation. *Chest* 1999;116:1416–1425.

Krauss B, Hess DR. Capnography for procedural sedation and analgesia in the emergency department. *Ann Emerg Med* 2007;50:172–181.

Landsverk SA, Hoiseth LO, Kvandal P, Hisdal J, Skare O, Kirkeboen KA. Poor agreement between respiratory variations in pulse oximetry photoplethysmographic waveform amplitude and pulse pressure in intensive care unit patients. *Anesthesiology* 2008;109: 849–855.

Lucangelo U, Bernabè F, Blanch L. Lung mechanics at the bedside: make it simple. *Curr Opin Crit Care* 2007;13:64–72.

Lucangelo U, Bernabé F, Blanch L. Respiratory mechanics derived from signals in the ventilator circuit. *Respir Care* 2005;50:55–67.

Lucangelo U, Blanch L. Dead space. *Intensive Care Med* 2004;30:576–579.

McMorrow RC, Mythen MG. Pulse oximetry. *Curr Opin Crit Care* 2006;12:269–271.

Owens RL, Hess DR, Malhotra A, Venegas JG, Harris RS. Effect of the chest wall on pressure-volume curve analysis of acute respiratory distress syndrome lungs. *Crit Care Med* 2008;36:2980–2985.

Owens RL, Stigler WS, Hess DR. Do newer monitors of exhaled gases, mechanics, and esophageal pressure add value? *Clin Chest Med* 2008;29:297–312.

Shapiro BA. Point-of-care blood testing and cardiac output measurement in the intensive care unit. *New Horizons* 1999;7:244–252.

Talmor D, Sarge T, Malhotra A, et al. Mechanical ventilation guided by esophageal pressure in acute lung injury. *N Engl J Med* 2008;359:2095–2104.

Thompson JE, Jaffe MB. Capnographic waveforms in the mechanically ventilated patient. *Respir Care* 2005;50:100–109.

Yem JS, Tang Y, Turner MJ, et al. Sources of error in noninvasive pulmonary blood flow measurements by partial rebreathing: a computer model study. *Anesthesiology* 2003;98: 881–887.

Use of Ultrasound in the ICU

Robin Guillory and Marc de Moya

Ultrasound imaging was introduced in the 1950s. As ultrasound technology has improved, physicians have recognized the potential of using it at the bedside of the critically ill or injured patient to assist with diagnosis and therapy. This chapter will provide an overview of the uses and limitations of point-of-care ultrasound and echocardiography in the ICU setting.

I. **Properties of ultrasound.** Although many properties of ultrasound technology make it an ideal modality for the critical care environment, there are also some barriers to point-of-care ultrasound use.

   A. **Pros.** Current ultrasound technology allows for **rapid** and **accurate** scanning at the bedside. In addition, an ultrasound examination can be quickly **repeated** if the clinical situation changes. Ultrasound also provides a **safety advantage** over many other imaging modalities, because it is noninvasive and does not require radiation, dye exposure, or patient transport. Bedside physician-performed ultrasound is not meant to replace or simulate a complete ultrasound evaluation. Rather, it is meant as an **extension of the physical examination** or as a tool to answer a clinical question. When used in this way, a substantial percentage of ultrasound examinations result in a change in treatment or workup.

   B. **Cons.** Establishing a bedside ICU ultrasound program requires an initial **investment** in both equipment and physician training. After machine acquisition and setup, the costs of ultrasound use are limited to machine cleaning, image archiving, and quality assurance tasks. Unfortunately, physician training can be a daunting task. **Formal training programs are limited** in many areas of ICU ultrasound, and the path to credentialing is often unclear. This is a problem that the point-of-care ultrasound community is actively addressing. Other barriers to ICU ultrasound use include **difficulty achieving good ultrasound windows** and images in an ICU population and concerns that the ultrasound probe could act as a **fomite.** Some worry that reliance on ultrasound guidance during procedures could result in a **loss of anatomic landmark-based technique.** There are no data, however, to support that ultrasound use increases infection rates or results in loss of landmark-based skills.

II. **Ultrasound physics.** A basic understanding of ultrasound physics and technology will help the user understand the limits and capabilities of ultrasound. In addition, it will help the user avoid misinterpreting artifacts.

   A. **Ultrasound** refers to sound waves with a frequency >20 kHz, too high for the human ear to hear.

   B. **Ultrasound probes** are made of arrays of piezoelectric crystal transducers. Piezoelectric crystals convert electrical energy (voltage) into mechanical energy (movement). As a result, stimulation of these crystals causes them to vibrate, producing high-frequency (2–10 MHz) sound waves, which propagate through tissue. Reflection of these sound waves occurs at tissue interfaces, and the returning signals are received by the ultrasound probe and integrated into an image.

C. **Echogenity.** Air and bone cause marked reflection of the ultrasound beam back to the probe. As a result, **air and bone produce a "bright" echogenic image**. Fluids allow transmission of the ultrasound wave without reflection, and thus **appear "dark" or hypoechoic**. Other tissues appear as differing levels of gray scale depending on their makeup. Highly reflective or echogenic tissues prevent visualization of deeper tissues, as the ultrasound beam is unable to penetrate the reflective tissue. In contrast, transmission through hypoechoic structures facilitates visualization of deep structures.

D. **Attenuation** (loss of energy) of the ultrasound beam occurs because of reflection, refraction, scattering, and absorption as the beam travels through tissue. As a result, waves reflected from deep tissues arrive at the ultrasound probe with less signal.

E. **Frequency.** The thickness of a piezoelectric crystal determines the frequency of the sound it emits. As a result, each ultrasound probe produces waves at a characteristic frequency, measured in hertz (cycles/second). Waves with higher frequency produce greater resolution. Need for resolution must be balanced against need for penetration to deep tissues, as lower-frequency beams undergo less attenuation and are thus able to travel further through tissue.

F. **Doppler** systems take advantage of the frequency change that occurs in the echoed signal when an object moves toward or away from the ultrasound source. Doppler ultrasound analyzes the scattered ultrasound waves generated by moving blood cells.

G. **Artifacts** occur in ultrasound images when physical processes alter the ultrasound beam in a way that is not predicted by the basic assumptions the operator makes about the beam. It is important to understand when these assumptions are violated so that artifacts are not misinterpreted as findings.

   1. **Basic assumptions**
      a. Sound waves travel in straight lines.
      b. Reflections occur from structures along the central axis of the beam.
      c. Intensity of reflection corresponds to the reflector scattering strength.
      d. Sound travels at exactly 1,540 m/s.
      e. Sound travels directly to the reflector and back.

   2. **Types of artifacts**
      a. **Reverberation** occurs when sound waves bounce back and forth between two tissue planes before returning to the receiver. Reverberation artifacts appear as multiple equally spaced lines. Reverberation artifacts can be reduced by changing the angle of the ultrasound probe.
      b. **Ring-down artifact** occurs when an object vibrates at a characteristic resonance frequency, producing an echogenic beam behind the object.
      c. **Mirror image artifact**. Smooth surfaces that are strong reflectors can reflect the ultrasound beam onto another surface. When this reflected beam returns to the probe, it produces a mirror image copy (a mirror image artifact) of the strong reflector in the image. This artifact is frequently produced by the diaphragm (**Fig. 3-1**).
      d. **Enhancement artifact** is brightness that occurs deep to a low-attenuation structure. For example, the ultrasound beam will travel through the fluid-filled gallbladder more easily than through the adjacent

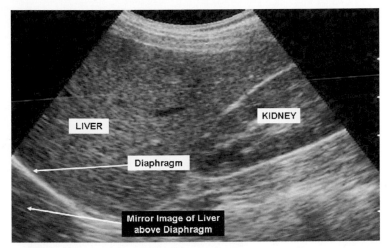

FIGURE 3-1 Normal ultrasound view of Morison's pouch. A mirror image artifact of the liver is visible above the hyperechoic diaphragm. Image courtesy of MGH Division of Emergency Ultrasound.

liver. As a result, more of the ultrasound beam will reach the tissue deep to the gallbladder, making this tissue appear abnormally bright.

   e. **Attenuation artifact (or acoustic shadowing)** is the opposite of enhancement artifact. Tissue deep to strongly attenuating objects appears abnormally dark. It is common to see attenuation artifact deep to gallstones.

III. Thoracic ultrasound

A. **Sensitivity/specificity.** Thoracic ultrasonography provides better sensitivity and specificity than do physical examination, auscultation, and plain radiography when evaluating for pleural effusion or pneumothorax, without subjecting the patient to the drawbacks of CT scanning (poor access, the need for irradiation, patient transport, and dye administration).

B. **Normal chest examination.** In a normal sonographic examination of the chest, the apposition of the parietal and visceral pleura produces a hyperechoic stripe that the lung parenchyma slides beneath. This generates the **"sliding lung sign"** as well as specific **"comet tail"** artifacts that are markers of normal lung parenchyma. In the face of chest pathology, these normal artifact findings are disrupted.

C. **Specific ultrasound findings in thoracic pathology**

   1. **Pneumothorax.** When a pneumothorax is present, the parietal pleura–visceral pleura interface is replaced by a parietal pleura–air interface. This results in horizontal reverberation artifact of the chest wall and elimination of lung sliding and the normal lung artifacts. Lack of lung sliding is common in critically ill patients but is nearly 100% sensitive for pneumothorax. Horizontal reverberation artifacts in the absence of lung sliding are 96.5% specific for the diagnosis of pneumothorax. Presence of lung sliding or comet tail artifacts provides a 100% negative predictive value for pneumothorax. This is far superior than plain radiography's ability to detect pneumothorax.

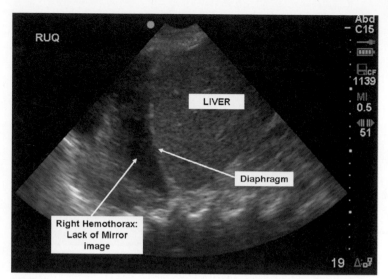

FIGURE 3-2 Hemothorax. A hypoechoic area is visible above the hyperechoic diaphragm, and the mirror image artifact of the liver is absent. Compare with **Fig. 3-1**. Image courtesy of MGH Division of Emergency Ultrasound.

2. **Pleural effusions** are visible as hypoechoic areas bordered by the chest wall, the lung parenchyma, and the diaphragm. The echogenicity of pleural effusion fluid is determined by the makeup of the effusion. Transudates are echo free. Exudates, hemothorax, and empyema are often echoic and loculated (**Fig. 3-2**). Ultrasound is superior to chest radiography in detection of pleural effusion (overall accuracy of 93.6%).

3. **Other chest pathology.** Use of chest ultrasonography to evaluate lung parenchyma for **consolidation, atelectasis, edema,** and **lung abscess** has been reported. Any process that reduces the aeration of the lung allows for greater ultrasound beam penetration and increased visualization of parenchymal structure.

IV. **Hemodynamic evaluation**
   A. **Goal-directed echocardiography.** Hemodynamic instability is common in the critically ill patient population, and rapid assessment and optimization are critical to patient care and survival. Traditional monitors of hemodynamic parameters (e.g., physical examination, central venous and pulmonary artery catheters) are of questionable utility and safety. Echocardiography allows for quick, reliable, accurate, and noninvasive diagnosis of a variety of cardiovascular pathologies. Physician-performed bedside echocardiography is not intended to be a replacement for a comprehensive echocardiographic evaluation. Multiple studies, however, have demonstrated the ability of novice sonographers to answer simple clinical hemodynamic questions using limited bedside echocardiography and ultrasound after 8 hours or less of training. When used as an extension of the physical examination, point-of-care goal-directed echocardiography

identifies the majority of cardiac causes of shock and provides valuable information that influences treatment in 63% of cases.

B. **Identifying the etiology of hemodynamic instability**
   1. **Assessment of ejection fraction**
      a. **Left ventricular ejection fraction** can be qualitatively assessed by visual inspection of echocardiographic images alone. A depressed left ventricular ejection fraction may suggest cardiac ischemia or a cardiomyopathy.
      b. **Right ventricular (RV) size and function** is generally evaluated by comparison with the left ventricle and evaluation of the interventricular septum. The right ventricle should be less than half the size of the left ventricle, and the interventricular septum should be convex toward the right ventricle. RV hypokinesis or dilation may be due to pulmonary embolism (PE), acute respiratory distress syndrome, excessive positive end-expiratory pressure, increased pulmonary vascular resistance, or RV ischemia. Acute regional RV wall dysfunction has a sensitivity of 77% and a specificity of 94% for the diagnosis of acute PE. Evidence of acute cor pulmonale in the setting of PE is associated with increased mortality and may have prognostic and therapeutic implications.
   2. **Pericardial effusion and tamponade.** Rapid diagnosis and treatment of cardiac tamponade are critical in both traumatic and nontraumatic patient populations. Physical examination evidence of tamponade is present in a minority of patients, while echocardiographic diagnosis of cardiac tamponade approaches a sensitivity of 100%, even in the hands of noncardiologist sonographers. Pericardial fluid, blood, or pus can usually be seen in either the subcostal (**Fig. 3-3**) or parasternal

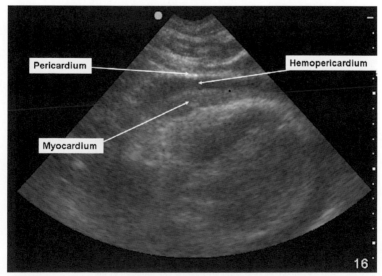

FIGURE 3-3 Even in this subcostal view obtained rapidly in the trauma bay, a pericardial effusion can be seen as a hypoechoic stripe between the myocardium and pericardium.

views, and diastolic right atrial or ventricular free wall collapse are consistent with tamponade physiology. Echocardiography can also facilitate safe and efficient pericardiocentesis.

3. **Volume status assessment.** Both ultrasound and echocardiography can provide insight into a patient's volume status.
   a. **Echocardiography.** Systolic obliteration of the left ventricular cavity during an echocardiographic examination is evidence of severe hypovolemia.
   b. **Ultrasound.** Normally the inferior vena cava (IVC) narrows during inspiration and distends with expiration. As venous pressure rises, however, the IVC distends and the normal cyclic variation in IVC diameter is lost. As a result, **IVC diameter and collapsibility** may be a noninvasive surrogate for central venous pressure (CVP). An IVC that collapses with respiration suggests decreased preload (CVP 0–5). A normally sized IVC with >50% decrease in diameter during respiration correlates with a CVP of 5 to 10. A normally sized IVC with <50% decrease in diameter during respiration correlates with a CVP of 10 to 15. A dilated (>2 cm) IVC with no or small change in diameter with respiration suggests a CVP >15. Studies suggest that a cutoff of >12% to 18% variation in IVC diameter with mechanical ventilation identifies the majority of patients that are volume responsive. In addition, lack of IVC dilation after fluid resuscitation may suggest ongoing blood loss in trauma patients.

4. **Other causes** of hemodynamic instability, including tension pneumothorax, intra-abdominal, and intrathoracic sources of blood loss, and infectious sources can also be diagnosed using point-of-care ultrasound. These ultrasound applications are discussed elsewhere in this chapter.

C. **Advanced echocardiography**
   1. **Advanced transthoracic echocardiography.** More experienced sonographers can use echocardiography to assess valvular function; to follow left ventricular end-diastolic area and volume for preload optimization; to measure stroke volume and cardiac output using Doppler imaging; to evaluate for diastolic dysfunction using transmitral and transpulmonary flow wave patterns; and to diagnose a patent foramen ovale, subtle wall motion abnormalities, and pulmonary hypertension.
   2. **Transesophageal echocardiography** (TEE) affords an even greater level of detail about cardiac structure and function. In addition, TEE allows for imaging of structures not visible with transthoracic echocardiography and in patients where adequate transthoracic sonographic windows cannot be obtained (severe obesity, COPD, dressings, high PEEP). Execution and interpretation of TEE, however, requires significant training and expertise beyond that required for bedside limited and goal-directed transthoracic echocardiography.

V. **Abdominal and retroperitoneal ultrasound**
   A. **Focused assessment with sonography for trauma (FAST). Hemorrhage** is the leading cause of potentially **preventable traumatic death.** As a result, traumatologists have searched for **rapid** and **accurate** methods for identifying bleeding sources in trauma patients in an effort to affect treatment more quickly. The FAST examination is one such method.
      1. **FAST involves real-time ultrasound examination of the**
         a. **Pericardium**
         b. **Perisplenic space (Fig. 3-4)**

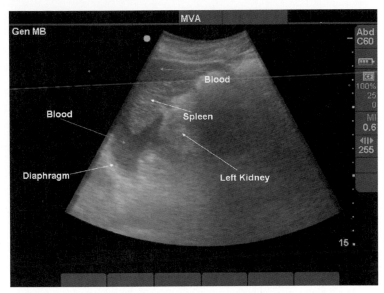

FIGURE 3-4 This FAST examination of the perisplenic space shows significant hemoperitoneum and suggests the need for urgent laparotomy.

    c. **Perihepatic space** (Morison's pouch)
    d. **Pelvic space** (Douglas' pouch)
    e. **Some authors** also advocate **supradiaphragmatic views**
  2. **The goal of the FAST examination** (see also **Chapter 9**) **is to identify significant bleeding** that must be treated rapidly, not to look for organ injury. A positive FAST examination may suggest the need for laparotomy, while a negative or minimally positive FAST examination in a hypotensive trauma patient directs the physician to look for other major sources of bleeding.
  3. FAST examination is accurate and expeditious in the hands of surgeons and radiologists.
  4. Use of the FAST examination in the emergency department results in **shorter time to operative intervention** and **reductions in hospital length of stay, complication rates, and cost of care.**
  5. **FAST examination has now become standard of care** in the evaluation of the trauma patient and has largely supplanted diagnostic peritoneal lavage for detection of significant hemoperitoneum.
 B. **Hepatobiliary ultrasound.** Ultrasound evaluation of the **liver** can reveal diffuse parenchymal pathology, masses, abscesses, cysts, congestion, lacerations, and ascites. Portal vein thrombosis can contribute to variceal bleeding. **Biliary system** examination can diagnose cholelithiasis and gallbladder polyps, suggest cholecystitis (in the presence of gallbladder wall thickening, sonographic Murphy sign, pericholecystic fluid, and other signs), and demonstrate biliary ductal dilation. The location of the **pancreas** can make it difficult to visualize with ultrasound. Pancreatic swelling and phlegmon,

mon, however, may be visible in severe pancreatitis, and free fluid may be visible after a pseudocyst rupture.

C. **Gastrointestinal ultrasound.** Ultrasound is more accurate in detecting free intraperitoneal air than is plain radiography (93% vs. 79% sensitivity). **Free air** appears as an echogenic area producing posterior reverberation artifact. Ultrasound has also been described in the evaluation of **prandial status.**

D. **Splenic ultrasound** can reveal splenic infarcts, hematomas, and abscesses, as well as splenomegaly. Splenic artery or vein involvement by pancreatitis is an important finding.

E. **Genitourinary ultrasound.** Ultrasound examination of the **kidneys** and **bladder** may reveal a distended bladder or hydronephrosis, suggesting a postrenal cause of renal failure. Doppler ultrasound may reveal poor **renal artery or vein** flow. Renal and perinephric abscesses and masses, as well as some traumatic renal injuries, may also be visible on ultrasound examination. Volumetric bladder scanning prior to transurethral urine collection improves first attempt success rate.

VI. **Ultrasound-guided procedures.** Need for vascular access and other procedures is common in the critically ill patient population. Traditionally, most procedures have been performed using palpation and landmark-based techniques. These techniques are flawed in the best of circumstances, and additional ICU challenges (e.g., difficult patient positioning, ventilator dependence, coagulopathy, and history of prior vascular access) increase both procedural risks and the chances for a failed procedure. **Ultrasound guidance may improve the efficacy and safety of many bedside procedures performed in the ICU.**

A. **Central venous line insertion.** Multiple randomized trials and two meta-analyses have found ultrasound-guided central venous line insertion to be safer, faster, and more efficacious when compared to traditional landmark-based techniques. These studies have evaluated a variety of practice settings and operators with varying levels of experience. Data exist for benefit at the internal jugular (**Figs. 3-5** and **3-6**), subclavian, and femoral vein positions, although the internal jugular site has been studied most extensively. This evidence has prompted several safety and quality assurance bodies to recommend ultrasound-guided central venous line insertion. **The technique is now standard of care in many hospitals.**

B. **Arterial line insertion.** When compared to the palpation technique, ultrasound-guided arterial line placement reduces procedural time, improves first-pass success rate, and reduces both the number of sites required and the incidence of hematoma formation.

C. **Peripheral intravenous (IV) cannulation.** Ultrasound guidance can facilitate placement of peripheral IVs in patients with difficult IV access.

D. **Thoracentesis.** Ultrasound-assisted thoracentesis and chest tube placement are well described. Ultrasound guidance improves the safety and efficacy of these procedures, especially in the presence of small or loculated effusions.

E. **Pericardiocentesis.** Ultrasound guidance improves the safety and efficacy of pericardiocentesis.

F. **Intra-abdominal procedures.** Critical illness is frequently complicated by intra-abdominal sepsis and the production of ascites. The safety and efficacy of a variety of ultrasound-guided abdominal procedures have been described (including **paracentesis; cholecystostomy tube placement; percutaneous nephrostomy tube placement; and drainage of subphrenic, hepatic, renal, abdominal, pelvic, and pancreatic abscesses**). Direct visualization during the

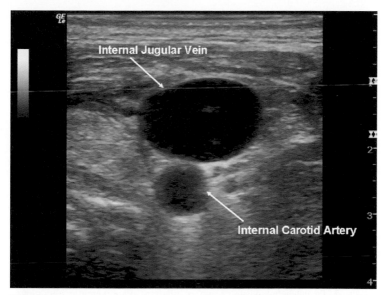

FIGURE 3-5 A transverse view of the right internal jugular vein and carotid artery allows for identification of both a patent vein and the relationship of the vein to the artery.

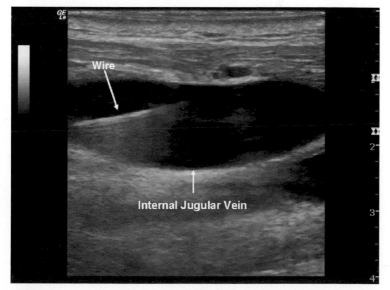

FIGURE 3-6 A longitudinal view of the internal jugular vein demonstrates intravenous placement of the wire.

procedure reduces the risk of damage to nearby structures, such as, the diaphragm, liver, spleen, kidneys, bowel, and epigastric arteries. Ultrasound-guided **feeding tube placement** has also been described. Many intensivists, however, do not have the training to perform these procedures.

VII. **Novel ultrasound applications**
 A. **Transcranial Doppler (TCD)** is a vital and evolving tool in neurocritical care. TCD can suggest the presence of **vasospasm** in post–subarachnoid hemorrhage patients. In addition, the TCD findings in **brain death** are well described, and TCD methods for determining **intracranial pressure, cerebral perfusion pressure,** and **intracranial vessel CO_2 reactivity/autoregulation** are being developed. These methods may assist in the management of patients with **traumatic brain injury,** as well as provide prognostic information.
 B. **Airway management**
    1. **Preintubation** measurement of anterior neck fat is a better predictor of difficult intubation than is body mass index, and ultrasound visualization of diaphragmatic excursion preextubation may predict extubation failure.
    2. **Intubation/tracheostomy.** Ultrasound-guided superior laryngeal nerve block may aid in awake intubation. Ultrasound, in conjunction with bronchoscopy, can improve the safety of bedside percutaneous tracheostomy by permitting visualization of the pretracheal veins, of the tracheal rings, and of the position of the endotracheal tube in the trachea.
    3. **Postintubation** visualization of bilateral diaphragmatic and pleural motions verifies endotracheal tube placement and rules out endobronchial intubation. This evaluation can assist with verifying lung isolation during dual-lumen tube placement as well. Ultrasound-measured tracheal width predicts proper dual-lumen tube size.
 C. **Search for an infectious source.** In addition to aiding in the diagnosis of pneumonia, pleural empyema, pericardial empyema, and intra-abdominal infection, as discussed previously, ultrasound can identify a variety of other infectious sources. Whole-body ultrasound examination of the critically ill patient has been shown to lead to a change in therapy in 22% of cases. The majority of therapy changes were due to identification of an infectious source.
    1. **Skin and soft tissue ultrasound** is a screening tool for necrotizing skin infection, retained foreign body, and soft tissue infection. It is superior to clinical evaluation in differentiating cellulitis from deep tissue abscess, and it can assist with soft tissue foreign body removal and abscess drainage.
    2. **Sinusitis** can be diagnosed on ultrasound.
    3. **Septic joint effusions** are visible and drainable with ultrasonography.
 D. **Ultrasound is also used** to guide nerve blocks for perioperative or peritrauma pain control; to diagnose aortic dissection, venous thrombosis, thrombophlebitis, and pseudoaneurysm; to place IVC filters at the bedside; to diagnose fascial dehiscence; to detect cardiac motion in cases of PEA arrest; and to diagnose sternal, long bone, and other fractures.

VIII. **The future of ultrasound in the ICU.** Bedside ultrasound is well suited to the critical care environment. It is an invaluable goal-directed adjunct to the physical examination, while being rapid, safe, accurate, available, and repeatable. Ultrasound also improves the safety and efficacy of many therapeutic interventions. Despite some remaining barriers, the use of bedside ultrasound is becoming increasingly widespread, and new applications are frequently reported. With time, the ultrasound will become a pocket tool used in every physical examination. A hypotensive patient will be rapidly evaluated for hypovolemia, tension pneumothorax, myocardial wall motion abnormalities, and pericardial effusion. The septic patient will be scanned, looking for a septic source, and the patient with new-onset renal failure will be examined for evidence of prerenal and postrenal etiologies. As the number of diagnostic and therapeutic uses of bedside ultrasound grows, its role is likely to expand until point-of-care ultrasound becomes a part of daily care in every intensive care unit.

Selected References

Abboud PAC, Kendall JL. Ultrasound guidance for vascular access. *Emerg Med Clin N Am* 2004;22:749–773.

Aldrich JE. Basic physics of ultrasound imaging. *Crit Care Med* 2007;35:S131–S137.

Arbelot C, Ferrari F, et al. Lung ultrasound in acute respiratory distress syndrome and acute lung injury. *Curr Opin Crit Care* 2008;14:70–74.

Beaulieu Y. Bedside echocardiography in the assessment of the critically ill. *Crit Care Med* 2007;35:S235–S249.

Beaulieu Y, Marik PE. Bedside ultrasonography in the ICU: part 1. *Chest* 2005;128:881–895.

Beaulieu Y, Marik PE. Bedside ultrasonography in the ICU: part 2. *Chest* 2005;128:1766–1781.

Beckh S, Bölcskei PL, Lessnau KD. Real-time chest ultrasonography: a comprehensive review for the pulmonologist. *Chest* 2002;122:1759–1773.

Bouhemad B, Zhang M, et al. Clinical review: bedside lung ultrasound in critical care practice. *Crit Care* 2007;11:205–213.

Feissel M, Michard F, et al. The respiratory variation in inferior vena cava diameter as a guide to fluid therapy. *Intensive Care Med* 2004;30:1834–1837.

Feller-Kopman D. Ultrasound-guided internal jugular access: a proposed standardized approach and implications for training and practice. *Chest* 2007;132:302–309.

Hudson PA, Promes SB. Abdominal ultrasonography. *Emerg Med Clin North Am* 1997;15:825–848.

Kirkpatrick AW. Clinician-performed focused sonography for the resuscitation of trauma. *Crit Care Med* 2007;35:S162–S172.

Lawrence JP. Physics and instrumentation of ultrasound. *Crit Care Med* 2007;35:S314–S322.

Lichtenstein DA. Ultrasound in the management of thoracic disease. *Crit Care Med* 2007;35:S250–S261.

Maecken T, Grau T. Ultrasound imaging in vascular access. *Crit Care Med* 2007;35:S178–S185.

Nicolaou S, Talsky A, et al. Ultrasound-guided interventional radiology in critical care. *Crit Care Med* 2007;35:S186–S197.

Ract C, Le Moigno S, et al. Transcranial Doppler ultrasound goal-directed therapy for the early management of severe traumatic brain injury. *Intensive Care Med* 2007;33:645–651.

Rose JS. Ultrasound in abdominal trauma. *Emerg Med Clin North Am* 2004;22:581–599.

Rozycki G, Ochsner MG, et al. A prospective study of surgeon performed ultrasound as the primary adjuvant modality for injured patient assessment. *J Trauma* 1995;39:492–500.

Saqqur M, Zygun D, Demchuk A. Role of transcranial Doppler in neurocritical care. *Crit Care Med* 2007;35:S216–S223.

Shiver S, Blaivas M, Lyon M. A prospective comparison of ultrasound-guided and blindly placed radial arterial catheters. *Acad Emerg Med* 2006;13:1275–1279.

Šustić A. Role of ultrasound in the airway management of critically ill patients. *Crit Care Med* 2007;35:S173–S177.

Tibbles CD, Porcaro W. Procedural applications of ultrasound. *Emerg Med Clin North Am* 2004;22:797–815.

Wang HP, Chen SC. Upper abdominal ultrasound in the critically ill. *Crit Care Med* 2007;35:S208–S215.

Yanagawa Y, Sakamoto T, et al. Hypovolemic shock evaluated by sonographic measurement of the inferior vena cava during resuscitation in trauma patients. *J Trauma* 2007;63:1245–1248.

4 Airway Management

Jonathan Charnin, Robert Goulet, and Richard Pino

Endotracheal intubation is indicated to treat respiratory failure by improving gas exchange and provide a patent airway when patients are at risk for aspiration, when airway maintenance by mask is difficult, and when prolonged mechanical ventilation is needed. This chapter discusses the evaluation of the airway, techniques for endotracheal intubation, and management of the chronically instrumented airway.

I. **Indications for endotracheal intubation**
   A. **Normal respiratory function** requires a patent airway, adequate respiratory drive, neuromuscular competence, intact thoracic anatomy, normal lung parenchyma, and the ability to cough, sigh, and defend against aspiration. Impairments in these parameters, singularly or in combination, may result in the need for endotracheal intubation and ventilatory support.
   B. **Endotracheal intubation**
      1. Provides a means for coupling the lungs to mechanical ventilators that apply positive airway pressures to improve gas exchange and treat respiratory failure.
      2. Provides relative protection against pulmonary aspiration, although microaspiration around the endotracheal tube (ETT) cuff does happen.
      3. Maintains a patent conduit for respiratory gas exchange.
      4. Establishes a route for clearance of respiratory secretions.

II. **Airway evaluation.** A systematic evaluation of the need for tracheal intubation is essential. The need for intubation can be immediate (e.g., cardiopulmonary arrest), emergent (e.g., impending respiratory failure), or urgent (e.g., decreased level of consciousness with inadequate airway control).
   A. **If cardiopulmonary resuscitation is underway,** bag–mask ventilation with 100% oxygen, followed by intubation, is required. Otherwise, perform a rapid evaluation to determine the need for intubation.
   B. **Apply oxygen by face mask.** The potential improvement in systemic oxygenation with supplemental oxygen may allow more time to evaluate the patient and consider options.
   C. **Assess level of consciousness.** Obtundation, stupor, or coma may be of respiratory origin (e.g., hypoxemia or hypercapnia) or arise from metabolic, pharmacologic, and neurologic causes. Depressed consciousness can lead to airway obstruction, pulmonary aspiration, atelectasis, and pneumonia. An absent gag reflex and/or the inability to maintain an adequate airway may indicate the need for intubation.
   D. **Integument.** Cyanosis occurs when deoxyhemoglobin is at least 5 g/dL. In anemia, cyanosis may be absent despite a low oxygen saturation in contrast to polycythemia in which small decreases in oxygen saturation may manifest as cyanosis. Cold, diaphoretic skin suggests intense autonomic stress or circulatory failure.

E. **Respiration**
 1. Respiratory efforts should be noted, with particular attention to the rate and depth of thoracic movements. **Slow, deep respirations** (<10/min) suggest opioid effect or central nervous system (CNS) disorder. **Tachypnea** (>35/min) is a nonspecific finding that can be present with disorders that cause decreased respiratory system compliance (e.g., pulmonary edema, consolidation, acute respiratory distress syndrome) or increased respiratory load (e.g., increased dead space, fever). It is a common finding in pulmonary embolism and with respiratory muscle fatigue.
 2. **Evaluation for upper airway obstruction** includes visual (laryngeal tug, chest wall retraction, chest/abdomen discoordination), tactile (air flow felt by placing a hand in front of the patient's mouth and nose, position of trachea in the neck), and auscultory (stridor, absent breath sounds) indicators of either complete or partial obstruction. In the absence of coexisting processes (e.g., cervical spine injury) and depending on the etiology of obstruction (e.g., depressed mental status), obstruction may be relieved by extending the head at the atlanto-occipital joint, performing a chin-lift, jaw thrust, and/or inserting an oral or nasal airway prior to intubation (see later discussion).
 3. **Examine respiratory excursions** for symmetry, timing, and coordination. A pneumothorax, splinting, or large bronchial obstruction can cause side-to-side asymmetry. Long inspiratory times suggest upper airway or other extrathoracic obstruction; a prolonged expiratory time suggests intrathoracic obstruction, bronchospasm, or both. Discordant breathing efforts or the use of accessory muscles suggests respiratory muscle weakness or fatigue. Long inspiratory or expiratory pauses (e.g., Cheyne-Stokes or apneustic breathing) are caused by brainstem or metabolic abnormalities and depressant drugs.
 4. **Auscultate** the chest for presence of symmetric breath sounds, bronchospasm, rhonchi, or rales suggestive of secretions or pulmonary edema.
 5. **Pulse oximetry** aids in assessing the adequacy of oxygenation.
F. **The etiology of respiratory failure** usually is apparent. Readily reversible causes may be addressed prior to intubation. Timely reversal of opioid- or benzodiazepine-induced respiratory depression, residual pharmacologic neuromuscular blockade, pneumothorax, acute pulmonary edema, or mucous plugging of the airway may circumvent the need for intubation. **Noninvasive ventilation** to avoid intubation may be useful during treatment for patients with reversible causes of respiratory failure.
G. **Arterial blood gas** (ABG) tensions and pH may help to measure disease severity, document changes in condition over time, and assess the efficacy of interventions. The use of ABGs should not substitute for clinical evaluation of the patient or delay needed interventions.

III. **Preparation for endotracheal intubation**
 A. **A focused history and physical examination,** which may be obtained quickly while preparing the equipment needed for intubation (see later discussion), includes
  1. **Assessment of airway anatomy.** A receding mandible (micrognathia), small oropharynx, protruding, prominent upper incisors, and a short, muscular "bull" neck are associated with potentially difficult laryngoscopy and intubation. Temporomandibular joint (TMJ) or cervical spine immobility can make visualization of the glottis difficult. Difficulty in subluxing the temporomandibular joint (TMJ) may be manifested in patients with diabetes mellitus. If these are recognized,

alternative or additional intubation techniques may be employed (**Section IV.G and following**). **Mask ventilation** will likely be more difficult in the obese patients, edentulous patients, and patients with facial hair.

2. **Allergies to medications.**
3. **Assessment of aspiration risk,** including time since last gastric intake, trauma, recent vomiting, upper gastrointestinal (GI) bleeding, hemoptysis, bowel obstruction, history of esophageal reflux, morbid obesity, and depressed mental status.
4. **Cardiovascular status,** angina–ischemia, infarction, dysrhythmias, congestive heart failure, aneurysms, and hypertension.
5. **Neurologic status,** increased intracranial pressure (ICP), ischemic symptoms, intracranial aneurysm, and hemorrhage.
6. **Musculoskeletal status,** neck and mandibular immobility or instability, neuromuscular disorders (especially recent cord denervation injuries, recent crush injuries, and burns).
7. **Coagulation status,** platelet count, anticoagulation therapy, or coagulopathy (especially if a nasal intubation is anticipated).
8. **Past intubation problems** including history of periglottic or subglottic stenosis. The prior history is not entirely reliable because many other factors, such as airway edema, trauma, and hemoptysis, may have intervened.

B. **Intubation method.** In an emergency, options are limited by the requirements for experience, expedience, and availability of specialized equipment. The most useful techniques are the following:

1. **Orotracheal intubation** is performed with direct laryngoscopy.
   a. **Advantages** include ease and minimal equipment needs. It is the most familiar technique, allowing ETT placement under direct vision.
   b. **Disadvantages.** Adequate mandible and neck mobility are necessary to allow direct visualization. Topical, regional (block), or general anesthesia is often required.
2. **Nasotracheal intubation** may be performed as a blind procedure guided by breath sounds or under direct vision with laryngoscope or fiberoptic bronchoscope.
   a. **Advantages.** Blind placement can be performed in a neutral head and neck position without general anesthesia or muscle paralysis. Nasotracheal intubation can be performed when the oral route is difficult or impossible (i.e., in a patient with limited mouth opening). A nasal tube also does not interfere with surgical repair of the mandible or oropharynx.
   b. **Disadvantages.** It is more difficult to place the tube quickly. Spontaneous respiration must be present to guide the tube for blind placement. Placement by direct vision with the laryngoscope, with or without the Magill forceps, has the same disadvantages as the orotracheal intubation method. Tube diameter is limited by nasal passage size. Severe nasal hemorrhage, which can be life threatening, can occur. Once placed, a nasally placed tube tends to soften and kink in the nasopharynx, which can increase airway resistance and make passage of a suction catheter more difficult. Nasal intubation is relatively contraindicated in the presence of suspected nasopharyngeal injury, nasal polyps, basilar skull fracture, epistaxis, coagulopathy, planned systemic anticoagulation or thrombolysis (i.e., the patient with an acute myocardial infarction), or immunocompromise. Sinusitis and otitis occur frequently with nasal intubation.
3. **Flexible fiberoptic intubation** can be used for oral or nasal intubations.
   a. **Advantages.** Very useful with distorted anatomy or in patients requiring maximal head–neck stability (i.e., unstable neck fractures).

b. **Disadvantages.** More skill is required than with other techniques. Fiberoptic intubation is not the technique of choice for emergency intubation of apneic patients. In patients with upper airway bleeding or vomiting, visualizing hypopharyngeal anatomy is difficult because of the limited capacity to clear secretions with the suction channel of the fiberscope.

4. **Rigid fiberoptic laryngosocopes** like the Bullard, Woo, or Upsher devices employ a rigid or semirigid fiberoptic bundle to transmit light and airway images that allow visualization of the larynx attached to a laryngoscope that is designed to expose the glottis to the fiberoptic apparatus. These laryngoscopes are designed to provide visualization of the glottis using a small mouth opening and with limited movement of the head. Malleable fiberoptic stylets like the Shikani Optical Stylet can allow visualization through the ETT during intubation. Video laryngoscopes employ a small video camera mounted on an laryngoscope blade to allow visualization of exposed pharyngeal and glottic structures as well as structures anterior to a typical laryngoscopic view on a video monitor. Although these are useful techniques, the expense to acquire these often precludes widespread usage for practice in nonemergent conditions.

5. **The laryngeal mask airway (LMA)** is an important adjunct for establishing an emergency airway, especially in patients in whom mask ventilation is difficult or impossible and traditional endotracheal intubation has been unsuccessful. Some LMA devices are specially designed to allow endotracheal intubation through the LMA after an airway has been established.

   a. **Advantages.** The LMA is a fast and reliable method of establishing an airway when other methods have failed and is the rescue airway of choice when mask ventilation and intubation have failed. Endotracheal intubation subsequently can be accomplished by placing an ETT through the lumen of the LMA with or without the assistance of a fiberoptic bronchoscope.

   b. **Disadvantages.** The LMA does not protect the airway against aspiration of gastric contents. The LMA may not be tolerated by an awake or agitated patient.

6. **Airway support devices** such as oral or nasopharyngeal airways do not prevent aspiration or guarantee continued airway patency. At best, they are temporary measures.

IV. Techniques for airway management

A. **Make thorough preparations for intubation prior to the initial attempt.** Time to establish the best possible intubating conditions usually is well spent. Equipment required for intubation is listed in **Table 4-1**.

1. **Essential equipment** includes a Yankauer-tipped suction, a laryngoscope with an appropriate blade (usually Macintosh 3 or Miller 2 for adults and Miller 1 for small children), and an appropriately sized ETT with a stylet inserted and the cuff checked by briefly inflating it with approximately 10 mL of air.

2. **Check that suction is available and functioning** in the form of a Yankauer or "tonsil tip" suction device.

3. **The appropriate size** for the ETT depends on the patient's age, body habitus, and indication for intubation. A 7.0-mm endotracheal tube is a reasonable choice for most women and an 8.0-mm endotracheal tube for most men. Suggested pediatric tube sizes are listed in **Table 4-2**. The absence of air leaking past the ETT during positive-pressure ventilation with the cuff down indicates too tight a fit at the laryngeal

or tracheal level. For an emergent intubation, a tube 0.5 mm smaller than usual will facilitate intubation.

4. **Position the patient**

   a. In the supine position, the pharyngeal and laryngeal axes of the patients are offset, making a good view of the glottis extremely difficult during direct laryngoscopy (**Fig. 4-1**). Positioning the patient in the "sniffing" position, with the occiput elevated by folded blankets and the head in extension, aligns the oral, pharyngeal, and laryngeal axes so that the pathway from the lips to the glottis is nearly a straight line.

   b. Move the bed away from the wall and remove the headboard to allow access to the patient's head. If the headboard is fixed, or for patients in unusual locations or traction, move the patient diagonally in the bed to afford access to the patient and airway. Adjust the height of the bed so that the patient's head is at your midchest level.

   c. **The trauma patient** presents special challenges. All patients with multiple trauma, head, or facial injury are presumed to have a cervical spine injury until excluded by a full evaluation. In such patients, excessive motion of the spine may produce or exacerbate a spinal cord injury. During airway manipulations, an assistant should stabilize the head and neck in a neutral position by maintaining in-line cervical stabilization. Note that **the greatest cervical**

TABLE 4-1	Suggested Contents of an Emergency Intubation Kit
Equipment	**Drugs**
Intravenous catheters (14–22 gauge)	Atropine
Laryngoscope blades	*cis*-atracurium
Endotracheal tubes (3–8 mm inner diameter)	Macintosh 2, 3, 4; Miller 0, 1, 2, 3
12-mL syringes	Ephedrine
Magill forceps	Epinephrine
Colorimetric end-tidal CO_2 detectors	Esmolol
Nasal airways	Topical anesthetic spray (lidocaine)
Oral airways	Etomidate
Tape	Glycopyrrolate
Yankauer suction catheters	Labetalol
Tube changers	Lidocaine (1% and 4%)
Guide wires	Lidocaine ointment
Cotton-tipped swabs	Midazolam
Nasogastric tubes	Naloxone (Narcan)
Jet ventilator	Oxymetazoline (Afrin) spray
	Pancuronium
	Phenylephrine
	Phenylephrine/lidocaine spray
	Propofol
	Propranolol
	Saline
	Succinylcholine
	Surgilube
	Viscous lidocaine

TABLE 4-2	Pediatric Endotracheal Tube Sizes
Age	**Size (mm)**
Premature infant	2.5
Term infant	3.0
1–4 mo	3.5
4 mo–1 y	4.0
1.5–2.0 y	4.5
2.5–3.5 y	5.0
4–6 y	5.5
7–9 y	6.0–7.0

Tube size should be adjusted to give airway leak pressures less than 25 cm H_2O; all tubes uncuffed.

displacement appears to occur during bag and mask ventilation, and that orotracheal intubation causes no more cervical displacement or neurologic sequelae than nasotracheal intubation.

B. **Ventilation** should be assisted (or maintained) and 100% oxygen administered by bag/valve as soon as the airway is clear. In the obtunded patient, the airway can be opened with a gentle chin-lift and the mask applied tightly over the patient's nose and mouth.

1. **An oropharyngeal airway (OPA)** may facilitate establishing a patent airway in the obtunded patient when proper head positioning and chin-lift/jaw thrust alone are ineffective. The adult sizes are 80, 90, and 100 mm (Guedel sizes 3, 4, and 5, respectively), which reflect the length from the flange to the distal tip. The size can be estimated by measuring the OPA from the ear lobe to the corner of the patient's lips. The device is normally inserted with the distal tip rotated upward along the hard palate and then rotated down into the posterior pharynx. Improperly placed, the OPA may obstruct the airway by pushing the tongue posteriorly or by pressing the epiglottis against the glottic opening. The OPA may induce vomiting or laryngospasm in an awake or semiconscious patient.

2. **A nasopharyngeal airway** should be considered as an adjunct to mask ventilation in patients with intact oropharyngeal reflexes, in away but obstructed patients, and in those in whom mouth opening is impossible. The adult sizes range from 6.0 to 9.0 mm, which indicate the internal diameter of the tube. The tube should be well lubricated and gently inserted through the naris, along the floor of the nasal cavity (parallel to the hard palate), until the flange rests against the outer naris. **Coagulopathy** is a relative contraindication to its use, as is the presence of a basilar skull fracture (especially involving the ethmoid bone). Although the risk is less than with an OPA, vomiting and laryngospasm may still occur in some patients.

C. **An intravenous line** should be freely running and its adequacy demonstrated prior to laryngoscopy. In cases of cardiac arrest, in which the administration of sedatives and paralytic agents is unnecessary, intubation may precede the establishment of adequate intravenous access.

D. **Monitoring during intubation** should include continuous electrocardiography (ECG), pulse oximetry, and frequent measurements of blood pressure. When available, continuous capnography is useful.

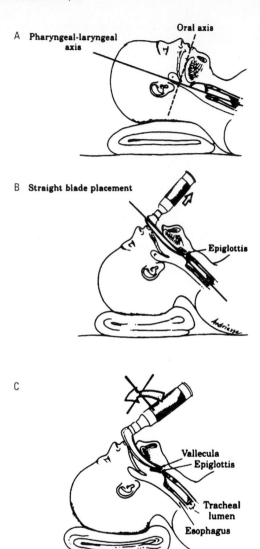

Curved blade placement

FIGURE 4-1 A. The "sniffing position" aligns the oral, pharyngeal, and laryngeal axes for visualization of the glottis during laryngoscopy. **B.** The handle of the laryngoscope should be lifted in the direction of the long axis of the handle to view the glottis. **C.** The laryngoscope should not be used as a lever, to prevent damage to teeth or the alveolar ridge.

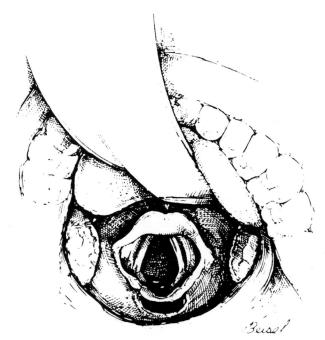

FIGURE 4-2 View of the glottis by direct laryngoscopy with a Macintosh blade. Notice that the tip of the blade has been placed in the vallecula (the tip of the Miller blade is placed under the epiglottis, lifting it to view the glottis).

E. **Orotracheal intubation**
   1. **The laryngoscope** is composed of a handle, which usually contains batteries for the light source, and a laryngoscope blade, which usually contains a light bulb in the distal one-third of the blade. The Macintosh and Miller blades are most commonly used.
      a. **The Macintosh blade** is curved, and the tip is inserted into the vallecula (the space between the base of the tongue and the pharyngeal surface of the epiglottis) (**Fig. 4-2**). Pressure against the hyoepiglottic ligament elevates the epiglottis to expose the larynx. The Macintosh blade provides a good view of the oro- and hypopharynx, thus allowing more room for ETT passage with diminished epiglottic trauma. Size ranges vary from No. 1 to No. 4, with most adults requiring a Macintosh No. 3 blade.
      b. **The Miller blade** is straight, and it is passed so that the tip lies beneath the laryngeal surface of the epiglottis. The epiglottis is then lifted to expose the vocal cords. This blade allows better exposure of the glottic opening but provides a smaller passageway through the oro- and hypopharynx. Sizes range from No. 0 to No. 3, with most adults requiring a Miller No. 2 or No. 3 blade.
   2. **A malleable stylet** inserted through the ETT (without extending past the tip) can be used to provide a 40- to 80-degree anterior bend 2 to 3 in from the tip of the ETT ("hockey stick" configuration). This will

allow passage of the tube along the posterior aspect of the epiglottis, facilitating intubation under difficult circumstances.

3. **Laryngoscopy.** Hold the laryngoscope in your left hand close to the junction of the blade and the handle. Open the patient's mouth with your right hand by applying a scissoring motion with your thumb and index finger on the patient's upper and lower premolars or gums. Insert the laryngoscope into the right side of the patient's mouth, taking care to avoid the teeth and pinching the lips between the blade and teeth. If using a Macintosh blade, insert it without resistance along the curve of the anterior pharynx. Once the blade is inserted, sweep the blade to the midline, utilizing the large flange of the blade to push the tongue out of the way. The epiglottis and vallecula will be visualized. Advance the blade into the vallecula and lift the handle in a direction parallel to its long axis to expose the vocal cords and laryngeal structures. If using a Miller blade, the tip of the blade is placed past the vallecula and is used to compress and elevate the epiglottis on lifting the handle. The laryngoscope blade should never be used as a lever with the upper teeth or maxilla as the fulcrum because damage to the maxillary incisors or gingiva may result.

4. **If the cords cannot be visualized**
   a. Secondary to vomitus or foreign material, suctioning or manual extraction is required.
   b. Because of an anterior position of the larynx, apply pressure to the thyroid or cricoid cartilages or change to a straight blade.
   c. Increase head flexion.
   d. Remove the laryngoscope and ventilate the patient with bag/valve mask. **Hypoxemia during a prolonged laryngoscopy must be avoided.**

5. **To insert the ETT,** hold it in your right hand as one would hold a pencil and advance it through the oral cavity from the right corner of the mouth and then through the vocal cords. Place the proximal end of the cuff just below the vocal cords, remove the stylet, and note the markings on the tube in relation to the patient's incisors or lips. In the average adult, the proper depth of insertion is approximately 21 cm for women, measured at the upper incisors, and 23 cm for men. Inflate the cuff just to the point of obtaining a seal in the presence of 20 to 30 cm H_2O positive airway pressure.

6. **Esophageal intubation** is one of the most common mistakes in airway management associated with a fatal outcome. No single technique for verifying endotracheal placement is foolproof.
   a. **Verification of proper ETT position** usually includes the persistent detection of carbon dioxide (CO_2) in end-tidal samples of exhaled gas and auscultation over the stomach and both lung fields.
   b. **The measurement of the CO_2 concentration** in exhaled gas has become a standard for verifying tracheal placement of an ETT. In the absence of a capnometer, disposable **colorimetric CO_2 detectors** can be used to confirm the presence of carbon dioxide. This technique is not foolproof; Co_2 will not be present if pulmonary circulation is absent (i.e., in a dead patient or in the absence of adequate chest compressions during cardiopulmonary circulation).
   c. Small concentrations of CO_2 may be detected after an esophageal intubation, especially if mask ventilation has insufflated the stomach. With an esophageal intubation, the amount of CO_2 detected in exhaled gas should decrease with repetitive breaths. With an endotracheal intubation, the end-tidal CO_2 concentration should be

stable during repetitive exhalations. If it is not, additional confirmation is necessary.

7. **Physical signs and symptoms** of a tracheal intubation include observation of the tube passing through the vocal cords and chest and abdominal movement with ventilation, the presence of breath sounds, and palpation of the ETT in the trachea as it is being inserted. Water vapor may be observed to fill the ETT on expiration and disappear on inspiration after proper placement. Other techniques for confirming correct placement include fiberoptic endoscopy, the use of a self-inflating bulb (the esophageal detector) or an airflow whistle on the proximal end of the ETT, and chest radiography. Although any or all of these tests may be performed, one must acknowledge that any single test lacks adequate predictive value to reliably exclude an esophageal intubation.

8. **In the absence of direct visualization** of the ETT passing between the vocal cords, a very high index of suspicion of incorrect tube placement must be maintained for the first several minutes following intubation. Only after adequate oxygenation and ventilation appears certain (i.e., after several minutes), it is safe to leave the patient under the care of others.

9. **If the tube position is uncertain** despite these maneuvers, or the patient is deteriorating without a readily explained cause (e.g., pneumothorax), **remove the tube** and reinstitute bag and mask ventilation prior to another intubation attempt. If the patient regurgitates through an ETT placed in the esophagus, some advocate leaving the esophageal tube in place to act as a conduit for vomitus. This is acceptable only if the tube does not interfere with repeat visualization of the cords.

10. **If the ETT has been advanced too far,** the right mainstem bronchus may be selectively intubated, resulting in absence of breath sounds over the left lung field and the right apex. Listening for breath sounds in the right lower thorax may decrease the chances of being misled by an intubation that has occluded the right upper lobe bronchus and transmitted breath sounds from the opposite lung.

11. **When the ETT is in good position,** securely fasten it with tape, preferably to taut skin overlying bony structures. Note the depth of the tube at the incisors or gums in the patient's chart along with a description of the procedure.

12. **Obtain a chest radiograph** following intubation to confirm tube position and bilateral lung expansion. The distal end of the tube should rest within the midtrachea, which is approximately 5 cm above the carina in the adult.

F. **Nasotracheal intubation**
  1. **Nasal mucosal vasoconstriction and anesthesia** are achieved with a solution of 0.25% phenylephrine and 3% lidocaine or 2% lidocaine with 1:200,000 epinephrine using cotton-tipped swabs. Even during general anesthesia, vasoconstriction with a topical solution such as oxymetazoline (Afrin) is advisable.
  2. **Common ETT size** is 6.0 to 6.5 mm for women and 7.0 to 7.5 mm for men. Insertion to a depth of 26 cm in women, measured at the naris, and 28 cm in men usually results in proper position.
  3. **General preparations** are as described for orotracheal intubation.
  4. **Nasal passage** of the tube. Generously lubricate the nares and tube. Initially probe the nasopharynx with a well-lubricated nasal airway to establish which naris has greater patency. If both nares are patent, the right naris is preferred because the bevel of most ETTs, when introduced through the right naris, faces the flat nasal septum, reducing

damage to the turbinates. Advance the tube in a direction that is perpendicular to the face and parallel to the hard palate. Inexperienced operators often tend to direct the tube cephalad, which tends to damage the turbinates. As the tube is passed into the nasopharynx, it may impact against the posterior nasopharyngeal wall. Retract the tube slightly, extend the patient's neck, and readvance. Forcible advancement of the tube at this point risks tearing the mucosa and creating a false passage. After passage through the naris into the pharynx, advance the tube through the glottic opening.

5. **Tracheal insertion** can be accomplished by several methods:

   a. **A Magill forceps** can be used to guide the tube into the trachea while direct laryngoscopy is performed. The laryngoscopic technique is the same as that used for oral intubation. The forceps is used to direct the tip of the ETT anteriorly and through the glottis. Grasp the tube with the forceps proximal to the ETT cuff. This reduces the chance of damaging the ETT cuff during insertion and permits the distal end of the tube to be inserted through the glottic opening. An assistant should advance the tube under the direction of the laryngoscopist.

   b. **Blind techniques** require a spontaneously breathing patient. While listening for breath sounds at the proximal end of the tube, advance the ETT during inspiration. A cough followed by a deep inhalation, condensate forming in the tube during exhalation, and loss of voice suggest tracheal entry. Sudden loss of breath sounds suggests passage into the esophagus, vallecula, or piriform recess:

      (1) Extending the neck or providing cricoid pressure may help direct the tube away from the esophagus.

      (2) Anterior flexion directs the tube away from the vallecula.

      (3) Tilting the head (not rotation) toward the side of the tube insertion and rotating the tube toward the midline directs the tube away from the piriform recess.

      (4) Inflating the cuff of the ETT may help lift it off the posterior wall of the pharynx and direct the tube through the cords in a patient with an anterior larynx. In this instance, the cuff is deflated as the tube passes between the cords.

   c. The **Endotrol** tracheal tube (Mallinckrodt, Inc., Glens Falls, NY) has a cord running up the concave side from the proximal end to the tip of the tube. Pulling on a ring attached to the proximal end of the cord flexes the tube anteriorly, which may direct the tip toward the glottis. It is sometimes useful for blind nasal intubation, especially when the neck cannot be manipulated.

   d. **A fiberoptic bronchoscope** can be used to direct the ETT into the trachea (see later discussion).

G. **Fiberoptic intubation** with a flexible bronchoscope can be used for both nasal and oral endotracheal intubation and should be considered as a first option in an anticipated difficult airway rather than as a last resort. Fiberoptic intubation should be considered for patients with known or suspected cervical spine pathology, head and neck tumors, morbid obesity, or a history of difficult ventilation or intubation. Facility with a fiberoptic bronchoscope should be obtained on mannequins and elective intubations prior to attempting emergency fiberoptic intubation.

   1. **Standard equipment** for oral or nasal fiberoptic intubation includes a sterile fiberoptic scope with light source, an oral bite block or Ovassapian airway, topical anesthetics and vasoconstrictors, and suction.

2. **Technique.** To perform a fiberoptic intubation, place an ETT over a lubricated fiberoptic scope, attach suction tubing to the suction port, and grasp the control lever with one hand and use the other hand to advance and maneuver the insertion tube. An assistant should sublux the mandible and protrude the tongue by grasping it with surgical gauze. An oral Ovassapian airway is helpful and well tolerated for oral laryngoscopy. Administration of an anticholinergic may help dry secretions that may obscure the view. After the administration of topical or general anesthesia, flex the tip of the insertion tube scope anteriorly and position it within the hypopharynx. Advance the scope toward the epiglottis. To avoid entering the piriform fossa, keep the insertion tube of the fiberoptic scope in the midline as it is advanced. If the view becomes impaired, retract the scope until the view clears or remove it and clean the lens, and then reinsert it in the midline. As the tip of the scope slides beneath the epiglottis, the vocal cords will be seen. Advance the scope with the tip in a neutral position until tracheal rings are noted. Then, stabilize the scope and advance the ETT over the insertion tube and into the trachea. Sometimes the tip of the ETT becomes caught against the arytenoids during advancement. If there is resistance, turning the ETT 90 degrees counterclockwise puts the bevel on the tip of the ETT in a more favorable position that may allow passage through the vocal cords.

3. **Nasal intubation** can be performed similarly. Anesthetize and vasoconstrict the nasal mucosa, as discussed previously. With the ETT loaded on the scope, pass the scope under direct vision through the nasopharynx and into the trachea. Tongue retraction is usually not needed, but may occasionally be helpful. Maintain the scope's position in the trachea while an assistant passes the ETT over the scope and through the nose.

4. **An alternate technique** involves passage of the nasotracheal tube into the oropharynx as in blind nasal intubation. Lubricate the scope, pass it through the ETT, and guide the tube's passage through the cords and position within the trachea under direct vision.

H. **The LMA** has assumed an important role in airway management in the operating room and as an emergency airway adjunct in other locations.

1. LMAs come in both pediatric and adult sizes (**Table 4-3**). The most common adult sizes are No. 4 and No. 5.

2. The LMA may be easily placed with minimal experience (**Fig. 4-3**) and an airway established in most patients. The most common causes of failure include the folding of the LMA cuff back on itself in the

TABLE 4-3	Laryngeal Mask Airway Sizes		
Patient Age/Size	**LMA Size**	**Cuff Volume (mL)**	**ETT Size (ID)**
Neonates/infants to 5 kg	1	4	3.5 mm
Infants 5–10 kg	1.5	7	4.0 mm
Infants/children 10–20 kg	2.0	10	4.5 mm
Children 20–30 kg	2.5	14	5.0 mm
Children 30 kg to small adults	3.0	20	6.0 cuffed
Average adults	4.0	30	6.0 cuffed
Large adults	5.0	40	7.0 cuffed

LMA, laryngeal mask airway; ETT, endotracheal tube; ID, inner diameter.

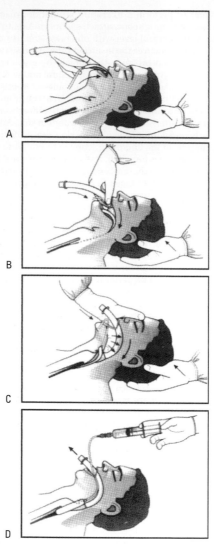

FIGURE 4-3 A. With the head extended and the neck flexed, carefully flatten the laryngeal mask airway (LMA) tip against the hard palate. **B.** The index finger pushes the LMA in a cranial direction following the contours of hard and soft palate. **C.** Maintaining pressure with the finger on the tube in the cranial direction, advance the mask until definite resistance is felt at the base of the hypopharynx. **D.** Inflation without holding the tube allows the mask to seat itself optimally. (From Brain AIJ, Denman WT, Goudsouzian N. *Laryngeal mask airway instruction manual.* San Diego, CA: Gensia, 1996. With permission).

oropharynx and the folding of the epiglottis down over the larynx by the tip of the LMA. These can be overcome by keeping the cuff pressed against the hard palate during insertion and using the correct size of LMA. The LMA should not be placed in patients with intact upper airway reflexes.

3. The LMA does not protect against the possibility of gastric aspiration and is not suitable for long-term mechanical ventilation. An ETT may be placed through the lumen of the LMA, either blindly or with the aid of a fiberscope. The *Fastrach LMA* is specially designed to permit subsequent endotracheal intubation through the LMA. The LMA also may be used as a temporary airway until a tracheostomy can be performed.

I. Other specialized techniques for endotracheal intubation include retrograde wire-guided intubation, use of a light-wand stylet, and tactile intubation.

J. Cricothyrotomy is performed as an emergency procedure when ventilation via mask or LMA is impossible and endotracheal intubation is unsuccessful.

1. **Technique.** Localize the cricothyroid notch (**Fig. 4-4**). Incise the skin and superficial subcutaneous tissues and pierce the cricothyroid membrane. Expand the membrane opening bluntly or with a scalpel and pass a small tracheostomy tube (No. 4 through No. 6) or a cut ETT (6.0- or 6.5-mm inner diameter [ID]) into the trachea.

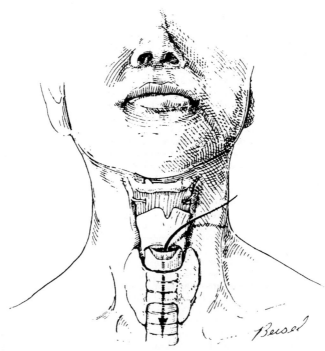

FIGURE 4-4 The cricothyroid membrane is the entry point of an artificial airway during cricothyrotomy.

2. **A needle cricothyrotomy** can be used to provide life-saving transtracheal jet oxygenation while other means are explored to secure the airway. A 14-gauge intravenous catheter attached to a syringe is used to puncture the cricothyroid membrane. Tracheal placement is confirmed by aspirating air from the catheter. The needle is removed and air is again aspirated from the catheter. Firmly maintaining the catheter in position, attach it by tubing to a jet ventilator or, if this is unavailable, to a wall oxygen flowmeter opened to its maximal setting. By cyclically interrupting the flow of oxygen, gas flow is delivered at a 1:2 ratio of inspiration to expiration (1 second on; 2 seconds off). The chest should be observed to rise and fall with each jet.

3. **Complications.** The flow from the wall at 50 psi can exceed 500 mL/s. Inadequate time for expiration can result in high airway pressures and barotrauma, leading to poor venous return and pneumothorax. Other complications of this technique are subcutaneous and mediastinal emphysema, tracheal mucosal trauma, bleeding, and misplacement of the catheter.

K. **Emergency tracheostomy** entails significant time and risk of bleeding, which usually precludes its use as an emergency airway technique.

V. **Pharmacologic aids to intubation** include **neuromuscular blocking drugs (NMBDs)**, sedatives, narcotics, and general and local anesthetics (see **Chapter 7**).

A. **NMBDs** induce complete respiratory arrest and abolish protective airway reflexes. Because laryngoscopy and intubation can be extremely painful and distressing, **patients who are chemically paralyzed must be either spontaneously or pharmacologically sedated.** When pharmacologic paralysis is required to secure the airway, patient survival depends on rapid and skillful laryngoscopy and intubation. NMBDs are slow in onset, and for that reason are quite dangerous for the patient who cannot tolerate even a few seconds of depressed ventilation.

1. **Succinylcholine** (1.0–1.5 mg/kg intravenously [IV]), with its rapid onset and brief duration of action, is the NMBD of choice for emergent endotracheal intubation in many patients. See **Chapter 7 for important contraindications.**

2. **Nondepolarizing muscle relaxants** typically have relatively slower onsets and longer durations of action. Rocuronium, an NMBD, also has a relatively rapid onset but can have a long duration of action. See **Chapter 7** for details.

3. **When rapid airway control is needed and succinylcholine is contraindicated,** large doses of *cis*-atracurium (>0.2 mg/kg IV) or **rocuronium** (1.2 mg/kg IV) can be used to decrease the onset of neuromuscular blockade from 1 to 1.5 minutes.

4. **All patients requiring emergent airway management are at risk for aspiration of gastric contents.** Thus, when paralysis is chosen, the intubation should follow a **"rapid sequence."** Administer the neuromuscular blocking agent immediately after rendering the patient rapidly unconscious with a drug such as propofol, etomidate, or ketamine. Apply cricoid pressure **(the Sellick maneuver)** with the onset of unconsciousness. To minimize gastric insufflation and the risk of regurgitation, under ideal circumstances, avoid positive-pressure ventilation until the airway is secured by an ETT. During rapid sequence intubation, a **stylet** should be used to support and help guide the ETT. If the intubation is not immediately successful, positive-pressure ventilation may be administered via bag and mask with maintenance of cricoid pressure or via an LMA.

B. **Sedative-hypnotics, analgesics, and amnestics** are used during airway manipulation primarily to blunt autonomic responses and to obtund consciousness, pain, and recall (**Chapter 7**).

C. **Benzodiazepines (Chapter 7)** are frequently employed for IV sedation and amnesia during endotracheal intubation. Onset is rapid (60–90 seconds), and duration is brief (20–60 minutes) following single-dose administration. Cardiovascular side effects are minimal. For sedation, incremental doses of **midazolam** 0.5 to 1.0 mg IV or lorazapam 2 mg IV may be repeated until the desired effect is achieved.

D. **Opioids. Fentanyl** and **morphine (Chapter 7)** are commonly employed for analgesia, sedation, and cough suppression during endotracheal intubation. Intravenous fentanyl has a rapid onset (1 minute) and in usual doses (50–500 μg) has a brief duration of action. Intravenous morphine (2–10 mg) has a longer peak onset time (5–10 minutes) and a longer duration of action (1–3 hours).

E. β-**adrenergic blocking drugs** such as **esmolol** (10–20 mg IV in the adult) may blunt the cardiovascular response to laryngoscopy and intubation. Doses should be titrated to effect.

F. **Lidocaine** (1.0–1.5 mg/kg IV) may augment anesthesia and blunt the hemodynamic response to intubation. Lidocaine must be administered several minutes prior to laryngoscopy to be maximally effective.

G. **Oropharyngeal topical anesthesia** can be provided with viscous lidocaine, aerosol anesthetic sprays, or inhalation of aerosolized lidocaine. Topical anesthesia with unmetered aerosol sprays poses a risk of overdose and toxicity.

H. Glossopharyngeal **nerve blocks,** superior laryngeal nerve blocks, and translaryngeal ("transtracheal") blocks are occasionally useful in selected patients. In general, these blocks diminish the ability to guard against aspiration. Nerve blocks are relatively contraindicated in patients with coagulopathy.

VI. **Special intubating situations**

A. **A difficult intubation** is defined as the inability to place an ETT after three attempts by an experienced laryngoscopist. Unfortunately, no single clinical examination is able to predict accurately those patients who will have difficult laryngoscopies.

1. The **American Society of Anesthesiologists (ASA) Difficult Airway Algorithm** (**Fig. 4-5**) outlines protocols to be used when a difficult airway is encountered. Although the algorithm was designed initially to aid the decision-making process when a difficult airway is encountered in the operating room, it is also useful for emergent airway situations in other locations such as the intensive care unit.

   a. For a patient with a recognized difficult airway and spontaneous respirations, the choices for establishing a secure airway include awake direct laryngoscopy, fiberoptic laryngoscopy, blind nasal intubation, or an elective surgical airway.

   b. When intubation attempts have failed and spontaneous or assisted ventilation is absent, quick action is required to establish oxygenation and ventilation by other means. Although the ASA Difficult Airway Algorithm lists the LMA, Combitube, and jet ventilation via a cricothyroidotomy as rescue techniques for ventilation of the failed airway at Massachusetts General Hospital only the LMA has been frequently used with success.

2. **Backup personnel** should be called if a difficult intubation is anticipated (e.g., in patients with severe facial injuries, airway burns, or unstable cervical spine injuries).

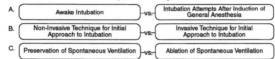

DIFFICULT AIRWAY ALGORITHM

1. Assess the likelihood and clinical impact of basic management problems:
   A. Difficult Ventilation
   B. Difficult Intubation
   C. Difficulty with Patient Cooperation or Consent
   D. Difficult Tracheostomy

2. Actively pursue opportunities to deliver supplemental oxygen throughout the process of difficult airway management

3. Consider the relative merits and feasibility of basic management choices:

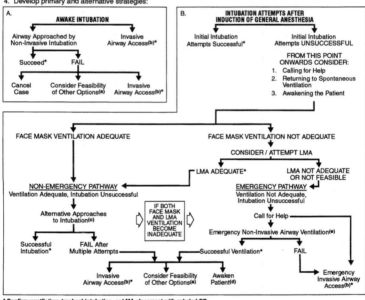

4. Develop primary and alternative strategies:

* Confirm ventilation, tracheal intubation, or LMA placement with exhaled CO₂

a. Other options include (but are not limited to): surgery utilizing face mask or LMA anesthesia, local anesthesia infiltration or regional nerve blockade. Pursuit of these options usually implies that mask ventilation will not be problematic. Therefore, these options may be of limited value if this step in the algorithm has been reached via the Emergency Pathway.

b. Invasive airway access includes surgical or percutaneous tracheostomy or cricothyrotomy.

c. Alternative non-invasive approaches to difficult intubation include (but are not limited to): use of different laryngoscope blades, LMA as an intubation conduit (with or without fiberoptic guidance), fiberoptic intubation, intubating stylet or tube changer, light wand, retrograde intubation, and blind oral or nasal intubation.

d. Consider re-preparation of the patient for awake intubation or canceling surgery.

e. Options for emergency non-invasive airway ventilation include (but are not limited to): rigid bronchoscope, esophageal-tracheal combitube ventilation, or transtracheal jet ventilation.

FIGURE 4-5 The American Society of Anesthesiologists Difficult Airway Algorithm. *Anesthesiology* 2003;98:1269–1277.

3. **The use of the LMA** should be considered when mask ventilation is inadequate and endotracheal intubation has failed.

4. **A surgical airway** should be considered if intubation has failed and the airway cannot be maintained with bag and mask or LMA. A surgical cricothyrotomy should be performed by personnel with training in the technique. In the absence of a physician specifically trained in

cricothyrotomy, a **needle or catheter percutaneous cricothyrotomy** should be considered when bag and mask or LMA ventilation and attempts at intubation have been unsuccessful. It should be noted that serious complications are common with this technique when performed under emergency conditions, including bleeding and subcutaneous emphysema, that may make a subsequent surgical cricothyrotomy impossible.

B. **A full stomach, vomiting, and airway bleeding** increase the hazards of pulmonary aspiration during intubation. If intubation is anticipated, oral and gastric feedings should be discontinued for 8 hours prior to intubation; however, this is seldom practical. If present, the nasogastric (NG) tube should be placed on suction. The elective placement of an NG tube to drain the stomach prior to intubation may be effective for liquid gastric contents, but its presence is not a guarantee of an empty stomach.

1. **With obtundation or neuromuscular incompetence,** the presence of oral foreign matter requires immediate oral intubation with laryngoscopic visualization. Suction with a Yankauer tip should be available. During intubation, estimate severity of aspiration and determine the pH of the suctioned material.

2. **In the conscious patient,** awake intubation is generally preferred unless contraindicated by cardiovascular or neurologic problems. Topical local anesthesia makes the procedure more comfortable, although its use decreases protective airway reflexes, increasing the risk of aspiration.

3. **A "rapid-sequence" intubation** is performed if general anesthesia is required. The technique is similar to a rapid-sequence induction.

4. **Increased intracranial pressure (ICP).** Pain or tracheal stimulation can increase ICP, even in comatose individuals. Intubation should be accomplished with minimal stimulation in any patient at risk for increased ICP. Adjuncts to consider include local anesthetic blocks, general anesthesia, including barbiturates, etomidate, or opioids, intravenous lidocaine, and the use of neuromuscular blockade to facilitate intubation.

C. **Myocardial ischemia or recent infarction** demands that heart rate and blood pressure should be maintained within a narrow range. Hypertension (or hypotension) and tachycardia can exacerbate myocardial ischemia. Pharmacologic adjuncts to consider during endotracheal intubation include deep opioid anesthesia, local anesthetic blockade of airway reflexes, and the use of adequate β-adrenergic blockade. A pharmacologic method of treating hypotension (e.g., phenylephrine) and hypertension (e.g., nitroglycerine) should be immediately available.

D. **Neck injury** with potentially unstable cervical vertebrae presents the risk of precipitating or aggravating spinal cord damage during intubation. The head, neck, and thorax should be maintained in a neutral position **(in-line stabilization).** Oral intubation is preferred during emergent situations. During intubation, a second individual should provide bimanual stabilization to maintain the head and neck in a neutral position. Flexion and anterior head motion pose the least risks for cord injury. If the intubation is difficult or the pharyngeal and vocal cord anatomy is not easily visualized, an awake fiberoptic intubation (oral or nasal), intubation through an LMA (with or without fiberoptic assistance), or proceeding to cricothyrotomy in more emergent situations is prudent.

E. **Oropharyngeal and facial trauma.** The nasal route is relatively contraindicated if there is a possibility of cranial vault disruption, because of the potential for tubes and catheters to penetrate the brain. Once the airway is secured, a fiberoptic nasal intubation can be performed electively, if needed, to facilitate operative repair. In the case of a massively disrupted face, a cricothyrotomy or tracheostomy may be preferable.

F. **Emergency neonatal and pediatric intubations.** Children generally are less cooperative than adults, making certain techniques (e.g., awake fiberoptic intubation) difficult. Hypoxemia occurs more rapidly during apnea in children than in adults. In addition, the tracheal cartilage in prepubertal individuals is not fully developed, predisposing them to tracheal malacia and stenosis. Cuffed ETTs are usually avoided because the cuff material requires a smaller tube size in already narrow airways and because of the risk of tracheal damage from mucosal ischemia due to compression by the inflated cuff. Tubes placed in pediatric patients should have a leak of air regurgitating back around the tube into the pharynx with positive-pressure ventilation. A leak at less than 25 cm H_2O of positive airway pressure is optimal. A greater leak makes ventilation more difficult, and a lesser leak is likely to cause tracheal edema on extubation and to increase the risk of tracheal damage.

G. **Complications of intubation.** Attempts at intubation may provoke serious hemodynamic alterations and expose the patient to profound hypoxemia. Hypertension and tachycardia may result from the stimulation of laryngoscopy and tracheal intubation. Conversely, patients with hypertension caused by respiratory distress may experience hypotension that may relate to relieving the discomfort of respiratory failure, loss of sympathetic tone with agents used to facilitate the intubation, and dynamic hyperinflation from zealous overventilation that will cause decreased venous return. Bradycardia is seen during attempted intubation and can be caused by many mechanisms, an example being a vagal response to laryngoscopy. Aspiration of gastric contents is possible especially when the patient has a full stomach and intubation is attempted when the patient is not fully paralyzed. Cardiac arrest is commonly associated with emergent intubation. Risk factors for increased complications during intubation include a suspected difficult airway, advanced age, more than two attempts at laryngoscopy, and a patient with significant respiratory distress.

VII. **Endotracheal and tracheostomy tubes**

A. Tube materials

1. **Polyvinyl chloride (PVC)** tubes are disposable, flexible, and transparent; they are the current standard tube. Siliconized PVC tracheostomy tubes are pliable and more easily conform to a patient's airway.

2. **Silicone** tubes are softer than PVC tubes but are more likely to kink.

3. **Armored or anode** tubes have metal-coil–reinforced bodies with a rubber, silicone, or PVC coating. They are less likely to kink than PVC tubes but are more flexible, usually requiring a stylet for placement.

B. **Cuff designs**

1. **High-pressure, low-compliance** cuffs have a small surface area of contact with the trachea and can produce tracheal damage more easily than low-pressure cuffs. High-pressure cuffs can be found on certain specialty tubes. Some low-pressure cuffs (such as those found on double-lumen endobronchial tubes) may generate high pressures if overinflated.

2. **Low-pressure, high-compliance** cuffs are found on standard disposable ETTs. They present a high surface area for tracheal contact at relatively low cuff pressures, preserving tracheal mucosal blood flow.

3. **Foam-filled** cuffs, as seen on **Kamen-Wilkinson** tubes or **Bivona** tubes, are sometimes used in patients with tracheal dilatation or in patients who require high cuff pressures to attain a seal (**Fig. 4-6**). The cuff is deflated for insertion, then left open to atmosphere and allowed to inflate

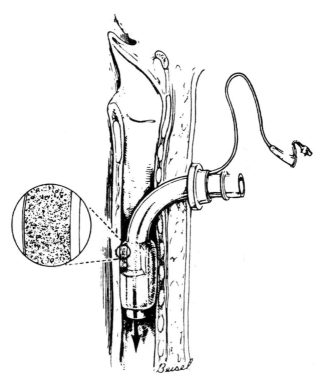

FIGURE 4-6 Kamen-Wilkinson tube (Fome-Cuf, Bivona Medical Technologies, Gary, IN).

passively within the trachea. A minimal cuff volume is required to ensure acceptable lateral wall pressures. Air and moisture are periodically aspirated from the cuff. If the cuff requires additional air to create a seal, the tube takes on the characteristics of the standard high-compliance tube.

4. **Lanz** cuffs have a balloon-within-a-shield pilot valve system to buffer the cuff pressure. The pilot system has a thick plastic guard surrounding a highly compliant inner balloon that distends at pressures above $28\ cm\,H_2O$, relieving high tracheal cuff pressure. The tracheal cuff is similar to the standard low-pressure, high-compliance cuffs found on other disposable tubes. Creating a seal at high airway pressures can be difficult.

C. **Tracheostomy tube designs.** Many tracheostomy tubes are available (**Fig. 4-7**). Representative tubes include the following:

1. **Portex disposable inner cannula (DIC).** The body of the DIC tube has a uniform radius of curvature, designed to accept a thin-walled, nonpliable inner cannula. With the inner cannula inserted, the inner diameter of the tube is reduced by 1 mm. This tube is available in fenestrated and nonfenestrated, cuffed and uncuffed versions.

2. **Portex blue line.** The body of this tube extends straight toward the anterior tracheal surface prior to initiating its curvature.

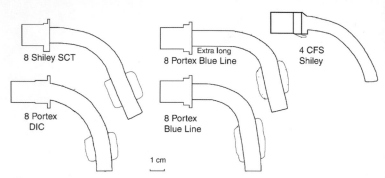

FIGURE 4-7 Tracheostomy tube designs.

3. **Portex extra long.** This tube is designed for the patient with a large neck. The distance between the tracheostomy tube flange and the initiation of curvature is longer than in the standard tracheostomy tube.

4. **Shiley single-cannula tube (SCT).** This tube is longer in vertical dimension (see **Table 4-4**) and has a larger-volume cuff than a Portex tube of equivalent internal diameter. The larger cuff usually allows the Shiley tube to seal at lower cuff pressure than a similarly sized Portex tube.

5. **Talking tracheostomy tube** or Communitrach (**Fig. 4-8**). A separate lumen within the body of the tube provides a dedicated air flow that exits just proximal to the tracheal cuff. The gas flow is patient-controlled by fingertip and passes retrograde through the glottis and pharynx, allowing

TABLE 4-4	Size Designations of Standard Tracheostomy Tubes		
Name	**ID (mm)**	**OD (mm)**	**Length (mm)**
Portex DIC[a]	6	8.2	64
	7	9.6	70
	8	10.9	73
	9	12.3	79
	10	13.7	79
Portex blue line	6	8.3	55
	7	9.7	75
	8	11.0	82
	9	12.4	87
	10	13.8	98
Shiley SCT	6	8.3	67
	7	9.6	80
	8	10.9	89
	9	12.1	99
	10	13.3	105

[a]Portex fenestrated tubes are made from the disposable inner cannula body. An inner cannula in place decreases the inner diameter by 1 mm.
DIC, disposable inner cannula; ID, inner diameter; OD, outer diameter; SCT, single-cannula tube.

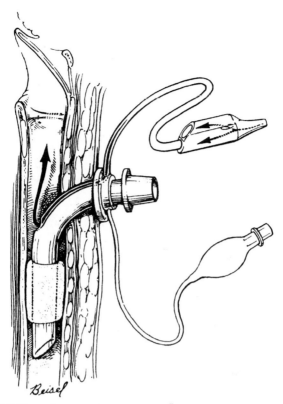

FIGURE 4-8 Talking tracheostomy tube.

intermittent phonation. Voice quality varies considerably, and secretions may occlude the gas flow port and prevent phonation.

6. **A fenestrated tracheostomy tube** (**Fig. 4-9**) is useful for patients who can spend some time off the ventilator. Designed to function in conjunction with a deflated cuff, the fenestration allows additional gas flow through the lumen of the tube to the pharynx. In conjunction with a one-way speaking valve (such as the Passy-Muir valve), excellent phonation is possible. A removable inner cannula blocks this fenestration and is used when the patient is receiving mechanical ventilation. An uncuffed fenestrated tube can be used for selected patients who do not require the tracheostomy to facilitate mechanical ventilation or protect the airway. Occlusion of the fenestration with secretions or by tissue of the tracheal wall due to tube malposition is a common problem. The size and pattern of fenestrations vary among tubes (**Fig. 4-10**).

7. **Sizes** of tracheostomy tubes vary depending on the manufacturer and style of tube (**Table 4-4**).

A   B

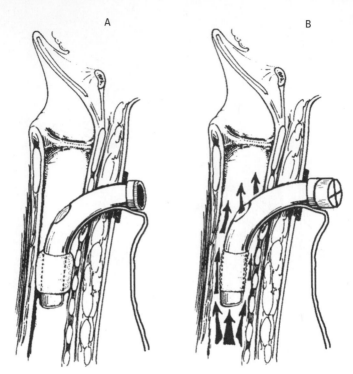

FIGURE 4-9   Fenestrated tracheostomy tube. **A.** With the cuff inflated and the long, hollow inner cannula in place, function is similar to that of the standard cuffed tracheostomy tube. **B.** With the inner cannula removed, the cuff deflated, and the occluder or one way speaking valve in place, gas flow is routed through the glottis and pharynx.

VIII. **Maintenance of endotracheal and tracheostomy tubes**
  A. **General care**
    1. **Suctioning.** The pharynx and trachea of intubated patients may require suctioning to clear secretions.
    2. **Cuff pressures** should be kept less than 30 cm H_2O and monitored routinely. Increased occlusion pressures may suggest the need for a larger tube or a similarly sized tube with a larger cuff.
    3. **Securing the tube.** Tape or a tube holder should be reapplied as needed. For an oral tube, avoid excessive pressure on the lips. Patients with **nasotracheal tubes** should be periodically assessed for sinusitis, otitis media, and necrosis of the nares.
  B. **Common endotracheal and tracheostomy tube problems**
    1. **Cuff leaks** are usually evident as audible pharyngeal gas flow diverted anteriorly around the cuff during positive-pressure ventilation. A large leak may prompt urgent reintubation with a new tube. Usually, however, addition of a small volume of air to the cuff temporarily restores a seal. Causes of persistent cuff leaks include
       a. **Supraglottic cuff position.** A cuff that holds air but does not seal the airway may be within or above the vocal cords. Cuff position

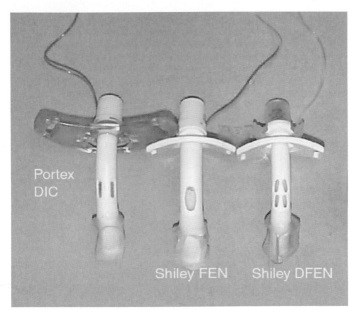

FIGURE 4-10 Fenestration patterns.

can be evaluated by chest radiograph or laryngoscopic examination. Deflate the cuff, advance the tube, and reconfirm intratracheal placement.

b. **Damaged cuff system.** A cuff unable to hold any air is likely to require immediate replacement. Slow cuff leaks allow time for further evaluation. Small leaks can occur from the pilot valve or balloon, the cuff, or the cuff–tube interface.

c. **Tracheal dilation** as a cause of persistent cuff leaks often can be diagnosed with the aid of a chest radiograph. The tissue–air interface at an inflated cuff is visible radiographically as a widened trachea. A larger tube or one with a larger cuff volume may be required. Alternatively, a foam cuff tube (e.g., Kamen-Wilkinson or Bivona) may be tried.

2. **Airway obstruction** is an emergency forewarned by the high-pressure-limit alarm during volume ventilation or by low-volume alarms during pressure ventilation. Quickly evaluate the airway. A kinked tube may allow manual ventilation but does not allow a suction catheter to pass. Manipulation of the head and neck may temporarily increase flow through a kinked tube. Inability to manually ventilate requires immediate tube replacement.

3. **Malpositioned tracheostomy tubes** (**Fig. 4-11**) can damage the tracheal mucosa, impede airflow, or predispose a patient to inadvertent decannulation.

C. **ETT changes** are indicated for mechanical tube failure or changing tube size or position (e.g., nasal to oral). Common techniques for tube changes include the following:

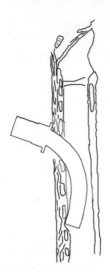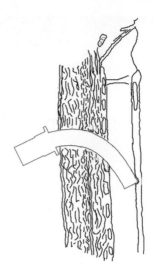

FIGURE 4-11 Malpositioned tracheostomy tubes.

1. Direct laryngoscopy.
2. Bronchoscopic change. With a new ETT loaded onto the fiberscope, the fiberscope is advanced to the cords. After the pharynx and superglottic areas are suctioned, an assistant deflates the cuff on the indwelling ETT and the fiberscope is advanced around the indwelling ETT and through the cords and into the trachea. While the endoscopist maintains intratracheal visualization of the fiberscope position, the assistant slowly withdraws the old ETT, and the new ETT is advanced over the fiberscope into the trachea. This technique is particularly useful in patients in whom direct laryngoscopy is contraindicated or technically difficult.
3. Specially designed long, malleable stylets (tube changers) can be used to perform tube changes blindly or under direct vision. Pass the stylet through the existing ETT and remove the tube, being careful not to dislodge the stylet. Then slip a new ETT into the trachea over the stylet. Many tube changers have a lumen for oxygen administration or, if necessary, jet ventilation. One caveat is that these tube changers are sufficiently long to pose a risk for pneumothorax.
4. When changing nasal tubes, change to an oral tube as an intermediate step rather than attempt placement of bilateral nasal tubes.

IX. **Tracheostomy** may be performed as an open surgical procedure or as a percutaneous, bedside procedure. The **bedside, percutaneous procedure is a safe procedure** that is gaining in popularity because it reduces the risk of transporting critically ill patients to the operating room, the cost of operating room resources, and the delay in scheduling encountered with today's busy operating room schedules. Most bedside tracheostomies are performed using a modification of the Ciaglia technique that employs wire-guided conical plastic or balloon tracheal dilators.

   A. **Advantages** of tracheostomy over translaryngeal intubation include the following:

1. Improved patient comfort.
2. Decreased risk of laryngeal dysfunction and/or damage.
3. Improved oral hygiene.
4. Improved ability to communicate, including the ability to phonate when the cuff can be deflated.

B. Disadvantages of tracheostomy include the following:
1. Possibility of tracheal stenosis at the stoma site.
2. Stomal infection, which may secondarily infect nearby open skin areas and vascular catheters.
3. Erosion of neighboring vascular tissue, which can lead to hemorrhage.
4. Operative complications.
5. Scarring and granulation tissue at the stoma site.

C. Deciding the appropriate time for conversion from ETT to tracheostomy is a controversial issue. It is generally accepted, but not proved, that incidence and severity of glottic damage are related to duration of intubation. In clinical practice, elective tracheostomy is considered after 2 to 3 weeks of translaryngeal intubation.

D. Replacement of tracheostomy tubes
1. **Changing a fresh tracheostomy tube.** The tract for the tracheostomy tube can be extremely difficult to cannulate in the initial postoperative period. If a tracheostomy change is required before the stoma is 7 to 10 days old, the tube should be changed over a malleable stylet and provisions for immediate orotracheal intubation should be immediately available in case the tract is lost. It is probably safe to change a percutaneous tracheostomy earlier. It is preferable for the surgeon who performed the tracheostomy to be present because exploration of the tract may be necessary.
2. **Tracheostomy tube changes.** Proper cleanliness, function, and mobility of the appliance should be assessed regularly and the appliance changed as needed.
   a. Be prepared to perform an orotracheal intubation, if necessary.
   b. Administer 100% oxygen.
   c. Clean the tracheostomy site and suction the patient.
   d. Check the new tube and test for cuff integrity. Insert the obturator through the lumen of the new tube to provide a smooth surface at the tip of the tracheostomy tube.
   e. Deflate the cuff and remove the existing tube. Expect some resistance to decannulation as the deflated cuff is pulled past the anterior tracheal wall.
   f. Visualize the stoma tract and insert the new tube. Inflate the cuff and be prepared to manually ventilate with 100% oxygen.
   g. Evaluate for proper intratracheal placement, as for any ETT (see Section **IV.E.6**).

E. Airway bleeding. Suctioning of blood from the airway requires prompt evaluation.
1. Commonly, this bleeding represents **mucosal erosion** from the repeated trauma of suctioning. Fiberoptic bronchoscopy is the most direct means of assessment. If the source is not obvious, pull the tube back with the bronchoscope in place to view the trachea underlying the cuff. If, after examination, the etiology of the persistent bleeding is in doubt, obtain a repeat examination by an otorhinolaryngologist. If bleeding is not significant, a period of healing without irritation is warranted. Alternatively, a tracheostomy tube or ETT can be placed distal to the area of erosion until healing occurs.

2. With tracheostomy, the risk of erosion into the mediastinal blood vessels exists. If this occurs, the patient can **exsanguinate.** If bleeding continues and is of sufficient quantity, there is a risk of clotting within the ETT and airway obstruction. Emergent orotracheal intubation and surgical exploration may be necessary.

F. **Decannulation** is considered once indications for airway support are no longer present. The patient should have adequate oxygenation and ventilation and be able to clear secretions and protect the lungs from aspiration.

1. **Vocal cord dysfunction and aspiration** can occur because of prolonged intubation. Such dysfunction may spontaneously resolve within several weeks following extubation.

   a. **Continued presence of a tracheostomy tube** can increase the chance of aspiration by mechanical interference with coordinated swallowing. Decreasing this potential problem may involve inserting a smaller uncuffed tracheostomy tube (such as a No. 4 Shiley) to decrease the mechanical stresses due to movement of the tracheostomy tube during swallowing. The smaller tube will maintain stomal patency and allow suctioning of the airway.

   b. **A NG tube** can contribute to decreased coordination during swallowing.

   c. **Protecting such patients from aspiration** may involve

      (1) **Tracheostomy.** A cuffed tracheostomy tube can be used to prevent gross aspiration until cord function improves.

      (2) **Extubation,** prohibiting oral intake, with enteral or parenteral feeding until the patient is no longer at risk. An enteral feeding tube should be located in the duodenum to decrease the chance of reflux and aspiration.

   d. **Consultation with a speech and swallowing therapist** is appropriate. Coordination of swallowing can be assessed by fiberoptic visualization or, radiographically, by a modified barium swallow. Patient education and training can reduce the risks of aspiration and improve swallowing.

2. The following airway appliances may be considered as the patient progresses toward decannulation:

   a. **Fenestrated tracheostomy tubes** allow breathing either through the tracheostomy or through the natural airway. The patient can speak normally when the inner cannula is removed, the cuff is down, and the opening of the tube is either occluded or fitted with a one-way speaking valve. A fenestrated tube provides no protection against aspiration when configured in this manner.

   b. **A small cuffless tracheostomy tube,** such as the No. 4 Shiley CFS (**Fig. 4-7**), is often the last airway appliance used prior to decannulation. Most often, it serves as a safety device and as a conduit for suction. Resistance to airflow around such tubes, even when the tube is capped, is seldom clinically significant.

Selected References

Benumof JL, Dagg R, Benumof R. Critical hemoglobin desaturation will occur before return to an unparalyzed state following 1 mg/kg intravenous succinylcholine. *Anesthesiology* 1997;87:979–982.

Bishop MJ, Weymuller EA Jr, Fink BR. Laryngeal effects of prolonged intubation. *Anesth Analg* 1984;63:335–342.

Brain AIJ, Denman WT, Goudsouzian N. *Laryngeal mask airway instruction manual.* San Diego, CA: Gensia, 1996:21–25.

Deutschman CS, Wilton P, Sinow J, et al. Paranasal sinusitis associated with nasotracheal intubation: a frequently unrecognized and treatable source of sepsis. *Crit Care Med* 1986;14: 111–114.

El-Gaqnzouri AR, McCarthy RJ, Tuman KJ, et al. Preoperative airway assessment: predictive value of a multivariate risk index. *Anesth Analg* 1996;82:1197–1204.

Fluck RR Jr, Hess DR, Branson RD. Airway and suction equipment. In: Branson RD, Hess DR, Chatburn RL, eds. *Respiratory care equipment*. Philadelphia, PA: Lippincott, 1995:116–144.

Jaber S, Amraoui J, Lefrant JY, et al. Clinical practice and risk factors for immediate complications of endotracheal intubation in the intensive care unit: a prospective multiple-center study. *Crit Care Med* 2006;34:2355–2361.

Hauswald M, Sklar DP, Tandberg D, et al. Cervical spine movement during airway management: cinefluoroscopic appraisal in human cadavers. *Am J Emerg Med* 1991;9:535–538.

Hurford WE. Orotracheal intubation outside the operating room: anatomic considerations and techniques. *Respir Care* 1999;44:615–629.

McKourt KC, Salomela L, Miraklew RK, et al. Comparison of rocuronium and suxamethonium for use during rapid induction of anaesthesia. *Anaesthesia* 1998;53:867–871.

Mehta S, Mickiewicz M. Pressure in large volume, low pressure cuffs: its significance, measurement, and regulation. *Intensive Care* 1986;31:199–201.

Mort TC. Complications of emergency tracheal intubation: hemodynamic alterations: part I. *J Intensive Care Med* 2007;22:157–165.

Mort TC. Complications of emergency tracheal intubation: immediate airway-related consequences: part II. *J Intensive Care Med* 2007;22:208–215.

Ovassapian A, Randel GI. The role of the fiberscope in the critically ill patient. *Crit Care Clin* 1995;11:29–51.

Roberts JT. *Clinical management of the airway*. Philadelphia, PA: Saunders, 1994.

Schmidt UH, Kumwilaisak K, Bittner E, George E, Hess D. Effects of supervision by attending anesthesiologists on complications of emergency tracheal intubation. *Anesthesiology* 2008;109:973–977.

Velmahos GC, Gomez H, Boicey CM, et al. Bedside percutaneous tracheostomy: prospective evaluation of the current technique in 100 patients. *World J Surg* 2000;24:1109–1115.

Whited RE. A prospective study of laryngotracheal sequelae in long term intubation. *Laryngoscope* 1984;94:367–377.

Wilson DJ. Airway appliances and management. In: Kacmarek RM, Stoller JK, eds. *Current respiratory care*. Philadelphia, PA: BC Decker, 1988:80–89.

Principles of Mechanical Ventilation

Claudia Crimi and Dean Hess

I. **Mechanical ventilation** provides artificial support of gas exchange.
  A. **Indications**
    1. **Hypoventilation**
      a. **Hypoventilation resulting in an arterial pH of less than 7.30** often is considered an indication for mechanical ventilation, but patient fatigue and associated morbidity must be considered and may prompt initiation of mechanical ventilation at a higher or lower pH.
    2. **Hypoxemia**
      a. **Supplemental oxygen** should be administered to all hypoxemic patients, regardless of diagnosis (e.g., appropriate oxygen therapy should not be withheld from hypercapnic patients with chronic obstructive pulmonary disease [COPD]).
      b. Patients with **hypoxemic respiratory failure** due to atelectasis and/or cardiogenic pulmonary edema may benefit from **continuous positive airway pressure (CPAP)** administered by face mask.
      c. **Endotracheal intubation and mechanical ventilation** should be considered for severe hypoxemia (arterial oxygen saturation by pulse oximetry [SpO_2] <90% at a fraction of inspired oxygen [FiO_2] equal to 1.0) unresponsive to more conservative measures.
    3. **Respiratory fatigue**
      a. Tachypnea, dyspnea, use of accessory muscles, nasal flaring, diaphoresis, and tachycardia may be an indication for mechanical ventilation before abnormalities of gas exchange occur.
    4. **Airway protection**
      a. Mechanical ventilation may be initiated in patients who require endotracheal intubation for airway protection, even in the absence of respiratory abnormalities (e.g., decreased mental status or increased aspiration risk).
      b. **The presence of an artificial airway** is not an absolute indication for mechanical ventilation. For example, many long-term tracheostomized patients do not require mechanical ventilation.
  B. **Goals of mechanical ventilation**
    1. Provide adequate oxygenation.
    2. Provide adequate alveolar ventilation.
    3. Avoid alveolar overdistension.
    4. Maintain alveolar recruitment.
    5. Promote patient–ventilator synchrony.
    6. Avoid auto-PEEP.
    7. Use the lowest possible FiO_2.
    8. When choosing appropriate goals of mechanical ventilation for an individual patient, consider the risk of ventilator-induced lung injury.

II. **The ventilator system**
  A. **The ventilator** is powered by gas pressure and electricity. Gas pressure provides the energy required to inflate the lungs (**Fig. 5-1**).

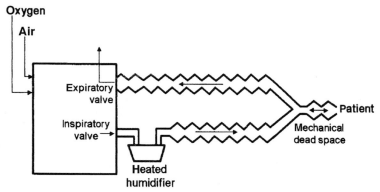

FIGURE 5-1 Simplified block diagram of a mechanical ventilator system.

1. Gas flow is controlled by **inspiratory and expiratory valves.** The micro-processor of the ventilator controls these valves such that gas flow is determined as per the ventilator settings.
   a. **The inspiratory valve** controls gas flow and/or pressure during the inspiratory phase. The expiratory valve is closed during the inspiratory phase.
   b. **The expiratory valve** controls PEEP. The inspiratory valve is closed during the expiratory phase.
B. **The ventilator circuit** delivers flow between the ventilator and the patient.
   1. Because of gas compression and the elasticity of the circuit, part of the gas volume delivered from the ventilator is not received by the patient. This **compression volume** is typically approximately 3 to 4 mL/cm H_2O. Some ventilators compensate for this; others do not.
   2. The volume of the circuit through which the patient rebreathes is **mechanical dead space.** Mechanical dead space should be as low as possible. This is particularly an issue when low tidal volumes are used as part of lung-protective ventilation strategies.
C. **Gas conditioning**
   1. **Filters** may be placed in the inspiratory and expiratory limbs of the circuit.
   2. **The inspired gas** is actively or passively humidified.
      a. **Active humidifiers** pass the inspired gas over a heated water chamber for humidification. Some active humidifiers are used with a **heated circuit** to decrease condensate within the circuit.
      b. **Passive humidifiers** (artificial noses or heat and moisture exchangers) are inserted between the ventilator circuit and the patient. They trap heat and humidity in the exhaled gas and return that on the subsequent inspiration. Passive humidification is satisfactory for many patients, but it is less effective than active humidification, increases the resistance to inspiration and expiration, and increases mechanical dead space.
      c. The presence of **water droplets** in the inspiratory circuit near the patient (or in the proximal endotracheal tube if a passive humidifier is used) suggests that the inspired gas is adequately humidified.

<u>Ventilator related</u>
• Ventilation mode
• Tidal volume
• Respiratory rate
• Duty cycle
• Inspiratory waveform
• Breath-triggering mechanism

<u>Device related - MDI</u>
• Type of spacer or adapter
• Position of spacer in circuit
• Timing of MDI actuation
• Type of MDI

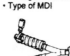

<u>Drug related</u>
• Dose
• Formulation
• Aerosol particle size
• Targeted site for delivery
• Duration of action

<u>Device related - Nebulizer</u>
• Type of nebulizer
• Fill volume
• Gas flow
• Cycling: inspiration vs. continuous
• Duration of nebulization
• Position in the circuit

<u>Patient related</u>
• Severity of airway obstruction
• Mechanism of airway obstruction
• Presence of dynamic hyperinfiation
• Patient-ventilator synchrony

<u>Circuit related</u>
• Endotracheal tube size
• Humidity of inhaled gas
• Density of inhaled gas

FIGURE 5-2 Factors affecting aerosol delivery during mechanical ventilation. MDI, metered-dose inhaler. From Dhand R. Basic techniques for aerosol delivery during mechanical ventilation. *Respir Care* 2004;49:611–622. With permission.

D. **Delivery of inhaled medications during mechanical ventilation**
  1. Inhaled medications can be delivered by **metered-dose inhaler** or **nebulizer** during mechanical ventilation. Dry-powder inhalers cannot be adapted to the ventilator circuit.
  2. A variety of factors influence aerosol delivery during mechanical ventilation (**Fig. 5-2**).
  3. With careful attention to technique, either inhalers or nebulizers can be used effectively during mechanical ventilation.

III. **Classification of mechanical ventilation**
  A. **Negative- versus positive-pressure ventilation**
    1. The **iron lung** and **chest cuirass** create negative pressure around the thorax during the inspiratory phase. Although useful for some patients with neuromuscular disease requiring long-term ventilation, these devices are almost never used in the ICU.
    2. **Positive-pressure ventilation** applies pressure to the airway during the inspiratory phase. Positive-pressure mechanical ventilation is used exclusively in the ICU.
    3. **Exhalation** occurs passively with both positive-pressure ventilation and negative-pressure ventilation.
  B. **Invasive versus noninvasive ventilation**
    1. **Invasive ventilation** is delivered through an endotracheal tube (orotracheal or nasotracheal) or a tracheostomy tube.
    2. Although mechanical ventilation through an artificial airway remains the standard in the most acutely ill patients, **noninvasive positive pressure ventilation (NPPV)** can be used successfully in many patients such those with an exacerbation of COPD, acute cardiogenic pulmonary edema, or immunocompromised patients with acute respiratory failure. NPPV is also useful to prevent postextubation

respiratory failure. There are many patients, however, in whom NPPV is not appropriate.

   a. NPPV can be applied with nasal mask, oronasal mask, nasal pillows, total face mask, or helmet. Oronasal masks are preferred in acutely ill dyspneic patients, in whom mouth leak is often problematic.

   b. Although bilevel ventilators are most commonly used for NPPV, any ventilator can be used to provide this therapy. Current generation ventilators designed for critical care have both invasive and noninvasive modes.

   c. **Pressure support ventilation (PSV)** is most commonly used for NPPV. For bilevel ventilators, this is achieved by setting inspiratory positive airway pressure **(IPAP)** and an expiratory positive airway pressure **(EPAP)**. The difference between IPAP and EPAP is the level of pressure support.

   d. An algorithm for use of NIV in the critical care setting is provided in **Fig. 5-3**.

C. Full versus partial ventilatory support

1. **Full ventilatory support** provides the entire minute ventilation with little interaction between the patient and the ventilator. This usually requires sedation and sometimes neuromuscular blockade. Full ventilatory support is indicated for patients with severe respiratory failure, patients who are hemodynamically unstable, patients with complex acute injuries while they are being stabilized, and all patients with paralysis.

2. **Partial ventilatory support** provides a variable portion of the minute ventilation, with the remainder provided by the patient's inspiratory effort. The patient–ventilator interaction is important during partial ventilatory support.

   a. Partial ventilatory support is indicated for patients with moderately acute respiratory failure or patients who are recovering from respiratory failure.

      (1) Advantages of partial ventilatory support include avoidance of muscle weakness during long periods of mechanical ventilation, preservation of the ventilatory drive and breathing pattern, decreased requirement for sedation and neuromuscular blockade, a better hemodynamic response to positive-pressure ventilation, and better ventilation of dependent lung regions.

      (2) Disadvantages of partial ventilatory support include a high work of breathing (WoB) for the patient and difficulty achieving adequate gas exchange.

IV. Gas delivery to the lungs

   A. Delivery of gas into the lungs is determined by the interaction between the ventilator, respiratory mechanics, and respiratory muscle activity, which is described by the **equation of motion** of the respiratory system:

$$P_{vent} + P_{mus} = V_T/C + \dot{V} \times R$$

where P_{vent} is the pressure applied by the ventilator, P_{mus} is the pressure generated by the respiratory muscles, V_T is tidal volume, C is compliance, $\dot{V}$ is gas flow, and R is airways resistance.

   1. Pressure generated from the respiratory muscles (spontaneous breathing), the ventilator (full ventilatory support), or both (partial ventilatory support) applied to the respiratory system result in gas flow into the lungs.

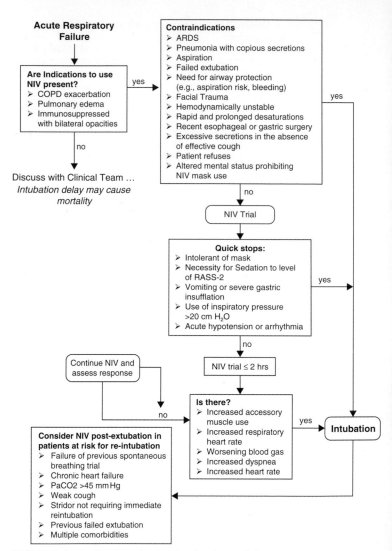

FIGURE 5-3 An algorithm for application of noninvasive ventilation.

2. For a given pressure, flow is opposed by airways resistance and the elastance (inverse of compliance) of the lungs and chest wall.

3. A larger tidal volume or higher flow requires a higher pressure.

V. Phase and control variables

  A. The **trigger variable** starts the inspiratory phase.

   1. The trigger variable is time when the ventilator initiates the breath.

2. When the patient triggers the breath, the ventilator detects either a pressure change **(pressure trigger)** or a flow change **(flow trigger)**.

3. The **trigger sensitivity** is set to prevent excessive patient effort but avoid Auto-triggering. Pressure trigger sensitivity is commonly set at 0.5 to 2 cm H_2O, and flow trigger sensitivity is commonly set at 1 to 3 L/min.

   a. Auto-trigger can be caused by artifacts such as cardiac oscillations and leaks. This is corrected by making the trigger less sensitive.

   b. Ineffective trigger is usually due to auto-PEEP. Neither flow trigger nor pressure trigger is effective with failed triggers due to auto-PEEP.

4. Pressure triggering and flow triggering are equally effective when sensitivity is optimized and closely monitored.

B. The **control variable** remains constant throughout inspiration. Most common are volume control, pressure control, and adaptive control **(Table 5-1)**.

1. **Volume control.** The term volume control is commonly used, although the ventilator actually controls flow (the time derivative of volume).

   a. With volume-controlled ventilation, **delivered tidal volume is constant** regardless of airways resistance or respiratory system compliance.

   b. A decrease in respiratory system compliance or an increase in airways resistance results in an increased peak inspiratory pressure during volume-controlled ventilation.

   c. With volume-controlled ventilation, the **inspiratory flow is fixed** regardless of patient effort. This unvarying flow may induce patient–ventilator dyssynchrony in patients making vigorous inspiratory efforts.

   (1) Inspiratory flow patterns during volume-controlled ventilation include **constant flow** (rectangular wave) **(Fig. 5-4)** or **descending-ramp flow** (**Fig. 5-5**).

   (2) Use of the constant-flow waveform results in a higher peak pressure, which is largely borne by the airways and not by the alveoli.

   (3) Use of a descending-ramp waveform results in maximal flow early in the breath when lung volume is minimal. This reduces peak pressures but decreases expiratory time, which may increase the risk of auto-PEEP and hemodynamic compromise.

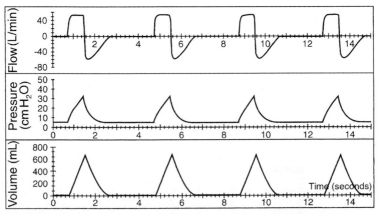

FIGURE 5-4 Constant-flow volume ventilation.

TABLE 5-1 Comparison of Several Breath Types During Mechanical Ventilation

	Pressure Control Ventilation	Volume Control Ventilation	Adaptive Control Ventilation	Pressure Support Ventilation	Proportional Assist Ventilation
Tidal volume	Variable	Set	Minimum set	Variable	Variable
Peak inspiratory pressure	Limited by pressure control setting	Variable	Variable	Limited by pressure support setting	Variable
Plateau pressure	Limited by pressure control setting	Variable	Variable	Limited by pressure support setting	Variable
Inspiratory flow	Descending; variable	Set; constant or descending ramp	Descending; variable	Variable	Variable
Inspiratory time	Set	Set (flow and volume settings)	Set for adaptive pressure control; variable for adaptive pressure support	Variable	Variable
Respiratory rate	Minimum set (patient can trigger)	Minimum set (patient can trigger)	Minimum set for adaptive pressure control; not set for adaptive pressure support	Variable; rate not set	Variable; rate not set

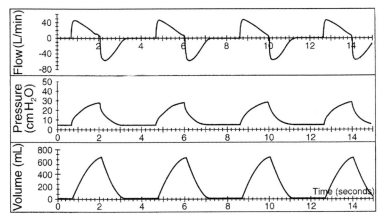

FIGURE 5-5 Descending-ramp volume ventilation.

    d. The **inspiratory time** during volume-controlled ventilation is determined by the inspiratory flow, inspiratory flow pattern, and tidal volume.

    e. Volume-controlled ventilation is preferred when an assured minute ventilation is desirable (e.g., avoidance of hypercarbia in patients with intracranial hypertension).

2. Pressure control

    a. With pressure-controlled ventilation (**Fig. 5-6**), **the pressure applied to the airway is constant** regardless of the airways resistance or respiratory system compliance.

    b. The inspiratory flow during pressure-controlled ventilation is exponentially descending and is determined by the pressure control setting, airways resistance, and respiratory system compliance.

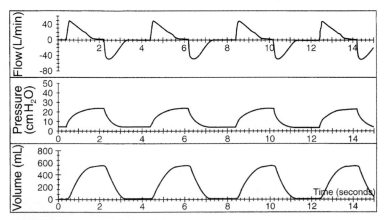

FIGURE 5-6 Pressure-controlled ventilation.

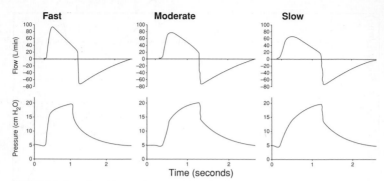

FIGURE 5-7 Examples of fast, moderate, and slow rise times during pressure ventilation.

With low respiratory system compliance (e.g., acute respiratory distress syndrome [ARDS]), flow decreases rapidly. With high airways resistance (e.g., COPD), flow decreases slowly.

  c. Some ventilators allow the adjustment of the **rise time,** which is the pressurization rate of the ventilator at the beginning of the inspiratory phase (**Fig. 5-7**). The rise time is the amount of time required for the pressure control level to be reached after the ventilator is triggered.

   (1) A rapid rise time delivers more flow at the initiation of inhalation, which may be useful for patients with a high respiratory drive.

  d. **Factors that affect tidal volume** during pressure-controlled ventilation are respiratory system compliance, airways resistance, pressure setting, rise time setting, and the inspiratory effort of the patient.

   (1) Increasing the inspiratory time will affect tidal volume during pressure-controlled ventilation only if the end-inspiratory flow is not 0. Once the flow decreases to 0, no additional volume is delivered.

  e. Unlike volume-controlled ventilation, **inspiratory flow is variable** during pressure-controlled ventilation. Increased patient effort will increase the flow from the ventilator and the delivered tidal volume.

  f. The variable flow with pressure-controlled ventilation may improve patient–ventilator synchrony in some patients.

  g. With pressure-controlled ventilation, **the inspiratory time is set** on the ventilator.

   (1) If the inspiratory time is set to be longer than the expiratory time, pressure-controlled inverse ratio ventilation (PCIRV) results. This strategy has been used to improve oxygenation in patients with ARDS.

   (2) Pressure-controlled ventilation can be used as an alternative to pressure support ventilation when a fixed inspiratory time is desired.

 3. **Adaptive control**

  a. With adaptive control, the breath is ventilator-triggered or patient-triggered, pressure-limited, and ventilator-cycled or patient-cycled. With adaptive pressure control, the pressure limit is not constant, but varies breath to breath based on a comparison of the set and delivered tidal volume.

b. Although the ventilator is capable of controlling only pressure or volume at any time, adaptive control combines features of pressure control (variable flow) and volume control (constant tidal volume) (**Table 5-1**).

c. **Pressure-regulated volume control (PRVC on Servo, Viasys), AutoFlow (Draeger), and VC+ (Puritan-Bennett)** are trade names used by different ventilator manufacturers to provide adaptive pressure control, in which the pressure limit increases or decreases in an attempt to deliver the desired tidal volume.

d. With **volume support (VS)**, the pressure support level varies on a breath-to-breath basis to maintain a desired tidal volume. If the patient's effort increases (increased tidal volume for the set level of PSV), the ventilator decreases the support for the next breath. If the compliance or patient effort decreases, the ventilator increases the support to maintain the set volume. This combines the attributes of PSV with the guaranteed minimum tidal volume. A concern with this mode is that the ventilator takes away support if the patient's respiratory demand increases and tidal volume exceeds the set tidal volume. This results in increased WoB for the patient.

e. The clinical utility of adaptive control is yet to be determined.

(1) If the patient makes a vigorous inspiratory effort, the tidal volume may exceed the desired tidal volume, which could result in overdistention lung injury.

(2) If the patient makes vigorous inspiratory efforts that cause the volume to exceed the target, the ventilator will decrease the level of pressure support, which may increase the patient's WoB.

(3) If the lungs become stiffer, the ventilator will increase the pressure, which could result in overdistention lung injury.

4. The choice of volume control, pressure control, or adaptive control usually is the result of clinician familiarity, institutional preferences or personal bias.

C. **Cycle** is the variable that terminates inspiration, which is commonly time (volume-controlled ventilation or pressure-controlled ventilation) or flow (PSV).

VI. **Breath types during mechanical ventilation**

A. **Spontaneous breaths** are triggered and cycled by the patient.

B. **Mandatory breaths** are triggered either by the ventilator or the patient (or both) and cycled by the ventilator.

VII. **Modes of ventilation.** The combination of the various possible breath types and phase variables determines the mode of ventilation (**Table 5-1**).

A. **Continuous mandatory ventilation (CMV) or assist-control (A/C) ventilation**

1. Every breath is a mandatory breath type (**Fig. 5-8**). Although CMV is more descriptive, the terms CMV and A/C are used interchangeably. Note that the term "*controlled* mechanical ventilation" has little meaning in the context of modern ventilators, which do not have modes that prevent patient-triggered breaths.

2. **The patient can trigger** at a rate greater than that set on the ventilator, but always receives at least the set rate.

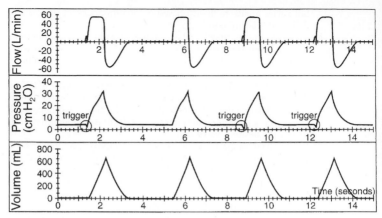

FIGURE 5-8 Continuous mandatory ventilation (assist-control ventilation).

    3. All breaths, whether ventilator triggered or patient triggered, are volume-control, pressure-control, or adaptive-control breaths.

    4. Triggering at a rapid rate may result in hyperventilation, hypotension, and dynamic hyperinflation.

  B. Continuous spontaneous ventilation. With continuous spontaneous ventilation modes, all breaths are triggered and cycled by the ventilator. There is no rate set.

    1. Continuous positive airway pressure (CPAP). With CPAP, the ventilator provides no inspiratory assistance.

      a. Strictly speaking, CPAP applies a positive pressure to the airway. Current ventilators, however, allow the patient to breath spontaneously without applying positive pressure to the airway (CPAP = 0).

      b. Modern ventilators offer little resistance to breathing and do not significantly increase the patient's WoB. This is particularly true with flow triggering.

      c. CPAP can be applied to an endotracheal tube (invasive) or to a face mask (noninvasive).

    2. Pressure support ventilation (PSV)

      a. The patient's inspiratory effort is assisted by the ventilator at a preset pressure with PSV. All breaths are spontaneous breath types **(Fig. 5-9)**.

      b. A pressure **rise time** can be set during PSV, similar to pressure control ventilation.

      c. Because the ventilator delivers breaths only in response to patient effort, appropriate apnea alarms must be set on the ventilator. The lack of a backup rate may result in apnea and sleep-disordered breathing in some patients.

      d. The ventilator cycles to the expiratory phase when the flow decreases to a ventilator-determined value (e.g., 5 L/min or 25% of the peak inspiratory flow). **If the patient actively exhales,** the ventilator may pressure cycle to the expiratory phase. The ventilator may not cycle correctly **in the presence of a leak** (e.g., bronchopleural fistula or mask leak with NPPV). A secondary time cycle will

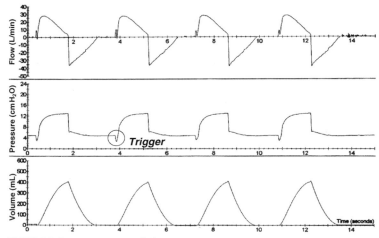

FIGURE 5-9 Pressure support ventilation.

terminate inspiration at 3 to 5 seconds (depending on the ventilator and adjustable on some).

e. Some ventilators allow the clinician to **adjust the flow cycle** criteria during PSV **(Fig. 5-10)**. This allows adjustment of the inspiratory time during pressure support to better coincide with the patient's neural inspiration (thus avoiding active exhalation or double triggering). If the ventilator is set to cycle at a greater percentage of peak flow, the inspiratory time is decreased. Conversely, if the ventilator is set to cycle at a lower percentage of the peak flow, the inspiratory time is increased. As a general rule, a higher flow cycle is necessary for obstructive lung disease and a lower flow cycle is necessary for restrictive lung disease (e.g., patients recovering from acute lung injury [ALI]).

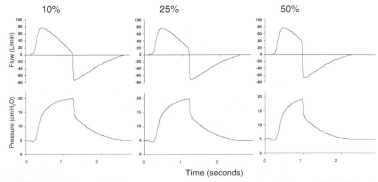

FIGURE 5-10 Examples of pressure support ventilation with termination flows of 10%, 25%, and 50% of peak flow.

> **f.** The tidal volume, inspiratory flow, inspiratory time, and respiratory rate may vary from breath to breath with PSV.
>
> **g. Tidal volume** is determined by the level of pressure support, rise time, lung mechanics, and the inspiratory effort of the patient.

3. Tube compensation (TC)

> **a.** TC is designed to overcome the flow resistive WoB imposed by the endotracheal tube or tracheostomy tube. It measures the patient's inspiratory flow and applies a pressure proportional to that flow, based on the size of the endotracheal tube or tracheostomy tube.
>
> **b.** The clinician can set the fraction of tube resistance for which compensation is desired (e.g., 50% compensation rather than full compensation).
>
> **c.** Although it has been shown that TC can effectively compensate for resistance through the artificial airway, it has not been shown to improve outcome.

4. Proportional assist ventilation (PAV)

> **a.** PAV provides ventilatory support in proportion to neural output of the respiratory center.
>
> **b.** The ventilator monitors respiratory drive as the inspiratory flow of the patient, integrates flow to volume, measures elastance and resistance, and then calculates the pressure required from the equation of motion.
>
> **c.** Using the pressure calculated from the equation of motion and the tidal volume, the ventilator calculates work of breathing (WoB): WoB $= \int P \times V$. These calculations occur every 5 ms during breath delivery.
>
> **d.** The ventilator estimates resistance and elastance (or compliance) by applying end-inspiratory and end-expiratory pause maneuvers of 300 ms every 4 to 10 seconds.
>
> **e.** The clinician adjusts the percentage of support (from 5% to 95%), which allows the work to be partitioned between the ventilator and the patient.
>
> > **(1)** Typically, the percentage of support is set so that the WoB is in the range of 0.5 to 1.0 J/L.
> >
> > **(2)** If the percentage of support is high, patient WoB may be inappropriately low and excessive volume and pressure may be applied (runaway phenomenon).
> >
> > **(3)** If the percentage of support is too low, patient WoB may be excessive.
>
> **f.** Because of changes in respiratory drive and the associated flow demand, PAV applies a pressure that varies from breath to breath, due to changes in patient's elastance, resistance and flow demand and within the breath. This differs from PSV, in which the level of support is constant regardless of demand, and VCV, in which the level of support decreases when demand increases.
>
> **g.** The cycle criterion for PAV is flow (adjustable by the clinician; similar to pressure support).
>
> **h.** PAV requires the presence of an intact ventilatory drive and a functional neuromuscular system.
>
> **i.** PAV is only available on one ventilator in the United States (PAV+, Puritan-Bennett 840), and cannot be used with NIV because leaks prevent accurate determination of respiratory mechanics.

5. **Neurally adjusted ventilatory assist (NAVA)**
   a. With NAVA, the ventilator is triggered, limited, and cycled by the electrical activity of diaphragm. The neural drive is transformed into ventilatory output (neuroventilatory coupling).
   b. The electrical activity of the diaphragm is measured by a multiple-array esophageal electrode, which is amplified to determine the support level (NAVA gain). The cycle-off is commonly set at 80% of peak inspiratory activity.
   c. The level of assistance is adjusted in response to changes in neural drive, respiratory system mechanics, inspiratory muscle function, and behavioral influences.
   d. Because the trigger is based on diaphragmatic activity rather than pressure or flow, triggering is not adversely affected in patients with flow limitation and auto-PEEP.
   e. NAVA is only available on the Servoi ventilator.

C. **Synchronized intermittent mandatory ventilation (SIMV)**
   1. With SIMV (**Fig. 5-11**), the ventilator is set to deliver both mandatory and spontaneous breath types.
   2. The mandatory breaths can be volume-control, pressure-control, or adaptive-control breaths.
   3. There is a set respiratory rate for the mandatory breaths and the mandatory breaths are synchronized with patient effort.
   4. Between the mandatory breaths, the patient may breathe spontaneously and the spontaneous breaths may be pressure supported (**Fig. 5-12**).
   5. The patient's inspiratory efforts may be as great during the mandatory breaths as the spontaneous breaths. Thus, it is a myth that SIMV rests the patient during the mandatory breaths and works the patient during the spontaneous breaths.
   6. The different breath types during SIMV may induce patient–ventilator dyssynchrony.
   7. Note that CMV and SIMV become synonymous if the patient is not triggering the ventilator (e.g., with neuromuscular blockade).

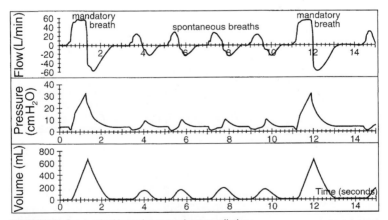

FIGURE 5-11 Synchronized intermittent mandatory ventilation.

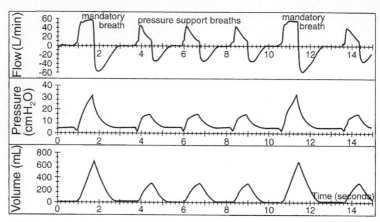

FIGURE 5-12 Synchronized intermittent mandatory ventilation with pressure support.

  D. Airway pressure release ventilation (APRV) produces alveolar ventilation as
     an adjunct to CPAP (**Fig. 5-13**). On some ventilators, APRV is achieved
     using modes called **BiLevel** (Puritan-Bennett) or **BiVent** (Maquet).
     1. Airway pressure is transiently released to a lower level, after which it is
        quickly restored to reinflate the lungs. The duration of the high-pres-
        sure level is greater than the duration of the low-pressure level.
     2. Minute ventilation is determined by lung compliance, airways resist-
        ance, the magnitude of the pressure release, the duration of the pres-
        sure release, and the magnitude of the patient's spontaneous breath-
        ing efforts.

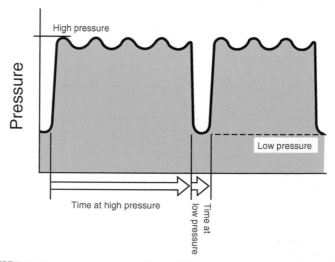

FIGURE 5-13 Airway pressure release ventilation (APRV).

3. Oxygenation is determined by the high-pressure setting. Spontaneous breathing by the patient may also provide recruitment of dependent lung regions.
4. Because the patient is allowed to breathe spontaneously at both levels of pressure, the need for sedation may be decreased. The patient is able to breathe at both levels of pressure due to an active exhalation valve.
5. **The potential advantage of APRV** is to provide lung recruitment at lower airway pressures than with traditional positive pressure ventilation by taking advantage of the spontaneous breathing efforts. This may increase Pao_2 while minimizing barotrauma, hemodynamic instability, and the need for sedation. However, it may be an uncomfortable breathing pattern for some patients.
6. A modification of APRV is the **PCV+** (available on the Drager Evita 4) or BiLevel mode (available on the Puritan-Bennett 840).
   a. Without spontaneous breathing, PCV+ is similar to PCV, and APRV is similar to PCIRV.
   b. PCV+ or BiLevel can be used to provide **sighs** during PSV or CPAP.
      (1) Several periods (2–4/min) of elevated airway pressure (20–40 cm H_2O) are used periodically (1–3 seconds at the higher pressure level) (**Fig. 5-14**).
      (2) The patient can breathe spontaneously at the higher pressure.
      (3) This strategy may be useful in spontaneously breathing patients prone to atelectasis.
E. **Adaptive support ventilation (ASV)** is a closed-loop mode that can provide pressure-limited time-cycled ventilation, add adaptive control of those breaths, allow for mandatory breaths and spontaneous breaths (SIMV + PSV), and switch to pressure support with adaptive control breath to breath.
   1. During ASV, the ventilator measures lung mechanics on a breath-to-breath basis and attempts to deliver 100 mL/min/kg of minute ventilation for an adult and 200 mL/min/kg for children.
   2. The target respiratory rate is calculated from the Otis Equation, striving for minimum WoB. V_T and respiratory rate cannot be set by the clinician.

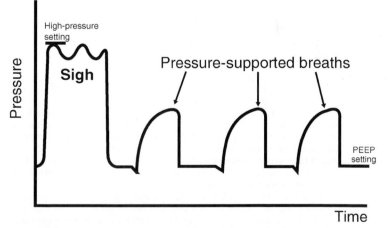

FIGURE 5-14 BiLevel or PCV+ used with pressure support ventilation to produce a sigh. PEEP, positive end-expiratory pressure.

3. The clinician sets the ideal body weight and the % minute volume that can vary from 20% to 200% to allow the ventilator's algorithm to choose a required minute volume and to adjusts its settings to meet the desired targets. This can be adjusted to provide full ventilatory support or encourage spontaneous breathing and facilitate weaning.

4. During mandatory breath delivery, the ventilator adjusts the inspiratory:expiratory (I:E) ratio and inspiratory time by calculating the expiratory time constant (compliance × resistance), and maintaining sufficient expiratory time to prevent auto-PEEP. Spontaneous and mandatory breaths can be combined to meet the minute ventilation target. Breath types are either pressure control or pressure support.

5. If the patient is not triggering, the ventilator determines the respiratory frequency, tidal volume, and pressure limit required to deliver the tidal volume, the inspiratory time, and the I:E ratio. If the patient is triggering, the number of mandatory breaths decreases and the ventilator chooses a pressure support that maintains a tidal volume sufficient to ensure alveolar ventilation based on a dead space calculation of 2.2 mL/kg.

F. Modes designed to facilitate weaning

1. **AutoMode** (Maquet ventilators).
   a. AutoMode provides automated weaning from pressure control to pressure support and automated escalation of support if patient effort diminishes.
   b. The ventilator provides PRVC if the patient is not breathing.
   c. If the patient triggers two consecutive breaths, the ventilator switches to VS.
   d. If the patient becomes apneic, the ventilator switches back to PRVC. AutoMode also switches between PCV and PSV or VCV and VS.

2. **SmartCare** (Draeger) is a closed-loop knowledge-based ventilator for PSV.
   a. SmartCare adapts the level of PSV to the patient's ventilatory needs, with the goal of keeping the patient within a comfort zone.
   b. Comfort is defined as a respiratory rate that can vary in the range of 15 to 30 breaths/min, a V_T above a minimum threshold, and an end-tidal CO_2 below a maximum threshold.
   c. PSV is adjusted in steps of 2 to 4 $cm H_2O$ to a minimum value, after which a spontaneous breathing trial is performed.
   d. If the spontaneous breathing trial is successful, a message on the screen recommends extubation.

VIII. High-frequency ventilation (HFV)

A. With HFV, the patient is ventilated with higher-than-normal rates (i.e., >60/min) and smaller tidal volumes (i.e., ,<5 mL/kg).

B. Potential advantages include a lower risk of alveolar overdistension due to smaller tidal volumes (thereby limiting peak alveolar pressure), and improved gas exchange $(\dot{V}/\dot{Q})$ due to more uniform distribution of ventilation, enhanced diffusion, and alveolar recruitment.

C. **High-frequency oscillatory ventilation (HFOV)** delivers small tidal volumes by oscillating a bias gas flow in the airway. The oscillator has an active inspiratory and an expiratory phase.

1. The determinants of CO_2 elimination are the pressure amplitude (ΔP) and frequency. Tidal volume and CO_2 elimination vary directly with ΔP. In contrast to conventional ventilation, CO_2 elimination varies inversely with frequency.
   a. ΔP is initially set at approximately 20 $cm H_2O$ above the $Paco_2$ or to induce wiggling that is visible to the patient's midthigh.

   b. The rate is adjustable from 3 to 15 Hz (180–900/min). Higher rates (12–15 Hz) are used in neonates and lower rates (3–6 Hz) are used in adults.

   2. The primary determinant of oxygenation during HFOV is mean airway pressure, which is essentially the level of PEEP. The ventilator oscillates the gas to pressures above and below (ΔP) the mean airway pressure.

   3. Available evidence suggests that arterial oxygenation is improved in some patients with ALI/ARDS, but evidence is lacking for better patient outcomes.

D. High-frequency jet ventilation delivers gas from a high-pressure source through a jet directed into the airway. Viscous shearing drags gas into the airway.

   1. Tidal volume is determined by the driving pressure, inspiratory time, catheter size, and respiratory system mechanics.

   2. Mean airway pressure is controlled by driving pressure, I:E ratio, and PEEP.

   3. High-frequency jet ventilation uses rates of 240 to 660 breaths/min.

   4. A jet ventilator is not available in the United States for adult use.

E. High-frequency percussive ventilation, also called volumetric diffusive respiration, uses a sliding nongated venturi to separate inspired and expired gases and provide PEEP. It is commercially available as the Percussionaire.

   1. Minute ventilation is controlled by respiratory rate and peak inspiratory pressure.

   2. Respiratory rates of 180 to 600 breaths/min are used.

   3. Oxygenation is determined by peak inspiratory pressure, I:E ratio, and PEEP.

   4. High-frequency percussive ventilation is popular in the care of patients with burn injury despite lack of evidence reporting better outcomes.

IX. Specific ventilator settings

A. A tidal volume target of 4 to 10 mL/kg predicted body weight is used. Ideal body weight is determined by the height and the sex of the patient.

Male patients : PBW = 50 + 2.3 × [height (inches) − 60]

Female patients : PBW = 45.5 + 2.3 × [height (inches)−60]

   1. Lower tidal volume targets decrease the risk of **ventilator-induced lung injury (VILI).**

   2. Use a tidal volume of 6 mL/kg (4–8 mL/kg) for patients with **ARDS and acute lung injury (ALI).**

   3. Use a tidal volume of 6 to 8 mL/kg with **obstructive lung disease.**

   4. Use a tidal volume of 8 to 10 mL/kg with **neuromuscular disease** or **postoperative ventilatory support.**

   5. Monitor the **plateau pressure** and consider tidal volume reduction if the plateau pressure is more than 30 cmH_2O.

   a. Because lung injury is a function of transalveolar pressure, a higher plateau pressure may be acceptable if chest wall compliance is decreased.

B. Respiratory rate

   1. The respiratory rate and tidal volume determine **minute ventilation.**

   2. Set the rate at 15 to 25/min to achieve a minute ventilation of 8 to 12 L/min.

   a. With low tidal volumes and a low pH, a higher respiratory rate may be necessary.

   b. A lower respiratory rate may be necessary to avoid air trapping and dynamic hyperinflation.

3. Adjust the rate to achieve the desired pH and $Paco_2$.
4. Avoid high respiratory rates that produce air trapping.
5. **A high-minute-ventilation** (>10 L/min) requirement is due to an increased carbon dioxide production or a high dead space.

C. **Inspiratory : expiratory (I : E) ratio**
1. **Inspiratory time** is determined by flow, tidal volume, and flow pattern during volume-controlled ventilation. Inspiratory time is set directly with pressure control ventilation.
2. **Expiratory time** is determined by the inspiratory time and respiratory rate.
3. The expiratory time generally should be longer than the inspiratory time (e.g., I:E of 1:2).
4. **The expiratory time should be lengthened** (e.g., higher inspiratory flow, lower tidal volume, lower respiratory rate) if the blood pressure drops in response to positive-pressure ventilation or if auto-PEEP is present. If air trapping is significant and accompanied by an acute drop in blood pressure, the patient may be temporarily disconnected from the ventilator (about 30 seconds), then reconnected.
5. **Longer inspiratory times** increase mean airway pressure and may improve arterial partial pressure of oxygen (Pao_2) in some patients.
   a. There is little role for an inverse I:E (i.e., inspiratory time longer than expiratory time).
   b. When long inspiratory times are used, hemodynamics and auto-PEEP must be closely monitored.

D. **Fio_2**
1. Initiate mechanical ventilation with an Fio_2 of 1.0.
2. Titrate the Fio_2 using pulse oximetry.
3. Inability to reduce the Fio_2 to less than 0.6 indicates the presence of shunt (intrapulmonary or intracardiac).

E. **PEEP**
1. **The use of appropriate levels of PEEP** increases the functional respiratory capacity, decreases intrapulmonary shunt, and improves lung compliance.
   a. Because lung volumes are typically decreased with acute respiratory failure, it is reasonable to use a PEEP of at least 5 cm H_2O with the initiation of mechanical ventilation for most patients.
   b. **Maintaining alveolar recruitment** in disease processes like ARDS may decrease the likelihood of Ventilator-induced lung injury.
   c. Although higher levels of PEEP often increase Pao_2, evidence has not shown that higher levels of PEEP (compared to modest levels of PEEP) decrease mortality.
2. A number of methods have been used to titrate the best level of PEEP in patients with ALI.
   a. PEEP can be titrated to a desired level of oxygenation, such as the level of PEEP that allows the Fio_2 to be decreased to 0.6 without hemodynamic compromise.
   b. PEEP can be set according to a table of Fio_2/PEEP combinations to achieve an Spo_2 of 88% to 95%, as was done in the ARDSNet trials.
   c. PEEP can be set 2 to 3 cm H_2O above the lower inflexion point of the pressure–volume curve. However, this is difficult to measure reliably in critically ill patients, and its role in the determination of appropriate PEEP setting remains to be determined.
   d. PEEP can be set to achieve the best respiratory system compliance. The best compliance can be determined from either an incremental

or a decremental PEEP trial. A decremental PEEP trial has the theoretical advantage or a greater lung volume for a level of PEEP.

  e. PEEP can be adjusted to the best stress index, as assessed from
the pressure-time curve during constant-flow volume ventilation.

  f. Improved oxygenation has been reported when PEEP is set at a
level greater than the end-expiratory esophageal pressure.

  g. Evidence is lacking that any approach to setting PEEP is superior to
another in terms of patient outcomes.

3. In patients with COPD, PEEP may be used to counterbalance auto-
PEEP and improve the ability to trigger the ventilator.

4. In patients with left ventricular failure, PEEP may improve cardiac performance by decreasing venous return and left ventricular afterload.

5. **Adverse effects of PEEP**

  a. PEEP may **decrease cardiac output**. Hemodynamics should be monitored during PEEP titration.

  b. High levels of PEEP may result in **alveolar overdistention** during the
inspiratory phase. It may be necessary to decrease the tidal volume
with high PEEP.

  c. PEEP may **worsen oxygenation with unilateral lung disease** because
it results in a redistribution of pulmonary blood flow from overdis-
tended lung units to the unventilated lung units. PEEP may worsen
oxygenation with cardiac shunt (e.g., patient foramen ovale).

X. Complications of mechanical ventilation
A. Ventilator-induced lung injury

1. **Overdistension injury** occurs if the lung parenchyma is subjected to an
abnormally high transpulmonary pressure.

  a. Overdistension injury produces inflammation and increased alveo-
lar-capillary membrane permeability.

  b. Tidal volume should be limited (e.g., 6 mL/kg in patients with
ALI/ARDS) to decrease the risk of overdistention lung injury.

  c. Plateau pressure should be maintained at less than or equal to
30 cm H_2O to prevent overdistension injury.

  d. A priority should be given to use of the lowest tidal volume *and*
plateau pressure possible to minimize the risk of lung injury during
mechanical ventilation.

  e. Because the risk of overdistension lung injury is related to transpulmonary pressure, higher plateau pressures may be acceptable if
chest wall compliance is reduced (e.g., abdominal distention, chest
wall burns, chest wall edema, obesity).

2. **Derecruitment injury**

  a. PEEP levels that are not high enough to maintain alveolar recruitment may result in alveolar opening and closing with each respiratory cycle. This may result in inflammation and increased alveolar-
capillary membrane permeability.

  b. This injury may be avoided by use of appropriate levels of PEEP
with ARDS: often 8 to 15 cm H_2O, and sometimes 15 to 20 cm H_2O.

3. **Oxygen toxicity**

  a. High concentrations of oxygen for long periods may cause lung
damage and may promote atelectasis.

  b. Although it is prudent to reduce the Fio_2 provided that arterial oxygenation is adequate (Spo_2 >90% in most patients; some patients
tolerate lower Spo_2), the precise role of oxygen toxicity in patients
with ALI is unclear.

   c. Appropriate levels of inspired oxygen should never be withheld for fear of oxygen toxicity.

B. Patient–ventilator dyssynchrony

1. **Dyssynchrony** can be the result of an insensitive trigger setting, auto-PEEP, incorrect flow setting during volume control ventilation, incorrect pressure or rise time during pressure control ventilation, an inspiratory time that is too short or too long during pressure control, or incorrect flow cycle during pressure support.

C. Auto-PEEP

1. **Auto-PEEP** is the result of gas trapping (dynamic hyperinflation) due to insufficient expiratory time and/or increased expiratory airflow resistance. The pressure exerted by this trapped gas is called auto-PEEP.

2. The increase in alveolar pressure due to auto-PEEP may adversely affect hemodynamics.

3. The presence of auto-PEEP can produce trigger dyssynchrony as discussed previously.

4. **Detection of auto-PEEP**

   a. Some ventilators allow auto-PEEP to be measured directly.

   b. In spontaneously breathing patients, auto-PEEP can be measured using an **esophageal balloon.**

   c. The **patient's breathing pattern** can be observed. If exhalation is still occurring when the next breath is delivered, auto-PEEP is present.

   d. Inspiratory efforts **that do not trigger the ventilator** suggest the presence of auto-PEEP.

   e. If flow graphics is available on the ventilator, it can be observed that **expiratory flow** does not return to 0 before the subsequent breath is delivered.

D. Factors affecting auto-PEEP

1. **Physiologic factors.** A high airways resistance or high respiratory system compliance increases the likelihood of auto-PEEP.

2. **Ventilator factors.** A high tidal volume, high respiratory rate, or prolonged inspiratory time will increase the likelihood of auto-PEEP. Reducing the minute ventilation decreases the likelihood of auto-PEEP.

E. Barotrauma

1. **Alveolar rupture** during positive-pressure ventilation may lead to air extravasation through the bronchovascular sheath into the pulmonary interstitium, mediastinum, pericardium, peritoneum, pleural space, and subcutaneous tissue. Sudden hemodynamic instability or sudden increase in peak inspiratory pressure in a mechanically ventilated patient should raise the suspicion of a **tension pneumothorax.**

F. Hemodynamic perturbations

1. Positive-pressure ventilation increases intrathoracic pressure and **decreases venous return**. Right ventricular filling is limited by the reduced venous return.

2. When alveolar pressure exceeds pulmonary venous pressure, pulmonary blood flow is affected by alveolar pressure rather than by left atrial pressure, producing an **increase in pulmonary vascular resistance**. Consequently, right ventricular afterload increases and right ventricular ejection fraction falls.

3. **Left ventricular filling is limited** by reduced right ventricular output and decreased left ventricular diastolic compliance.

4. Increased right ventricular size affects left ventricular performance by shifting the interventricular septum to the left.

5. **Intravascular volume replacement** counteracts the negative hemodynamic effects of PEEP.
6. Increased intrathoracic pressure may **improve left ventricular ejection fraction and stroke volume.** This beneficial effect may be significant in patients with poor ventricular function.
G. **Nosocomial pneumonia:** see **Chapter 29**

Selected References

Branson RD, Chatburn RL. Should adaptive pressure control modes be utilized for virtually all patients receiving mechanical ventilation? *Respir Care* 2007;52:478–488.

Brower RG, Lanken PN, MacIntyre N, et al. Higher versus lower positive end-expiratory pressures in patients with the acute respiratory distress syndrome. *N Engl J Med* 2004;351: 327–336.

Chatburn RL. Classification of ventilator modes: update and proposal for implementation. *Respir Care* 2007;52:301–323.

Dhand R, Guntur VP. How best to deliver aerosol medications to mechanically ventilated patients. *Clin Chest Med* 2008;29:277–296.

Fan E, Needham DM, Stewart TE. Ventilatory management of acute lung injury and acute respiratory distress syndrome. *JAMA* 2005;294:2889–2896.

Fessler HE, Derdak S, Ferguson ND, et al. A protocol for high-frequency oscillatory ventilation in adults: results from a roundtable discussion. *Crit Care Med* 2007;35:1649–1654.

Fessler HE, Hess DR. Does high-frequency ventilation offer benefits over conventional ventilation in adult patients with acute respiratory distress syndrome? *Respir Care* 2007;52: 595–608.

Garpestad E, Brennan J, Hill NS. Noninvasive ventilation for critical care. *Chest* 2007;132: 711–720.

Hess DR. The evidence for noninvasive positive-pressure ventilation in the care of patients in acute respiratory failure: a systematic review of the literature. *Respir Care* 2004;49: 810–829.

Hess DR. Ventilator waveforms and the physiology of pressure support ventilation. *Respir Care* 2005;50:166–186.

MacIntyre NR. Is there a best way to set positive expiratory-end pressure for mechanical ventilatory support in acute lung injury? *Clin Chest Med* 2008;29:233–239.

MacIntyre NR. Is there a best way to set tidal volume for mechanical ventilatory support? *Clin Chest Med* 2008;29:225–231.

Masip J. Noninvasive ventilation in acute cardiogenic pulmonary edema. *Curr Opin Crit Care* 2008;14:531–535.

Meade MO, Cook DJ, Guyatt GH, et al. Ventilation strategy using low tidal volumes, recruitment maneuvers, and high positive end-expiratory pressure for acute lung injury and acute respiratory distress syndrome: a randomized controlled trial. *JAMA* 2008;299: 637–645.

Mercat A, Richard JC, Vielle B, et al. Positive end-expiratory pressure setting in adults with acute lung injury and acute respiratory distress syndrome: a randomized controlled trial. *JAMA* 2008;299:646–655.

Myers TR, MacIntyre NR. Does airway pressure release ventilation offer important new advantages in mechanical ventilator support? *Respir Care* 2007;52:452–460.

NIH/NHLBI ARDS Network. Ventilation with lower tidal volumes as compared with traditional tidal volumes for acute lung injury and the acute respiratory distress syndrome. *N Engl J Med* 2000;342:1301–1308.

Siau C, Stewart TE. Current role of high frequency oscillatory ventilation and airway pressure release ventilation in acute lung injury and acute respiratory distress syndrome. *Clin Chest Med* 2008;29:265–75.

Sinderby C, Beck J. Proportional assist ventilation and neurally adjusted ventilatory assist-better approaches to patient ventilator synchrony? *Clin Chest Med* 2008;29:329–342.

6

Hemodynamic Management

Jonathan Fox and Edward Bittner

I. **Hemodynamic perturbations** are common during intensive care unit admission. Both hypotensive and hypertensive emergencies threaten the goal of our cardiovascular system, which is the provision of oxygen and metabolic substrates in sufficient supply to meet the demands of the body's tissues. In the event that supply is insufficient for demand, predictable pathophysiologic patterns emerge, and a patient's clinical presentation is the manifestation of progressive end-organ damage, be it neurologic, cardiovascular, pulmonary, renal, gastrointestinal, hematologic, or musculocutaneous. The goal of the hemodynamic management of such patients is to maintain end-organ oxygenation and perfusion in order to preserve function.

II. **Shock** is a state of generalized inadequate tissue perfusion, the effects of which are tissue hypoxia and organ dysfunction. In its early stages, shock may be *nonprogressive* or *compensated*: potent neurohumoral reflexes, including activation of the sympathetic nervous system and the renin–angiotensin–aldosterone system, act to maintain a supply of oxygen sufficient to meet cellular demands. With the failure of these reflexes, however, shock becomes *progressive* and, ultimately, *irreversible*: as demand for intracellular energy outstrips supply, anaerobic metabolism predominates and lactic acid production rises; membrane-associated ion transport pumps fail; the integrity of cell membranes is compromised; and cell death ensues. Pathophysiologically, shock has been historically classified according to one of four mechanisms: hypovolemic, cardiogenic, obstructive, or distributive. The first three mechanisms may be categorized as states of *hypodynamic* shock, while the last may be categorized as a state of *hyperdynamic* shock.

A. **Types of shock**

1. **Hypovolemic shock** occurs with the depletion of effective intravascular volume, due to insufficient intake, excessive loss, or to a combination thereof. Common causes include dehydration, acute hemorrhage, gastrointestinal and renal losses, and interstitial fluid redistribution occurring in the context of severe tissue trauma, burn injuries, and pancreatitis. Hemorrhage is the most common cause of shock in trauma patients and has been categorized by the American College of Surgeons into four classes, providing a correlation between the percent of total blood volume lost and the expected attendant physiologic changes in mental status, blood pressure, heart rate, respiratory rate, and urine output (**Table 6-1**). Hemodynamically, hypovolemic shock is characterized by **decreased cardiac output, decreased filling pressures** (see **Chapter 1**), and increased systemic vascular resistance.

2. **Cardiogenic shock** is defined as persistent hypotension and inadequate tissue perfusion due to primary cardiac dysfunction occurring in the context of adequate intravascular volume and adequate or elevated left ventricular filling pressures. It may be caused by any number of changes in heart rate, rhythm, or contractility, although it occurs most

TABLE 6-1	American College of Surgeons Hemorrhage Classification[a]			
	Class			
	I	**II**	**III**	**IV**
Blood loss (mL)	<750	750–1500	1500–2000	>2000
Blood loss (%)	<15	15–30	30–40	>40
SBP	Normal	Normal	Decreased	Decreased
HR (beats/min)	<100	100–120	120–140	>140
RR (breaths/min)	14–20	20–30	30–40	>35
UOP (mL/h)	>30	20–30	5–15	Negligible
Mental status	Slightly anxious	Mildly anxious	Anxious, confused	Confused, lethargic

SBP, systolic blood pressure; HR, heart rate; RR, respiratory rate; UOP, urine output.
[a]Based on 70-kg individual.

commonly after extensive acute myocardial infarction (AMI) or ischemia leading to left ventricular failure. Other etiologies of cardiogenic shock include acute (e.g., tako-tsubo) and chronic cardiomyopathies, myocarditis, and **myocardial contusion.** Hemodynamically, cardiogenic shock is characterized by **decreased cardiac output, increased filling pressures,** and increased systemic vascular resistance.

3. **Obstructive shock** occurs as a result of an impediment to the normal flow of blood either to or from the heart, producing impairment of venous return or arterial outflow. Common causes include **tension pneumothorax, abdominal compartment syndrome, pulmonary embolism, pericardial tamponade,** auto-PEEP, severe aortic stenosis, dissecting aortic aneurysm, and severe aortic coarctation. Hemodynamically, obstructive shock is characterized by **decreased cardiac output, increased filling pressures,** and increased systemic vascular resistance.

4. **Distributive shock,** unlike hypovolemic, cardiogenic and obstructive shocks, tends to represent a *hyperdynamic* state characterized by a **normal or high cardiac output** and a low systemic vascular resistance. In the critical care setting, it is most commonly caused by sepsis (infection) or a systemic inflammatory response syndrome (inflammation). Other etiologies include neurogenic shock, anaphylaxis, adrenal insufficiency, hepatic failure, and arteriovenous fistulae. Hemodynamically, distributive shock is characterized by normal or increased cardiac output, decreased filling pressures, and decreased systemic vascular resistance. The hemodynamic and metabolic profiles of the various types of shock are summarized in **Tables 6-2 and 6-3.**

TABLE 6-2	Hemodynamic Parameters in Shock			
Type of Shock	**MAP**	**CO**	**PAOP**	**SVR**
Hypovolemic	↓	↓	↓	↑
Cardiogenic	↓	↓	↑	↑
Obstructive	↓	↓	↔/↑	↑
Distributive	↓	↔/↑	↔/↓	↓

MAP, mean arterial blood pressure; CO, cardiac output; PAOP, pulmonary artery occlusion pressure; SVR, systemic vascular resistance.

B. Clinical presentation of shock reflects the macro- and microvascular consequences of inadequate tissue perfusion and oxygenation.
1. **Neurologic:** Altered mental status, manifested as anxiety, disorientation, delirium, and frank obtundation.
2. **Cardiac:** Chest pain, hypotension, electrocardiographic and enzymatic evidence of myocardial damage, echocardiographic wall motion abnormalities.
3. **Respiratory:** Increased respiratory rate and minute ventilation, respiratory muscle failure.
4. **Renal:** Renal ischemia, acute tubular necrosis, decreased urine output, uremia.
5. **Gastrointestinal:** Hepatic centrilobar necrosis and transaminitis, stress ulceration, bacterial translocation.
6. **Hematologic:** Coagulopathy, thromboses, thrombocytopenia, disseminated intravascular coagulation.
7. **Musculocutaneous:** Weakness, fatigue, vasoconstriction, cool limbs, poor capillary refill, weak pulses.
C. Monitoring in shock should be directed toward detecting if not preventing the progression of tissue hypoperfusion as well as toward assessing the adequacy of resuscitation.
1. **Standard monitors** (continuous electrocardiography, pulse oximetry, noninvasive blood pressure, urinary output, temperature) should not preclude the vigilance of the clinician in performing a comprehensive history and serial physical examinations.
2. **Monitors of tissue perfusion** include both hemodynamic and metabolic indices, the utility of which are likely greater when followed over time rather than when examined at discrete time points.
   a. **Hemodynamic indices.** Measurement of systemic blood pressure allows for a global rather than a regional assessment of the adequacy of tissue perfusion. Given the desire for continuous arterial pressure monitoring and the need for frequent blood draws to track trends in arterial blood gases and serum lactate levels (see later), most patients in shock will have an **indwelling arterial cannula** placed for systemic blood pressure measurement (see **Chapter 1**). The need to monitor central filling pressures, establish large volume access, infuse potent vasoactive medications, and draw serial central blood samples (see later) frequently requires placement of a **central venous catheter**. Placement of a **pulmonary artery (PA) catheter** may further assist in the differential diagnosis of shock when the hemodynamic profile is not clear from peripheral assessment and may aid in the monitoring of global (e.g., mixed venous oxygen saturation, see below) and cardiac (e.g., PA occlusion pressure, cardiac output) responses to therapeutic interventions. Additional monitors are now available to allow

TABLE 6-3	Metabolic Parameters in Shock	
Type of Shock	**Svo_2, $Scvo_2$**	**Lactate**
Hypovolemic	↓	↑
Cardiogenic	↓	↑
Obstructive	↓	↑
Distributive	↔/↑	↑

Svo_2, mixed venous oxygen saturation; $Scvo_2$, central venous oxygen saturation.

less-invasive assessment of cardiac output, stroke volume, and systemic vascular resistance (**Chapter 1**).

b. Metabolic indices

(1) **Serum pH.** Metabolic acidemia may reflect a state of increased anaerobic metabolism and endogenous acid production occurring with progressive tissue hypoperfusion. It may also signal worsening renal compromise and an inability to clear the increasing endogenous acid load.

(2) **Serum lactate.** In the absence of sufficient cellular levels of oxygen, cellular demand for energy sources such as ATP exceeds cellular supply, the citric acid cycle and oxidative phosphorylation fail, and pyruvate generated by glycolysis is increasingly reduced to lactate.

(3) **Mixed venous (Svo_2) or central venous ($Scvo_2$) oxygen saturation** reflects the balance between systemic oxygen delivery (DO_2) and systemic oxygen consumption (VO_2). When supply is insufficient to meet demand or demand exceeds supply, Svo_2 falls below the normal range of 65% to 75%. Given that Svo_2 reflects the balance between DO_2 and VO_2, it depends on the variables determining them in turn, including body temperature, metabolic rate, hemoglobin concentration, arterial oxygen partial pressure, and cardiac output (**Fig. 6-1**).

D. Management of shock

1. **General principles.** If shock is defined as a state of inadequate tissue perfusion and oxygenation, it makes sense that treatment should be aimed at increasing DO_2 while minimizing VO_2.

a. **Supplemental oxygen** should be supplied and the institution of endotracheal intubation with controlled mechanical ventilation should be considered early.

b. **Circulation.** Delivery of well-oxygenated blood to the tissues depends on an adequate cardiac output and driving pressure. Thus, fluid resuscitation plays an integral role in the treatment of shock. In the event that infusion of crystalloid, colloid, or blood products is insufficient to establish and maintain adequate systemic oxygen delivery, pharmacologic therapy with inotropes and/or vasopressors may be required.

Central/Mixed Venous Oxygen Saturation

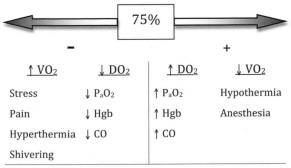

↑ VO_2	↓ DO_2	↑ DO_2	↓ VO_2
Stress	↓ P_aO_2	↑ P_aO_2	Hypothermia
Pain	↓ Hgb	↑ Hgb	Anesthesia
Hyperthermia	↓ CO	↑ CO	
Shivering			

FIGURE 6-1 Factors affecting central and mixed venous oxygen saturation. After Rivers EP, Ander DS, Powell D. Central venous oxygen saturation monitoring in the critically ill patient. *Curr Opin Crit Care* 2001;7(3):204–211. VO_2, systemic oxygen consumption; DO_2, systemic oxygen delivery; PaO_2, arterial oxygen partial pressure; Hgb, hemoglobin concentration; CO, cardiac output.

2. **Volume replacement** is the cornerstone of the treatment of hypotension and shock. Its aim is both to increase effective circulating intravascular volume and, through the Frank-Starling mechanism, to increase cardiac output. Unfortunately, it is often difficult to predict whether, and by how much, the **cardiac output will increase with volume loading.** While inadequate fluid replacement may result in continued tissue hypoperfusion and the progression of shock, **overly aggressive resuscitation may produce heart failure** and pulmonary and tissue edema, which themselves will further compromise tissue perfusion. The fluids available for resuscitation include crystalloids, colloids, and blood products, however, the optimal choice of fluid remains controversial.

    a. **Crystalloids.** The most commonly used crystalloid solutions are **lactated Ringer's** and **normal saline solutions,** which are inexpensive, easily stored, and readily available. Because these fluids readily leave the intravascular space, however, they require a volume equal at least to three to four times the intravascular deficit to restore circulating volume. In addition, by expanding the interstitial volume, they have the potential to create tissue edema and worsen tissue perfusion, thus providing an at least theoretical argument for the use of colloids in fluid resuscitation instead.

    b. **Colloids** include both natural and synthetic solutions. Because of their high molecular weight and increased osmotic activity, colloids remain in the intravascular space longer than crystalloids and thus require less volume to achieve the same hemodynamic goals.

        (1) **Human albumin** is derived from pooled human plasma and is available as 5% and 25% solutions in normal saline. Heat treatment eliminates the risk of transmission of viral infections. Although there is no evidence of harm from the use of albumin as a resuscitation fluid (except perhaps in head injury victims), no clear benefit has been shown either and its relatively high cost limits its widespread use.

        (2) **Synthetic colloids** include **dextran** and **hydroxyethyl starch (HES).** Because of their antigenicity and high incidence of anaphylactic and anaphylactoid reactions, the dextrans have largely been replaced by starch-based compounds. **HES** are high-polymeric glucose compounds available with a variety of mean molecular weights and molar substitution patterns and dissolved in normal saline or sodium lactate. Less expensive than albumin, HES are nonantigenic, and anaphylactoid reactions are rare. High- and medium-molecular-weight compounds in particular may produce significant decreases in the plasma concentrations of factor VIII and von Willebrand factor and may **impair platelet reactivity**. A maximum dose less than 20 mL/kg/d has been recommended. Recent data also suggest that HES **may be nephrotoxic in patients with septic shock.** Until further evidence is available, we discourage the use of HES in such patients and consider albumin a safe alternative.

    c. **Blood products.** While not recommended for pure volume expansion due to their potential for disease transmission, immunosuppression, transfusion reaction, and transfusion-related acute lung injury as well as their limited availability and high cost, administration of packed red blood cells may be indicated to improve systemic oxygen delivery when infusion of crystalloid or colloid and institution of vasoactive agents have proven insufficient to halt the progression of shock. The choice of a transfusion trigger for any given patient in any given situation remains unclear. However, general agreement exists that the Hb level in stable anemic patients needs not to be increased above a concentration of 10 mg/dL.

3. **Specific considerations**
   a. **Hypovolemic shock.** Since hypovolemic shock entails a reduction in effective intravascular volume, it would seem logical that its treatment would involve rapid volume resuscitation. However, in the case of hemorrhagic shock with ongoing blood loss, aggressive fluid administration prior to definitive hemostasis may increase bleeding from disrupted vessels and promote the progression of tissue hypoperfusion. As such, delayed and initially limited rather than immediate and vigorous fluid resuscitation may be beneficial. It must also be kept in mind that massive hemorrhage also involves loss of platelets and coagulation factors, such that balanced infusions of packed red blood cells and fresh frozen plasma may be required. As is the case with any massive transfusion, care must be taken to guard against development of the lethal triad of cold, coagulopathy, and acidemia.

   b. **Cardiogenic shock.** The abnormalities in rate, rhythm, contractility, and valvular mechanics associated with cardiogenic shock may require a host of specialized interventions, ranging from pacemaker and defibrillator placements to antithrombotic therapy, percutaneous coronary intervention with angioplasty, stenting, open coronary revascularization, mechanical support with intra-aortic balloon counterpulsation devices, and even left ventricular assist devices (see **Chapter 18**). Despite such sophisticated treatments, the initial approach to the management of patients in cardiogenic shock adheres to the same basic principles of rectifying the imbalance between systemic oxygen delivery and systemic oxygen consumption until definitive treatment can be obtained.

   c. **Obstructive shock** requires specific interventions targeted to the cause of blood flow impairment. Tension pneumothorax is treated with needle decompression followed by tube thoracostomy; abdominal compartment syndrome is treated with surgical decompression; pulmonary embolism is treated with supportive care and may involve the use of thrombolysis or surgical embolectomy; cardiac tamponade is treated with pericardiocentesis; auto-PEEP requires temporary suspension of mechanical ventilation and adjustment of ventilatory parameters.

   d. **Distributive shock.** In the critical care setting, distributive shock is most commonly caused by *sepsis* (infection) or a *systemic inflammatory response syndrome* (inflammation). Guidelines for the management of **severe sepsis** and **septic shock** are reviewed in **Chapter 30**. In brief, appropriate initial management rests upon the triad of antimicrobial management, hemodynamic resuscitation, and source control. **Anaphylactic shock** is another form of distributive shock resulting from an acute, immunoglobulin E (IgE)–mediated reaction involving the release of multiple inflammatory mediators from mast cells and basophils. Initial management requires immediate identification and discontinuation of the suspected antigen, prompt provision of ventilatory and cardiovascular support, and pharmacologic therapy directed at the immune mediators of the symptomatology, including epinephrine, the histamine H_1- and H_2-receptor blockers diphenhydramine and ranitidine, and corticosteroids.

III. **Pharmacologic therapies of hypotension and shock.** When appropriate fluid replacement fails to restore adequate blood pressure and tissue perfusion, pharmacologic therapy with vasopressors and/or inotropes is required. Even with the return of physiologic systemic filling and perfusion pressures (e.g., CVP 8–12 mm Hg, MAP 65–90 mm Hg), regional perfusion abnormalities may cause refractory tissue hypoperfusion. Persistent metabolic acidemia, elevated serum lactate levels, and depressed $Scvo_2$ suggest the need for further pharmacologic intervention, although the choice of a specific agent will depend on the clinical context. **Tables 6-4 and 6-5** summarize the common vasopressor and inotropic agents, including their receptor binding affinity and major hemodynamic effects and side effects. Specific informations, including dosage, of the drugs described in the following sessions, are also available in the **Appendix**.

A. **Non–catecholamine sympathomimetic agents** are synthetic drugs used primarily as vasopressors. They are classified according to their affinity for activation of **α- and/or β-adrenergic receptors**.

1. **Phenylephrine** is a selective α_1 adrenergic agonist that causes arterial vasoconstriction. By increasing systemic vascular resistance, it rapidly raises mean arterial pressure, although reflex bradycardia may effect a reduction in cardiac output. Because of its rapid onset, its ease of titration, and its ability to be administered through a peripheral intravenous (IV) line, phenylephrine is often used as a first-line, temporizing agent to treat hypotension. Its indications include hypotension secondary to peripheral vasodilatation, such as following the administration of potent hypnotic drugs or epidural local anesthetic drugs, or hypotension occurring in the presence of a mild to moderate infection. Because of its pure vasoconstrictive effect, phenylephrine may be poorly tolerated in patients with compromised left ventricular function.

2. **Ephedrine** is a direct and indirect **α- and β-adrenergic agonist** that causes an increase in heart rate and cardiac output with modest vasoconstriction. As such, its hemodynamic profile is similar to that of epinephrine, although much less potent.

3. **Arginine vasopressin (AVP)** (antidiuretic hormone, ADH) is a nona-peptide hormone endogenously synthesized in the hypothalamus and stored in

TABLE 6-4	Commonly Used Vasopressor and Inotropic Agents: Receptor Selectivity					
Drug	α_1	α_2	β_1	β_2	**DA**	**Other**
Phenylephrine	+ + + + +	+	+	0	0	
Ephedrine	+ + +	0	+ + +	+ +	0	
Vasopressin						V_1/V_2
Dopamine[a]	+ + +	+ + +	+ + + +	+ +	+ + + + +	
Norepinephrine	+ + + +	+ + +	+ + +	+	0	
Epinephrine	+ + + + +	+ + +	+ + + +	+ + +	0	
Isoproterenol	0	0	+ + + + +	+ + + + +	0	
Dobutamine	+	0	+ + + + +	+ + +	0	
Milrinone						N/A
Levosimendan						N/A

α_1, α_1 receptor; α_2, α_2 receptor; β_1, β_1 receptor; β_2, β_2 receptor; DA, dopamine receptors; V_1/V_2, vasopressin receptors; 0, zero receptor affinity; + through + + + + +, minimal to marked receptor affinity.
[a]Effects of dopamine vary with dose, from predominantly DA agonism at low doses to predominantly α agonism at high doses.

the posterior pituitary. In addition to its roles in osmoregulation and volume regulation, which are mediated through the **V$_2$ receptors**, AVP also acts through **V$_1$ receptors** to increase arteriolar smooth muscle tone and thus systemic vascular resistance while remaining chronotropically and inotropically neutral. While vasopressin levels in hypovolemic (hemorrhagic) and cardiogenic shock are appropriately elevated, serum levels in patients with septic shock have been found to be inappropriately low. Given this relative vasopressin deficiency in septic shock, **low-dose infusions in the range of 0.01 to 0.04 U/min** may produce V$_1$-mediated vasoconstriction while potentiating the effects of other vasoactive and inotropic agents. While pharmacologic doses (>0.1 U/min) may cause potentially deleterious vasoconstriction of splanchnic, renal, pulmonary, and coronary vascular beds, physiologic infusions (0.01–0.04 U/min) do not.

B. **Catecholamines** include both the endogenous compounds **dopamine, norepinephrine** and **epinephrine** and the synthetic compounds such as **isoproterenol** and **dobutamine**.

   1. **Endogenous**

      a. **Dopamine** is the immediate precursor to norepinephrine and epinephrine. Its actions vary with its dosing. At low doses, it affects primarily dopaminergic receptors in splanchnic, renal, coronary, and

TABLE 6-5	Commonly Used Vasopressor and Inotropic Agents: Hemodynamic Effects and Major Clinical Side Effects					
Drug	**HR**	**MAP**	**CO**	**SVR**	**Renal Blood Flow**	**Side Effects**
Phenylephrine	↓	↑↑↑	↓	↑↑↑	↓↓↓	Reflex bradycardia, HTN, peripheral and visceral vasoconstriction
Ephedrine	↑↑	↑↑	↑↑	↑	↓↓	Tachycardia
Vasopressin	0	0	0	↑	↑	Peripheral and visceral vasoconstriction
Dopamine[a]	↑↑	↑	↑↑↑	↑	↑↑↑	Arrhythmias
Norepinephrine	↓	↑↑↑	↑/↓	↑↑↑	↓↓↓	Arrhythmias
Epinephrine	↑↑	↑	↑↑	↓/↑	↓↓	HTN, arrhythmias, cardiac ischemia
Isoproterenol	↑↑↑	↓	↑↑↑	↓↓	↓/↑	Arrhythmias
Dobutamine	↑	↑	↑↑↑	↓	↑	Tachycardia, arrhythmias
Milrinone	0	↓	↑↑	↓↓↓	↓	Arrhythmias, hypotension
Levosimendan	0	↓	↑↑	↓↓↓	↓	Tachycardia, hypotension

HR, heart rate; MAP, mean arterial pressure; CO, cardiac output; SVR, systemic vascular resistance; 0, zero receptor affinity; ↓↓↓ through ↑↑↑, decrease through increase in effect; HTN, hypertension.
[a]Effects of dopamine vary with dose, from predominantly DA agonism at low doses to predominantly α agonism at high doses.

cerebral vascular beds leading to vasodilatation and increased blood flow. At intermediate doses, dopamine increasingly stimulates β_1-adrenergic receptors producing positive inotropic and chronotropic effects. At high doses, α_1-adrenergic effects predominate causing an increase in systemic vascular resistance. While dopamine is frequently chosen as a first-line agent for shock because of its potentially beneficial effects on the renal circulation and cardiac contractility and its ability to be administered peripherally, its predictable chronotropic and arrhythmogenic effects limit its use in many patients. Furthermore, dopamine has not been shown in randomized clinical trials to confer any clinically significant renal protection in patients at risk for renal failure.

b. **Norepinephrine** is an endogenous catecholamine with both α- and β-adrenergic activity. Norepinephrine's potent vasoconstrictive and inotropic effects frequently make it the drug of choice to treat hemodynamically unstable patients who require the support of both vascular tone and myocardial contractility. Typical examples are patients in septic shock who have preexistent or acute myocardial dysfunction. Compared to epinephrine, norepinephrine lacks β_2 activity.

c. **Epinephrine** is the primary endogenous catecholamine produced by the adrenal medulla. As mentioned earlier, epinephrine demonstrates potent α as well as β_1 and β_2 effects, which together act to increase heart rate and cardiac contractility. It is a mainstay of cardiopulmonary resuscitation (**Chapter 34**). Its effect on BP is due to positive inotropic and chronotropic effects and to vasoconstriction in vascular beds, especially the skin, mucosae, and kidney. Its strong β_2 effect promotes bronchodilation and blocks mast cell degranulation, making it the drug of choice for **anaphylaxis**.

2. **Synthetic**

a. **Isoproterenol** is a pure β-adrenergic agonist whose β_1 effects increase heart rate, contractility, and cardiac output. Because of its β_2 activation, both diastolic and mean arterial pressures may fall slightly. The combination of increased cardiac work and decreased diastolic pressures may compromise coronary perfusion and lead to myocardial ischemia, particularly in patients with preexisting coronary artery disease. Despite these limitations, isoproterenol may be useful in cases of cardiogenic shock in heart transplant recipients, where the donor organ is denervated and will respond appropriately only to direct-acting sympathomimetic agents.

b. **Dobutamine** is a second synthetic catecholamine with predominantly β activity. With its high affinity for β_1 receptors, dobutamine is a potent inotrope with more moderate chronotropic effects. The β_2 effects of dobutamine produce a modest decrease in systemic vascular resistance. Taken together, dobutamine's potent inotropic and slight vasodilatory effects make it a choice agent for patients with cardiogenic shock with depressed left ventricular function, elevated filling pressures, and increased systemic vascular resistance.

c. **Dopexamine** is a synthetic derivative of dopamine with marked β_2 activity and modest dopaminergic agonism, but little β_1 and no significant α-adrenergic effects. While dopexamine's decreased β_1 effect provides for a lower arrhythmogenic potential than dopamine, in practice the use of higher doses of the agent is limited by the development of tachycardia. Dopexamine is not approved for clinical use in the United States, and its use in Europe is somewhat hindered by its high cost.

C. **Phosphodiesterase-III (PDE-III) inhibitors. Amrinone** and **milrinone** exert their hemodynamic effects through the inhibition of PDE-III, an enzyme especially rich in vascular smooth muscle and cardiac tissues, where it increases cAMP levels, with consequent increases in chronotropy and inotropy. Amrinone has been largely replaced by milrinone due to its shorter duration of action, easier titratability, and the propensity for amrinone to produce clinically significant thrombocytopenia. Milrinone is indicated for IV administration in patients with acute heart failure and may be of some benefit to patients with right heart failure secondary to elevated PA pressures. Milrinone is administered as a load of 50 μg/kg followed by a continuous infusion of 0.25 to 1.0 μg/kg/min. Its elimination half-life is 30 to 60 minutes. Hypotension and tachycardia are the main side effects that limit its use.

D. **Calcium sensitizers.** The calcium sensitizer **levosimendan** stabilizes the conformational change in troponin C as it binds to calcium, thus facilitating myocardial cross-bridging and augmenting contractility. Given its ability to increase cardiac output while lowering central filling pressures, levosimendan has been approved in Europe for treatment with acute heart failure, but is not available in the United States.

IV. **Hypertension.** As was the case with shock, hypertensive crises may also compromise blood flow and the delivery of oxygen to tissues, complicating the care of patients and necessitating their treatment in a higher acuity critical care setting. According to the seventh report of the Joint National Committee on Prevention, Detection, Evaluation, and Treatment of High Blood Pressure, patients with blood **pressures higher than 180/120 mm Hg** and with evidence of acute or progressive end-organ damage are classified as having a **"hypertensive emergency"** and require immediate blood pressure reduction, albeit not necessarily to normal ranges, to limit target-organ damage.

A. The **clinical presentation** of hypertensive emergencies largely reflects the macro- and microvascular consequences of compromised tissue perfusion and oxygenation.

1. **Neurologic:** Encephalopathy with the symptoms and signs of increased intracranial pressure secondary to cerebral hyperperfusion, including headache, nausea, vomiting, visual disturbances, papilledema, altered mental status, confusion, obtundation, localized or generalized seizure activity, stroke.

2. **Cardiovascular:** Angina, acute coronary syndrome with electrocardiographic and enzymatic evidence of ischemia and/or AMI, acute aortic dissection.

3. **Respiratory:** Dyspnea, acute pulmonary edema, respiratory failure.

4. **Renal:** Oliguria, acute renal failure.

5. **Obstetric:** Severe pre-eclampsia, HELLP (**h**emolysis, **e**levated **l**iver enzymes and **l**ow **p**latelets) syndrome, eclampsia.

6. **Hematologic:** Hemolytic anemia, coagulopathy.

B. **Management. The goal of therapy** is to limit end-organ damage and restore the balance between supply and demand of tissue oxygen. In the case of hypertensive emergencies not complicated by recent ischemic cerebrovascular accident or acute aortic dissection, a general goal is to reduce blood pressure by not more than 25% within an hour and then to 160/100 to 110 mm Hg within the succeeding 2 to 6 hours, provided the patient remains clinically stable. If these changes are well-tolerated, further reduction toward a normal blood pressure can be made over the course of the next 24 to 48 hours. Too rapid a reduction in blood pressure may cause organ blood flow to become pressure dependent and precipitate cerebral, coronary, or renal ischemia.

1. **Acute ischemic stroke.** In patients who have suffered an acute ischemic stroke, higher pressures may be tolerated in an attempt to improve perfusion to metabolically compromised tissues. For patients not eligible for thrombolytic therapy (see **Chapter 31**) and lacking evidence of other end-organ involvement, the American Stroke Association recommends pharmacologic intervention for systolic pressures >220 mm Hg and/or diastolic pressures >140 mm Hg, aiming for a 10% to 15% reduction in blood pressure. Patients eligible for thrombolytic therapy require intervention for systolic pressures >185 mm Hg and diastolic pressures >110 mm Hg.

2. **Acute aortic dissection.** For patients with acute aortic dissections, various consensus guidelines published in 2001 recommend achieving a systolic blood pressure between 100 and 120 mm Hg, provided that symptoms and signs of neurological and/or renal compromise do not develop. In general, the goals of pharmacologic intervention are to reduce the force of left ventricular contraction and to decrease the rate of rise of the aortic pulse pressure wave (i.e., the "dP/dT") while maintaining the blood pressure as low as possible without compromising organ function. If the strength of left ventricular contraction can be reduced and the rate of rise of arterial pressure as function of time mitigated, the risk of dissection extension and rupture may be minimized.

C. **Pharmacologic therapies**
  1. **Vasodilators**
      a. **Sodium nitroprusside** is a potent arterial and (to a less extent) venous vasodilator. The rapid onset and short duration of action make it ideal for continuous infusion. **Central administration** is preferred. The normal dose range is 20 to 200 μg/min. Because sodium nitroprusside is photodegradable, protection with foil wrapping is necessary. **Adverse effects** include **cyanide toxicity**—free cyanide ions (CN^-) bind to cytochrome oxidase and uncouple oxidative metabolism, causing tissue hypoxia. At low infusion rates, cyanide can be converted to thiocyanate (by thiosulfate and rhodanase), which is less toxic than CN^-. The risk of cyanide and thiocyanate toxicity is dose dependent and increases with renal impairment. **Signs of cyanide toxicity** include tachyphylaxis, increased mixed venous Po_2, and metabolic acidosis. Pharmacologic treatment depends on facilitating cyanide metabolism through two nontoxic pathways by providing **sodium nitrite** to increase production of methemoglobin or **sodium thiosulfate** to provide additional sulfur donors. In addition, **hydroxocobalamin** may be given, which combines with cyanide to form cyanocobalamin (vitamin B_{12}), which is excreted in the kidneys. Other potentially adverse effects of nitroprusside infusion include increased intracranial pressure with cerebral vasodilatation, intracoronary steal with coronary vasodilatation, and impairment of hypoxic pulmonary vasoconstriction. **Rebound hypertension** may occur when SNP is abruptly discontinued.
      b. **Nitroglycerine** is a venous and (to a lesser extent) arterial vasodilator. By dilating venous capacitance vessels, nitroglycerine reduces preload and offloads the heart, decreasing ventricular end-diastolic

pressure, myocardial work, and myocardial oxygen demand. At the same time, nitroglycerine dilates large coronary vessels and relieves coronary artery vasospasm, promotes the redistribution of coronary blood flow to ischemic regions, and decreases platelet aggregation, all of which serve to improve myocardial oxygen supply. Nitroglycerine's salutary effects on the balance between supply and demand of myocardial oxygen render it of particular use in hypertensive emergencies associated with acute coronary syndromes or acute cardiogenic pulmonary edema. **IV administration** of NTG is easy to titrate to effect, and is the preferred route for critically ill patients. Common rates of infusion range from 25 to 1,000 μg/min. Because NTG is absorbed by polyvinyl chloride IV tubing, its dose may decrease after 30 to 60 minutes, once the IV tubing is fully saturated. **Hypotension, reflex tachycardia,** and **headache** are common. Nitroglycerine administration may **worsen hypoxemia** during acute respiratory failure by increasing pulmonary blood flow to poorly ventilated areas of the lung, which can worsen ventilation–perfusion mismatch and shunt. **Tachyphylaxis** is common with continuous exposure to the drug.

c. **Nicardipine** is a second-generation dihydropyridine calcium channel blocker that causes vascular and coronary vasodilation through relaxation of vascular smooth muscle. The reduction in afterload and cardiac work accompanied by coronary vasodilatation and increased coronary blood flow make nicardipine useful in hypertensive crises associated with angina and coronary artery disease. The normal dose range is 5 to 15 mg/h. The development of reflex tachycardia may limit its benefit in some patients. A newer, third-generation dihydropyridine, **clevidipine,** has recently received FDA approval for treatment of perioperative hypertension. An ultra-short-acting and selective arteriolar vasodilator, clevidipine reduces afterload and increases cardiac output without causing reflex tachycardia. It is metabolized by erythrocyte esterases so that its clearance is not prolonged in cases of renal or hepatic dysfunction.

d. **Fenoldopam** is an arteriolar vasodilator acting primarily as a δ_1 dopamine receptor agonist. At low doses (up to 0.04 μg/min), it results in renal vasodilation and natriuresis without systemic hemodynamic effects. At higher doses, it is a potent antihypertensive. Its onset is within 5 minutes and its duration of action is 30 to 60 minutes. In addition to its antihypertensive effects, fenoldopam has been shown to improve creatinine clearance in severely hypertensive patients with and without impaired renal function. Its administration may lead to increased intraocular pressure and so should proceed with caution in patients with glaucoma.

e. **Hydralazine** is an arteriolar vasodilator with a not well-understood mechanism of action. Its delayed onset of action (5–15 minutes) makes it difficult to titrate in most hypertensive emergencies. It is often used on an as-needed basis (10–20 mg IV) as an additional means of controlling BP high points. High doses may be accompanied by immunologic reactions, including a lupuslike syndrome with arthralgias, myalgias, rashes, and fever.

2. **Adrenergic inhibitors**

a. **Labetalol** is a selective β_1- and nonselective α-antagonist with an **α- to β-blocking ratio of 1:7** following IV administration. With this receptor profile, labetalol reduces arterial pressure and systemic vascular resistance while largely maintaining heart rate, cardiac output, coronary and cerebral blood flow. Initial IV doses of 5 to 10 mg can be increased to 15 to 20 mg in 5-minute intervals and followed by a continuous infusion of 1 to 5 mg/min.

b. Esmolol is an ultrashort-acting β_1-selective antagonist with a rapid onset of action lending to its ease of titratability. As is the case with clevidipine, it contains an ester linkage that is rapidly hydrolyzed by erythrocyte esterases. In cases of hypertensive emergencies complicating and complicated by acute aortic dissection, esmolol is frequently the α-blocker of choice to combine with a vasodilator such as nitroprusside to achieve hemodynamic control.

Selected References

Annane D, Vignon P, Renault A, et al. Norepinephrine plus dobutamine versus epinephrine alone for management of septic shock: a randomised trial. *Lancet* 2007;370(9588):676–684.

Aronson S, Dyke CM, Stierer KA, et al. The ECLIPSE trials: comparative studies of clevidipine to nitroglycerin, sodium nitroprusside and nicardipine for acute hypertension treatment in cardiac surgery patients. *Anesth Analg* 2008;331(17):1105–1109.

Bickell WH, Wall MJ Jr, Pepe PE, et al. Immediate versus delayed fluid resuscitation for hypotensive patients with penetrating torso injuries. *N Engl J Med* 1994;331(17):1105–1109.

Chobanian AV, Bakris GL, Black HR, et al. Seventh report of the Joint National Committee on Prevention, Detection, Evaluation, and Treatment of High Blood Pressure. *Hypertension* 2003;42(6):1206–1252.

Dellinger RP, Levy MM, Carlet JM, et al. Surviving sepsis campaign: international guidelines for management of severe sepsis and septic shock: 2008. *Crit Care Med* 2008;36(1):296–327.

Dutton RP. Current concepts in hemorrhagic shock. *Anesthesiol Clin* 2007;25(1):23–34.

Lacroix J, Hébert PC, Hutchison JS, et al. Transfusion strategies for patients in pediatric intensive care units. *N Engl J Med* 2007;356(16):1609–1619.

Marik PE, Varon J. Hypertensive crises: challenges and management. *Chest* 2007;131(6):1949–1962.

Mebazaa A, Nieminen MS, Packer M, et al. Levosimendan vs dobutamine for patients with acute decompensated heart failure: the SURVIVE Randomized Trial. *JAMA* 2007;297(17):1883–1891.

Reynolds HR, Hochman JS. Cardiogenic shock: current concepts and improving outcomes. *Circulation* 2008;117(5):686–697.

Russell JA, Walley KR, Singer J, et al. Vasopressin versus norepinephrine infusion in patients with septic shock. *N Engl J Med* 2008;358(9):877–887.

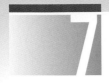

Sedation and Analgesia

Houman Amirfarzan, Ulrich Schmidt, and Luca Bigatello

The discomfort that patients experience in the ICU is multifactorial, and it includes a number of unpleasant sensations such as pain, dyspnea, anxiety, fear, and delirium. Surveys of ICU survivors acknowledge poor control of anxiety and pain. On the other hand, excessive use of sedatives and analgesics contributes to prolonged ventilation and ICU stay.

I. **Analgesia**
   A. **Assessment of pain.** Pain can be communicated directly or with the aid of visual or numeric scoring tools. In patients with altered levels of consciousness, pain assessment is complicated by the lack of subjective reporting, and requires experienced evaluation of indirect signs.
      1. **The visual analogue scale (VAS)** consists of a 10-cm line bounded by extremes of pain such as "no pain" and "pain that could not be more severe" and represents a continuum on which patients place their current pain level. Although the VAS has been tested in many non-ICU populations and is regarded as the standard analgesic assessment tool, its validity in ICU patients has not been confirmed.
      2. The **numeric rating system** is an assessment tool similar to the VAS that also uses discrete numbers to quantify the intensity of pain. The rating scale (typically from 0 to 10) can be administered verbally or in writing and requires minimal motor coordination. It has been independently validated and it correlates well with the VAS in cardiac surgical patients. Hence, it may be preferable to the VAS in critically ill patients.
      3. **Face scales** (happy to frowning, **Fig. 7-1**) are immediate to understand and are used more frequently in the pediatric than in the adult ICU population.
   B. **Treatment of pain**
      1. **Nonpharmacological** approaches can lessen analgesic and sedative requirements. Proper positioning of patients and attention to sources of pain and irritation such as catheters and tubes can enhance patient comfort.
      2. **Regional analgesia**
         a. **Continuous epidural analgesia** is the most commonly used regional technique in the ICU. It provides superior pain relief in selected categories of ICU patients, such as those who are recovering from thoracotomies, upper laparotomies, or those who have sustained multiple rib fractures. In addition to the direct effect on pain, benefits of continuous epidural analgesia include facilitation of deep breathing and coughing, clearance of secretions, early ambulation, and resumption of bowel function. Despite these objective advantages, epidural analgesia has not consistently demonstrated a beneficial effect in outcomes such as the incidence of postoperative respiratory failure or the duration of ICU stay.

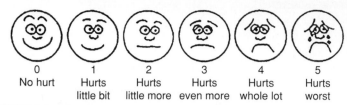

0	1	2	3	4	5
No hurt	Hurts little bit	Hurts little more	Hurts even more	Hurts whole lot	Hurts worst

FIGURE 7-1 Example of a face scale.

Patient-controlled epidural analgesia has been recently introduced in the ICU setting.

(1) A combination of a local anesthetic and an opioid continuously infused epidurally is the most effective regimen of analgesia in many postoperative patients. Common combinations include **bupivacaine** in a concentration of **0.1%** and **fentanyl (2–5 μg/mL)** or **hydromorphone (1–20 μg/mL)**. Fentanyl is often preferred in elderly patients, since it may have less central spread and might therefore cause less respiratory depression. For epidural analgesia in thoracic surgery patients, see **Chapter 40**.

(2) Common **complications** associated with epidural placement are the result of both the local anesthetic and the opioid medication administered.

   (a) **Hypotension** secondary to sympathetic blockade is common, and can be approached in different ways depending on the individual patient. Reasonable treatment options include the administration of **fluids**, the initiation of a low-dose vasopressor (e.g., **phenylephrine, 10–50 μg/min**), the decrease of the rate of infusion, or the **discontinuation of the local anesthetic** from the mix.

   (b) Lower extremities **weakness** is commonly due to inhibition of motor neurons. However, the occurrence of an **epidural abscess** and **hematoma,** although rare, must always be considered in the differential diagnosis of an ICU patient with new-onset weakness or paralysis of the lower extremities. A careful physical examination, a neurology consultation, and the performance of a spine CT or MRI scan must be promptly considered.

   (c) **Respiratory depression** secondary to the sytemic absorption of epidural opiates may occur and can be corrected by reducing or eliminating the narcotic in the epidural solution.

b. **A number of other regional analgesia techniques** can be performed in the ICU, including intercostal, femoral, paraspinal, and brachial plexus blocks. Many of these nerve blocks can be prolonged in time by inserting a catheter within the plexus sheath allowing continuous delivery of analgesia. In reality, very few of these techniques are implemented on a regular basis in the ICU, because of obstacles such as coagulopathy, systemic infection, and because patients who stay in the ICU for prolonged periods of time beyond their operation are often intubated and receive systemic sedation/analgesia. For peripheral block techniques, see *Clinical Anesthesia Procedures of the Massachusetts General Hospital*, 7th Edition, Chapter 17.

    c. **Anticoagulation and epidural catheters.** Prophylaxis for deep vein thrombosis and therapeutic anticoagulation impact the placement and removal of epidural catheters. It is generally accepted that epidural catheters can be safely placed and removed in patients receiving prophylactic doses of subcutaneous heparin and in patients with a platelet count of $\geq 100,000/mm^3$ of functioning platelets. More controversial situations include the administration of aspirin 325 mg/d, and the presence of platelet counts somewhat lower than 100,000. When low-molecular-weight heparin is used for prophylaxis (see **Chapter 26**), catheters should not be manipulated within at least 12 hours of administration. The IIb/IIIa platelet inhibitors have long half-lives that necessitate epidural removal prior to starting these drugs in the postoperative period. Guidelines from the American Association of Regional Anesthesia are periodically updated on the Web site *http://www. asra.com/consensus-statements/2.html*.

3. Systemic treatment of pain

    a. **Opioids** are the most effective analgesics for use in the ICU. Opioids also have well-known side effects of high relevance to the ICU population, including ventilatory depression, bradycardia and hypotension, nausea, constipation, urinary retention, pruritus, tachyphylaxis, and physical addiction. Both analgesia and the side effects herein listed are largely mediated through the activation of μ-receptors. Comparative trials of opiates are lacking in ICU patients, and specific agents are chosen based on pharmacological profile as well as local practice. **Continuous infusions** can provide a constant level of analgesia, but can also result in higher cumulative doses administered and consequent overnarcotization. **Patient-controlled analgesia** provides excellent analgesia, reduces opioid consumption and complications compared to continuous infusions, but needs an awake and cooperative patient to be effective. Individual opioids commonly used in the ICU include: (see **Table 7-1** and **Appendix**)

TABLE 7-1	Intravenous Opioids Commonly Used in the ICU				
	Single Dose (mg)	Infusion Rate (mg/h)	Onset (min)	Duration of Effect of One Dose	Comments
Remifentanil	0.025–0.25	0.025–0.25	2	10 min	Bradycardia, tachyphylaxis
Fentanyl	0.025–0.25	0.025–0.25	5	0.5–2 hr	Prolonged infusion increases duration
Morphine	1–10	1–50	5	2–4 hr	Active metabolites with renal insufficiency
Hydromorphone	0.25–2	0.25–5	10	4–6 hr	Predictable duration in renal insufficiency

(1) **Morphine** has an onset of 5 minutes and a peak effect between 10 and 40 minutes after IV administration, with a variable duration of action of 2 to 5 hours. When administered as a bolus injection, morphine induces the release of histamine, which increases the likelihood of hypotension. An active metabolite, morphine-6-glucuronide is excreted in the urine and may accumulate in renal insufficiency.

(2) **Hydromorphone** is five- to sevenfold more potent than morphine, with a peak onset time of 10 to 20 minutes and a duration of action of 4 to 6 hours. Hydromorphone does not significantly accumulate in fat tissues and does not have active metabolites. Therefore, it is well suited for continuous infusions even in patients with moderate renal insufficiency.

(3) **Fentanyl** is approximately 100-fold more potent than morphine and has an almost immediate onset of action and an average duration of 30 to 60 minutes. During prolonged infusions, its duration of action may be prolonged due to its high lipid solubility.

(4) **Meperidine** is rarely used in the ICU other than for the treatment of shivering. Meperidine tends to cause tachycardia and has an active metabolite, normeperidine, which accumulates with renal insufficiency and lowers the seizure threshold.

(5) **Methadone** is approximately equipotent to morphine when administered parenterally and one-half as potent when given orally. It has a duration of 15 to 40 hours, although it often seems to wear off earlier in ICU patients. Methadone is used primarily in patients who are chronic users of intravenous (IV) opioids.

(6) **Remifentanil** is an extremely short-acting opioid, suitable to provide analgesia for procedures such as dressing changes and bronchoscopies. A rapidly occurring tolerance and a high cost limit its use for prolonged infusion.

b. **Acetaminophen** is an analgesic and an antipyretic that can provide relief from mild to moderate pain, particularly as an adjunct to opioids. Acetaminophen should be used carefully in patients with hepatic dysfunction. **Acetaminophen with oxycodone or codeine** is an oral analgesic that is useful when parenteral narcotics are no longer needed. As with parenteral opioids, **respiratory depression** and **sedation**, especially in the elderly, is possible. The maximum doses of acetaminophen should not exceed 4 g/d.

c. **Nonsteroidal anti-inflammatory drugs (NSAIDs)** provide effective analgesia through nonselective inhibition of cyclooxygenase.

(1) **Ketorolac** is the most potent parenteral NSAID currently available. The dose of ketorolac is **15 to 30 mg every 6 to 8 hours**. The analgesic effect of 30 mg is similar to 10 mg of morphine. The use of ketorolac is associated with an increased risk of gastrointestinal bleeding, renal failure, and platelet dysfunction. Elderly patients and those with a tenuous volume status are particularly susceptible to its renal toxicity. To minimize adverse effects, ketorolac should be given for 3 days or less.

(2) **Ibuprofen** is the most commonly used enteral NSAID in the United States. Although effective, it seems less potent than ketorolac. The analgesic dose is **200 to 600 mg every 6 to 8 hours**. Ibuprofen has a similar toxicologic profile as ketorolac.

(3) **Diclofenac** is commonly used in Europe. In the United States, it is contraindicated by the Food and Drug Administration (FDA)

in the postoperative setting of coronary artery bypass because of the increased risk of cardiovascular thrombotic events. Its analgesic, anti-inflammatory, and side-effects profile is similar to ibuprofen. The parenteral formulation is not available in the United States.

    (4) Naproxen is in all respects (efficacy and toxicity) similar to diclofenac.

  d. Anticonvulsants and tricyclic antidepressants may be particularly helpful in treating neuropathic pain. In the ICU setting, the most common drug used is **gabapentin,** a γ-aminobutyric acid (GABA)–receptor agonist with unremarkable antiseizure properties but a potent modulator of neuropathic pain. Its main side effects are sedation and dizziness. It is usually started at relatively low doses, **100 mg 3 times a day**, and increased as needed every 2 to 3 days to **300 mg** per dose or even more, watching for excessive sedation.

  e. **Ketamine** is a potent analgesic and an anesthetic structurally related to phencyclidine. In the doses used for analgesia in the ICU (**0.25–1 mg/ kg IV boluses, or 0.25–1 mg/kg/h in continuous infusion**) ketamine preserves pharyngeal–laryngeal reflexes and ventilatory drive, and does not significantly affect cardiovascular function. Although known to produce hallucinations and nightmares, it is unclear whether this occurs at low doses, and it is difficult to sort it out in ICU patients, where delirium and subsequent nightmares are frequent. Ketamine can be an effective analgesic for procedures such as debridement and dressing changes, and can also be used as an opioid-sparing analgesic adjunct.

  f. **Parenteral lidocaine** in doses of **1.0 to 1.5 mg/kg/h after a 1.0 to 1.5 mg/kg bolus** can provide effective analgesia and reduce the need for opioids. Sedation, myocardial depression, arrhythmia, and seizures are potential but rare side effects. The efficacy of parenteral lidocaine is variable, and it has not been documented in the ICU in controlled studies.

II. **Sedation.** Pharmacological sedation of ICU patients may be indicated both for their comfort and to facilitate interventions such as mechanical ventilation or invasive procedures. However, excessive sedation is associated with an increased duration of mechanical ventilation, ICU stay, and morbidity. Hence, clinicians need to strike the right balance between what is necessary and what may eventually be counterproductive. Protocols aimed to provide targeted sedation, particularly those including **daily interruption of all sedative medications,** have been successful in decreasing the amount of sedatives administered and may improve outcomes.

  A. **Assessment of sedation.** Numerous scales exist to aid clinicians to objectively describe the level of sedation, both as it is assessed in real time and as it is targeted. In many ICUs, a sedation scale is displayed on the patient's flow sheet, and objective goals of sedation are charted for the current and upcoming shifts.

  1. **The Ramsay Sedation Scale** scores six levels of agitation, from anxious and restless to unarousable. The main limitation of this scale is that the individual categories are not all mutually exclusive.

  2. The **Richmond Agitation–Sedation Scale** (**RASS, Fig. 7-2**) is commonly used in the United States. In the RASS, 10 individual categories are equally distributed above (agitation) and below (sedation) a 0 point of normal response. The RASS is also part of the Confusion Assessment

+4	Combative, violent, of immediate danger to himself and staff
+3	Very agitated, aggressive, pulls or removes tubes or catheters
+2	Agitated frequent non-purposeful movement, dyssynchronous with the ventilator
+1	Restless, anxious but not aggressive
0	Alert and calm
-1	Drowsy, not fully alert, but has sustained eye-opening/eye contact to *voice* (**>10s**)
-2	Light sedation- briefly awakens with eye contact to *voice* (**<10 s**)
-3	Moderate sedation- moves or opens eyes to *voice* (**but no eye contact**)
-4	Deep sedation. No response to voice. Movement or eye opening to *physical* stimulation
-5	Unarousable. No response to *voice or physical* stimulation

FIGURE 7-2 The Richmond Agitation and Sedation Scale (RASS).

Method-ICU (CAM-ICU), an instrument designed to diagnose delirium in ICU patients (see **Section III.C.1**).

3. Objective monitoring of sedation via some form of **processing of the electroencephalogram (EEG)** is commonly used during general anesthesia, and occasionally in the ICU. None of these devices has been properly validated in ICU patients, where the levels of sedation and the drugs administered are different than during general anesthesia, where these monitors have been validated. Nevertheless, their use has been advocated by some in patients who are pharmacologically paralyzed and hence more difficult to monitor from a standpoint of comfort and possible awareness (see **Section IV.B**).

B. **Treatment: sedative, anxiolytic, and hypnotic** medications (**Table 7-2**; see also Appendix)

1. **Benzodiazepines** are **potent anxiolytic** and **sedative** medications. They act on GABA receptors and have a dose-dependent pharmacodynamic and toxicological profile. At low doses, their main effect is anxiolysis and mild sedation; at increasing doses, benzodiazepines induce deeper sedation, as well as respiratory depression and hypotension. **Tachyphylaxis** is common,

TABLE 7-2   Sedative/Hypnotic Medications Commonly Used in the ICU

	Bolus Dose	Infusion Rate	Onset Time	Duration	Comments
Midazolam	1–2 mg	0.5–5 mg/h	0.5–2 min	1–3 hr	Rapid tachyphylaxis
Lorazepam	0.25–2 mg	0.25–3 mg/h	2–5 min	4–10 hr	Duration too long for effective infusions
Propofol	0.2–2 mg/kg	0.5–3 mg/kg/h	Few seconds	10–20 min	Hypotension
Dexmedetomidine	1 μg/kg	0.2–0.7μg/kg/h	15 min	2 hr	Minimal ventilatory depression, predictable hypotension, bradycardia

and **withdrawal** symptoms can occur when interrupting both chronic outpatient intake and acute, prolonged administration in the ICU. Benzodiazepines can cause **paradoxical agitation** and confusion, particularly in the elderly, and have been repeatedly associated with the development of delirium in the ICU. Benzodiazepines are also anticonvulsants (**Chapter 31**) and are the mainstay of the treatment of **alcohol withdrawal** (**Chapter 33**). Benzodiazepines commonly used in the ICU include (also see **Appendix**)

a. **Midazolam.** This is currently the shortest-acting drug in its class, which makes it suitable for continuous infusion. However, accumulation does occur during prolonged infusions, particularly in patients with increased fat stores (morbid obesity). Midazolam also seems to develop **tachyphylaxis** more rapidly than other benzodiazepines.

b. **Lorazepam** is possibly the most commonly used sedative in the ICU setting. When administered IV, its onset is rapid, and its duration of action varies widely in critically ill patients, ranging from a few hours to as long as 8 to 12 hours. Its duration of action after a bolus injection is slightly longer than midazolam and, like all benzodiazepines, is affected mostly by liver function, as it does not have active metabolites. Characteristics that have made lorazepam very popular in the ICU include its fairly predictable kinetics, side-effects profile, and low cost. However, it has also been reproducibly associated with the onset of delirium, and its unfavorable comparison with shorter-acting sedatives such as propofol and dexmedetomidine may decrease its overall use.

c. **Diazepam** is the oldest of the IV benzodiazepines. Its long half-life and presence of active metabolites have made it essentially expendable in the ICU.

2. **Propofol** is a **potent sedative-hypnotic** drug. After a single IV dose of 0.5 to 2.0 mg/kg, its onset of action is nearly immediate, and its effect is brief (context sensitive half life is 10–15 minutes) because of rapid central nervous system penetration and subsequent redistribution. These pharmacokinetic characteristics make it an ideal drug for continuous infusions. Upon discontinuation of an infusion, patients become arousable very rapidly, allowing reliable examination and rapid reinstitution of sedation if needed. Like benzodiazepines, propofol is a GABA-receptor agonist, but its relationship with the onset of delirium is unknown. Like benzodiazepines, propofol is a potent **amnestic** and has no analgesic effect. Long-term infusion propofol results in accumulation within lipid stores and prolongation of its duration of action, although not as significantly as with midazolam. Propofol requires a **dedicated IV line** when administered as a continuous infusion because of the potential for drug incompatibility. Propofol causes significant, dose-dependent respiratory depression and its use in the surgical ICU at the Massachusetts General Hospital is limited to intubated patients. **Hypotension** is also common with propofol, generally due to vasodilation, and, in high doses and unstable patients, due to myocardial depression as well. Other adverse effects of propofol include

a. **Bacterial contamination** can occur due to their high-concentration (10%) lipid emulsion. To avoid bacterial contamination, our pharmacy recommends discarding ampules and vials after single use, discarding admixed containers and tubing every 6 hours, and discarding infusions directly from bottles every 12 hours.

b. **Hypertriglyceridemia** and occasionally **elevation of pancreatic enzymes** can also occur due to the lipid emulsion. We recommend checking triglycerides, amylase, and lipase serum levels periodically during prolonged propofol administration. The amount of propofol administered over 24 hours needs to be kept in account in ordering total parenteral nutrition solutions (see **Chapter 11**).

c. **Propofol infusion syndrome (PRIS)** is a rare but possibly fatal complication of prolonged propofol infusion, characterized by myocardial depression and shock, profound metabolic acidosis, rhabdomyolysis, and renal failure. PRIS is seen only at very high doses of propofol—4 to 5 mg/kg/h for at least 48 to 72 hours, and its etiology is unknown. The highest-risk group among critically ill patients is children, particularly those with traumatic brain injury, receiving high doses not only of propofol, but also of catecholamines and/or corticosteroids. However, PRIS has been reported in adults as well. Given the clear relationship with the administration of very high doses, we recommend to avoid reaching 4 mg/kg/h by using multimodal sedation regimens that may include opioids, benzodiazepines, antipsychotics, or α_2-receptors agonists, depending on the need of each individual patient.

3. **α_2-Receptors agonists** have specific sedative and hemodynamic effects.

a. **Clonidine** is the longest used α_2-agonist. Although primarily prescribed as an antihypertensive, clonidine has been used as an adjunct to general and regional anesthesia, as well as a sedative in the ICU. Hemodynamically, clonidine consistently decreases arterial blood pressure and heart rate. Its most common use in the ICU is as an adjunct to benzodiazepines or opioids to ameliorate withdrawal syndromes from alcohol or opioids. It is available for parenteral, transdermal, and intravenous use. If abruptly discontinued, rebound hypertension and tachycardia may develop.

b. **Dexmedetomidine** is a selective α_2-receptor agonist with more predictable sedative effects than clonidine and a short duration of action, which make it suitable for continuous infusion. Its use is currently limited by the FDA to a low dose (**0.2–0.7 µg/kg/h**) for a short period of time, for the indication of providing sedation to intubated patients. Accordingly, its most common indication is to provide short-term sedation to patients who are otherwise ready to be extubated but cannot safely be weaned off other sedative-hypnotics. In recent controlled trials where higher doses were allowed, dexmedetomidine was safe and at least as effective as lorazepam and midazolam in providing targeted sedation, and was associated with a lower incidence of delirium and fewer days on the ventilator and in the ICU. What limits the dose of dexmedetomidine is the predictable onset of **hypotension** and **bradycardia**. The latter seems to have an incidence as high as 40%, but rarely (less than 5%) requires treatment.

C. **Daily interruption of all sedative medications** may decrease time on the ventilator, the need for additional neurological workup (e.g., head CT scans), and ICU stay. The combination of **daily interruption of sedation** and performance of a **spontaneous breathing trial** (see **Chapter 23**) may add further outcome benefit. These observations have markedly influenced the way sedation is delivered in the ICU. It is now clear that sedation per se should not be a goal but a treatment of a specific need, such as to facilitate mechanical ventilation, relieve dangerous agitation, and so on. Whether the actual interruption of sedation is necessary, is a source of debate. In the surgical ICU at the Massachusetts General Hospital, we do not routinely interrupt all sedation daily, but we set a **daily RASS target** aimed at providing the lowest possible level of sedation compatible with patient comfort and physiological needs.

III. **Cognitive and behavioral changes** commonly seen in ICU patients include anxiety, fear, agitation, confusion, restlessness, and delirium. These changes occur often together, and can be difficult to precisely diagnose and quantify.
   A. **Anxiety** and fear are common, given that very few patients know in advance what to expect when they are admitted to an ICU. Behavioral interventions that include reassurance and explanation, often repetitive over time, can be helpful. Coaching of patients with the inclusion of family members can also be of help. The pharmacologic mainstay of treatment of anxiety is the administration of **benzodiazepines**.
   B. **Agitation, restlessness,** and **confusion** are common among ICU patients. Like all changes in mental status, **possible organic etiologies** must always be considered, such as hypoxemia and withdrawal syndromes. However, in most cases no specific etiology is found. Interventions that may improve these complex behaviors include the restoration of a day/night cycle with sufficient sleep at night, the reduction of noise, and possibly the administration of sedatives and antipsychotics (see below for delirium). In most cases, these symptoms subside as the patient's general condition improves.
   C. **Delirium** is a combination of several of the symptoms described earlier. It is defined as an **acute and fluctuating change in mental status** characterized by an impairment of cognition, attention, and behavior. Most commonly, delirium is associated with psychomotor agitation (**hyperactive** delirium), during which the patient can be of danger to the self. Less frequently, delirium may be of the quiet (or **hypoactive**) variety, which is harder to diagnose and may be undertreated. Delirium is prevalent among surgical and medical ICU patients, particularly in the elderly and mechanically ventilated patients. It is associated with a prolonged duration of ventilatory support, increased ICU stay, and increased morbidity. **Delirium tremens** is specifically related to withdrawal from alcohol, and is described in **Chapter 33**.
      1. **Assessment of delirium** is a relatively simple matter when delirium is associated with severe psychomotor agitation (hyperactive delirium). Yet, even in this case, not all clinicians assess it and treat it in a consistent way. For this reason, and to allow diagnosing less obvious forms of delirium (hypoactive delirium), objective diagnostic instruments of delirium have been designed. Two scales have been extensively validated: the Confusion Assessment Method for the ICU (**CAM-ICU**) and the Intensive Care Delirium Screening Checklist (**ICDSC**). The CAM-ICU (**Fig. 7-3**) is more common in the United States, while the ICDSC is used preferentially in Canada.
      2. **Treatment of delirium. Behavioral interventions** of the type described in **Sections III.A** and **B** can be of help to delirious patients. Correcting metabolic abnormalities, treating pain, and favoring sleep at night can also facilitate managing delirious patients. However, pharmacologic control is commonly needed. Although no specific medication has been demonstrated to be superior to another or even to no treatment, **antipsychotic agents** are the mainstay of treatment of delirium.
         a. **Haloperidol**, a butyrophenone antipsychotic, is the most common drug administered to treat delirium in ICU patients. Haloperidol is available IV and can be administered in a wide range of doses.

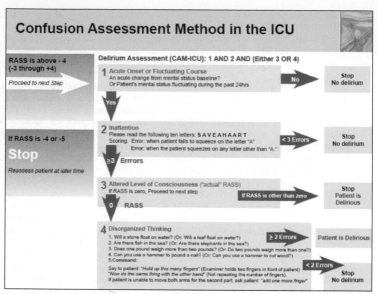

FIGURE 7-3 The Confusion Asessment Method-ICU (CAM-ICU) flow sheet, modified: Harvard CAM-ICU Flowsheet © 2007 by Houman Amirfarzan, MD All rights reserved.

However, a cautious approach is recommended, as the drug has a slow onset and long duration of action, and can accumulate. Particularly in elderly patients, we recommend to start from very low doses (**1–2 mg IV every 8 hours**) and use other interventions (ideally behavioral) while the drug starts taking effect. In younger and healthier patients, **2 to 5 mg IV** at shorter time intervals can be safely administered, but vigilance for side effects must always be used. In addition to age and severity of illness, the effect and duration of action of all antipsychotics is increased with liver insufficiency, as all these drugs undergo extensive hepatic metabolism. **Side effects** of haloperidol include

(1) **Sedation** is predictable and dose-dependent. Age and severity of illness can enhance it. Intubated patients allow more latitude in respect to this side effect, but excessive sedation may result in prolonged time on the ventilator and increase morbidity.

(2) **Extrapyramidal** movements, particularly tardive dyskinesia, occur at all doses, particularly, it seems, when haloperidol is administered orally. The reason for this observation is unclear.

(3) **Severe ventricular arrhythmia** and **sudden death** have been consistently documented with haloperidol. The classical arrhythmia is **torsades de pointes ventricular tachycardia** (**Chapter 28**). This is generally preceded by a prolongation of the **QT interval** on the electrocardiogram (ECG, **Fig. 7-4**). Hence, daily monitoring of the ECG is recommended in all ICU patients who are on more than a minimal or increasing dose of haloperidol. The QT interval, corrected for the length of the RR interval, is generally automatically

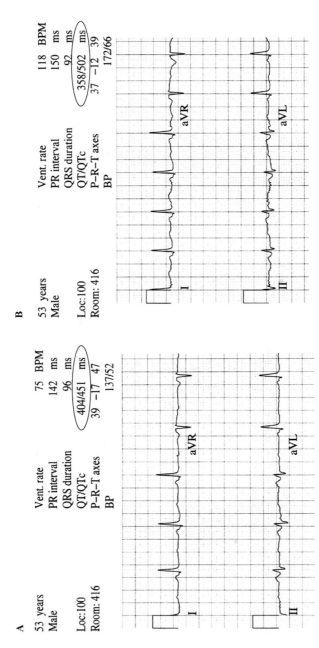

A

53 years		
Male		
	Vent. rate	75 BPM
	PR interval	142 ms
	QRS duration	96 ms
	QT/QTc	404/451 ms
	P–R–T axes	39 –17 47
Loc:100		
Room: 416	BP	137/52

I

aVR

II

aVL

B

53 years		
Male		
	Vent. rate	118 BPM
	PR interval	150 ms
	QRS duration	92 ms
	QT/QTc	358/502 ms
	P–R–T axes	37 –12 39
Loc:100		
Room: 416	BP	172/66

I

aVR

II

aVL

FIGURE 7-4 Prolongation of the QT interval on the ECG. The two ECGs were taken on the same patient, at approximately 24 hours interval. On panel A, the corrected QT interval is within normal limits (451 ms) and on panel B it is abnormally prolonged (502 ms). Note that the absolute duration of the QT interval is actually shorter on panel B, due to the significantly faster heart rate. Also note the consistency of the QRS complex duration between the two traces. ECG, electrocardiogram.

123

calculated by ECG monitoring algorithms. However, we encourage caution in confiding on the automated reading, particularly in the presence of arrhythmia and of prolongation of the QRS complex, such as a bundle branch block. A simple rule of thumb is that **the QT interval should not be longer than half of the RR interval.** The exact range of duration of normal QT interval is not known. Most use an upper limit of 490 to 500 ms (slightly lower in females) or an increase from baseline higher than 20%. When a significant increase of the QT interval occurs, haloperidol should be discontinued, and every effort made to prevent ventricular irritability (e.g., correct hypokalemia, hypomagnesemia, etc). In addition, a number of drugs commonly used in the ICU can increase the risk of QT prolongation, and should be avoided if possible when using haloperidol (e.g., amiodarone, methadone, quinolone antibiotics, etc—see **Chapter 19, Table 19-2**).

(4) **Neuroleptic malignant syndrome** is a rare complication of butyrophenones and other antipsychotics, described in **Chapter 32**.

b. **Atypical antipsychotics** are currently available in the United States orally or sublingually. Their efficacy in treating delirium, as well as safety profile, compared to haloperidol, has not been fully elucidated. Although a number of medications exist in this family, we will refer here only to **quetiapine** and **olanzapine**, which are the most commonly used atypical antipsychotics for this indication in the United States. Both drugs have a similar **toxicologic profile. Extrapyramidal movements** seem to be reduced in comparison to haloperidol. **Sedation** is marked, possibly more than with haloperidol. These drugs seem not to have a safer profile than haloperidol in regard to their most severe side effect—**ventricular arrhythmia** and **death**. Recent data suggest that, at least in the general population, atypical antipsychotics may have a higher incidence of sudden death than the traditional antipsychotics. Like typical antipsychotics, these drugs undergo extensive metabolism in the liver, and their dosage must be adjusted in patients with liver insufficiency.

(1) **Quetiapine** is available only orally, and is initiated at low doses, given its marked sedative effect and its tendency to cause hypotension; **12.5 to 25 mg two or three times a day** is a reasonable initial dose, and incrementally it can be increased to as high as 300 to 600 mg daily. These high doses, however, are seldom used in the ICU setting.

(2) **Olanzapine** is structurally related to quetiapine. It comes in an oral, an **orally absorbable**, and an intramuscular form. The orally dissolvable form has a fast onset of action. Similarly to quetiapine, we recommend to start at low doses, such as **2.5 to 5.0 mg every 12 hours**, and progressively increase, if needed, to a maximum of 20 to 30 mg daily.

IV. **Nouromuscular blockade (NMB,** see *Clinical Anesthesia Procedures of the Massachusetts General Hospital*, 7th Edition, Chapter 12, for a more comprehensive review)

A. **NMB** is currently used in less than 10% of ICU patients. Most common indications include

1. To facilitate **mechanical ventilation.**

a. **Severely hypoxemic patients** may benefit from NMB in two ways. *First*, NMB eliminates the patient's contribution to ventilation, which, in conditions of severe failure, may be ineffective and generate dys-synchrony with the ventilator. *Second*, it will decrease oxygen con-sumption, which, in selected patients such as those who have a high core temperature or are shivering, may contribute to the gen-esis of hypoxemia.

b. **Patients with acute lung injury/acute respiratory distress syndrome (Chapter 20)** may require heavy sedation and ultimately NMB to be able to receive lung-protective, low tidal volume ventilation. Whether the need to institute NMB may be a relative contraindica-tion to implement a strict lung-protective strategy is still a matter of debate.

2. **Endotracheal intubation** (see **Chapter 4**).

3. **Procedures/diagnostic studies** such as tracheostomy, percutaneous endoscopic gastrostomy, and an MRI scan may require NMB. It is unclear whether such time-limited use constitutes a risk factor for the development of polyneuropathy of critical illness (**Chapter 32**).

B. **Complications** of NMB include

1. **Awareness.** Monitoring the level of awareness during NMB is difficult because the typical signs of agitation and pain are lost, and clinicians must rely on autonomic signs of inappropriate sedation, which can be blocked by medications. **Processed EEG signal** monitors are frequently used to provide evidence that a patient is adequately sedated. Although the absence of muscular interference may increase the valid-ity of such technology, there is still no satisfactory validation of their performance.

2. **Prolonged weakness** (see **Chapter 32**) may result from the use of NMB and may increase hospital length of stay and morbidity.

3. **Delay in diagnoses.** The absence of elicited and spontaneous move-ments, appropriate response to stimuli, and so on pose a significant limitation to the effectiveness of the physical examination, particularly the neurological examination, and the abdominal examination when an acute process is suspected.

C. **Neuromuscular blocking agents** (see also **Appendix**)

1. **Succinylcholine** is a non-depolarizing NMB agent with the fastest onset of action of all that are currently available (less than 1 minute), and is primarily used to facilitate endotracheal intubation (see **Chapter 4**). Succinylcholine is **contraindicated in patients with denervation and crush injuries, burns,** and **immobility,** because of the risk of **hyperkalemia** and **death** secondary to the massive release of potassium from abnormal neuromuscular receptors that develop under these circumstances.

2. **Cisatracurium** is a curare derivative that is particularly useful in criti-cally ill patients because of its **dependable pharmacokinetics** due to its independence of both hepatic and renal metabolism. A useful **starting dose is 0.15 mg/kg,** followed by an infusion titrated to effect.

3. **Rocuronium** is a steroid derivative with a very fast onset of action (60–90 seconds) and basically the best alternative to succinylcholine when a rapid sequence intubation is planned (see **Chapter 4**). Other steroid-based NMB agents include **vecuronium** and **pancuronium.** Although very appealing from a cost-saving standpoint, neither drug should have a place for continuous infusions in modern critical care, because of their long half-life, that can be further and significantly pro-longed in the presence of renal and hepatic failure.

D. **Monitoring** the level of NMB is sensible, and may avoid overdosing and unnecessary prolongation of the block. The **"train of four"** is the most commonly employed method to monitor the extent of NMB. In the train of four, a known stimulation (60–70 mA) is repeated four times at a standard interval transcutaneously at the ulnar nerve, and its response is visually quantified at the *adductor pollicis* muscle. Ample anesthesia literature supports the observation that the presence of at least one weak "twitch" at the *adductor pollicis* is compatible with a less than complete receptor occupancy by the relaxant, and the consequent ability to reverse the block pharmacologically. However, unfamiliarity with the technique, improper placement of the electrodes, cold extremities, neuropathy, and edema will contribute to inaccurate assessments.

Selected References

Cabello B, Thille AW, Drouot X, et al. Sleep quality in mechanically ventilated patients: comparison of three ventilatory modes. *Crit Care Med* 2008;36:1749–1755.

Ely EW, Shintani A, Truman B, et al. Delirium as predictor of mortality in mechanically ventilated patients in the intensive care unit. *JAMA* 2004;291:1753–1762.

Girard TD, Kress JP, Fuchs BD, et al. Efficacy and safety of a paired sedation and ventilator weaning protocol for mechanically ventilated patients in intensive care (Awakening and Breathing Controlled trial): a randomised controlled trial. *Lancet* 2008;371:126–134.

Herroeder S, Pecher S, Schonherr ME, et al. Systemic lidocaine shortens length of hospital stay after colorectal surgery: a double-blinded, randomized, placebo-controlled trial. *Ann Surg* 2007;246:192–200.

Himmelseher S, Durieux ME. Ketamine for perioperative pain management. *Anesthesiology* 2005;102:211–220.

Kam PCA, Cardone D. Propofol infusion syndrome. *Anaesthesia* 2007;62:690–671.

Kress JP, Pohlman AS, O'Connor M, Hall JB. Daily interruption of sedative infusions in critically ill patients undergoing mechanical ventilation. *New Eng J Med* 2000;342:1471–1472.

Pandharipande PP, Pun BT, Herr DL, et al. Effect of sedation with dexmedetomidine vs lorazepam on acute brain dysfunction in mechanically ventilated patients: the MENDS randomized controlled trial. *JAMA* 2007;298:2644–2653.

Riker RR, Shehabi Y, Bokesh PM, et al. Dexmedetomidine vs. midazolam for sedation of critically ill patients. *JAMA* 2009;301:489–499.

Sessler CN, Gosnell MS, Grap MJ, et al. The Richmond Agitation-Sedation scale: validity and reliability in adult intensive care unit patients. *Am J Respir Crit Care Med* 2002;166: 1338–1344.

R. Phillip Dellinger MD, Mitchell M, Levy, MD, Jean M. Carlet, MD, et al. Surviving sepsis campaign: international guidelines for management of severe sepsis and septic shock: 2008. *Crit Care Med* 2008;36:296–327.

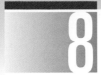

Fluids, Electrolytes, and Acid–Base Management

Cosmin Gauran and David Steele

Optimal management of fluids, electrolytes, and acid–base status in critically ill patients requires a general understanding of their normal composition and regulation. Disease processes, trauma, and surgery can all affect the manner by which the body controls its fluid balance and electrolytes.

I. **Fluid compartments.** There are multiple fluid compartments in the body, separated by semipermeable membranes and structures.
   A. **The total body water (TBW)** ranges from 50% to 70% of the body mass and is determined by lean body mass, gender, and age (**Table 8-1**). There is an inverse relationship between TBW and percentage body fat due to the low water content of adipose tissues.
   B. **Compartments of TBW**
      1. The **intracellular** compartment is approximately 66% of TBW (approximately 40% of body mass).
      2. The **extracellular** compartment is approximately 34% of TBW (approximately 20% of body mass), and can be further divided:
         a. The **intravascular** compartment is comprised of plasma, and is approximately 5% of total body mass.
         b. The **extravascular** compartment is comprised of lymph, interstitial fluid, bone fluid, fluids of the various body cavities, and mucosal/secretory fluids. The extravascular compartment represents approximately 15% of total body mass.
   C. **Ionic composition of the fluid compartments.** Various physiologic terms describe the concentrations of ions in a solution:
      1. **Molarity:** Moles of solute per liter of solution.
      2. **Molality:** Moles of solute per kilogram of solvent.
      3. **Osmolarity:** Osmoles per liter of solution. The number of osmoles is determined by multiplying the number of moles of solute by the number of freely dissociated particles from one molecule of solute. For example, 1 mole of NaCl will yield 2 osmoles (Osm) in solution.
      4. **Osmolality:** Osmoles per kilogram of solvent.
      5. **Electrical equivalence:** Moles of ionized substance multiplied by its valence. For example, **1 mole of calcium is equal to 2 equivalents in solution.** For a calcium solution to be electrically neutral, it has to combine with 2 moles of opposite charge, such as chloride.
      6. Electrolytes in physiology are generally described in terms of milliequivalents per liter (mEq/L). The fluids of each compartment are electrically neutral. Average concentrations of each electrolyte in various compartments are given in **Table 8-2.**
         a. Serum osmolality (S_{osm}) can be estimated using the equation

$$S_{osm} \text{ (mOsm/kg } H_2O) = (2 \times [\text{Na}] + ([\text{BUN}]/2.8) + ([\text{glucose}]/18))$$

         with blood urea nitrogen (BUN) and glucose concentration expressed in milligrams per deciliter and sodium concentration expressed in

TABLE 8-1	Total Body Water as a Percentage of Body Weight (%)	
	Male	**Female**
Thin	65	55
Average	60	50
Obese	55	45
Neonate	75–80	
First year	65–75	
Ages 1–10 y	60–65	
Ages 10 y to adult	50–60	

milliequivalent per liter. In general, this estimate is within 10% of measured osmolality.

b. In the setting of unequal distribution of nonpermeable proteins between compartments, the **Gibbs-Donnan effect** allows for unequal concentrations of small diffusible ions between the compartments.

D. Movement of water in the body

1. Water is generally readily permeable through cell membranes and moves freely throughout the different fluid compartments. Movement of water is largely determined by **osmotic pressure** and **hydrostatic pressure**. The osmotic pressure is dependent on the number of osmotically active molecules in the solution and is much greater than hydrostatic pressure. In normal states, all fluid compartments are essentially iso-osmolar. Water diffuses down an osmotic gradient to keep the extracellular and intracellular milieus iso-osmolar.

2. The movement of water between extracellular interstitial and intravascular compartments is described by **Starling's equation**:

$$Q_f = K_f[(P_c - P_i) - \sigma(\pi_c - \pi_i)]$$

where Q_f is the fluid flux across the capillary membrane, K_f is a constant, P_c and P_i are the hydrostatic pressures in the capillary and the interstitium, respectively, σ is the *reflection coefficient* (see later discussion), and π_c and π_i are the colloid osmotic pressures in the capillary and interstitium, respectively.

a. Large, negatively charged intravascular proteins to which vascular membranes are impermeable are responsible for the osmotic pressure gradient between intravascular and interstitial compartments. This component of osmotic pressure, known as the **oncotic pressure** or **colloid osmotic pressure,** contributes a small amount to the total osmotic pressure of the fluids. The positive ions that are associated with the negatively charged proteins also contribute to the osmotic pressure. **Albumin** is the predominant type of protein responsible for the oncotic pressure, accounting for approximately two-thirds of the total oncotic pressure. Cells do not contribute to the oncotic pressure.

b. The **reflection coefficient** σ describes the permeability of a substance through a specific capillary membrane. Its value ranges from 0 (completely permeable) to 1 (impermeable), and varies in different disease states; it is approximately 0.7 in healthy tissues.

c. Basic dynamics at the capillary. Fluids exit the capillary at the arteriolar end, where the hydrostatic pressure is greater than the oncotic

TABLE 8-2	Fluid Electrolyte Composition of Body Compartments		
	Plasma (mEq/L)	Interstitial (mEq/L H_2O)	Intracellular[a] (mEq/L H_2O)
Cations			
Na	142	145	10
K	4	4	159
Ca	5	5	<1
Mg	2	2	40
Anions			
Cl	104	117	3
HCO_3	24	27	7
Proteins	16	<0.1	45
Others	9	9	154

[a]Intracellular electrolytes are difficult to measure and most of the measurements are from myocytes, which might or might not be applicable to other cell types.

pressure. This increases the oncotic pressure of the plasma. As the plasma flows down the capillary, the hydrostatic pressure dissipates. Toward the venous end of the capillary, fluid is reabsorbed because the oncotic pressure is greater than the hydrostatic pressure. Perturbations in this balance can lead to increased interstitial fluid. **Edema** occurs when the rate of interstitial fluid accumulation is greater than the rate of removal of interstitial fluids by the lymphatic system.

II. **Fluid deficits and replacement therapy**
  A. **Fluid volume deficits** and appropriate fluid therapy are dependent on the source and type of fluid loss. Because all membranes are permeable to water, fluid deficits in one compartment will affect all other compartments. Fluid losses can be broadly classified based on the initial source of loss. Fluid losses also lead to electrolyte abnormalities.
    1. **Intracellular fluid (ICF) compartment** deficits arise from **free water loss**.
       a. **Sources of free water loss** include
          (1) **Insensible losses** through skin and respiratory tract.
          (2) **Renal losses** secondary to inability to recollect water, such as in neurogenic or nephrogenic diabetes insipidus (see **Section III.C**).
       b. With free water loss, both intracellular and extracellular volumes decrease in proportion to their volumes in the body; therefore, two-thirds of the loss will be intracellular. Similarly, **free water replacement** will be distributed in proportion to their volumes in the body, and only one-third of the administered free water will end up in the extracellular space.
       c. Therapy includes replacement of water with either **hypotonic saline** (5% dextrose in water with 0.45% sodium chloride solution) or **free water** (5% dextrose in water). Electrolytes (especially sodium) must be monitored with therapy.
    2. **Extracellular fluid (ECF) compartment** deficit
       a. In general, ECF losses are isotonic. Losses may occur in each compartment, and fluid losses from one compartment are rapidly reflected in others.

   b. Clinical manifestations include the following:
      (1) From 3% to 5%: Dry mucous membranes and oliguria.
      (2) From 6% to 10%: Tachycardia and orthostatic hypotension.
      (3) From 11% to 15%: Hypotension.
      (4) Greater than 20%: Anuria and circulatory collapse.
   c. Causes of ECF losses include **blood loss, vomiting, diarrhea,** and **distributional changes.**
      (1) Distributional change of ECF volume is due to the transudation of isotonic fluids from a functional interstitial fluid compartment to a nonfunctional compartment. This results in intravascular volume depletion. Examples include tissue injury from surgery or trauma ("third spacing"), burn injuries, ascites formation, fluid accumulation inside an obstructed bowel, and pleural effusions.
      (2) Replacement of ECF volume loss usually requires isotonic salt solutions. Volumes required to replace ECF deficits can vary considerably among patients based on the inciting event and comorbid processes.
 3. Intravascular fluid (plasma volume) deficit
   a. Intravascular volume deficits will lead to interstitial fluid depletion as the two compartments equilibrate.
   b. Manifestations include the following:
      (1) From 15% to 30% of intravascular volume: Sinus tachycardia while supine.
      (2) Greater than 30% loss of intravascular volume: Decreased arterial blood pressure, decreased central venous pressures.
B. Fluid replacement therapy (see also **Chapter 35**)
 1. Crystalloid solutions (Table 8-3)
   a. Maintenance fluids are used to replace constitutive losses of fluids and electrolytes.
      (1) Insensible water losses include normal losses by skin and lungs, and total approximately 600 to 800 mL/d. **Sensible losses** of water include losses from the kidneys and gastrointestinal (GI) tract. The obligate minimal urine output is 0.3 mL/kg/h and the average urine output is 1 mL/kg/h in an average 70-kg person (approximately 1,700 mL/d).
      (2) Electrolytes. Daily loss of sodium is approximately 1 to 2 mEq/kg. Daily loss of chloride and potassium is approximately 1 to 1.5 mEq/kg. A total of 1 mEq/kg of each electrolyte should be replaced each day.

TABLE 8-3 Composition of Crystalloid Solutions

	Na	Cl	K	Ca	Buffer	Dextrose	pH	Osmolarity
D$_5$W	0	0	0	0	0	5	4.5	252
D$_5$ 0.45% NaCl	77	77	0	0	0	5	4.0	406
0.9% NaCl	154	154	0	0	0	0	5.0	308
7.5% NaCl	1283	1283	0	0	0	0	5.0	2567
Lactated Ringer's	130	109	4	3	28[a]	0	6.5	273

Na, Cl, K, Ca, and buffer concentrations are in milliequivalent per liter; dextrose is in grams per 100 mL.
D$_5$W, 5% dextrose in water; D$_5$ 0.45% NaCl, 5% dextrose in water with 0.45% sodium chloride solution.
[a]Lactate.

(3) **Glucose** supplement as a caloric source should range from 100 to 200 mg/kg/h. However, glucose should not be a routine part of replacement fluids in critically ill patients because of the potential metabolic and neurologic imbalances caused by its rapid administration. Enteral or parenteral nutrition provides the needed dietary glucose (see **Chapter 11**).

(4) **General guidelines for hourly maintenance fluid replacement** based on body weight
   i. 0 to 10 kg: 4 mL/kg/h
   ii. 11 to 20 kg: 40 mL + 2 mL/kg/h for each kilogram above 10 kg
   iii. >20 kg: 60 mL + 1 mL/kg/h for each kilogram above 20 kg

(5) **Maintenance fluid composition.** In general, **hypotonic maintenance fluids** are used to replace insensible losses. Additional losses from other sources are often present in critically ill patients (e.g., through drains, fistulas, etc) and require **isotonic fluid repletion**.

b. For **ECF repletion,** isotonic solutions are used.

(1) Because electrolytes are permeable through capillary membranes, crystalloids will rapidly redistribute from the intravascular compartment throughout the entire ECF, in the normal distribution of 75% extravascular to 25% intravascular.

(2) **0.9% sodium chloride (normal saline [NS])** contains sodium and chloride (both 154 mEq/L) and has an osmolarity of 308 mOsm/L and a pH of 5.0. Thus, NS is hypertonic and more acidic than plasma, has a high chloride content, and can cause hyperchloremic acidosis.

(3) **Lactated Ringer's** (LR) solution contains sodium (130 mEq/L), potassium (4 mEq/L), calcium (3 mEq/L), chloride (109 mEq/L), and lactate (28 mEq/L). LR has an osmolarity of 272.5 mOsm/L and a pH of 6.5. LR is slightly hypotonic and does not cause hyperchloremia.

c. Isotonic crystalloid solutions can be used to replace volume deficits from **blood loss.** Replacement volumes of 2 to 5 mL of isotonic solution are infused per 1 mL of blood loss.

2. **Colloid solutions** (**Table 8-4**). Colloid solutions are most commonly used for intravascular volume expansion. Unlike crystalloid solutions, the colloid elements do not freely cross-intact capillary membranes and therefore do not redistribute as readily into the entire ECF compartment. In general, it takes two to six times less colloid solutions than crystalloid solutions to achieve the same level of intravascular volume expansion.

a. **Albumin** is a natural blood colloid and the most abundant plasma protein. Albumin infusions can maintain plasma oncotic pressure

TABLE 8-4	Physiologic and Chemical Characteristics of Colloid Solutions		
Fluid	Weight–Average Molecular Weight (kd)	Oncotic Pressure (mm Hg)	Serum Half-Life (h)
5% albumin	69	20	16
25% albumin	69	70	16
6% hetastarch	450	30	2–17

and hence may be more effective than crystalloid in expanding intravascular volume. However, the use of albumin as a means of expanding intravascular volume has been shown to have an equivalent effect as crystalloids on the outcome of critically ill patients. **5%** (5 g/dL) and **25%** (25 g/dL) **albumin** solutions are commercially available. They are prepared in isotonic saline, with the 25% albumin preparation in small volumes (called "salt-poor" due to the relatively lower salt load). The oncotic pressure of 5% albumin is similar to that of plasma; 25% albumin has a higher oncotic pressure, and can expand plasma volume by four to five times of infused volume.

   b. **Hetastarch** is a high-molecular-weight synthetic colloid (hydroxyethyl starch, branched glucose polymers). Hetastarch is available in the United States as **6% solution in NS and in LR.** The oncotic pressure of these preparations is approximately 30 mm Hg. The increased plasma oncotic pressures after infusion can last for 2 days. Side effects include elevation in serum amylase, anaphylactoid reactions, and **coagulopathy.** Use of hetastarch in coagulopathic states is controversial, and maximum dose of 20 mL/kg/d is recommended.

3. **Transfusions** of blood and blood components are important for maintaining the oxygen-carrying capacity of blood and for coagulation. A detailed discussion of transfusions as a part of fluid management can be found in **Chapter 35.**

III. Electrolytes and electrolyte abnormalities: Sodium

   A. The normal range of serum (plasma) sodium concentration is 136 to 145 mEq/L. Abnormalities in serum sodium suggest abnormalities in both water and sodium balance. The adult requirement for sodium ranges from **1 to 2 mEq/kg/d**. The requirement is higher in infants. The kidneys of healthy individuals precisely control sodium balance by excreting the exact amount of intake (range, 0.25–6 + mEq/kg/d). This process is modulated by neurohumoral systems, including the renin-angiotensin-aldosterone system, atrial natriuretic peptide, antidiuretic hormone (ADH), parathyroid hormone (PTH), and the sympathetic nervous system.

   B. **Hyponatremia** is defined by a serum sodium of less than 136 mEq/L. Severe hyponatremia can cause central nervous system (CNS) and cardiac abnormalities, such as seizures and dysrhythmias. Hyponatremia can be classified based on concomitant plasma tonicity.

   1. **Isotonic hyponatremia** (approximately 290 mOsm/kg H_2O) occurs when there are elevated levels of other ECF constituents such as protein and lipids. This form of hyponatremia is also known as **pseudohyponatremia** and is an artifact of measurement due to lipid and protein displacement of volume for a given volume of plasma. Therapy for this hyponatremia is not required.

   2. **Hypertonic hyponatremia** is due to the movement of intracellular water into the ECF compartment under the influence of **osmotically active substances** (e.g., glucose, mannitol) with consequent dilution of ECF sodium. A common example of hypertonic hyponatremia is seen with **hyperglycemia,** which can decrease serum sodium concentration by approximately 1.6 mEq/L for each 100 mg/dL of blood glucose. Removal of the osmotically active etiologic substance and restoration of volume are goals of therapy.

   3. **Hypotonic hyponatremia** is the most common form of hyponatremia. This true type of hyponatremia is due to higher TBW relative to total body

sodium. Hypotonic hyponatremia is further classified based on the ECF volume status (hypovolemic, hypervolemic, and isovolemic). In all three scenarios, the extracellular compartment volume status does not always correlate with the intravascular or effective arterial volume status.

a. **Hypovolemic hypotonic hyponatremia** can result from renal or nonrenal sources. In either case, water and salt are lost, but the loss of sodium is greater than the loss of water.

    (1) Renal causes include the use of diuretics (particularly thiazide diuretics), mineral corticoid deficiency, hypothyroidism, and, rarely, renal salt-wasting nephropathy, cerebral salt wasting, and certain types of renal tubular acidosis (RTA).

    (2) Nonrenal causes include fluid losses from the GI tract and intravascular volume depletion via third spacing.

    (3) Renal and nonrenal causes can be distinguished by urine electrolytes. A urine sodium of greater than 20 mEq/L suggests a renal source, while a urine sodium of less than 10 mEq/L suggests a nonrenal etiology.

    (4) The goal of therapy is to replace extracellular volume with isotonic sodium solutions and to allow for appropriate renal-free water excretion.

b. **Hypervolemic hypotonic hyponatremia** is associated with congestive heart failure (CHF), renal failure with nephritic syndrome, and cirrhosis.

    (1) Mechanism: In these disease processes, the effective *arterial* intravascular volume is low even if the *total* intravascular volume is normal or increased. The activation of the renin-angiotensin-aldosterone system and the sympathetic nervous system, and the release of ADH lead to oliguria and salt retention. The result is expansion of ECF volume.

    (2) Manifestations include edema, elevated jugular venous pressures, pleural effusions, and ascites.

    (3) The goal of therapy is to control the primary disease process. Fluid and salt restriction and the use of proximal and loop diuretics may also be appropriate.

c. **Isovolemic hypotonic hyponatremia**

    (1) Causes: Syndrome of inappropriate ADH secretion (**SIADH**), psychogenic polydipsia, medications (e.g., oxytocin), physiologic nonosmotic stimulus for ADH release (e.g., nausea, anxiety, pain), hypothyroidism, and adrenal insufficiency.

    (2) Despite an absence of volume deficit or osmotic stimuli, ADH is increased, which causes an increase in free water retention.

    (3) Therapy depends on the primary cause and the clinical presentation. In general, treatment involves water restriction. In some cases, **demeclocycline** is used to induce a nephrogenic diabetes insipidus to balance the effect of the excess ADH secretion.

    (4) The **vaptans** are active **nonpeptide vasopressin receptor antagonists** that are newly available. Their benefit in the treatment of euvolemic and hypervolemic hyponatremia including patients with chronic heart failure, cirrhosis, SIADH, or hyponatremia from other causes has been shown in clinical study. **Conivaptan** is a V1a/V2 nonselective vasopressin-receptor antagonist that has been approved by the Food and Drug Administration as an intravenous (IV) infusion for in-hospital treatment. **Tolvaptan** is an oral V2-receptor antagonist. Experience with these agents is limited.

d. **General guidelines** for managing **hypotonic hyponatremia**. **NS** should be used for patients who are hypovolemic or who have hyponatremia induced by diuretic use. If the patient is euvolemic, treatment will vary depending on presentation. Often, euvolemic patients are best treated with water restriction. Hypervolemic patients are treated with diuretics along with free water restriction.

e. **Urgent intervention** is required in patients with symptomatic hyponatremia (nausea, vomiting, lethargy, altered level of consciousness, and seizures). The **sodium deficit** can be calculated:

$$\text{Sodium deficit} = \text{TBW} \times (140 - [\text{Na}]_{\text{serum}})$$

The rate of correction of the serum sodium is important and must be tailored to the individual patient. Both delayed and rapid correction can be associated with neurologic injury. Safe correction can be achieved with **hypertonic saline (3% NaCl)** in euvolemic patients and with infusion of NS in hypovolemic patients. The rate of infusion should result in a correction of serum sodium of 1 to 2 mEq/L per hour for the first 24 hours or until serum sodium reaches a level of 120 mEq/L and then be reduced to a correction rate of 0.5 to 1 mEq/L/h.

C. **Hypernatremia** is defined by serum sodium of greater than 145 mEq/L. Hypernatremia is also a description of total body sodium content relative to TBW and can exist in hypovolemic, euvolemic, and hypervolemic states. In all cases, the serum is hypertonic. Clinical manifestations of hypernatremia include tremulousness, irritability, spasticity, confusion, seizures, and coma. Symptoms are more likely to occur when the rate of change is rapid. When the change is gradual and chronic, cells in the CNS will increase the cellular osmolality, thereby preventing cellular water loss and dehydration. This process starts approximately 4 hours after the onset and stabilizes in 4 to 7 days. This change in CNS cellular osmolality is an important concept when considering therapy.

1. **Hypovolemic hypernatremia**
   a. Caused by the loss of hypotonic fluids through extrarenal (e.g., excessive sweating and osmotic diarrhea) or renal (e.g., osmotic diuresis and drug-induced) sources. There is loss of water and salt, with a greater proportion of water loss, which results in a decrease in the ECF volume and the effective arterial intravascular volume.
   b. It is recommended that isotonic saline be used for initial volume repletion, followed by hypotonic crystalloid solutions, such as 0.45% NS.

2. **Euvolemic hypernatremia**
   a. Caused by the loss of free water through extrarenal (e.g., excessive insensible loss through skin or respiration) or renal (e.g., diabetes insipidus) sources.
   b. Measuring urine osmolality (Uosm) is important. Extrarenal processes cause a high Uosm (>800 mOsm/kg H_2O), whereas renal processes cause a low Uosm (approximately 100 mOsm/kg H_2O).
   c. In most cases of hypernatremia from free water loss, the intravascular and extracellular fluid **volumes appear normal.**
   d. Therapy involves replacement of free water.
   e. **Central** and **nephrogenic diabetes insipidus (DI;** see also **Chapter 27)** are among the renal causes of euvolemic hypernatremia. Evaluation of Uosm and the response to ADH may help to determine the site of the lesion.

(1) Central (neurogenic) DI can be caused by pituitary damage from tumor, trauma, surgery, granulomatous disease, and idiopathic causes. Central DI is treated with desmopressin (intranasal, 5–10 μg daily or twice daily).

(2) Nephrogenic DI can be caused by severe hypokalemia with renal tubular injury, hypercalcemia, chronic renal failure, interstitial kidney disease, and drugs (e.g., lithium, amphotericin, demeclocycline). Therapy includes correcting the primary cause if feasible, and possibly free water repletion.

3. **Hypervolemic hypernatremia** is caused by addition of excess sodium and usually results from the infusion or intake of solutions with high sodium concentration. The acute salt load leads to intracellular dehydration with ECF expansion, which can cause edema or CHF. The goal of therapy is to remove the excess sodium; this can be accomplished by using non–medullary gradient disrupting diuretics (e.g., thiazides).

4. **Free water deficit** and correction of hypernatremia

$$\text{Free water deficit} = \text{TBW} \times \{1 - (140/[\text{Na}])\}$$

The correction of hypernatremia should occur at approximately 1 mEq/L/h. Approximately one-half of the calculated water deficit is administered during the first 24 hours and the rest over the following 1 to 2 days. Aggressive correction is dangerous, especially in chronic hypernatremia, where rapid correction can cause cerebral edema. Rapid correction is reasonable if the hypernatremia is acute (<12 hours). Neurologic status should be carefully monitored while correcting hypernatremia, and the rate of correction should be decreased if there is any change in neurologic function.

IV. Electrolyte abnormalities: Potassium

A. In an average adult, the total body potassium is approximately 40 to 50 mEq/kg. Most of the potassium is in the ICF compartment. In general, intake and excretion of potassium are matched. **Average daily intake is approximately 1 to 1.5 mEq/kg.** Although the serum potassium is used as a marker for total body potassium, potassium can have dynamic transcellular redistribution depending on the acid–base status, tonicity, and levels of insulin and catecholamines. The electrocardiogram (**ECG**) is useful in diagnosing true potassium imbalance because the level of polarization of an excitable cell and the ability for repolarization are determined by the extracellular and intracellular potassium concentrations.

B. **Hypokalemia:** Serum potassium concentration of less than 3.5 mEq/L. A general rule is that a 1 mEq/L decrease in serum potassium represents approximately a total body potassium deficit of 200 to 350 mEq.

1. **Causes** of hypokalemia
   a. Transcellular redistribution
      (1) Alkalemia (a 0.1–0.7 mEq/L change per 0.1 U change in pH).
      (2) Increased circulating **catecholamines.**
      (3) Increased **insulin.**
   b. Renal-associated causes
      (1) Without hypertension
         i. With **acidosis**
            (a) Diabetic ketoacidosis (DKA) and renal tubular acidosis (RTA) types 1 and 2.
         ii. With **alkalosis**
            (a) Diuretics
            (b) Vomiting

      (c) Nasogastric suction (leading to hyperaldosteronism)

      (d) Transport defects

        ■ Thick ascending limb: Bartter's syndrome

        ■ Cortical collecting duct: Gitelman's syndrome

    (2) With hypertension

      i. Renal artery stenosis

      ii. Hyperaldosteronism due to tumor (Conn's syndrome, adrenal adenoma)

      iii. Glucocorticoid-mediated hyperadrenalism

      iv. Pseudo-hyperadrenalism

        (a) Licorice ingestion

        (b) Cushing's syndrome

        (c) Liddle's syndrome

  c. Hypomagnesemia

  d. Acute leukemia

  e. Excessive GI losses

  f. Dietary deficiency

  g. Lithium toxicity

  h. Hypothermia

2. Manifestations of hypokalemia include myalgias, cramps, weakness, paralysis, urinary retention, ileus, and orthostatic hypotension. **ECG manifestations,** in order of progression of worsening hypokalemia, are decreased T-wave amplitude, prolonged QT interval, U wave, dragging of ST segment, and increased QRS duration. **Arrhythmias** are common, including atrial fibrillation, premature ventricular beats, supraventricular and junctional tachycardia, and Mobitz-I second-degree atrioventricular block **(Chapter 19).**

3. Therapy: IV potassium replacement is appropriate in patients who have severe hypokalemia or who cannot take oral preparations. The rate of replacement should be governed by the clinical signs. The recommended maximal rate of infusion is 0.5 to 0.7 mEq/kg/h, with continuous ECG monitoring. Oral potassium preparations include immediate- and slow-release preparations. Serum potassium levels should be monitored carefully during repletion. Potassium-sparing diuretics are sometimes used to treat renal losses of potassium. **Hypomagnesemia** should be corrected prior to potassium repletion (see **Section V.C**).

C. Hyperkalemia: Serum potassium of greater than 5.5 mEq/L.

  1. Causes of hyperkalemia

    a. Hemolysis of sample.

    b. Leukocytosis (white blood cell count $>50,000/mm^3$).

    c. Thrombocytosis (platelet count $>1,000,000/mm^3$).

    d. Transcellular redistribution:

      (1) Acidemia.

      (2) Insulin deficiency.

      (3) Drugs (digitalis, β-blockers, succinylcholine).

    e. Malignant hyperthermia.

    f. Cell necrosis (rhabdomyolysis, hemolysis, burns).

    g. Increased intake via replacement therapy and transfusions.

    h. Decreased renal potassium secretion.

      (1) Renal failure.

      (2) Hypoaldosteronism.

      (3) Drugs: Heparin, angiotensin-converting enzyme inhibitors, and potassium-sparing diuretics.

2. **Manifestations** of hyperkalemia include muscle weakness and cardiac conduction disturbances. **ECG changes** include atrial and ventricular ectopy (serum potassium of 6–7 mEq/L), shortened QT interval, and peaked T waves. Worsening hyperkalemia will lead to widening of the QRS, and eventually **ventricular fibrillation**.

3. **Therapy** for hyperkalemia is emergent in the presence of ECG changes, particularly when serum potassium is >6.5 mEq/L. Continuous ECG monitoring is recommended.

   a. **Calcium chloride** or **calcium gluconate** should be given to stabilize the cellular membrane and to decrease excitability of the cells. Calcium does not have an effect on the extracellular potassium. The duration of calcium therapy is approximately 60 minutes, so repeat dosing may be necessary.

   b. Emergency measures to shift extracellular potassium intracellularly, and thereby restore the polarized state of the cell include the use of **sodium bicarbonate** and **insulin with glucose** (insulin, 1 U IV for 2 g of dextrose).

   c. Total body potassium can be reduced by using loop diuretics (e.g., **furosemide**) or exchange resins such as sodium polystyrene sulfonate (**Kayexalate** either orally or rectally; time for effect orally is 120 minutes and rectally is 60 minutes).

   d. **Hemodialysis** should be initiated if hyperkalemia is not controlled adequately with these measures.

V. **Electrolyte abnormalities: Calcium, phosphorus**, and **magnesium**

A. **Calcium** acts as a key signaling element for many cellular functions and is the most abundant electrolyte in the body. Most calcium is stored in bones, but the intestine and kidneys play crucial roles in calcium homeostasis (see **Chapter 28**). Normal values of total serum calcium range from 8.5 to 10.5 mg/dL (4.5–5.5 mEq/L). However, because calcium is bound to protein (approximately 40%), the appropriate range of total serum calcium that can provide for adequate ionized calcium is dependent on the total serum calcium and the amount of serum protein (particularly albumin). The **ionized calcium** provides a better functional assessment, with **normal values ranging from 4 to 5 mg/dL (2.1–2.6 mEq/L, 1.05–1.3 mmol/L)**. Ionized calcium can be affected by the pH of the serum, with acidemia leading to higher ionized calcium and alkalemia to lower ionized calcium. Modulators of calcium homeostasis include PTH and 1,25-vitamin D, which increase calcium levels, and calcitonin, which decreases calcium levels.

1. **Hypercalcemia** (see also **Chapter 28**): A total serum calcium greater than 10.5 mg/dL or ionized calcium greater than 5.0 mg/dL (2.6 mEq/L or 1.29 mmol/L).

   a. **Causes** of hypercalcemia

      (1) Primary hyperparathyroidism.

      (2) Immobilization.

      (3) Malignancy.

      (4) Granulomatous diseases (tuberculosis, sarcoidosis), secondary to increased 1,25-vitamin D production by the granulomatous tissue.

      (5) Thyrotoxicosis.

      (6) Primary bone reabsorption abnormalities (Paget's disease).

      (7) Adrenal insufficiency.

      (8) Pheochromocytoma.

      (9) Milk-alkali syndrome: High intake of calcium (>5 g/d).

      (10) Drugs (thiazides, vitamin D, lithium, estrogens).

    b. Diagnosis

       (1) PTH levels: Low in malignancy-associated hypercalcemia, high in primary, secondary, and tertiary hyperparathyroidism.

       (2) 1,25-Vitamin D levels: Elevated in granulomatous disease.

       (3) PTH-related protein: Elevated in malignancy-associated hypercalcemia (breast, lung, thyroid, renal cells).

       (4) Protein electrophoresis: Monoclonal band associated with myeloma.

       (5) Thyroid-stimulating hormone (TSH).

       (6) Chest radiographs: Evaluate for malignancy and granulomatous disease.

    c. Manifestations of hypercalcemia include GI symptoms, arthralgias, weakness, bone pain, lethargy, shock, and coma. **ECG abnormalities** include shortened QT interval, increased PR and QRS intervals, T-wave flattening, and atrioventricular block. **Polyuria and dehydration** occur due to an inability of the kidneys to concentrate urine.

    d. Treatment is described in detail **in Chapter 28.** Here we summarize the main considerations from a nephrologic standpoint. Treatment should be initiated if neurologic symptoms are present, total serum calcium is >12 to 13 mg/dL, or calcium/phosphate product is >75.

       (1) Immediate **hydration** with NS to restore volume status and decrease serum calcium concentration by dilution.

       (2) After establishing euvolemia, a loop diuretic can be added to NS with the goal of generating a **urine output** of 3 to 5 mL/kg/h.

       (3) Other electrolytes should be repleted.

       (4) Hemodialysis, if the above therapy is ineffective.

       (5) The use of **pamidronate, calcitonin, and glucocorticoids** is described in detail in **Chapter 28. Calcium channel blockers** can also be used to treat the cardiotoxic effects of hypercalcemia.

2. Hypocalcemia (see also **Chapter 28**): An ionized calcium of less than 4 mg/dL.

    a. Causes of hypocalcemia:

       (1) Sequestration of calcium can be caused by hyperphosphatemia (from renal failure), pancreatitis, intravascular citrate (from packed red blood cells), and alkalemia.

       (2) PTH deficiency: PTH deficiency can be caused by surgical excision of parathyroid gland, autoimmune parathyroid disease, amyloid infiltration of parathyroid gland, severe hypermagnesemia, hypomagnesemia, HIV infection, and hemochromatosis.

       (3) PTH resistance: PTH resistance is due to congenital abnormality or secondary to hypomagnesemia.

       (4) Vitamin D deficiency is caused by malabsorption, poor nutritional intake, liver disease, anticonvulsants (phenytoin), inadequate sunlight, and renal failure.

       (5) Inappropriate calcium deposition can be due to formation of complex with phosphorus in hyperphosphatemic states (rhabdomyolysis), acute pancreatitis, and postparathyroidectomy.

       (6) Sepsis and toxic shock syndrome.

    b. Manifestations of hypocalcemia include generalized excitable membrane irritability leading to paresthesias and progressing to tetany and seizures. The classic physical examination findings include **Trousseau's sign** (spasm of the upper extremity muscles that causes flexion of the wrist and thumb with the extension of the fingers, can be elicited by occluding the circulation to the arm) and **Chvostek's**

sign (contraction of ipsilateral facial muscles elicited by tapping over the facial nerve at the jaw). **ECG changes** include prolonged QT and heart block.

  c. Diagnosis
    (1) Confirm true hypocalcemia by checking ionized calcium and pH.
    (2) Rule out hypomagnesemia.
    (3) Check PTH level; if low or normal, hypoparathyroidism may be involved; if high, check a phosphorus level. A low phosphorus level is indicative of pancreatitis or vitamin D deficiency, while a high phosphorus level suggests rhabdomyolysis and renal failure.
  d. Therapy of hypocalcemia: Infusion of calcium at 4 mg/kg of elemental calcium with either **10% calcium gluconate** (93 mg of calcium/10 mL) or **10% calcium chloride** (272 mg of calcium/10 mL). A bolus should be followed by an infusion because the bolus will increase the ionized form of calcium for 1 to 2 hours. To avoid precipitation of calcium salts, **IV calcium solutions should not be mixed with IV bicarbonate solutions.** Calcium chloride is caustic to peripheral veins and should be given via central venous access if possible. Suspected vitamin D or PTH deficiency is treated with calcitriol (0.25 µg, up to 1.5 µg PO once a day). Oral calcium repletion with at least 1 g of elemental calcium a day should be given together with vitamin D therapy.

B. Phosphorus exists mainly as a free ion in the body. Approximately 0.8 to 1 g of phosphorus is excreted in the urine per day. Phosphorus excretion is affected by PTH (which inhibits proximal and distal nephron phosphorus reabsorption), vitamin D, high dietary phosphorus intake, cortisol, and growth hormone.

  1. Hypophosphatemia occurs in 10% to 15% of hospitalized patients.
    a. Causes
      (1) GI: Malnutrition, malabsorption, vitamin D deficiency, diarrhea, and use of aluminum-containing antacids.
      (2) Renal losses: Primary hyperparathyroidism, renal transplantation, ECF expansion, diuretics (acetazolamide), Fanconi's syndrome, post–obstructive and post–acute tubular necrosis (ATN), glycosuria, DKA.
      (3) Redistribution: Alkalosis, postalcohol withdrawal, parenteral hyperalimentation, burns, and continuous venovenous hemofiltration.
    b. Clinical symptoms usually occur when phosphorus is less than 1.0 mg%.
      (1) Neurologic: Metabolic encephalopathy.
      (2) Muscular: Myopathy, respiratory failure, cardiomyopathy.
      (3) Hematologic: Hemolysis, white blood cell dysfunction.
    c. Diagnosis
      (1) Urinary phosphorus less than 100 mg/d implies GI losses.
      (2) Urinary phosphorus more than 100 mg/d suggests renal wasting.
      (3) Elevated serum calcium suggests hyperparathyroidism.
      (4) Elevated PTH suggests primary or secondary hyperparathyroidism or vitamin D–resistant rickets.
    d. Treatment
      (1) Increase oral intake to 1,000 mg/d.
      (2) Elemental phosphorus, 450 mg per 1,000 kcal of hyperalimentation.
      (3) Dose of IV phosphorus should not exceed 2 mg/kg (0.15 mmol/kg) of elemental phosphorus.

2. **Hyperphosphatemia**
   a. **Causes**
      (1) **Renal:** Decreased glomerular filtration rate (GFR), increased tubular reabsorption, hypoparathyroidism, pseudohypoparathyroidism, acromegaly, thyrotoxicosis.
      (2) **Endogenous:** Tumor lysis, rhabdomyolysis.
      (3) **Exogenous:** Vitamin D administration, phosphate enemas.
   b. **Clinical symptoms** are related to hypocalcemia due to calcium phosphate deposition and decreased renal production of 1,25-vitamin D.
   c. **Treatment**
      (1) Phosphate binders to reduce GI absorption.
      (2) Volume expansion and dextrose 10% in water with insulin may reduce acutely elevated phosphorus levels.
      (3) Hemodialysis and peritoneal dialysis.
C. **Magnesium:** Serum magnesium is maintained between 1.8 and 2.3 mg/dL (1.7–2.1 mEq/L); 15% is protein bound.
   1. **Hypermagnesemia** is rare in patients with normal renal function.
      a. **Causes**
         (1) Acute and chronic renal failure.
         (2) Magnesium administration for toxemia of pregnancy, magnesium-containing antacids and laxatives.
      b. **Signs and symptoms**
         (1) Cardiac dysrhythmias.
         (2) Decreased neuromuscular transmission.
         (3) CNS dysfunction: Confusion, lethargy.
         (4) Hypotension.
         (5) Respiratory depression.
         (6) Death at higher levels.
      c. **Treatment**
         (1) IV calcium.
         (2) Hemodialysis to remove magnesium in renal failure.
   2. **Hypomagnesemia** is defined as serum magnesium less than 1.8 mg/dL.
      a. **Causes**
         (1) **GI**
            i. Decreased intake (chronic alcoholism).
            ii. Starvation.
            iii. Magnesium-free enteral feedings.
            iv. Decreased GI intake due to nasogastric suction and malabsorption.
         (2) **Renal losses**
            i. Diuretic therapy.
            ii. Postobstructive diuresis.
            iii. Recovery (polyuric phase) from ATN.
            iv. DKA.
            v. Hypercalcemia.
            vi. Primary hyperaldosteronism.
            vii. Barter's syndrome.
            viii. Aminoglycoside, cisplatin, and cyclosporine nephrotoxicity.
         (3) **Manifestations**
            i. Hypokalemia and hypocalcemia; hypokalemia is the result of excess urine losses, which can only be corrected with magnesium repletion.
            ii. ECG changes mimic hypokalemia.
            iii. Digoxin toxicity is magnified by hypomagnesemia.

    iv. Neuromuscular fasciculations with Chvostek's and Trousseau's signs may be present.

  (4) Treatment for hypomagnesemia should be initiated when ECG changes and/or tetany are present.

    i. IV: With $MgSO_4$, 6 g in 1 L of 5% dextrose in water over 6 hours.

    ii. Oral: With magnesium oxide, 250 to 500 mg four times a day.

VI. Standard approach to acid–base physiology. The normal extracellular hydrogen ion (H^+) concentration is 40 nEq/L (one-millionth the milliequivalent-per-liter concentrations of sodium, potassium, and chloride). Maintenance of acid–base homeostasis depends on the presence of buffers. The standard approach to acid–base balance is based on the bicarbonate buffer system:

$$H^+ + HCO_3^- \Leftrightarrow H_2CO_3 \Leftrightarrow H_2O + CO_2$$

Although other buffers are present in the plasma (e.g., H^+ + protein$^-$ $\Leftrightarrow$ HProtein and other fixed acids), the bicarbonate buffer is the most significant because the acid and the conjugate base can be regulated by the lungs and kidneys, respectively. The H_2CO_3 species is in equilibrium with dissolved CO_2; therefore, the **Henderson–Hasselbalch equation** to describe weak acids and its conjugate base is as follows:

$$pH = 6.1 + \log\{[HCO_3^-]/(0.03 \times Paco_2)\}$$

Because $pH = -\log[H]$, the equation can be rearranged:

$$[H^+] = 24 \times (Paco_2/[HCO_3^-])$$

and used to calculate the bicarbonate for a specific $Paco_2$ at a specific pH. The hydrogen ion concentration can be quickly estimated when the pH is near 7.4 by adding or subtracting 10 nEq/L per change in 0.1 pH units from 40 nEq/L. Although buffers maintain acid–base homeostasis in the short term, compensatory changes in CO_2 and bicarbonate are responsible for continued maintenance of pH. Basic aspects of simple acid–base disorders and compensatory changes are included in **Table 8-5**. In general, the pH, $Paco_2$, and bicarbonate are used to determine the primary disorder. The adequacy of compensation is then determined (see **Table 8-5**). If there is inadequate compensation, then there is likely to be a mixed acid–base disturbance.

A. Metabolic acidosis causes a primary decrease in serum bicarbonate due to one of three mechanisms: (a) a strong acid is generated either by endogenous production or by exogenous intake/administration and is buffered by bicarbonate; (b) bicarbonate is lost from the GI tract or is underproduced or lost by the kidney; and (c) there is ECF dilution due to high-dose administration of non–bicarbonate-containing IV fluids (large infusions of NS). Metabolic acidoses are classified as anion-gap and non–anion-gap types (**Table 8-6**).

  1. Anion-gap metabolic acidosis: The anion gap is based on the presence of unmeasured anions and is calculated as $Na - (Cl^- + HCO_3^-)$, with normal values between 7 and 14 mEq/L. **Albumin** is the largest constituent of the unmeasured anions. If albumin is low, the presence of other unmeasured anions, such as lactic acid, will be falsely low based on the calculated anion gap. If the albumin concentration is less than 4 g/dL, the normal anion-gap range should be corrected by subtracting 2.5 mEq/L for every 1 g/dL of albumin less than 4 g/dL.

    a. Lactic acidosis occurs when there is inadequate tissue O_2 delivery.

      (1) Causes. Septic, cardiogenic, and hypovolemic shock, seizures.

TABLE 8-5 Simple Acid–Base Disorders and Compensatory Changes

Disorder	Mechanism	Primary Disturbance	Compensation	Compensatory Change
Metabolic acidosis, pH <7.37	H^- retention or production; HCO_3^- loss	$\downarrow HCO_3^-$ from 24 mEq/L	$\downarrow Pa_{CO_2}$	$\Delta Pa_{CO_2} = 1.2 \times \Delta HCO_3^-$
Metabolic alkalosis, pH >7.43	HCO_3^- retention or production; H^+ loss	$\uparrow HCO_3^-$ from 24 mEq/L	$\uparrow Pa_{CO_2}$	$\Delta HCO_3^- = 0.7 \times \Delta Pa_{CO_2}$
Respiratory acidosis, pH <7.37	Pa_{CO_2} retention	$\uparrow Pa_{CO_2}$ from 40 mm Hg	$\uparrow HCO_3^-$	Acute: $\Delta HCO_3^- = 0.1 \times \Delta Pa_{CO_2}$; $\Delta pH = 0.08/10$ mm Hg ΔPa_{CO_2} Chronic: $\Delta HCO_3^- = 0.4 \times \Delta Pa_{CO_2}$; $\Delta pH = 0.03/10$ mm Hg ΔPa_{CO_2}
Respiratory alkalosis, pH >7.43	Excessive Pa_{CO_2} reduction	$\downarrow Pa_{CO_2}$ from 40 mm Hg	$\downarrow HCO_3^-$	Acute: $\Delta HCO_3^- = 0.2 \times \Delta Pa_{CO_2}$; $\Delta pH = 0.08/10$ mm Hg ΔPa_{CO_2} Chronic: $\Delta HCO_3^- = 0.5 \times \Delta Pa_{CO_2}$; $\Delta pH = 0.03/10$ mm Hg ΔPa_{CO_2}

(2) **Treatment.** The primary goal is to restore tissue perfusion. Bicarbonate therapy may not be effective because it produces only a transient rise in pH and causes increased local CO_2 production, which may exacerbate intracellular acidemia. Bicarbonate therapy may also reduce endogenous hepatic lactate utilization. However, in severe acidemia, small amounts of sodium bicarbonate are often infused to maintain arterial pH above 7.20.

b. **Diabetic ketoacidosis (DKA, Chapter 27).** Insulin deficiency and glucagon excess lead to hepatic production of ketoacids. Administration of insulin stops ketoacid production. DKA is treated with IV infusion of insulin and saline to replace fluid losses from the glycosuria-driven osmotic diuresis. Again, small amounts of bicarbonate are often infused intravenously to maintain arterial pH above 7.20.

c. **Starvation ketosis.** Ketones are present in serum and urine. Treatment includes refeeding and correction of associated metabolic and electrolyte abnormalities such as hypophosphatemia and hypokalemia.

d. **Alcoholic ketoacidosis.** This condition is caused by chronic alcoholism and binge drinking. Serum alcohol and lactate levels are increased. Treatment should include hydration with saline, glucose with 100 mg of thiamine, and IV phosphorus.

e. **Salicylate intoxication (see Chapter 31).** Manifestations include respiratory alkalosis secondary to stimulation of the respiratory center and metabolic acidosis secondary to interference with oxidative metabolism.

f. **Ethylene glycol ingestion (Chapter 31),** a component of automobile antifreeze, causes renal failure. Patients present with an anion and osmolar gap and calcium oxalate crystals in the urine.

g. **Methanol ingestion (Chapter 31)** produces an acidosis with an elevated anion gap and osmolar gap.

 TABLE 8-6   Classification of Metabolic Acidoses

Anion-gap metabolic acidosis
Endogenous
    Diabetic ketoacidosis; severe ketoacidosis (alcohol, starvation); uremia; lactate
Exogenous
    Toxins
        Ethylene glycol, methanol, salicylate

Non–anion-gap metabolic acidosis
Gastrointestinal losses
    Diarrhea; pancreatic, biliary, and enterocutaneous fistulas; ostomies
    Ureterosigmoidostomy
Infusion and ingestion of chloride-containing salts: total parenteral nutrition; cholestyramine
RTA
    Distal RTA
    Proximal RTA
    Type IV RTA
Metabolic acidosis of renal failure

RTA, renal tubular necrosis.

2. **Non–anion-gap metabolic acidosis.** The **urine anion gap (UAG)** is a useful tool in the differential diagnosis of non–anion-gap acidosis:

$$UAG = (Na_{urine} + K_{urine}) - Cl_{urine}$$

UAG is negative if the cause of the acidosis is nonrenal (e.g., GI losses) and the unaccounted-for cation in the urine is NH_4^+, and it is positive if the cause of the acidosis is renal in origin.
   a. **Nonrenal non–anion-gap acidosis**
      (1) **Metabolic acidosis associated with GI losses.** Bicarbonate wastage and consequent non–anion-gap metabolic acidosis are frequently seen with diarrhea, ileus, enterocutaneous fistulas, ostomies, laxative abuse, and villous adenoma of the rectum. Therapy includes bicarbonate replacement. In patients with volume contraction and avid renal sodium retention, decreased distal renal sodium delivery may impair the ability of the distal nephron to excrete hydrogen ions. Thus, volume repletion is also crucial.
      (2) **Ureterosigmoidostomy.** The diversion of urine through intestinal segments can cause a non–anion-gap metabolic acidosis, hypokalemia, and occasionally hypocalcemia and hypomagnesemia. Given the frequency of these abnormalities when urine is diverted into the sigmoid colon, urinary diversions are now preferentially done with ileal conduits (which has a lower frequency of causing hyperchloremic acidosis).
   b. **Renal tubular acidosis (RTA)**
      (1) **Type 1 RTA**
         i. **Mechanisms:** Direct impairment of apical membrane H^+/ATPase and decreased ability to excrete protons distally; increased permeability of the apical membrane or tight intercellular junctions to protons allowing hydrogen ions back diffusion; or decreased Na absorption in principal cells, which may result in a reduction in luminal electronegativity and impede hydrogen ions excretion in adjacent intercalated cells.
         ii. **Diagnosis:** Positive UAG, urine pH greater than 5.5, percentage filtered bicarbonate excreted less than 10, low serum potassium, and possible nephrocalcinosis and nephrolithiasis.
         iii. **Therapy:** Bicarbonate replacement (1–2 mEq/kg/24 h) and potassium supplements.
      (2) **Type 2 (proximal) RTA**
         i. **Mechanism:** Impaired **proximal bicarbonate** reabsorption with transient bicarbonate loss in urine.
         ii. **Diagnosis:** UAG is an unreliable measure due to the presence of additional anion (bicarbonate) in the urine, urine pH less than 5.5, percentage filtered bicarbonate greater than 15, low serum potassium. If it is associated with a generalized tubular absorption disorder, urine phosphate, amino acids, and glucose are present (Fanconi's syndrome).
         iii. **Therapy:** High doses of bicarbonate (10–25 mEq/kg/24 h), aggressive potassium supplementation, and calcium and vitamin D supplementation.
      (3) **Hyperkalemic (type 4) RTA**
         i. **Mechanisms:** Selective aldosterone deficiency (common in patients with types 1 and 2 diabetic nephropathy) and hyporeninemic hypoaldosteronism. This RTA is frequently

encountered in patients with tubulointerstitial disease with mild to moderate renal insufficiency.

ii. **Diagnosis:** Positive UAG, urine pH less than 5.5, percentage filtered bicarbonate less than 10, high serum potassium.

iii. **Therapy:** Exchange resins (Kayexalate) for hyperkalemia (which will also enhance ammonium excretion and hence acid secretion), and loop diuretics.

(4) Renal failure

i. **Mechanism of acidosis.** With nephron loss, net acid excretion is maintained by increased ammonium production per functioning nephron; however, when GFR falls to less than 30 to 40 mL/min, ammonium production falls below the level required to excrete the daily acid load. The retained acid (hydrogen ions) is buffered in the ECF by bicarbonate and in the tissues by cells and bone, and bicarbonate levels fall concomitantly.

ii. **Therapy.** Oral sodium bicarbonate (650 mg PO two to three times daily; 30–45 mEq bicarbonate) to maintain a serum bicarbonate level of greater than 20 mEq/L may be appropriate to reduce the adverse effects of prolonged acidosis (muscle wasting and bone demineralization).

B. Metabolic alkalosis

1. Causes

a. **GI losses.** There are proton losses from the upper GI tract due to nasogastric suctioning and vomiting.

b. **Diuretics.** These cause a contraction alkalosis and chloride and potassium wasting, which disturb normal renal handling of protons and bicarbonate. **Contraction alkalosis** refers to the reduction in ECF volume around a fixed quantity of bicarbonate as is seen when diuretics cause ECF depletion by the excretion of bicarbonate-free urine.

c. **Hyperaldosteronism** generates a metabolic alkalosis by increasing distal hydrogen ions excretion.

d. **Others**

(1) Posthypercapneic alkalosis.

(2) Hypokalemia by cellular translocation of protons.

(3) Bicarbonate or citrate administration.

2. Metabolic alkalosis may be characterized based on urine chloride concentrations and responsiveness to chloride infusion (either as NaCl or as KCl).

a. **Chloride-unresponsive** metabolic alkaloses are due to endogenous overproduction of aldosterone or mineralocorticoid derivatives.

b. **Chloride-responsive** metabolic alkaloses are reversible with chloride repletion, and a number of factors play a role in the maintenance of an established chloride-responsive metabolic alkalosis:

(1) Effective circulating volume depletion.

(2) Chloride depletion and a low urine chloride.

(3) Potassium depletion.

C. Respiratory acidosis is a primary increase in $Paco_2$ due to inadequate excretion of CO_2. Increased CO_2 results in increased carbonic acid production that is buffered by tissue buffers. Renal compensation results in a net increase in bicarbonate production. Full compensation usually takes more than 24 hours.

D. Respiratory alkalosis is a primary decrease in $Paco_2$ that usually results from alveolar hyperventilation. The alkalemia is buffered with intracellular protons. Renal compensation over a period of days causes a net excretion of bicarbonate. Clinical manifestations are perioral paresthesia, muscle cramps and hyperreflexia, seizures, and cardiac arrhythmias.

E. **Mixed acid–base disorders.** In contrast to emergency room and operating room patients (who generally start out with a normal acid–base status), critically ill patients frequently develop multiple acid–base abnormalities over time, of different and coexisting etiologies. The diagnosis of mixed acid–base disturbances highlights the need for a systematic approach to the analysis of acid–base disorders. Historical information should be sought, including drug and toxin exposure and the use of medications, such as diuretics, that may affect acid–base homeostasis. The presence of underlying disease of major organ systems such as cardiac, pulmonary, hepatic, or renal disease should be considered. The presence of diarrhea and the use of parenteral nutrition are examples of other relevant information. Laboratory data should include electrolytes, BUN and creatinine, urine electrolytes, the anion gap, and arterial blood gas. While the ratios of pH, $Paco_2$, and bicarbonate vary in a fixed way in simple acid–base disorders (see **Table 8-5**), these ratios do not behave according to these properties in mixed acid–base disturbances. The following general rules must be considered:

1. **Overcompensation does not occur** in primary disorders. Therefore if the change in ratio of $Paco_2$ to bicarbonate or of bicarbonate to $Paco_2$ is out of the ranges outlined in **Table 8-5**, a mixed acid–base disorder is present.

2. **A low bicarbonate** is due to either primary acidosis or respiratory alkalosis. A bicarbonate of less than 15 mEq/L is usually due to a metabolic acidosis.

3. **An elevated bicarbonate** is due either to metabolic alkalosis or respiratory acidosis. A bicarbonate of greater than 40 mEq/L is usually due to a metabolic alkalosis.

4. **Severe acidemia can result from a combination** of metabolic and respiratory acidoses in which $Paco_2$ and bicarbonate may not be markedly abnormal, but the pH may be very low.

5. **In mixed metabolic acidosis and respiratory alkalosis,** bicarbonate and $Paco_2$ are both reduced, and the $Paco_2$ will be lower than predicted based on the expected respiratory compensation for metabolic acidosis.

6. **Mixed metabolic acidosis and alkalosis** primarily affects bicarbonate; pH, and bicarbonate may be high, low, or normal; an elevated anion gap suggests an underlying anion-gap acidosis; vomiting is a frequent component of this mixed disorder.

7. **Combined metabolic alkalosis and respiratory acidosis** occurs with a high bicarbonate and $Paco_2$. The elevation in bicarbonate will be greater than predicted for primary compensation of a respiratory acidosis. This disorder is frequently seen in patients with a combination of pulmonary and cardiac diseases who are on diuretics.

8. **Mixed metabolic and respiratory alkalosis causes a severe alkalemia;** a mixed disorder of this type is noted when a respiratory alkalosis is not accompanied by an appropriate decrease in bicarbonate or metabolic alkalosis is not accompanied by an appropriate increase in $Paco_2$; mechanical ventilation and diuretic use often underlie this disorder.

9. **A triple acid–base disorder** with metabolic acidosis and alkalosis and either respiratory acidosis or alkalosis can be seen in alcoholic or diabetic patients who present with lactic acidosis or ketoacidosis, vomiting, and respiratory alkalosis due to sepsis or cirrhosis.

VII. Physicochemical systems approach to acid–base physiology

A. The Henderson–Hasselbach equation offers only a partial image of a complex system. Although changes in bicarbonate can be used as an indicator of nonrespiratory acid–base disturbances, changes in bicarbonate are not primary, but instead result from the cumulative effects of multiple processes, both metabolic and respiratory. Therefore, the standard approach to acid–base analysis requires the calculation of compensation, anion gap, subsequent manipulation of the anion gap in states of low or high weak acids, and bicarbonate (Δ-Δ) calculations to reveal all the acid–base disturbances found in the system. An alternative, more rigorous method is to first define the system, all its components, and the laws that govern the interactions of the components. Components that can be primarily and individually affected are independent variables, and components of the system that are changed due to changes in the independent variables are the dependent variables. The **Stewart physicochemical model** for acid–base physiology dissects and describes mathematically the determinants of acid–base balance in aqueous solutions. The system is based on three independent variables: (a) the **strong ion difference (SID)**, (b) the **total weak acids (A_{tot})**, and (c) the **$Paco_2$**. The constraints that control the interaction of the variables are set by the law of mass action (dissociation equilibrium must be accounted for both strong ions and weak acids), the law of mass conservation, and maintenance of electroneutrality in solution. Other changes in the system, including changes in hydrogen ions and bicarbonate, are the result of changes in one or more of the independent variables.

1. **SID.** Strong ions are ions derived from compounds with an equilibrium dissociation constant K greater than 10^{-4} (acids) or less than 10^{-12} (bases) and are fully dissociated at the system's pH ([HA] = [H$^+$] + [A$^-$]). SID is the difference between the sum of concentrations of all completely dissociated cations and all completely dissociated anions: SID = [Na] + [K] + [Ca] + [Mg] − [Cl] − [other unmeasured strong anions, noted XA$^-$]. In normal conditions, other strong anions do not exist, and the contributions of Ca and Mg are minimal; therefore, SID is approximated by [Na] + [K] − [Cl] and is roughly equal to 40 mEq/L. SID is a concept related to the AG and is based on respecting electroneutrality. It can be represented graphically under the from of the "gamblegram" (**Fig. 8-1**). Accumulation of unmeasured fully dissociated anions (and corresponding protons) would result in an SID value lower than 40 mEq/L and represents metabolic acidosis. Conversely, an increase in the SID above 40 mEq/L signifies accumulation of weak acids (i.e. buffers [A_{tot}]) and represents metabolic acidosis.

2. **A_{tot}.** Weak acids are compounds with equilibrium dissociation constants between 10^{-4} and 10^{12} that are only partially dissociated at body pH, (k × [HA$_{tot}$] = [H$^+$] × [A_{tot}^-]). These compounds represent the buffer activity of the system and include proteins (albumin being the predominant buffer species in plasma), sulfates, and phosphates.

3. **$Paco_2$** provides the link between metabolic and respiratory processes within the system. Dissolved plasma CO_2 is regulated by ventilation.

B. With the system defined, one can evaluate the independent variables to determine the type of acid–base disturbance present (**Table 8-7**). The following rules apply:

1. **Metabolic alkalosis**
   a. Low A_{tot}: Secondary to low albumin from nephrotic syndrome and cirrhosis.

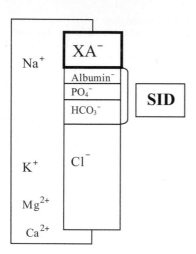

FIGURE 8-1 The "Gamblegram": The sum of the anions is equal to the sum of the anions in solution. XA^-: unmeasured strong ions; SID: strong ions difference.

    b. High SID: From chloride loss secondary to vomiting, villous adenoma, or increased Na from hyperaldosteronism, Barter's syndrome, and Na load from total parenteral nutrition.
  2. Metabolic acidosis
    a. Low SID due to increased chloride or decreased sodium.
    b. High A_{tot} due to increases in albumin or phosphates.
  3. To further detail the **metabolic acidosis** diagnosis, one can calculate the **strong ion gap (SIG)**, starting from the equation of electroneutrality:

$$[Na] + [K] + [Mg] + [Ca] = [Cl] + [HCO_3] + [albumin] + [PO_4] + [XA^-].$$

Rearranging, this results in

$$[Na] + [K] + [Mg] + [Ca] - [Cl] = [albumin] + [PO_4] + [HCO_3] + [XA^-].$$

$[Na] + [K] + [Mg] + [Ca] - [Cl]$ is called the **apparent SID (SID$_{app}$)**, and $[protein] + [PO_4] + [HCO_3]$, is called the **effective SID (SID$_{eff}$)**.

TABLE
8-7   Acid–Base Disorders According to Stewart's Physicochemical Model

	Acidosis	Alcalosis
I. Respiratory	↑CO_2	↓CO_2
II. Metabolic		
1. Abnormal SID		
a. Water excess/deficit	↓SID ↓Na^+	↑SID ↑Na^+
b. Strong anions imbalance		
i. Chloride excess/deficit	↓SID ↑Cl^-	↑SID ↑Cl^-
ii. Unidentified anions	↓SID ↑XA^-	—
2. Nonvolatile weak acids		
a. Albumin	↑Albumin	↓Albumin
b. Phosphate	↑Phosphate	↓Phosphate

Therefore, the SIG $= SID_{app} - SID_{eff} = [XA^-]$.

If SIG is greater than 0 mEq/L, then there are elevated unaccounted-for anions causing the acidosis (e.g., lactic acid, ketones, formate, methanol, and salicylates); if SIG is 0, then the acidosis is due to Cl^- retention (secondary to RTA, rapid saline infusion, and anion exchange resins).

4. Respiratory disturbances are similarly described by the traditional method, which relies on the independent variable $Paco_2$.

C. **The Stewart model is controversial.** Proponents feel that complex acid–base disorders are easier to understand, explain, and rationalize using the Stewart model, and that the Stewart model is mathematically valid. Using current technology, all the variables described can be provided directly by the laboratory for ease of interpretation. Detractors note that the model adds little clinically as studies show no difference in outcomes in patients treated with either method. Implementing the Stewart model in the daily clinical practice would require a significant effort and change in culture.

Selected References

Adrogue HJ, Madias NE. Management of life-threatening acid-base disorders. First of two parts. *N Engl J Med* 1998;338(1):26–34.

Adrogue HJ, Madias NE. Management of life-threatening acid-base disorders. Second of two parts. *N Engl J Med* 1998;338(2):107–111.

Adrogue HJ, Madias NE. Hypernatremia. *N Engl J Med* 2000;342:1493–1499.

Adrogue HJ, Madias NE. Hyponatremia. *N Engl J Med* 2000;342:1581–1589.

Choi PT, Yip G, Quinonez LG, et al. Crystalloids vs. colloids in fluid resuscitation: a systematic review. *Crit Care Med* 1999;27:200–210.

Fencl V, Jabor A, et al. Diagnosis of metabolic acid-base disturbances in critically ill patients. *Am J Respir Crit Care Med* 2000;162:2246–2251.

Fencl V, Leith DE. Stewart's quantitative acid-base chemistry: applications in biology and medicine. *Respir Physiol* 1993;91:1–16.

Finfer S, Bellomo R, Boyce N, et al. A comparison of albumin and saline for fluid resuscitation in the intensive care unit. *N Engl J Med* 2004;350:2247–2256.

Gunnerson K, Kellum J. Acid base and electrolyte analysis in critically ill. *Curr Opp Crit Care* 2003;9:468–473.

Jones NL. A quantitative physicochemical approach to acid-base physiology. *Clin Biochem* 1990;23:189–195.

Morgan HG. Acid-base balance in blood. *Brit J Anaesth* 1969;41:196–212.

Narins RG, Emmett M. Simple and mixed acid-base disorders: a practical approach. *Medicine* 1980;59:161–186.

Sirker AA, Rhodes A, et al. Acid-base physiology: the 'traditional' and the 'modern' approaches. *Anaesthesia* 2002;57:348–356.

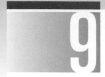

Critical Care of the Trauma Patient

Jeffrey Ustin and Hasan Alam

INTRODUCTION

In the United States, traumatic injury is the leading cause of death among individuals between the ages of 1 and 44 years. It kills more individuals between the ages of 1 and 34 years in the United States than all other causes combined. Injury accounts for approximately one out of six hospital admissions, with almost 20% of trauma admissions being admitted to the ICU. It is therefore crucial for intensivists to be familiar with the care of trauma patients. Although many of the principles used to treat other critically ill patients apply, there are aspects that are unique to traumatized patients. This chapter will cover the pathophysiology, evaluation, and treatment of these conditions. Injuries to the **brain** and **spinal cord** as well as cervical spine clearance are covered in **Chapter 10**.

I. **Trauma evaluation**
   A. **Primary survey (ABCs)**. This is a quick examination that aims to identify the most immediately life-threatening injuries.
      1. **Airway with C-spine control:** Evaluation of airway patency and determination of need to establish a definitive and secure airway.
      2. **Breathing:** Examination of quality of air movement with treatment of tension or open pneumothorax, flail chest, or massive hemothorax.
      3. **Circulation:** Assessment of the hemodynamic status with the establishment of vascular access, and electrocardiogram (ECG) monitoring.
      4. **Disability:** Examination neurologic status including gross movement of extremities and Glasgow Coma Scale (**Chapter 10**).
      5. **Exposure/environmental control:** Undressing the patient for full evaluation while preventing hypothermia.
   B. **Secondary survey.** This is a head-to-toe examination that includes the back and spine. Every part of the patient is examined for injury, deformity, and pain. The Focused Assessment with Sonography for Trauma **(FAST) examination** is usually included at this point in the evaluation.
   C. **Tertiary survey.** Unrecognized injuries may occur in up to 65% of patients and are clinically significant in 15% of patients. Therefore, an additional thorough survey is done typically within 24 hours of admission.

II. **Specific injuries**
   A. **Neurotrauma**: see **Chapter 10**.
   B. **Facial trauma** occasionally presents with life-threatening **airway** obstruction from swelling or massive bleeding. Intubation, tracheostomy, or anterior and posterior nasal packing may be necessary.
      1. **Fractures** may affect any region including mandible, zygoma, nose, orbit, and sinuses. Patterns of injury are often seen including zygomatic-maxillary complex (ZMC or tripod fracture) and **Le Fort I** (maxillary separation), **II** (nasomaxillary separation), and **III** (craniofacial separation, **Fig. 9-1**).

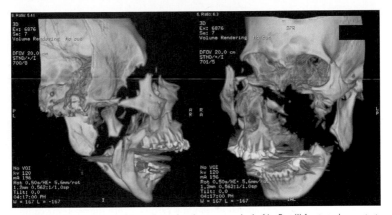

FIGURE 9-1 CT scan images (three-dimensional reconstruction) of Le Fort III fracture demonstrating craniofacial separation. CT, computerized tomography.

   2. Specific **treatment** considerations include
      a. Vigilance for nasal septal hematomas, which need drainage
      b. Avoidance of all nasal intubations (nasotracheal, nasogastric, etc) in cases of skull base fractures
      c. Evaluation for ophthalmologic emergencies including foreign bodies, globe entrapment, retrobulbar hemorrhage, hyphema (anterior chamber blood), ruptured globe, corneal abrasions and lacerations, and lacrimal duct injuries
      d. Consideration for computed tomography (CT) angiogram studies in Le Fort II and III injuries
      e. Careful examination of cranial nerves V and VII
   C. **Neck trauma** frequently mandates immediate intervention during the primary survey to secure the airway or control bleeding. The neck is an anatomically rich region containing major respiratory, digestive, vascular, endocrine, and neurologic structures in a small cross-sectional area.
      1. From a surgical standpoint, the neck is divided into **three anatomic zones.** Zone I is between the clavicles and cricoid cartilage. Zone II is between the cricoid and the angle of the mandible. Zone III is between the angle of the mandible and the skull base.
      2. There is ongoing debate as to which injuries require surgical exploration, other diagnostic evaluation, or close monitoring. "Hard signs" of major injury including active bleeding, expanding hematoma, bruit or thrill, hoarseness, subcutaneous emphysema, sucking wound, and dysphagia require emergent exploration. Otherwise, consideration is made for angiography, laryngoscopy, bronchoscopy, and esophagoscopy.
      3. **Cervical spine injuries:** see **Chapter 10.**
   D. **Chest trauma**
      1. **Myocardial injury**
         a. **Penetrating.** Any penetrating injury to the precordium should be suspected of having injured the heart until proven otherwise. The **right ventricle** is at the greatest risk of injury. Stab wounds more commonly present with tamponade, whereas gunshot wounds tend

to create larger defects and present with bleeding and hypovolemic shock.

(1) **Evaluation.** Patients may present with the classic Beck's triad of pericardial tamponade (muffled heart sounds, hypotension, and distended neck veins). Hemodynamically stable patients should undergo echocardiography to assess for pericardial fluid. If the results are equivocal, a subxiphoid pericardial window should be performed in the operating room.

(2) **Treatment.** Resuscitation should utilize the ATLS guidelines with volume resuscitation via large-bore intravenous (IV) lines. Stable patients with positive pericardial fluid should be expeditiously transported to the operating room. Unstable or borderline patients should undergo an emergent thoracotomy to relieve tamponade and then be transported to the operating room. Pericardiocentesis has no role in the diagnosis of tamponade because of a high false-negative rate. Very rarely it can have a therapeutic role in a setting where thoracotomy cannot be performed expeditiously.

b. **Blunt cardiac injury (BCI),** formerly referred to as cardiac contusion, occurs in 8% to 71% of all patients with blunt chest trauma. It can encompass a variety of injuries, including myonecrosis, valvular disruption, coronary artery dissection, and/or thrombosis.

(1) Unfortunately, BCI has few reliable **signs and symptoms.** One must therefore maintain a high index of suspicion in patients with an appropriate mechanism of injury or in patients who have an inappropriate cardiovascular response to the level of their injury.

(2) **Evaluation.** All patients with suspected BCI should have a 12-lead **ECG** performed on admission that has a negative predictive value of greater than 95%. If the ECG is abnormal (arrhythmia, ST changes, heart block), the patient should be admitted for continuous ECG monitoring for 24 to 48 hours. Measurement of cardiac enzymes is controversial. Creatine kinase (CK) and CK-MB fraction tend to have poor sensitivity and specificity. Measurements of **troponin I and T** have shown an improved specificity and sensitivity. The ideal timing for measuring troponin has not been determined and a second set may need to be repeated in 4 to 6 hours after injury. Echocardiogram should be used as a complementary test in those patients with abnormal results on physical examination and in those with persistent symptoms for more than 12 hours or in hemodynamically unstable patients.

(3) **Treatment.** BCI is managed mostly symptomatically in stable patients. If there is evidence of pericardial fluid on echocardiogram and the clinical picture is consistent with tamponade, the patient should have a subxiphoid pericardiotomy in the operating room or an anterolateral thoracotomy if in extremis. Severe cardiac dyskinesis may require hemodynamic support with inotropes and/or intra-aortic balloon pump.

2. **Traumatic aortic disruption (TAD)** is the second most common cause of death after motor vehicle accidents. Most commonly, it occurs at the aortic isthmus (90%), where the descending aorta is relatively fixed to the main pulmonary artery by the *ligamentum arteriosum.* Transection may be partial thickness, similar to a tear in aortic dissection, or full thickness and equivalent to a ruptured aneurysm (**Fig. 9-2**).

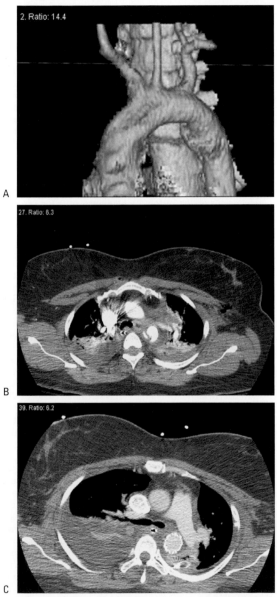

FIGURE 9-2 Traumatic aortic disruption. Panel **A:** Three-dimensional CT scan reconstructed image showing aortic injury just distal to the left subclavian artery takeoff. Panel **B:** Cross-sectional CT scan of the same injury before repair. Panel **C:** Cross-sectional CT scan of the injury after repair with an endoluminal stent. CT, computed tomography.

a. **Evaluation.** TAD should be suspected in any patient with severe head trauma, multiple extremity fractures, multiple rib fractures, and/or a mechanism of injury that involves rapid deceleration. Symptoms are nonspecific, with chest pain, back pain, and dyspnea being the most frequent. Physical findings are also nonspecific. External chest trauma is evident in 70% to 90% of patients, but less than one-third of patients will have unequal pulses or blood pressures in extremities. Evaluation should begin with a **chest radiogram** demonstrating widening of the mediastinum. Other potential findings include loss of the aortic knob, depression of left main bronchus, lateral deviation of the trachea, apical pleural hematoma, left hemothorax, scapular fractures, and fractures of the first and second ribs. A normal chest radiogram does not rule out the diagnosis of TAD. **Angiography** has been replaced at most centers with helical **CT scan** as a primary screening test. The CT scan can show either the absence of a mediastinal hematoma, thus ruling out TAD, or clear signs of disruption. An equivocal situation can occur with an isolated mediastinal hematoma without other signs of aortic injury and these patients should undergo **transesophageal echocardiogram** (TEE), if the expertise exists.

b. **Treatment.** Initial resuscitation follows ATLS guidelines. However, volume resuscitation is limited to maintaining systolic blood pressure around 100 mm Hg. Invasive hemodynamic monitoring should be instituted with a right radial a-line. **IV β-blockade** and a vasodilator such as **sodium nitroprusside** should be used to keep the systolic arterial blood pressure less than 100 mm Hg and the heart rate around 60. Adequate analgesia and sedation are also important. **Prompt surgical therapy** is the best approach, if the general conditions of the patient allow it. Operative treatment may be delayed in multitrauma patients while other injuries are being stabilized. A subset of patients who are elderly or have comorbidities that prohibit emergency thoracic surgery such as sepsis, extensive burns, or severe central nervous injury may be managed medically with strict antihypertensive therapy that is transitioned from parenteral to enteral. The favored repair for stable patients is **percutaneous aortic stent grafting**. Postoperatively, the patient should be closely observed for possible **paraplegia** related to occluding the anterior spinal artery (see also **Chapter 39**).

3. **Pulmonary injuries**

a. **Pneumothorax** occurs when air becomes trapped within the pleural cavity outside the lung, causing the lung to collapse. Chest tube placement is standard initial treatment for pneumothorax, although close observation of minimal pneumothoraces seen on CT only is acceptable. Recent data show that for a pneumothorax <3 cm in maximal length from the lung to chest wall on CT scan, there is a 95% likelihood of spontaneous resolution. Once the pneumothorax has been evacuated and there is no air leak for 24 hours, the chest tube is put to water seal. If no pneumothorax develops on water seal, the tube may be removed.

b. **Hemothorax** occurs when blood from a chest wall or lung injury accumulates in the pleural cavity. Hemothorax should be treated promptly. Return of greater than 1,000 cm^3 of blood upon placement or continuous output of greater than 200 cm^3/h for 4 hours suggests the need for operative evaluation. If evacuation is not complete by 48 to 72 hours, strong consideration should be given for further intervention including instillation of **tissue plasminogen activator (TPA)** or **video-assisted thoracic surgery (VATS)** intervention. All efforts should be made to fully evacuate the hemothorax by day 7 since around this time the clot organizes with increased difficulty in evacuation and increased rate of empyema and fibrothorax.

c. **Pulmonary contusion** is common with chest trauma. The treatment involves judicious fluid resuscitation in conjunction with pain control and lung protective ventilation (**Chapter 20**) for intubated patients.

d. **Pulmonary laceration** occurs with penetrating and blunt injuries resulting in hemothorax, pneumothorax, or pneumatocele (pockets of air trapped within the lung parenchyma). Most lacerations are managed by tube thoracostomy and heal without further operative intervention, but those involving the most proximal bronchi may require surgical repair.

e. **Bronchopleural fistula** occurs when air leaks from a larger, more proximal airway, and should be suspected with large and persistent air leaks in chest tube. Immediate treatment requires bronchoscopic evaluation with surgical intervention.

4. **Diaphragmatic rupture** can at times be easily noted on chest radiogram, but is often more subtle and only detected by having a high index of suspicion. Fine cut CT and contrast studies may be helpful (**Fig. 9-3**). The left side is involved more frequently than the right side. Diaphragmatic paralysis may result from the injury and cause significant respiratory compromise.

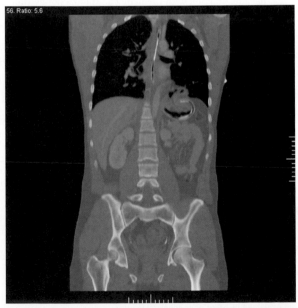

FIGURE 9-3 Computed tomography scan showing left diaphragmatic injury with partial gastric herniation in the left chest.

5. **Chest wall** injuries can involve any part of the bony structure or soft tissue of the thorax.
   a. **Rib fractures** commonly complicate blunt thoracic trauma.
      (1) The first and second rib fractures indicate a high-energy mechanism of injury and a greater association with underlying pulmonary, neurologic, and vascular injuries.
      (2) Fractures of the lower chest (ribs 8–12) should raise the suspicion for diaphragmatic, hepatic, splenic, or renal injury.
      (3) With multiple fractures, there may be mechanical instability (flail chest) resulting in respiratory compromise or even failure. Positive-pressure ventilation acts like a splint in these cases. Pain tends to be significant and can also cause significant respiratory compromise. For multiple rib fractures, **epidural analgesia** provides excellent relief. Multiple intercostals blocks can be used to provide early temporary relief and to break the cycle of pain while systemic analgesia is achieved. For multiple fractures with extensive displacement of the bone, internal fixation can expedite healing and recovery.
      (4) **Scapular fractures** also indicate a high-energy mechanism of injury. They do not typically require surgical intervention, unless the fracture extends into the glenoid fossa.
   b. **Clavicular fractures** occur commonly, do not tend to have associated injuries, and are most often treated with a figure-of-eight sling.
E. **Abdomen**
   1. **Solid organs**
      a. The management of solid-organ injury has evolved over the last decade. Starting with the pediatric trauma population, there has been a gradual shift toward **nonoperative management** of a select group of patients with both liver and spleen injuries. Recent consensus from the Eastern Association for the Surgery of Trauma (EAST) has concluded that there are sufficient class II data to support the nonoperative management of blunt hepatic and splenic injuries in hemodynamically stable patients (**Table 9-1**).
      b. **Evaluation/management:** Most trauma centers now use the **FAST examination** instead of peritoneal lavage to evaluate for the presence of intraperitoneal blood. Hemodynamically unstable patients with a positive examination should undergo operative exploration. Stable patients with a positive FAST examination should undergo CT of the abdomen with IV contrast to further identify and assess the severity of injury. However, the grade of injury and the degree of hemoperitoneum cannot fully predict the outcome of nonoperative management (**Table 9-2**). The hemodynamic status of the patient is

TABLE 9-1	Criteria for Nonoperative Management of Solid-organ Injury

Hemodynamic stability
Documentation of injury by computed tomography scan
No active contrast extravasation or pooling on computed tomography scan
Absence of other injuries requiring laparotomy
Absence of ongoing blood transfusion requirement or a persistently decreasing hematocrit that is not explained by other nonabdominal injuries
Ability to perform serial abdominal examinations

TABLE 9-2		American Association for the Surgery of Trauma Hepatic Injury Scale
Grade		**Injury Description**
I	Hematoma	Subcapsular, nonexpanding, <10 surface area
	Laceration	Capsular, nonbleeding, <1 cm depth
II	Hematoma	Subcapsular, nonexpanding, 10%–50% surface area
		Intraparenchymal, nonexpanding, <2 cm diameter
	Laceration	Capsular, active bleeding, 1–3 cm depth, <10 cm length
III	Hematoma	Subcapsular, expanding, or >50 surface area
		Ruptured subcapsular with active bleeding
		Intraparenchymal >2 cm diameter or expanding
	Laceration	>3 cm depth
IV	Hematoma	Ruptured central hematoma with active bleeding
	Laceration	25%–50% of lobe parenchymal disruption
V	Hematoma	>50% of lobe parenchymal disruption
	Laceration	Venous disruption: major hepatic veins, retrohepatic inferior vena cava
VI	Hepatic avulsion	

the most reliable criterion for deciding on operative versus nonoperative management. Another predictor is contrast pooling or active contrast extravasation on CT, which indicates active bleeding (**Fig. 9-4**). CT scans can, however, miss hollow viscous injury in 2% to 15% of patients. **Angiography** has been increasingly used to both diagnose and treat (by **embolization**) bleeding in both hepatic and splenic injuries.

c. **The liver** is the most commonly injured solid abdominal organ in both penetrating and blunt trauma. The incidence of rebleeding following hepatic injury is less than 3% of all patients managed

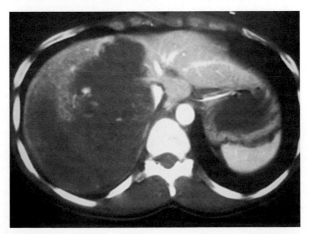

FIGURE 9-4 Large liver injury with contrast "blush" on the computed tomography scan suggesting active hemorrhage.

nonoperatively. In addition, if bleeding recurs, it does not follow the pattern of catastrophic bleeding that can be associated with splenic injuries. Transfusion requirement has been shown to be actually higher in operative cases than in nonoperative ones. Other potential complications include liver abscess and biliary tract injury with bilomas and hemobilia. These are rare and will usually manifest by physical signs and symptoms.

   d. **Spleen.** In contrast to hepatic trauma, the nonoperative management of splenic injuries has a 5% to 10% failure rate and bleeding can be brisk, potentially causing hemodynamic instability. Rebleeding most often occurs within days after injury, but may be delayed till several weeks later. A second peak in frequency occurs around 7 days after injury. Patients with splenic injuries should have frequent hematocrit checks. A continued transfusion requirement may indicate the need for an operation or angiography and embolization. Patients who undergo splenectomy may have a transient **thrombocytosis** of 600,000 to 1,000,000. **Aspirin, 325 mg/d,** is recommended if the count is higher than 1,000,000 to try to minimize thrombosis. Patients should also receive **vaccination** against *Pneumococcus, Haemophilus influenzae,* and *Meningococcus,* although the timing of vaccination is controversial. Some advocate immediate postoperative vaccination (trauma patients do not always reliably return for follow-up) and others prefer to wait 2 weeks. Antibiotics for these patients should be given at first signs of infection and with invasive procedures rather than as a daily prophylactic dose.

   e. **Follow-up.** Patients with both hepatic and splenic trauma should have serial abdominal examinations and hematocrit checks. Follow-up CT scans are not routinely indicated unless there is a change in clinical status or an unexplained drop in hematocrit, which may represent ongoing bleeding. There is no evidence that bed rest is necessary; however, the time to resuming normal activity is variable and depends on the extent and severity of injury.

2. **Pancreatic injuries** are often seen in conjunction with duodenal injuries and with upper lumbar fractures. These carry a high rate of complications and mortality. It is important to keep a high index of suspicion with elevations in amylase and lipase. CT scans can be used to look for fracture of the pancreas, peripancreatic fluid, or fluid in the lesser sac (**Fig. 9-5**).

3. **Hollow viscus** injuries occur with both blunt and penetrating trauma. There is a high association with other injuries. The **small bowel** is the most commonly injured viscus in penetrating trauma. Seat belts, when not appropriately worn across the iliac wings, can cause rupture of the small bowel or colon. Free air requires surgical exploration. Free fluid on CT scan is most often blood and not enteric contents. However, free fluid without solid-organ injury must raise the clinician's level of suspicion. In this situation, serial abdominal examinations with careful evaluation of the patient's vital signs, arterial blood gases, and complete blood count is crucial. Likewise, penetrating injuries, especially low-energy mechanisms such as stab wounds, are being followed nonoperatively more frequently. The expectant approach requires a high level of vigilance by the clinician looking for changes on the physical examination or on laboratory tests. A missed bowel injury will typically declare itself within 12 to 18 hours.

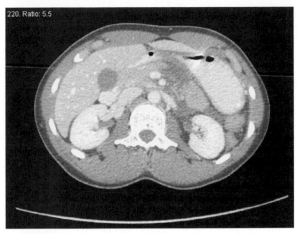

FIGURE 9-5 Pancreatic injury. Cross-sectional computed tomography scan of the abdomen demonstrating a complete transection of the pancreas just lateral to the superior mesenteric vessels. This is the classic location for this injury following blunt trauma.

   F. **Urologic injuries** occur with both penetrating and blunt trauma. It is useful to consider whether the upper (ureter and kidneys) or lower (bladder and urethra) organs are involved.
      1. **Evaluation.** Macroscopic **hematuria** and persistent microscopic hematuria require CT examination, which can elucidate a renal injury or bladder injury with evidence of extravasation. If neither is found, a cystogram is more sensitive than CT for bladder injury and a retrograde urethrogram can demonstrate a urethral injury.
      2. **Renal injuries** are usually handled expectantly unless the patient is hemodynamically unstable. Subsequent urinomas that may develop can be handled percutaneously.
      3. **Ureteral injuries** are rare in blunt trauma and typically found at the time of exploration for penetrating trauma.
      4. **Bladder disruptions** are divided into intraperitoneal and extraperitoneal injuries. The mechanism of injury is either direct laceration of the bladder typically adjacent to the pubic symphysis or rupture related to a sudden increase in intra-abdominal pressure with a full bladder. Intraperitoneal injuries require operative repair while extraperitoneal injuries require bladder catheterization and drainage.
      5. **Urethral injuries** typically result from pelvic fractures or straddle injuries. The urethra in the man is longer, and therefore it is more vulnerable to injury. The injury most commonly occurs at the junction of the prostatic and membranous urethra. Urethral injuries can be suspected on the clinical examination. Signs include blood at the meatus, perineal or scrotal hematoma, and a high-riding prostate. These signs mandate a retrograde urethrogram prior to placement of a urinary catheter. Initial treatment is long-term catheterization.
   G. **Pelvic fractures** are often associated with other major trauma, especially brain injuries. High-volume blood loss is common and requires aggressive resuscitation with multiple large-bore IV access and massive transfusion

protocol activation. **Pelvic injuries are categorized** by the mechanism of injury into anterior-posterior compression, lateral compression, and shear. Severe anterior-posterior and shear injuries cause the greatest damage by increasing the volume of the pelvis and disrupting the extensive plexus of retroperitoneal veins. Initial treatment involves decreasing the volume by externally or internally fixating the pelvis. This can be accomplished with a binder, external fixator, or internal plating. Other treatment options include angiographic embolization and preperitoneal packing.

H. **Extremity injuries** frequently involve bone, muscle, nerves, and blood vessels.

1. The bones require stabilization through splinting followed by external fixation and ultimately internal fixation. Open fractures require urgent operative intervention with irrigation, debridement, and coverage. Long bone fractures can lead to large-volume blood loss, even if the fracture is closed. A femur fracture can lead to loss of 1 L of blood in the thigh. Additionally, long bone fractures can result in **fat emboli syndrome (FES)** either directly related to the fracture or following reaming and manipulation of the bone during repair. FES is believed to result from deposition of fat globules into the venous system from the bone marrow. The globules deposit in the pulmonary and cerebral circulation causing an inflammatory response. The inflammation causes tachycardia, which is worsened by hypoxia from an increased ventilation/perfusion mismatch. A careful examination demonstrates petechial hemorrhages in the upper body as well as subconjunctival and retinal hemorrhages. Neurologic symptoms include delirium, seizure, or altered level of consciousness with worsening Glasgow Coma Scale scores.

2. As soon as the clinical situation permits, a careful neurologic examination should be completed to look for occult neurologic injury. **Table 9-3** includes a list of fractures and nerve injuries commonly seen with the fracture.

3. Any suspicion of vascular compromise should be screened with measurement of an ankle-brachial index (ABI) or brachio-brachial index (BBI). An ABI of less than 0.9 or a BBI of less than 1 should prompt an angiographic evaluation of the vasculature of the extremity in question.

4. Soft tissue injuries can carry a high morbidity in terms of long-term loss of function as well as having profound immediate systemic effects.

   a. **Crush injury** is the most severe form of soft tissue injury. This can manifest as crush syndrome with cell membrane injury and release of intracellular contents producing systemic hypotension, circulatory shock, muscle swelling, and acute myoglobinuric renal failure. Renal failure occurs secondary to shock and precipitation of myoglobin, urate, and phosphate in the distal convoluted tubules and form tubular casts.

   b. **Evaluation** for patients with crush injury includes monitoring **serum CK levels**. Peak CK level has been shown to correlate with the

TABLE 9-3	Common Fractures and Associated Nerve Injuries
Humeral neck fracture	Axillary nerve
Proximal humerus fracture	Radial nerve
Elbow fracture or dislocation	Ulnar nerve
Proximal tibial fracture	Peroneal nerve

development of renal failure, with the highest risk in patients with CK levels greater than 75,000.

c. **Management.** After the initial trauma evaluation, patients with crush injury should have a urinary catheter placed to measure hourly urine production. Prevention of renal failure requires maintenance of urine output (>0.5 mL/kg/h) and consideration for alkalinizing the urine with 2 to 3 ampoules of bicarbonate per liter of IV fluids and following the urine pH.

III. Special considerations

A. Abdominal compartment syndrome (ACS)

1. Although commonly associated with damage control laparotomy, ACS is not uniquely associated with trauma. It can be seen in patients with ruptured abdominal aortic aneurysms, pancreatitis, neoplasms, massive ascites, liver transplantation, retroperitoneal hemorrhage, pneumoperitoneum, massive fluid resuscitation, or circumferential abdominal burns. ACS is defined as elevated intra-abdominal pressure (IAP) associated with organ dysfunction. Normal IAP is atmospheric pressure. The level at which IAP causes ACS is not well defined, but pressure above 15 mm Hg is associated with physiologic changes, and vascular congestion probably occurs around 25 mm Hg.

2. **Pathophysiology.** ACS causes many derangements in normal physiology.
   a. **Cardiac output** is decreased secondary to decreased venous return from the inferior vena cava (IVC). Extracardiac intrathoracic pressure also increases and impairs ventricular diastolic filling, further decreasing stroke volume and cardiac output. Central venous pressure and pulmonary artery wedge pressure both are elevated. Cardiac imaging will reveal a small but hyperdynamic left ventricle.
   b. **Pulmonary.** The lungs are compressed by the elevated diaphragms, causing reduced lung volumes, atelectasis, and hypoxemia. Pulmonary compliance is reduced and airway pressures are increased.
   c. **Renal** perfusion and glomerular filtration progressively decrease as IAP increases. A decline in urine output occurs with oliguria at IAP of 15 to 20 mm Hg, and anuria occurs at IAP greater than 30 mm Hg. This occurs secondary to the decreased cardiac output and direct compression of the renal parenchyma. Elevated levels of renin, antidiuretic hormone, and aldosterone further contribute to the low urine output.
   d. **Perfusion to all abdominal viscera** is compromised. This can lead to abnormalities in gut mucosal barrier function, bacterial translocation, and eventually gut ischemia.

3. **Evaluation.** IAP can be measured indirectly via an indwelling urinary catheter. The easiest method is to instill 50 to 100 mL of sterile saline into the bladder connected to a T-connector. The catheter is then clamped and intravesical pressure can be measured using a pressure transducer or a manometer connected to the other arm of the T-connector. The symphysis pubis is used as a zero reference point.

4. **Treatment.** Initial treatment involves pharmacological paralysis, which relaxes the abdominal wall musculature and is often sufficient to decrease the pressure. The next step is to reduce the intra-abdominal volume by removal of peritoneal blood, foreign bodies such as laparotomy pads, fluid, or tumor. Commonly, the abdomen is left open with a sterile silo or vacuum dressing in place. Treatment should be instituted

on an urgent basis. Relief of elevated pressure should produce almost an immediate improvement in cardiopulmonary parameters. Renal and visceral impairments will improve as long as irreversible ischemic damage had not already occurred.

B. **Extremity compartment syndrome** is caused by an increase in intracompartmental pressure, with obstruction of the venous outflow and capillary beds in the extremity. It results from a crush injury, a vascular injury with subsequent limb ischemia and reperfusion, or secondary to massive resuscitation following another injury.

1. **Signs and symptoms.** Compartment syndrome is marked by **pain** (out of proportion to injury) and **paresthesia.** On examination, one or all of the compartments **are swollen, there is sensory loss and pain on passive movement of the muscle.** Loss of pulses is a late sign. Unfortunately, most of the signs and symptoms cannot be easily assessed in the sedated ICU patient and a high index of suspicion is necessary. Any question of elevated compartment pressure should prompt measurement using some form of manometry. The normal pressure is between 0 and 8 mm Hg in resting muscle. The critical pressure for diagnosis of compartment syndrome is debated. Typically, sustained pressures greater than 25 mm Hg or a difference between the diastolic pressure and the ICP of less than 30 mm Hg prompts surgical intervention. Of note, the clinical examination is notoriously insensitive.

2. **Treatment.** The primary treatment is by decompression with **fasciotomies** of all compartments in the affected extremity. The fasciotomy wounds are usually left to heal by secondary intention or undergo delayed skin closure several days after decompression.

C. **Damage control surgery**

1. **Introduction.** Over the last 15 to 20 years, definitive initial operative intervention with repair of all injuries has been abandoned in favor of damage control surgery. The goal of a damage control operation is **to control bleeding and enteric contamination.** The patient is then resuscitated in the ICU with the goals of restoring physiologic reserve and avoiding the development of hypothermia, coagulopathy, and metabolic acidosis. The patient is subsequently brought back to the operating room, sometimes on several occasions, for further therapy. The critical care team must be ready to address the consequences of massive bleeding and peritoneal contamination, to allow for as early as possible definitive repair of injuries.

2. **Hypothermia.** Studies have shown that trauma patients with core temperatures of less than 32°C have 100% mortality. Hypothermia has an inhibitory effect on both the coagulation cascade and platelet function that is underestimated by the usual laboratory tests, because most laboratories rewarm the plasma to 37°C before measuring clotting times. External rewarming techniques such as blankets or convective hot air can help to decrease heat loss, but are not very efficient in transferring heat back to the patient. Pleural or peritoneal lavage with warm fluid can result in significant heat transfer, but large amounts of fluid are required. Administration of warm IV fluids and especially rewarming blood products, which are stored at 4°C, is critical. Cardiopulmonary bypass and continuous arteriovenous rewarming are the most rapid methods available.

3. **Coagulopathy.** Trauma patients can develop clotting factor depletion leading to a consumption coagulopathy and activation of fibrinolysis. Shock itself can lead to a dilutional thrombocytopenia that is independent of blood loss. Treatment should begin with transfusions

of fresh frozen plasma, clotting factors, and platelets. Early initiation of **massive transfusion protocols** (see **Chapter 35**) offers the best opportunity to avoid coagulopathy. The precise ratios of red cells to plasma to platelets is unknown, but it appears that early administration of 1 U of plasma to 2 U of blood and a 10-pack of platelets for every 10 U of product administered improves coagulopathy and reduces mortality. It is important to treat early and aggressively, which often means initiating massive transfusion protocols prior to return of laboratory values.

4. **Acidosis.** Hypovolemic shock can result in tissue hypoperfusion and metabolic acidosis. This in turn can lead to decreased cardiac output, hypotension, and arrhythmias, further worsening the shock state. Failure to timely resuscitate the patient and correct the acidosis leads to a higher incidence of multisystem organ failure and death.

D. **Resuscitation considerations**

1. **Permissive hypotension.** There is evidence to suggest that hypotension is an adaptive response to decrease bleeding and allow clot formation. Therefore, in the non–head-injured patient, many clinicians are recommending resuscitating to a systolic blood pressure of 70 to 80 mm Hg until the bleeding is controlled.

2. **Albumin versus crystalloid.** No data have definitely shown the superiority of albumin versus crystalloid for resuscitation of trauma patients. However, data exist to **discourage the use of albumin in the head-injured patient.**

3. **Lactated Ringer's (LR) solution versus saline.** For patients with closed head injuries, saline is the fluid of choice to help maintain plasma sodium concentrations. Otherwise, **LR solution is preferred** because saline tends to contribute to hyperchloremic metabolic acidosis. However, there is an increasing body of literature suggesting that all crystalloid fluids have side effects and they should be used carefully and in modest doses. Most importantly, aggressive fluid resuscitation can worsen bleeding, making early hemorrhage control even more important.

4. **Line placement considerations.** The traumatized patient offers several additional points of consideration when placing IV lines. Trauma lines placed emergently should be changed within 24 hours of placement, if complete sterile precautions were not maintained. The subclavian position has a lower rate of infection than does the femoral or internal jugular, and should be used preferentially. Care should be taken to not place IV cannulas in injured extremities and to not administer fluids distal to a repaired or ligated vessel. Likewise, efforts should be made to avoid passing a catheter through a repaired vessel.

IV. **Procedures**

A. **Percutaneous tracheostomy** is done commonly under bronchoscopic guidance. The tissue overlying the trachea is anesthetized and a vertical incision is made. The tissues are spread and Seldinger's technique is used to dilate a tracheal hole and eventually pass a tracheostomy tube. The technique has been demonstrated to be as safe as an open tracheostomy. The track is mature by day 5 and the tube may be changed or downsized. Optimal timing for tracheostomy in trauma patients is debated. There is evidence to suggest that early tracheostomy (within the first week) reduces pneumonia and length of ventilation. However, no survival difference has been demonstrated.

B. **Percutaneous endoscopic gastrostomy** can be completed under ultrasound guidance or with direct visualization via a gastroscope. Complications include infection, often at the skin level, intra-abdominal injury, or displacement of the tube.

V. Deep vein thrombosis (DVT) prophylaxis (see also **Chapter 13**). Trauma patients are at increased risk for DVT due to immobility, altered vascular function secondary to injury and inflammation, and decreased blood flow. **Low-molecular-weight heparin** has been demonstrated in the elective orthopedic surgery population to be superior to unfractionated heparin for the prevention of DVT. The studies in the trauma population, however, have produced mixed results. **Sequential compression devices** are widely used but the evidence demonstrating effectiveness is lacking. Current EAST guidelines suggest using **low-molecular-weight heparin** with consideration of compression devices as a supplement only. In most cases, the low-molecular-weight heparin should be started as soon possible, preferably within 24 hours of admission. **IVC filter** placement is also controversial. While Class I data demonstrating long-term benefit in prevention of PE or survival are lacking, it has become a common procedure in the trauma population, with the accumulation of Class II and III data. IVC filters should be placed in patients who develop new emboli or who propagate old thrombus while anticoagulated, as well as patients with emboli or proximal thrombus in whom anticoagulation is contraindicated. The use of prophylactic filters in patients who are high risk but are not anticoagulation candidates is controversial.

VI. Shock in the trauma patient
   A. Hypovolemic. Sources of hemorrhage include external, intrathoracic, intraperitoneal, or retroperitoneal bleeding, and bleeding into extremities with long bone fractures. Additional, soft tissue shear injuries can create large spaces, which can be filled with massive volumes of blood. The treatment entails establishing multiple large-bore IV accesses and initiating massive transfusion protocols. Blood products should be warmed and administered in the ratios described earlier (**Section III.C.3**). Most importantly, the source of bleeding must be addressed.
   B. Obstructive. Pericardial tamponade with a cardiac injury or tension pneumothorax with rotation of the heart and blockage of the venous return can produce hypotension and shock.
   C. Cardiogenic. Shock can result from cardiac pump failure related to direct myocardial injury or injury to the coronary arteries. Treatment is most frequently supportive in nature. Rarely, there is an injury to the heart itself to address.
   D. Distributive. Spinal cord injury can cause loss of vascular tone with subsequent inability to maintain blood pressure and perfusion. This is most commonly caused by a cervical injury, above the level of C5, but can occur even with thoracic injuries as low as T4. Treatment involves increasing the circulating volume through resuscitation and then using vasopressors to improve organ perfusion.

Selected References

Alam HB, Rhee P. New developments in fluid resuscitation. *Surg Clin North Am* 2007; 87(1):55–72.

Cameron JL. *Current surgical therapy.* 9th ed. St. Louis: Mosby, 2008.

Demetriades D, Velmahos GC, Scalea TM, et al; American Association for the Surgery of Trauma Thoracic Aortic Injury Study Group. Operative repair or endovascular stent graft in blunt traumatic thoracic aortic injuries: results of an American Association for the Surgery of Trauma Multicenter Study. *J Trauma* 2008;64(3):561–570.

Eastern Association for the Surgery of Trauma (2009). Trauma practice guidelines. Chicago, IL. http://www.east.org/Portal/Default.aspx?tabid=57.

Feliciano D, Mattox K, Moore E. *Trauma*. 6th ed. New York: McGraw-Hill, 2007.

Hoffman JR, Mower WR, Wolfson AB, et al. Validity of a set of clinical criteria to rule out injury to the cervical spine in patients with blunt trauma. *N Engl J Med* 2000;343:94–99.

Lee JC, Peitzman AB. Damage-control laparotomy. *Curr Opin Crit Care* 2006;12:346–350.

MacKenzie EJ, Rivara FP, Jurkovich GJ, et al. A national evaluation of the effect of trauma-center care on mortality. *N Engl J Med* 2006;354:366–378.

Maerz L, Kaplan LJ. Abdominal compartment syndrome. *Crit Care Med* 2008; 36(suppl): S212–S215.

Neschis DG, Scalea TM, Flinn WR, Griffith BP. Blunt aortic injury. *N Engl J Med* 2008; 359:1708–1716.

Velmahos GC, Alam HB. Advances in surgical critical care. *Curr Probl Surg* 2008;45(7):453–516.

Wilson WC, Grande CM, Hoyt DB. *Trauma*. New York: Informa Healthcare, 2007.

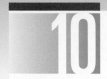

Critical Care of the Neurologic Patient

Kevin Sheth and Lee Schwamm

I. **Neuroprotection** is the goal of neurocritical care.
  A. **Common presenting symptoms** that require neurocritical care intervention include weakness, cognitive dysfunction, reduced alertness with or without impaired airway reflexes, uncontrolled seizures, and respiratory muscle failure.
  B. **Diagnoses** likely to produce these symptoms include subarachnoid, subdural, or intracerebral hemorrhage; ischemic stroke; brain tumor; infectious or inflammatory meningoencephalitis; traumatic brain or spinal cord injury; status epilepticus, toxic-metabolic encephalopathy; amyotrophic lateral sclerosis; myasthenia gravis and acute myopathies; and polyneuropathies.
  C. Because cerebral ischemia and hypoxemia are the most common mechanisms of secondary brain injury, a thorough understanding of the regulation of **cerebral blood flow (CBF)** is necessary. Familiarity with the neurologic examination of the critically ill patient is required for early recognition of secondary brain injury and subsequent evaluation of the efficacy of therapeutic interventions.
  D. Three aspects distinguish hemodynamic management in neurocritical care from that of other critically ill patients:
    1. Assessment of end-organ perfusion is at times more difficult to determine.
    2. Because of the lack of local energy reserves, the interval to end-organ failure under adverse conditions is more rapid.
    3. Unlike most other organs, injury to even small regions of brain can have devastating consequences.

II. **Intracranial hemodynamics**
  A. **Intracranial compliance.** The skull is a rigid box filled with incompressible brain parenchyma. When the volume inside the skull increases, there is evacuation of cerebrospinal fluid (CSF) into the extracranial subarachnoid space followed by a rapid rise in **intracranial pressure (ICP; Fig. 10-1)**. **ICP** is normally less than 10 mm Hg; transient elevations up to 30 mm Hg are well tolerated. When ICP rises above 20 mm Hg (or **cerebral perfusion pressure [CPP]** falls below 60 mm Hg), CBF may be inadequate. In addition, the anatomy of various vaults and dural reflections can allow for compartmentalization of pressures. Pressure gradients may exist between compartments and lead to clinical herniation even though measured or global ICP may not be significantly elevated.
  B. **ICP monitoring devices and potential complications**
    1. The most common device is an **external ventricular drain (EVD)** in which a ventricular catheter is connected to a transducer. The setup involves an external fluid column and is analogous to those used for arterial and central venous pressure (CVP) monitoring. The risk of complications is greatest with this device, especially intracranial hemorrhage

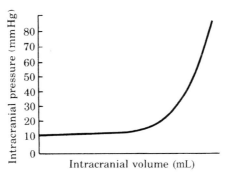

FIGURE 10-1 Intracranial compliance curve. In the normal ICP range; increases in intracranial volume produce minimal changes in ICP initially. Further small increases in intracranial volume at the "elbow" of the curve, however, can produce an abrupt increase in ICP. ICP, intracranial pressure.

upon insertion, and infection increases with duration of EVD presence. The great advantage is that this allows for drainage of CSF and can be recalibrated as needed. This also is least susceptible to false readings.

2. Less invasive are the transducer-tipped **fiberoptic intraparenchymal catheters** which can be placed through a mini-craniotomy. These devices have essentially replaced the prior subarachnoid screw known commonly as an "ICP bolt" that transduced the pressure via a diaphragm that was directly in contact with the subarachnoid fluid. The modern fiberoptic device is placed several millimeters into the cortex but cannot be recalibrated once it has been placed. This requires special signal transducing monitors and may not be compatible with the available monitoring systems if patients are transferred between institutions. External transducers require periodic recalibration to remain accurate, sometimes called "zeroing" because of the task of zero calibrating to the level of the foramen of Monro. Antibiotic therapy as indicated and monitoring for coagulopathy are essential.

C. **CBF** equals CPP divided by the cerebrovascular resistance (CVR), according to Ohm's law. CPP is the difference between the mean intracerebral artery pressure (hard to measure) and the mean ICP (easy to measure). CVR (hard to measure) is the ability of the precapillary arterioles to dilate and constrict in response to changes in pressure or metabolic factors. Because CBF is cumbersome to measure directly and is held relatively constant over a mean arterial pressure (MAP) between 50 and 150 mm Hg in healthy, young individuals, a CPP of 60 to 90 mm Hg likely provides appropriate CBF (**Fig. 10-2**).

D. **Autoregulation of CBF is often impaired** in patients with acute cerebral injury. In this setting, reductions in CPP below 60 mm Hg may decrease CBF and cause cerebral ischemia. Increases in CPP above 80 mm Hg may increase CBF and cause vasogenic edema and increased ICP. An optimal CPP goal should therefore include both a minimum and a maximum range.

E. **Tissue oxygen delivery.** Because brain energy metabolism is dependent on continuous tissue oxygen influx, the primary focus should be optimal tissue oxygen delivery. Over a wide range of temperature and pH, oxygen delivery is proportional to the oxygen saturation, hemoglobin content, and cardiac output. Cardiac output may be compromised due to

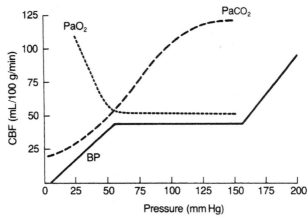

FIGURE 10-2 Autoregulation maintains a constant level of CBF over a wide range of carotid artery mean BPs. Independent of this effect, CBF is elevated by hypercarbia ($PaCO_2$) and hypoxemia (PaO_2); hypocarbia diminishes CBF. BP, blood pressure; CBF, cerebral blood flow.

hypovolemia, sepsis, and impaired myocardial contractility or cardiac dysrhythmia as a complicating factor of brain or spinal cord injury.

F. **Oxygen extraction.** The immense energy requirements of the brain demand a system for oxygen delivery that can tolerate sudden increases in demand (e.g., seizures) or decreases in supply (e.g., hypotension and hypoxemia). Unlike other organs, a system of "oxygen reserve" exists in which the brain can vary its oxygen extraction from a baseline of approximately 30% to an extreme of 70% under conditions of oligemia (CBF 20–30 mL/100 g/min) or hypoxemia. It is only when CBF decreases below 20 mL/100 g/min that electrical and chemical cellular functions are interrupted and ischemic symptoms develop. Increased oxygen extraction can be demonstrated with radiolabeled oxygen species using positron emission tomography (PET) or single photon emission computed tomography (SPECT) imaging (not practical in the management of most critically ill patients), or as a decrease in **cerebral mixed venous oxygen saturation** via cerebral venous jugular bulb sampling (**$SjvO_2$**).

G. **Medications that influence ICP**
  1. **Vasodilators** such as **hydralazine, sodium nitroprusside (SNP), nitroglycerin,** and, to a lesser degree, **nicardipine** can induce cerebral vasodilation. In patients with poor intracranial compliance, this can increase ICP.
  2. **β-Adrenergic blockers** such as **labetalol** or **propranolol** have minimal direct effect on CBF or ICP and are easily titrated. Because labetalol also blocks α-adrenergic tone, it may reduce sympathetically mediated large-vessel vasoconstriction. This better simulates the endogenous mechanisms of lowering blood pressure and helps to prevent regional ischemia as blood pressure is lowered pharmacologically.
  3. **Barbiturates** such as **thiopental** and **pentobarbital,** although typically administered to lower ICP, are also potent antihypertensive agents, decreasing venous tone and cardiac contractility. This usually undesirable side effect may require the use of α- and/or β-adrenergic agonists such as **phenylephrine** and **norepinephrine** to maintain adequate CPP.

4. **Catecholamines** have an unpredictable potential to increase cerebral metabolic rate and CBF. These effects are likely to be more pronounced as BP is increased above normal and in the presence of blood–brain barrier disruption.

5. **Hypo-osmolar and iso-osmolar solutions** such as lactated Ringer's solution and half normal saline in 5% dextrose (D_5 ½ NS) may exacerbate brain edema in the setting of osmotic diuretic therapy. **Glucose-containing solutions** may produce hyperglycemia and may lead to neurologic worsening after brain ischemia.

H. **Other factors that influence ICP**

1. ICP is increased by many of the complications of **central venous access** including pneumothorax, carotid puncture, painful stimulation, and body position (e.g., Trendelenburg, lateral head rotation, jugular compression). Patients should be kept in optimal position for ICP management until the last possible moment prior to puncture.

2. **Noxious stimuli** can increase ICP, CBF, and cerebral metabolic rate and should be prevented and treated aggressively.

III. **Extracranial hemodynamics.** The primary goal of systemic blood pressure management is defined by the type of central nervous system (CNS) injury or systemic injury present. An optimal CPP must be maintained at all times. Because the MAP decreases to the same extent ($<20\%$) between the aortic root and the distal middle cerebral arteries or the radial arteries, conventionally measured systemic MAP is a reasonable surrogate for mean intracerebral artery pressure.

A. **Reduced CPP.** In the case of reduced CPP, the primary objective should be the lowering of ICP, but systemic MAP may need to be pharmacologically augmented while the ICP reduction strategies are initiated. The first choice in patients with adequate myocardial contractility should be a pure α-adrenergic agonist such as **phenylephrine** because it is well tolerated and causes minimal cerebrovascular vasoconstriction. If this does not produce sufficient blood pressure elevations or there is inadequate contractility to support the increased systemic vascular resistance, then additional inotropic support is required.

B. **Excessive CPP.** When there is evidence of excessive CBF because of severe hypertension or impaired autoregulation or blood–brain barrier permeability (e.g., eclampsia, brain neoplasm), MAP should be reduced in a reliable and highly titratable manner. Hypertension alone in the absence of excessive CBF or myocardial dysfunction should not be treated because it often reflects a homeostatic response to acute cerebral ischemia. Reductions in blood pressure can provoke cerebral ischemia in this setting.

1. **Sympathetic antagonists** such as **labetalol** reduce the systemic effects of the high-catecholamine-output states frequently associated with CNS injury, including arterial hypertension, tachycardia, cardiac irritability, neurogenic pulmonary vascular injury, and large-vessel vasoconstriction.

2. Often, additional agents are necessary, and **nicardipine** and **SNP** provide a reliable and titratable response. Both agents may lead to significant cerebral vasodilation and therefore raise ICP.

3. **Avoid sublingual administration** of short-acting calcium channel blockers, which lower pressure unpredictably without reducing sympathetic output.

C. **Cardiac dysrhythmias**

1. In large strokes and subarachnoid hemorrhage, **ST-segment changes** may be seen on the electrocardiogram (ECG), but these do not predict

future cardiovascular morbidity. Electrocardiographic changes may be diffuse or confined to a cardiovascular territory. Myocardial ischemia should always be excluded.

2. **Sympathetic outflow** associated with brain injury may provoke ventricular dysrhythmias in patients with coronary artery disease, and **Guillain-Barré syndrome** may produce an autonomic cardioneuropathy.

3. **Cervical spine injury** may cause sympathetic cardiac denervation and unopposed vagal tone, leading to bradydysrhythmias.

IV. Airway and ventilation

A. **Indications for endotracheal intubation.** Impairment of airway reflexes occurs frequently in the brain-injured patient and predisposes to aspiration and poor clearance of secretions. **Neuromuscular respiratory failure** may be seen in amyotrophic lateral sclerosis, myasthenia gravis, acute inflammatory demyelinating polyneuropathy, and critical care myopathy or polyneuropathy. **Transient apnea** in the setting of a self-limited generalized convulsion is not an indication for intubation or assisted ventilation.

B. **Complications of endotracheal intubation** (see also **Chapter 4**) include hypotension, reduced CBF, and paradoxically increased ICP due to increased transthoracic pressures. An experienced anesthesiologist should be present at the intubation of a patient with intracranial hypertension or hemorrhage.

C. **Considerations in extubation.** The ability to prevent aspiration and protect the airway is of utmost concern when extubating a neurologically ill patient. After confirming adequate cuff leak, oxygenation and ventilation exist to support independent respiratory function, the clinician should additionally evaluate the capacity for adequate airway protection. Ideally a cough and gag should be present, pharyngeal suctioning to keep the airway clear should be less frequent than hourly and not increasing. In addition, careful evaluation of the swallowing and oral function should occur, especially in patients with facial weakness. Ask the patient to protrude the tongue, lick the lips, pucker the lips, and cough volitionally. While the patient does not need to be neurologically intact for a successful extubation, poor oral control may lead to rapid failure of extubation. In addition, since hypercapnia may be poorly tolerated in patients with significant brain edema or disturbed autoregulation, the patient should be able to maintain normocapnia without ventilatory assistance and the period of peak anticipated brain swelling should have passed.

D. **Permissive hypercapnia** (see **Chapter 20**) is generally contraindicated in patients with intracranial hypertension or blood–brain barrier injuries because hypercapnia may result in unacceptable elevations of the ICP.

E. **Spontaneous or induced hyperventilation** causes acute cerebral vasoconstriction in a brain in which CO_2 reactivity is preserved. This decreases **cerebral blood volume (CBV)** and thereby ICP. If pressure autoregulation is preserved, the increased CPP may restore CBF.

1. **The brain quickly equilibrates** to changes in P_{CO_2}. A new steady state is established within 3 to 4 hours in most patients. This is accomplished by both carbonic anhydrase and nonbicarbonate buffer systems.

2. **With excessive hypocapnia,** excessive vasoconstriction may produce regional or generalized cerebral ischemia.

3. **A rapid return to baseline P_{CO_2}** may produce cerebral vasodilation, causing increased CBV and a further deleterious rise in ICP. Therefore, hyperventilation should be used as a temporizing measure until more effective and durable measures can be initiated.

4. **Lack of response to hyperventilation** is a poor prognostic sign.

F. **Neurogenic pulmonary edema.** Within minutes to hours of CNS injury, there can be increased pulmonary interstitial and alveolar fluid. This entity can be clinically difficult to distinguish from aspiration; however, fever and focal infiltrates are often absent. The alveolar fluid is usually a transudate, favoring a change in interstitial hydrostatic pressure as the culprit mechanism. It is felt by some that a massive sympathetic surge at the time of acute CNS injury may cause dramatically elevated pulmonary artery pressures and lead to capillary fracture with subsequent pulmonary edema even though the pressures at the later time of measurement are no longer elevated; however the precise pathophysiology is not completely understood. Supportive care and careful fluid management are required.

V. **Sodium and water homeostasis**
   A. The goal of fluid resuscitation in the brain-injured patient is to maintain **hyperosmolar euvolemia.** This is accomplished with the use of osmotic diuretics (e.g., **mannitol**) and hyperosmolar solutions (e.g., **hypertonic saline**). It is important to note that the distinction between 23.4% NaCl as an osmotic diuretic rather than a hyperosmolar intravenous fluid replacement is due to the predominant diuretic action of 23.4% NaCl when given as a bolus. Brain injury may disturb sodium balance in several different ways, sometimes simultaneously. Rapid shifts in subacute plasma sodium may produce demyelination or aggravate cerebral edema.
      1. **Hyponatremia**
         a. Cerebral injury may cause release of **natriuretic factors,** leading to profound **salt wasting,** that may require up to 200 mL/h of normal saline replacement or use of 3% solution in continuous infusion in addition to fludrocortisone (0.1–0.3 mg by mouth once or twice a day). This is seen most often in vasospasm after subarachnoid hemorrhage.
         b. **Syndrome of inappropriate antidiuretic hormone (SIADH)** release should be treated aggressively with normal or hypertonic saline (3%) solution and loop diuretics when intravascular volume repletion is essential and fluid restriction is contraindicated.
         c. **High-dose osmotic diuretic administration** (mannitol ≥50 g intravenously [IV] every 4 hours) rarely may demand renal solute excretion to such a degree that it causes paradoxical free water retention. This is easily treated with small doses of loop diuretic to degrade the renal-concentrating ability.
         d. **Intravascular volume depletion** remains the most common cause of hyponatremia in the neurocritical care unit. Bladder catheterization and monitoring of CVP and plasma sodium are essential.
      2. **Hypernatremia due to diabetes insipidus (DI)** may be seen after pituitary tumor resection, traumatic brain injury, central herniation syndromes, and, occasionally, vasospasm following subarachnoid hemorrhage. **Hypotonic fluids** and **vasopressin** therapy may be indicated, and hourly monitoring of urine output and specific gravity is required.
   B. **Osmotic balance**
      1. **Plasma osmolality** $= (2 \times [Na^+]) + [BUN]/2.8 + [Glucose]/18$, where BUN is blood urea nitrogen, and is normally 280 to 290 mOsm/kg.
      2. When plasma osmolality is increased above normal for more than 48 hours, intracellular osmotic particles are generated (idiogenic osmoles) and a new steady state is achieved to restore cell volume. Any rapid correction of plasma osmolality after this will result in a shift of free water into the intracranial compartment. Therefore, once osmotic agents have been initiated with sustained osmolality, they must be

withdrawn gradually to permit excretion of these idiogenic osmoles. This is true regardless of the osmotic agent.

3. **Mannitol** (0.5–1.0 g/kg IV bolus every 4–6 hours) should be given to attain the minimum osmolality sufficient to produce the desired effects, which often results in a stepwise increase in osmolar gap (osmolar gap = measured mOsm − calculated mOsm; normal ≤10). The goal of therapy is to continue until the osmolality gap is equal to or greater than 15. Osmolality in excess of 320 mOsm/kg with mannitol does not produce incremental benefits and is often associated with an increased osmolar gap and acute renal failure.

4. **Hypertonic saline** may also be used to reach a desired osmolality by directly affecting plasma sodium levels. When administering hypertonic saline solutions, frequent serum Na assessments are required to avoid a rapid change in plasma Na concentration. Hypertonic saline solutions may exacerbate or contribute to the development of congestive heart failure and should be used with caution in patients at risk; **3% NaCl** can be given as either a bolus of 150 mL every 4 to 6 hours or as a continuous infusion of 0.5 to 1.0 mL/kg/h. One administers **23.4% NaCl** as a 30- to 60-mL IV bolus every 6 hours.

5. While **corticosteroids** are useful in the management of vasogenic edema associated with brain tumors or other conditions that disrupt the blood–brain barrier, their utility in treating increased ICP is quite limited. Studies of steroids in stroke, intracerebral hemorrhage, and head injury have not demonstrated benefit.

VI. Glucose control
A. Elevated blood glucose levels after acute brain and spinal cord injuries increases tissue acidosis and edema in and around injured tissue and impairs endogenous antiinflammatory mechanisms of repair. **Hyperglycemia** (≥200 mg/dL) has been shown to be a predictor of poor outcome in the intensive care unit (ICU) population and in many forms of acute brain injury. Hypoglycemia (<60 mg/dL) can also lead to focal neurologic deficits, and glucose levels should be acutely restored with a bolus of **50% dextrose solution (D_{50})** along with 100 mg IV **thiamine** to avoid the complication of Wernicke's encephalopathy. Overall, the goal for care is to achieve normoglycemia (80–140 mg/dL) with the administration of insulin.

VII. Temperature regulation
A. The occurrence of **hyperthermia** after brain injury is very common and has been shown to increase the release of excitatory neurotransmitters, further the breakdown of the blood–brain barrier, and worsen the clinical outcome. Once the source of fever has been properly investigated and appropriate therapy initiated, antipyretic measures, such as the administration of acetaminophen 650 mg every 4 to 6 hours, surface cooling (cooling blankets, ice packs), and/or intravascular cooling catheters, should be instituted. **Normothermia** (temperature 37°C) should be the goal for all patients in the neuro-ICU.

B. **Induced hypothermia** has been shown to be neuroprotective in global ischemic brain injury after cardiac arrest but not in focal brain injury, such as traumatic brain injury, ischemic stroke, and intracerebral hemorrhage. Because of the potentially significant adverse effects, including electrolyte disturbances, cardiac arrhythmias, and coagulopathy, induced hypothermia has limited application.

VIII. Hypothesis-driven neurologic examination

A. **The neurologic examination** of the critically ill patient should document cortical, brainstem, and spinal cord function in a simple and easily reproducible manner that can be recognized by a colleague at a later point in time.

1. **Avoid confusing acronyms** and empty summaries (e.g., "MS nonfocal").
2. **Report the neurologic examination** in the following order: cognitive functions (alertness, orientation, attention, language), cranial nerves, strength, sensation, deep tendon reflexes, and other.
3. **Use a minimal stimulus** first, then escalate as needed (e.g., speak before yelling, yell before pinching).
4. **Coma** is produced by bilateral cortical or bilateral brainstem dysfunction.

B. **Cortical function. Language and attention** are lateralized in the human brain, and essentially all right-handed individuals and 85% of left-handed individuals process language in the left hemisphere and attention in the right hemisphere. The **motor cortex** (precentral gyrus) controls the contralateral limbs and directs voluntary gaze (saccades) to the contralateral field. **Sensation** is processed in the postcentral gyrus of the contralateral hemispheres. **Inattention** is common in critically ill patients (a hallmark of delirium) and often is due to medication or metabolic insults. However, the presence of a lateralizing hemiparesis, sensory loss, or gaze deviation should trigger urgent investigation. Cortical injury often produces face and arm weakness due to their large area of representation on the brain's surface.

C. **Brainstem function.** The brainstem controls involuntary eye movements, pupillary function, facial sensation, and vital functions. Knowledge of its functions is critical in the evaluation of the comatose patient and the posterior circulation acute stroke syndromes (see **Table 10-1**).

D. **Spinal cord function.** In contrast to brainstem and cortical injuries, spinal cord injury of any type (vascular, traumatic, demyelinating) often produces bilateral, symmetric impairment of the limbs but never facial weakness. Always distinguish anterior column function (strength, sensation of pin/temperature) from posterior column function (sensation of vibration, proprioception) and document sacral functions (anal sphincter tone, bulbocavernosus reflex). The **anterior spinal artery** receives contributions from

TABLE 10-1	Common Findings in Brainstem Lesions	
Lesion Level	**Common Findings**	**Anatomic Pathway**
Midbrain	Midposition fixed pupils	Light reflex pathways
	Ophthalmoplegia	Oculomotor nuclei
	Hemiparesis, Babinski sign	Cerebral peduncles
High pons	Pinpoint, reactive pupils	Sympathetic fibers
	Internuclear ophthalmoplegia	Medial longitudinal fasciculus
	Facial weakness	Facial nerve
	Reduced corneal sensation	Trigeminal nerve
Low pons	Horizontal reflex gaze paralysis	Abducens nerve, horizontal gaze center
	Hemiparesis, Babinski sign	Corticospinal, corticobulbar tracts
Medulla	Disordered breathing	Respiratory center
	Hypotension, hypertension, dysrhythmias	Vasomotor center

the vertebral arteries in the cervical region and the artery of Adamkiewicz (a branch of the abdominal aorta) in the thoracolumbar region. This anatomy creates a "watershed" vascular territory, which is prone to hypoperfusion, in the high thoracic cord.

1. **Brown-Séquard syndrome** of hemicord dysfunction is characterized by ipsilateral loss of motor and proprioceptive functions and contralateral loss of pain and temperature.

2. **Central cord syndrome** is characterized by weakness in arms more than legs and variable sensory, bladder, and bowel dysfunction. This predilection for arm involvement is due to the medial lamination of arm fibers in the descending corticospinal tracts.

3. **Anterior spinal artery syndrome** is characterized by bilateral symmetric motor weakness and disassociated sensory loss, with impairments in pain and temperature sensation and preservation of proprioception and vibration.

4. **Cauda equina syndrome** is characterized by variable degrees of bilateral lower motor neuron weakness in the legs (sparing the arms), sensory loss of the lower extremities and sacrum, and dysfunction of bowel and bladder.

5. **Mixed tract syndromes** occur commonly in traumatic injury of the spinal cord. The aim of localization is to identify the highest level of injury.

IX. **Neuroimaging.** Advances in **computed tomography (CT)** and **magnetic resonance (MR)** make it possible to noninvasively image neurovascular structures and identify sites of venous sinus thrombosis, arterial occlusion, nonocclusive dissection, focal tissue ischemia, and diffuse axonal injury (**Fig. 10-3**). Areas of mismatch between tissue hypoperfusion (oligemia) and tissue ischemia can be identified to measure tissue at risk. Spinal cord compression or ischemia can also be rapidly evaluated. With appropriate planning, MR imaging can be performed in the presence of a halo vest or invasive monitoring. Extra lengths of rigid tubing can pass from the patient, through a small hole placed in the

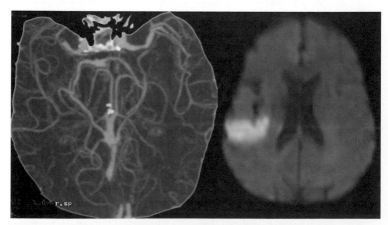

FIGURE 10-3 Computed tomography angiographic image (*left*) demonstrates an acute occlusion of the right middle cerebral artery. Diffusion-weighted magnetic resonance image (*right*) identifies an area of hyperintensity reflecting hyperacute ischemia. These techniques have revolutionized acute stroke management by providing rapid identification of vascular occlusion and early tissue injury.

shielding wall, and to monitoring equipment and infusion pumps located in the MR control room. **Nuclear medicine blood flow imaging** is useful for assessing cerebral perfusion in cases of suspected brain death, especially when factors that confound the clinical evaluation are present. **Transcranial Doppler ultrasound imaging** can identify regions of increased blood flow velocity consistent with focal arterial narrowing (e.g., atherosclerosis, vasospasm), retrograde flow (which provides information about collateral circulation), or absent blood flow (which may indicate complete occlusion).

X. **Physiologic monitoring.** Even with frequent, careful neurological examinations, changes in the patient's condition may occur which are not detectable by bedside examination. In addition, physiologic and multimodality monitoring may offer opportunities to anticipate early detection of ischemia.
   A. **Continuous EEG.** Seizures are often brief and paroxysmal. Continuous EEG monitoring can help detect clinical events that may easily be missed with a routine EEG. For those patients who are encephalopathic or sedated, subclinical seizures and nonconvulsive status epilepticus may also be identified. Quantitative EEG, utilizing Fourier transform analysis, may also aid in detecting small changes in the EEG that may correlate with changes in ICP or impending ischemia.
   B. **Jugular bulb oxygen tension.** Continuous jugular bulb oxygenation saturation may provide information regarding brain tissue oxygen extraction when compared to arterial oxygen saturation. Patients with jugular saturations below 50% tend to have poor outcomes.
   C. **Brain tissue oxygenation.** Oxygen partial pressure measurements can be made using fiberoptic catheters placed within the brain tissue, usually as part of ICP monitoring catheters. This type of monitoring provides information about local brain tissue oxygen. Additional catheters can measure temperature and pH. Adjustments in cerebral perfusion, systemic oxygenation, temperature management, and transfusion strategies can be made as indicated.
   D. **CSF microdialysis.** CSF microdialysis probes can be inserted into brain tissue and allow for serial sampling of physiological markers such as glucose, lactate, pyruvate, amino acids as well as drug concentrations. These measurements may provide information regarding impending cerebral ischemia and also allow for more precise adjustments in medications such as antibiotic or insulin therapy. Both this and the use of brain probes for temperature, pH, and oxygenation are gradually making their way from the bench to the bedside as research studies begin to explore their benefits.

XI. **Coagulation disturbances.** Because of the release of large quantities of brain tissue thromboplastin, massive brain injury may be associated with activation of the clotting cascade, disseminated intravascular coagulation, and subsequent clinical hemorrhage or clotting. Fresh frozen plasma and recombinant coagulation factors (factors VII and IX) may be administered to treat coagulopathies in the setting of intracerebral hemorrhage.

Selected References

Adams RD, Victor M. *Principles of neurology.* New York: McGraw-Hill, 1993.
Arieff AI, Kerian A, Massry SG, et al. Intracellular pH of brain: alterations in acute respiratory acidosis and alkalosis. *Am J Physiol* 1976;230:804–812.
Fisher CM. The neurological examination of the comatose patient. *Acta Neurol Scand* 1969;45(suppl 36):1–56.

Guarantors of Brain. *Aids to the examination of the peripheral nervous system*. London: Bailliere Tindall, 1986.

Paulson OB, Standgaard S, Edvinsson L. Cerebral autoregulation. *Cerebrovasc Brain Metab Rev* 1990;2:161–192.

Plum F, Posner JB. *Diagnosis of stupor and coma*. 3rd ed. Philadelphia: FA Davis, 1982.

Ropper AH. *Neurological and neurosurgical intensive care*. 4th ed. New York: Raven Press, 2003.

Schwamm LH, Koroshetz WJ, Sorensen AG, et al. Time course of lesion development in patients with acute stroke: serial diffusion- and hemodynamic-weighted magnetic resonance imaging. *Stroke* 1998;29:2268–2276.

Suarez JI, ed. *Critical care neurology and neurosurgery*. New York: Humana Press, 2004.

Wijdicks EF. *The clinical practice of critical care neurology*. New York: Lippincott-Raven, 1997.

Nutrition

Elizabeth Sailhamer and Hasan Alam

I. **Introduction.** The gastrointestinal (GI) tract has important nutritional and immune functions, and early **enteral nutrition (EN)** provides significant benefits for surgical and critically ill patients. When EN is not possible, **total parenteral nutrition (TPN)** is provided intravenously, although at higher costs, higher complication rates, and less clear benefits.

II. **Pathophysiology of nutrition in critical illness.** Postsurgical and critically ill patients are at risk for protein-calorie malnutrition. The body responds to illness (trauma, burns, inflammation, or surgery) with increased energy expenditure (hypermetabolism), and increased secretion of counterregulatory hormones (glucagon, glucocorticoids, and catecholamines), inflammatory mediators (cytokines and acute phase proteins), and other hormonal regulators such as vasopressin.
   A. Fluid shifts and edema occur due to water retention and increased vascular permeability.
   B. Hyperglycemia results from increased hepatic glycogenolysis, gluconeogenesis, and peripheral resistance of tissues to insulin.
   C. Skeletal muscle protein is preferentially used for gluconeogenesis during stress (particularly glutamine and alanine).
   D. Increased lipolysis (fat becomes the primary energy source).

III. **Estimation of calorie and protein requirements.** Assessment of a patient's nutritional status should include clinical information (medical history, nutritional intake history, and physical examination), as well as laboratory data and basic bedside tests. Reassessment and monitoring of nutritional support should occur on a weekly basis.
   A. **Clinical history**
      1. Pre-existing conditions (severe weight loss/cachexia, chronic disease, drug or alcohol abuse) increase a patient's risk for protein-calorie malnutrition.
      2. Severity of current illness (burns, sepsis, trauma, organ failure, or fever) is associated with hypermetabolism and increased nutritional requirements.
      3. Other acute care problems alter nutritional requirements (acid–base status, cardiopulmonary problems, electrolyte imbalance, etc) and if possible, should be corrected prior to initiation of nutritional support.
   B. Body weight measurements
      1. **Body mass index (BMI)** $=$ weight (kg)/height (m^2)
         a. Normal $=$ 18.5 to 24.9 kg/m^2
         b. Overweight $=$ 25 to 29.9 kg/m^2
         c. Obese $=$ 30 kg/m^2 and above
      2. **Ideal body weight (IBW)**
         a. IBW in men (kg) $=$ 50 + 2.3 [height (inches) − 60]
         b. IBW in women (kg) $=$ 45.5 + 2.3 [height (inches) − 60]

3. **Adjusted body weight (ABW)** (kg) = IBW + 0.4 (actual weight − IBW)
   a. Calculate ABW if actual body weight is >30% of IBW

C. **Nutritional laboratory indices**
   1. Albumin: Long-term marker of nutritional status (half-life, 21 days).
   2. Prealbumin and transferrin: Serum proteins with short half-lives (2–3, and 8 days, respectively), and are useful for monitoring nutritional support.
   3. Chemistries, glucose, liver function tests (LFTs) for baseline levels.

D. **Resting energy expenditure (REE).** Various methods exist for estimating daily caloric requirements, and these requirements should be fulfilled with both protein and "nonprotein calories" (carbohydrate and fat). Protein requirements are calculated separately (**Section IV.A**)
   1. **Indirect calorimetry** ("metabolic cart"). Measures oxygen consumption (**VO_2**) and carbon dioxide productions (**VCO_2**) over a 10- to 30-minute period to calculate the **respiratory quotient (RQ)**. To be reliable, indirect calorimetry needs to be performed in an intubated patient, breathing at a relatively low inspired oxygen fraction (FiO_2 <0.6), without leaks from a chest tube or patient agitation.
      a. $RQ = VO_2/VCO_2$
      b. $REE = (3.94\ [VO_2] + 1.1\ [VCO_2])\ 1.44 - (2.17\ [UUN])$
   2. **Harris–Benedict** equation. Estimates **basal metabolic rate (BMR)** using a calculation based on gender, weight (kg), height (cm), and age (years).
      a. **BMR in men** (kcal/d) = 66 + 13.7 (weight) + 5 (height) − 6.8 (age)
      b. **BMR in women** (kcal/d) = 665 + 9.6 (weight) + 1.8 (height) − 4.7 (age)
      c. **REE** = (BMR) × (activity factor) × (stress factor)
         (1) *Activity factor* is 1.2 to 1.3 for most hospitalized patients (non-ambulatory and ambulatory patients, respectively).
         (2) *Stress factor* depends on degree of critical illness:
            i. Postoperative/trauma = 1.2 to 1.3
            ii. Sepsis = 1.6 to 1.7
            iii. Severe burns = 2.0 or more
   3. In many patients, REE can be estimated by 25 kcal/kg/d. Multiply by *stress factor* for critically ill patients.

E. **Protein requirements.** Nitrogen balance can be calculated by measuring 24-hour urine urea nitrogen (UUN) to assess adequacy of protein intake.
   1. Nitrogen loss (g/d) = 1.2 [UUN (g/dL) × urine output (mL/d) × (1 g/1,000 mg) × (1 dL/100 mL)] + 2 g/d.
   2. Nitrogen balance (g/d) = [total protein intake (g/d)/6.25 (g protein/g nitrogen)] − [Nitrogen loss (g/d)]
   3. Goal is a positive nitrogen balance (anabolic state). Negative nitrogen balance indicates muscle breakdown (catabolic state), and protein intake should be increased.
   4. An estimate calorie-to-nitrogen ratio is 150:1, and is provided in most isotonic enteral formulas. This may need to be supplemented in critical illness (**Table 11-1**).

IV. **Components of nutrition (Table 11-1)**
   A. **Protein** provides 4 kcal/g of calories, with an RQ of 0.8. Adequate protein intake (both essential and nonessential amino acids) is critical for muscle building and maintenance of a positive nitrogen balance (anabolic state), especially during critical illness. The following guidelines should be used when calculating protein requirements:
      1. Normal patient = 0.8 to 1.0 g/kg
      2. Postsurgical, mild trauma = 1.25 to 1.5 g/kg
      3. Severe trauma, sepsis, organ failure = 1.5 to 2.0 g/kg
      4. Burn (>20% TBSA) or severe head injury ≥2.0 g/kg

Component	Calorie Conversion	RQ	Maximum Daily Administration	% Total Calories
Amino acids	4 kcal/g	0.8	0.8–1.0 g/kg (normal) 1.25–1.5 g/kg (post-surgery, mild trauma) 1.5–2.0 g/kg (severe trauma, sepsis, organ failure) ≥2.0 g/kg (>20% TBSA burn, severe head injury)	15%–25%
Dextrose	3.4 kcal/g	1.0	5–7 g/kg (350–500 g or 1190–1700 kcal in 70 kg)	40%–60%[b]
Lipids	9 kcal/g	0.7	2.5 g/kg[a] (175 g or 1575 kcal in 70 kg)	20%–30%[b]
Total calories	—	—	25 kcal/kg plus stress factor (~1750+ kcal in 70 kg)	—
Fluid/volume	—	—	30 mL/kg (~2100 mL in 70 kg)	—

RQ, respiratory quotient; TBSA, total body surface area.
[a]Critically ill patients may not be able to oxidize more than 1–1.5 g/kg/d.
[b]70:30 ratio of nonprotein calories (carbohydrate:lipid).

B. Carbohydrates provide 4 kcal/g (IV dextrose = 3.4 kcal/g) with an RQ of 1.0. Between 40% and 60% of total caloric needs (or 70% of nonprotein calories) should be fulfilled with carbohydrates.
C. Fat provides 9 kcal/g with an RQ of 0.7. Between 20% and 30% of total caloric requirements (or 30% of nonprotein calories) should be derived from fat. Polyunsaturated fats (ω-6 and ω-3) are essential fatty acids and must be obtained from dietary sources.

V. Evidence-based guidelines in nutrition
   A. Indications for initiation of nutritional support
      1. A previously healthy, well-nourished patient who has been without nutrition for 7 days (i.e., postsurgical).
      2. Patients whose expected illness duration without nutrition will exceed 7 days.
      3. Critically ill patients (i.e., severe trauma, sepsis, burns, pancreatitis, or organ dysfunction).
      4. Patients with pre-existing malnourishment or severe weight loss (>15% of usual weight).
   B. EN versus TPN (Fig. 11-1)
      1. EN is superior to TPN in patients with a functional GI tract, and reduces infectious complications, improves wound healing, decreases GI mucosal permeability, and reduces patient costs. TPN is associated with immune suppression and an increased infectious risk.
      2. If TPN is the primary source of nutrition, "trophic" tube feeds (10–20 mL/h) help maintain GI mucosal integrity and immune function. Enterocytes preferentially metabolize **glutamine** as their primary fuel source.

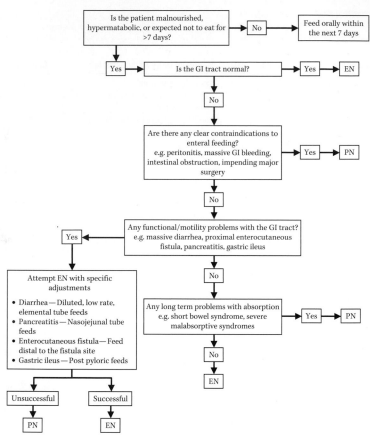

FIGURE 11-1 Algorithm for enteral nutrition (EN) vs. parenteral nutrition (PN). GI, gastrointestinal.

    3. Contraindications to EN include hemodynamic instability, abdominal distension (ileus or obstruction), intestinal perforation, massive GI bleed, severe diarrhea, or high-output enterocutaneous fistula.
C. Early versus delayed enteral nutrition
    1. In critically ill patients, EN should be initiated within 24 hours via a nasogastric or nasojejunal tube. Even low rate (trophic feeds) may decrease **subsequent gastroparesis and feeding intolerance.**
D. Delivery route of EN
    1. Nasogastric or nasoenteric tubes may be used for short-term enteral nutritional support (<1 month).
    2. Postpyloric tubes may be helpful if gastroparesis prevents tolerance of gastric feeds, but do not have proven lower rates of aspiration compared to gastric feeding. They may be placed blindly or with endoscopic or fluoroscopic guidance. Blind **placement of stiletted postpyloric tubes** must be done cautiously and by experienced physicians. When

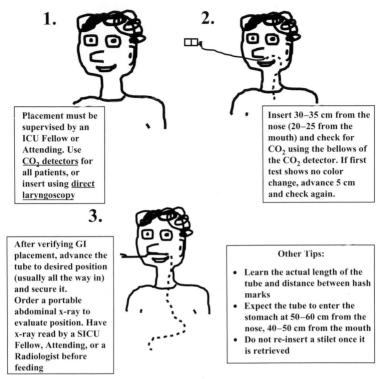

1.

Placement must be
supervised by an
ICU Fellow or
Attending. Use
<u>CO$_2$ detectors</u> for
all patients, or
insert using <u>direct
laryngoscopy</u>

2.

Insert 30–35 cm from the
nose (20–25 from the
mouth) and check for
CO$_2$ using the bellows of
the CO$_2$ detector. If first
test shows no color
change, advance 5 cm
and check again.

3.

After verifying GI
placement, advance the
tube to desired position
(usually all the way in)
and secure it.
Order a portable
abdominal x-ray to
evaluate position. Have
x-ray read by a SICU
Fellow, Attending, or a
Radiologist before
feeding

Other Tips:

• Learn the actual length of the
  tube and distance between hash
  marks
• Expect the tube to enter the
  stomach at 50–60 cm from the
  nose, 40–50 cm from the mouth
• Do not re-insert a stilet once it
  is retrieved

FIGURE 11-2 Diagram for the safe placement of a stiletted soft feeding tube. Courtesy of
Jonathan Charnin, MD.

inserted in sedated, mechanically ventilated patients, these soft and
sharp-tipped tubes may enter the airway instead of the GI tract.
Complications may then include perforation of the lung with pneumothorax, and lung infection/abscess secondary to infusion of feedings into the airway. The algorithm shown in **Fig. 11-2** is used in our ICU
to guide the safe placement of stiletted feeding tubes in intubated
patients.

3. Surgical placement of gastric or jejunal feeding tube is indicated for
   long-term nutritional support (>1 month), or if a patient is already
   undergoing laparotomy for another reason.

4. Keep head of bed >30 degrees to prevent aspiration.

E. **Immune-enhancing diets** have been shown to be beneficial in trauma
   patients with severe torso injuries (ISS >18) and malnourished elective
   GI surgical patients (albumin <3.5 mg/dL for upper GI and <2.8 mg/dL
   for lower GI surgery), but should be avoided in septic patients (data are
   conflicting but may increase mortality). When indicated, initiation of
   immunonutrition 5 to 7 days preoperatively may be more beneficial than
   postoperative administration alone. Other patient populations may

benefit from immunonutrition, but the evidence is inconclusive. Current immune-enhancing formulas may include the following nutrients:

1. **Glutamine** is a conditionally essential amino acid and may become deficient in patients under stress/hypermetabolism. It is the primary substrate for enterocytes and T lymphocytes, and may protect the integrity of the GI mucosa and immune system. Parenteral supplementation is challenging because of low solubility and instability in solution. Enteral administration decreases infections and length of hospital stay, and a high dose of glutamine may decrease mortality.

2. **Arginine** is a conditionally essential amino acid during periods of stress, and has important roles in nitrogen metabolism and formation of nitric oxide. Administration of arginine decreases infections and length of hospital stay and ventilator days, but has mixed results in respect to mortality.

3. **Ω-3 polyunsaturated fatty acids (fish oils)** are incorporated into cell membranes and compete with the usual substrate (ω-6 fatty acids, or arachidonic acid) for cyclo-oxygenase. Therefore, ω-3 fatty acids prevent the metabolism of arachidonic acid to prostaglandins, prostacyclins, leukotrienes, and thromboxanes, which are proinflammatory mediators. Long-term benefits of ω-3 fatty acids have been demonstrated (reduce heart disease), and also may have beneficial anti-inflammatory effects in the acute setting.

4. **Nucleotides** can be synthesized de novo or recycled by the body to be incorporated into DNA and RNA. During periods of stress, administration of nucleotides in the diet may prevent their depletion in rapidly dividing cells such as the GI mucosa and lymphocytes. However, evidence of its clinical efficacy is lacking.

VI. Parenteral nutrition

A. Parenteral nutrition is indicated in patients who require aggressive nutritional support but cannot tolerate enteral nutrition (nonfunction GI tract).

B. **Peripheral parenteral nutrition (PPN)** versus **TPN**

1. **PPN** provides partial nutritional support and can be administered through a peripheral vein due to lower osmotic solutions (<900 mOsm/L). Dextrose, lipids, and proteins can all be given peripherally, but require a large volume of infusion and will not meet total metabolic demands.

2. **TPN** contains higher concentrations of dextrose and amino acids to meet total metabolic demands, and is therefore hypertonic (requires central venous access).

3. The risk–benefit ratio of PPN has been questioned because it is associated with the same risk of immunosuppression and increased risk of infections as TPN, but without the benefit of total nutritional support.

C. Components of TPN (**Table 11-1**)

1. **D-glucose (dextrose)** is the major source of nonprotein calories (3.4 kcal/g). Maximum daily administration is 5 to 7 g/kg/d. Exceeding this maximum rate of glucose oxidation may result in lipid synthesis with CO_2 accumulation and hepatic steatosis.

2. **Lipid emulsion** is another source of nonprotein calories (9 kcal/g), and also provides essential fatty acids (ω-6 and ω-3 polyunsaturated fats). Maximum administration of lipid emulsion is 2.5 g/kg, and should comprise <30% of total calories. Lipid emulsions provide 1.1 kcal/mL (for 10% IV emulsion), 2.0 kcal/mL (for 20% IV emulsion), and 3.0 kcal/mL for 30% IV emulsion). Avoid infusion >110 mg/kg/h because of neutrophils and monocytes impairment and worsening gas exchange.

	Additives to Total Parenteral Nutrition (TPN)

Additive	Recommended or Usual Daily Dose
Electrolytes	
Sodium	100–150 mEq/d
Potassium	60–120 mEq/d
Calcium gluconate	10–20 mEq/d
Phosphate	15–30 mM/d
Magnesium	8–24 mEq/d
Chloride or acetate	Anion for sodium and potassium
Vitamins	
Vitamin C (ascorbic acid)	75–70 mg/d
Vitamin A	3300 IU/d
Vitamin D	400 IU/d
Thiamine (B_1)	1.1–1.2 mg/d
Pyridoxine (B_6)	1.3–1.7 mg/d
Riboflavin (B_2)	1.1–1.3 mg/d
Niacin	14–16 mg/d
Pantothenic acid	5 mg/d
Vitamin E	15 mg/d
Biotin	30 μg/d
Folic acid	400 μg/d
Vitamin B_{12}	2.4 μg/d
Vitamin K	90–120 μg/d
Trace Elements	
Zinc	8–11 mg/d
Copper	900 μg/d
Manganese	1.8–2.3 mg/d
Chromium	20–35 μg/d
Selenium	55 μg/d

[a]Chloride can produce a metabolic acidosis; use acetate for patients with metabolic acidosis (converted to bicarbonate in the liver).

       3. Amino acids (essential and nonessential) are needed to build muscle and maintain a positive nitrogen balance, but also are a source of calories (4 kcal/g). As in EN, protein requirements should be calculated based on stress level, and monitored with weekly UUN and nitrogen balance.

   D. Calculation of TPN formulation

       1. Calculate total calorie requirements (**Section III.D, Table 11-1**)

       2. Estimate protein requirements (**Sections III.E and IV.A, Table 11-1**)

       3. Calculate maximum carbohydrate and lipid amounts (**Sections IV.B and IV.C, Table 11-1**), and provide these "nonprotein calories" in a ratio of 70:30 (ideal).

       4. Fluid/volume requirements average 30 mL/kg/d, but daily weight and strict measurement of fluid losses (urine, stool, insensible losses) help monitor fluid status.

       5. Electrolytes, minerals, vitamins, and trace elements should be added according to usual or recommended doses (**Table 11-2**). Adjustments may be needed in critical illness, or with certain disease states (i.e., renal failure or high-output fistula), and serum levels should be monitored routinely.

6. Other TPN additives
   a. **Glutamine** is difficult to solubilize safely for intravenous administration, but feeds enterocytes and protects GI mucosa even when given parenterally.
   b. **Insulin** can be added directly to TPN solution (up to half of daily sliding scale insulin requirement).

VII. **Enteral formulas.** Common enteral formulas used at the Massachusetts General Hospital are shown in **Table 11-3.** These vary by proportion of carbohydrate, protein, and fat, as well as caloric concentration, osmolality, elemental components, and various additives. Several formulas are particularly designed for certain patient populations (i.e., pulmonary or renal disease).

VIII. **Nutritional modifications in disease**
   A. **Diabetes.** Low simple sugar, high fiber, and high fat to minimize hyperglycemia.
   B. **Renal failure.** High calorie, low protein, and low electrolytes (phosphorus, potassium) to prevent volume overload, hyperammonemia, and electrolyte imbalance. However, in patients on dialysis, protein requirements may actually increase.
   C. **Liver failure.** Low protein, high branch chain amino acids to prevent encephalopathy.
   D. **Respiratory failure.** High calorie, high fat (low carbohydrate) to prevent CO_2 accumulation.
   E. **Pancreatitis.** Enteral, postpyloric (nasojejunal) feeding is superior to TPN.
   F. **Other GI diseases.** If nonfunctional GI tract, may require TPN.
   G. **Trauma.** Consider immune-enhancing diet.

IX. **Monitoring of nutrition.** After initiation of nutritional support, basic laboratory values should be monitored to assess adequacy of nutrition and detect potential complications.
   A. Glucose
      1. Blood glucose measurement with sliding scale insulin (SQ or IV drip) to prevent hyperglycemia and related complications (infection and poor wound healing).
      2. Tight glucose control (blood glucose <150 mg/dL) reduces mortality.
   B. Serum electrolytes and LFTs should be measured routinely.
   C. Albumin, prealbumin, transferrin, and UUN: To ensure adequacy of protein intake and prevent catabolic state (muscle breakdown).
   D. Triglyceride levels in patients receiving fat emulsions (IV). Decrease rate of infusion or hold if serum levels >500 mg/dL.
   E. Gastric residuals.
      1. If feeding by nasogastric tube, check for gastric residuals every 4 hours. If more than 200 to 250 mL (or 50% of volume administered), then hold feeds and recheck in 1 hour. If residuals still high, then decrease rate by 25 mL/h until residuals are acceptable.
      2. Initiate prokinetic agents (metoclopramide or erythromycin).
      3. If unable to reach goal nutrition through gastric feeds within 24 hours, consider placing a postpyloric or nasojejunal tube for intestinal feeding.
      4. Changing to elemental formula may improve tolerance.

TABLE
11-3

Massachusetts General Hospital Enteral Formulary

	Osmolite	Osmolite HN	Jevity Plus	Ensure Plus HN	Twocal HN	Glucerna	Promote with Fiber
Calories/mL	1.06	1.06	1.2	1.5	2.0	1.0	1.0
Protein (g/L) (% cal)	37.1 (14.0%)	44.3 (16.7%)	55.5 (18.5%)	62.6 (16.7%)	83.7 (16.7%)	41.8 (16.7%)	62.5 (25%)
Fat (g/L) (% cal)	34.7 (29%)	34.7 (29%)	39.3 (29.0%)	50 (30%)	89.1 (40.1%)	54.4 (49%)	28.2 (25%)
Carbohydrate (g/L) (% cal)	151.1 (57%)	143.9 (54.3%)	172.7 (52.5%)	199.9 (53.3%)	216.1 (43.2%)	95.6 (34.3%)	138.3 (50%)
Osmolality (mOsm)	300	300	450	650	690	355	380
Comments	Isotonic	Isotonic	Moderate protein, 12 g/L fiber	High calorie, high protein	Hypermetabolic fluid restricted patients	Low carbohydrates, 14.4 g/L fiber	High protein, low fat, 14.4 g/L fiber

	Pulmocare	Suplena	Nepro	Peptamen	Alitraq	Tolerex	Vital HN	Vivonex Plus
Calories/mL	1.5	2.0	2.0	1.0	1.0	1.0	1.0	1.0
Protein (g/L) (% cal)	62.6 (16.7%)	30.0 (6%)	69.9 (14%)	40.0 (16%)	52.5 (21%)	21 (8.0%)	41.7 (16.7%)	45 (18%)
Fat (g/L) (% cal)	93.3 (55.1%)	95.6 (43%)	95.6 (43%)	39 (33%)	15.5 (13%)	1.5 (1.0%)	10.8 (9.5%)	6.7 (6%)
Carbohydrate (g/L) (% cal)	105.7 (28.2%)	255.2 (51%)	222.3 (43%)	127 (51%)	165 (66%)	230 (91%)	185.0 (73.8%)	190 (76%)
Osmolality (mOsm)	475	600	665	380	575	550	500	650
Comments	High protein, high fat, low carbohydrate (to minimize CO_2 production)	Renal failure—predialysis (low protein, low electrolyte), high calorie.	Renal failure—on dialysis (moderate protein, low electrolyte)	Peptide based, gluten free, glutamine (3 g/L)	Elemental, glutamine (14.2 g/L)	Elemental, low protein	Elemental, higher protein	Elemental, glutamine (10 g/L)

X. Complications of parenteral nutrition
A. Catheter-placement complications (pneumothorax, hemothorax, or arrhythmia).
B. Catheter infection.
C. Other infections (immune suppression from TPN).
D. Metabolic derangements (hyperglycemia, hypoglycemia, electrolyte imbalances, fluid overload).

Selected References

Heyland DK, Dhaliwal R, Drover JW, et al. Canadian clinical practice guidelines for nutritional support in mechanically ventilated, critically ill adult patients. *JPEN J Parenter Enteral Nutr* 2003;27:355–373.

Kalfarentzos F, Kehagias J, Mead N, et al. Enteral nutrition is superior to parenteral nutrition in severe acute pancreatitis: results of a randomized prospective trial. *Br J Surg* 1997;87:695–707.

Kieft H, Roos AN, van Drunen JDE, et al. Clinical outcome of immunonutrition in a heterogeneous intensive care population. *Intensive Care Med* 2005;31:524–532.

Koretz RL, Avenell A, Lipman TO, Braunschweig CL, Milne AC. Does enteral nutrition affect clinical outcome? A systematic review of the randomized trials. *Am J Gastroenterol* 2007;102:412–429.

Marik PE, Zaloga GP. Gastric versus post-pyloric feeding: a systematic review. *Crit Care* 2003;7:R46–R51.

Matarese L, Steiger E. Parenteral nutrition support. In: Hark L, Morrison G, eds. *Medical nutrition and disease: a case-based approach.* 3rd ed. Maulden, MA: Blackwell Publishing Company, 2003:378–391.

Mazaki T, Ebisawa K. Enteral versus parenteral nutrition after gastrointestinal surgery: a systematic review and meta-analysis of randomized trials in the English language [published online ahead of print]. *J Gastrointest Surg* 2007 Oct 16.

Novak R, Heyland DK, et al. Glutamine supplementation in serious illness: a systematic review of the evidence. *Crit Care Med* 2002;30:2022–2029.

Peter JV, Moran JL, Phillips-Hughes J. A metaanalysis of treatment outcomes of early enteral versus early parenteral nutrition in hospitalized patients. *Crit Care Med* 2005;33:213–220.

Proceedings from the summit on immune-enhancing enteral therapy. *JPEN J Parenter Enteral Nutr* 2001;25(suppl):S1–S63.

Rolandelli RH, Gupta D, Wilmore DW. Chapter 24: nutritional support. In: *ACS surgery: principles and practice.* WebMD, Inc., 2003:1–22.

Simpson F, Doig GS. Parenteral vs enteral nutrition in the critically ill patient: a meta-analysis of trials using the intention to treat principle. *Intensive Care Med* 2005;31:12–23.

The Veteran Affairs TPN Cooperative Study Group. Perioperative TPN in surgical patients. *N Eng J Med* 1991;325:525–532.

Thomson C, Sarubin-Fragakis A. Vitamins, minerals, and phytochemicals. In: Hark L, Morrison G, eds. *Medical nutrition and disease: a case-based approach.* 3rd ed. Maulden, MA: Blackwell Publishing Company, 2003:39–74.

Van Den Berghe G, Wouters P, Weekers F, et al. Intensive insulin therapy in critically ill patients. *N Eng J Med* 2001;345:1359–1367.

Velmahos GC, Alam HB. Advances in surgical critical care. *Curr Probl Surg* 2008;45(7):453–516.

Zaloga GP. Parenteral nutrition in adult inpatients with functioning gastrointestinal tracts: assessment of outcomes. *Lancet* 2006;367:1101–1111.

Infectious Disease—General Considerations

Laura Leduc and Judith Hellman

I. Introduction

A. The **diagnosis of infection** in ICU patients can be complicated by the fact that patients often develop clinical signs of infection such as fever and hemodynamic instability from noninfectious causes. In addition, there are multiple potential sites of infection (**Table 12-1**). A thorough evaluation is essential to localize sites of infection and to exclude noninfectious etiologies so that appropriate interventions can be initiated.

B. **Nosocomial infections** are hospital-acquired infections that occur after 48 hours of hospitalization. They are frequently caused by organisms with increased antimicrobial resistance. Risk factors for development of serious infections in the ICU are outlined in **Table 12-2**.

C. Infections can be caused by a variety of microorganisms including bacteria, fungi, viruses, and parasites. Common organisms are listed in **Table 12-3**.

II. Antibacterial agents

A. **β-Lactam** antimicrobial agents interfere with bacterial cell wall synthesis. The spectrum of various β-lactams varies widely. β-Lactams have bactericidal activity against susceptible organisms. However, they have only bacteriostatic activity against *Enterococcus* species (spp). A synergistic combination of a β-lactam (or vancomycin) plus an aminoglycoside is necessary for bactericidal activity against *Enterococcus* spp. **Resistance to β-lactams** results from production of β-lactamase, altered binding to penicillin-binding proteins, and/or decreased antibiotic penetration into the bacteria. Treatment of *Enterobacter* spp, *Citrobacter* spp, and *Acinetobacter* spp with β-lactams, especially cephalosporins, may be complicated by rapid development of resistance because they harbor an inducible chromosomal β-lactamase.

1. **Penicillins** (penicillin, nafcillin, ampicillin, ticarcillin, piperacillin)

    a. **Spectrum**

    (1) **Penicillin** and **nafcillin** are active against aerobic and anaerobic gram-positive bacteria. **Penicillin** is active against gram-positive cocci such as *Streptococcus* spp, gram-positive rods such as *Listeria monocytogenes,* and many anaerobes. *Staphylococcus aureus* and *Staphylococcus epidermidis* are often resistant. **Nafcillin** is effective against *S. aureus,* excluding methicillin-resistant *S. aureus* (**MRSA**). Nafcillin is less active than penicillin against *Streptococcus* spp.

    (2) **Ampicillin** is active against many gram-positive cocci and enteric gram-negative bacilli, including *Escherichia coli, Proteus* spp, and *Serratia* spp. The addition of the β-lactamase inhibitor **sulbactam** to ampicillin (**Unasyn**) increases the activity against *S. aureus* (not MRSA), β-lactamase–producing gram-negatives, and anaerobes.

    (3) **Ticarcillin** and **piperacillin** are active against gram-positive, gram-negative, and anaerobic bacteria. Their resistance to β-lactamase

TABLE 12-1	Potential Sites of Infection in Intensive Care Unit Patients
Site	**Infection**
Surgical	Superficial and deep wound infection, anastomotic breakdown, abscess
Chest	Pneumonia, tracheobronchitis, mediastinitis, lung abscess, empyema, endocarditis
Abdomen	Peritonitis, abscess, cholecystitis, cholangitis, urinary tract infection, *Clostridium difficile* colitis
Head and neck	Sinusitis, parotitis, central nervous system infection, peritonsillar abscess
Indwelling catheters, drains, and monitors	Urinary catheter, intravascular catheter, epidural catheter, cerebrospinal fluid drain, intracranial pressure monitor
Central nervous system	Meningitis, encephalitis, epidural abscess, brain abscess

confers broader gram-negative coverage than ampicillin and can include *Pseudomonas* and *Enterobacter* spp. **Piperacillin** is also active against some species of *Klebsiella*. Although these antipseudomonal penicillins are active against many gram-positives, *Staphylococcus aureus* is often resistant. The addition of the β-lactamase inhibitor clavulanate to ticarcillin **(Timentin)** and the addition of tazobactam to piperacillin **(Zosyn)** broaden the spectrum to include *Staphylococcus aureus* (except MRSA), *Bacteroides fragilis*, and some aerobic β-lactamase–producing gram-negatives.

   b. **Adverse reactions** to penicillins include hypersensitivity reactions ranging from rash to anaphylaxis, bleeding due to impaired platelet function (ticarcillin), volume overload or hypernatremia due to a large salt load (ticarcillin, piperacillin), interstitial nephritis (especially nafcillin), neutropenia (nafcillin at high doses), fever, and central nervous system (CNS) toxicity. A history of **"allergy"** to penicillin is often elicited in patients without clear documentation that an actual allergic reaction has occurred. **Skin testing** may be useful in diagnosing true allergy to β-lactams. **Desensitization** may be an option if a β-lactam is essential for optimal treatment of a

TABLE 12-2	Risk Factors for Infections in the Intensive Care Unit

1. Age >70 years
2. Shock
3. Major trauma
4. Coma
5. Prior antibiotics
6. Mechanical ventilation
7. Drugs affecting the immune system (steroids, chemotherapy)
8. Indwelling catheters
9. Prolonged intensive care unit stay (>3 days)
10. Acute renal failure

TABLE 12-3	Classification of Microorganisms Causing Infections in the Intensive Care Unit
General Groups	**Specific Microorganisms**
Bacteria: gram-positive aerobes	*Staphylococcus aureus*, *S. epidermidis* (coagulase-negative staphylococcus), *Streptococcus* spp, *Enterococcus* spp
Bacteria: enteric gram-negative aerobes and facultative anaerobes	*Escherichia coli*, *Klebsiella pneumoniae*, *Proteus mirabilis*, *Enterobacter* spp, *Acinetobacter* spp, *Citrobacter* spp, *Serratia marcescens*, *Salmonella* spp
Bacteria: nonenteric gram-negative aerobes and facultative anaerobes	*Pseudomonas aeruginosa*, *Burkholderia cepacia*, *Neisseria* spp, *Haemophilus influenzae*, *Haemophilus parainfluenzae*
Bacteria: anaerobes (gram-positive and gram-negative)	*Bacteroides fragilis* and other *Bacteroides* spp, *Clostridium difficile* and other *Clostridium* spp, *Peptostreptococcus* spp
Fungi	*Candida* spp, *Aspergillus* spp, *Histoplasma capsulatum*, *Pneumocystis carinii*
Viruses	Varicella-zoster virus (VZV), herpes simplex virus (HSV) I and II, cytomegalovirus (CMV), Epstein-Barr virus (EBV)

life-threatening bacterial infection in a patient with a history of a severe β-lactam allergy. Rapid desensitization may be achieved by intravenous administration of escalating doses of the desired antibiotic in a carefully monitored setting. The process of desensitization can result in serious complications and should be performed by a specially trained physician.

2. **Cephalosporins**

   a. **Spectrum**

      (1) **First-generation cephalosporins,** such as **cefazolin,** are active against many gram-positive and some gram-negative bacteria. Enteric gram-negative rods such as *E. coli,* some *Klebsiella* spp, and gram-positive oral anaerobes are often susceptible. Organisms that are resistant to first-generation cephalosporins include *Enterococcus* spp, methicillin-resistant *Staphylococcus epidermidis* (MRSE) and gram-negative anaerobes such as *Bacteroides* spp.

      (2) **Second-generation cephalosporins** are more active against gram-negatives and less active against gram-positives as compared with the first-generation agents. There are two major subgroups of second-generation cephalosporins. One group, which includes **cefuroxime,** is active against *Haemophilus influenzae.* The other group, which includes **cefoxitin** and **cefotetan,** is active against anaerobes such as *Bacteroides* spp.

      (3) **Third-generation cephalosporins** have greater activity against gram-negative bacilli than do second-generation agents. They are active against most enteric and some nonenteric (*H. influenzae* and *Neisseria* spp) gram-negative bacilli. *Enterobacter* spp, *Citrobacter* spp, and *Acinetobacter* spp often become resistant to third-generation cephalosporins because of the inducible production of β-lactamase. **Ceftazidime** has strong activity against

Pseudomonas spp, but is poorly active against gram-positive organisms. **Ceftriaxone** and **cefotaxime** have activity against some gram-positives, (not *Enterococcus* spp, *L. monocytogenes*, MRSA, or MRSE) but are often ineffective against *Pseudomonas* spp. The third-generation cephalosporins have good CNS penetration and are often used in the treatment of bacterial meningitis.

    (4) Fourth-generation cephalosporins, such as **cefepime,** have a similar spectrum to ceftriaxone against gram-positive cocci, but broader gram-negative coverage that includes bacteria with inducible β-lactamase, such as *Enterobacter* spp, and *Citrobacter* spp. Cefepime may also be active against some ceftazidime-resistant *Pseudomonas aeruginosa.*

  b. **Adverse reactions** to cephalosporins include hypersensitivity reactions (5%–10% incidence of cross-reactivity with penicillin allergy) and bleeding due to inhibition of vitamin K–dependent coagulation factor synthesis (cefotetan).

3. **Carbapenems** have broad antibacterial activity. They offer the advantage of extensive coverage of gram-positives, gram-negatives, and anaerobes. It is prudent to reserve carbapenem agents for treating documented or highly suspected nosocomial infections due to antibiotic-resistant bacteria.

  a. **Spectrum. Imipenem/cilastatin** and **meropenem** have similar spectra. They are active against most gram-negatives, many gram-positives, and anaerobes. Although they have the broadest spectrum of the β-lactams, some pathogenic strains do develop resistance. Resistant gram-negatives have included *Stenotrophomonas maltophilia, Burkholderia* (previously known as *Pseudomonas*) *cepacia*, and occasionally *P. aeruginosa, Enterobacter cloacae,* and *Serratia marcescens.* Resistant gram-positives have included some *Enterococci* spp, MRSA, *Corynebacterium* spp, and *Bacteroides* spp. **Ertapenem** has a spectrum similar to the above carbapenems except that it has limited activity against *Pseudomonas* and *Acinetobacter* spp. Therefore, ertapenem is not recommended for use as empiric therapy in nosocomial infections. It is better suited to treat a pathogen that is known to be sensitive. The advantages to ertapenem are that it does not require dose adjustment for renal insufficiency and can be administered once daily.

  b. **Adverse reactions** include seizures and hypersensitivity reactions. Safety data from clinical trials using meropenem suggest that it may be less frequently associated with seizures than imipenem/cilastatin. Ertapenem also has a reported decreased incidence of seizure activity relative to imipenem/cilastatin.

4. **Monobactams**

  a. **Spectrum. Aztreonam** is active against many gram-negative bacteria. It is not active against gram-positive bacteria or anaerobes. Some nonenteric gram-negatives can be resistant, including *S. maltophilia, Acinetobacter* spp, and *P. aeruginosa.*

  b. **Adverse reactions** include hypersensitivity reactions. Despite the β-lactam structure, aztreonam seems to have very little cross-reactivity with other β-lactams and is often used in patients who have had minor allergic reactions to β-lactams. There is a theoretical concern that patients with an anaphylactic response to ceftazidime may also react to aztreonam because both drugs have a side chain in common; however, clinical data supporting this are sparse.

B. Glycopeptides, including **vancomycin** and **teicoplanin,** interfere with bacterial cell wall synthesis.

1. **Spectrum.** Glycopeptides are bactericidal for most gram-positive bacteria. They are active against the highly resistant staphylococcal strains, MRSA, and MRSE, as well as *Enterococcus* spp and *Streptococcus* spp. As with the β-lactams, vancomycin is not bactericidal for *Enterococcus* spp, and should be combined with an aminoglycoside for synergistic coverage if bactericidal activity is required.

2. **Adverse reactions** to vancomycin include "red man syndrome," rash, ototoxicity, nephrotoxicity, and neutropenia. "Red man syndrome" is a histamine-release syndrome characterized by flushing of the face, neck, and trunk with varying degrees of hypotension. It is not a true allergy in that it is not immunoglobulin E mediated. This syndrome occurs frequently, and can be minimized or prevented by delivering the drug in a large volume of fluid, reducing the dose, slowing the rate of infusion, and premedicating with an antihistamine. The other adverse reactions listed are rare. Ototoxicity is often irreversible and may be associated with a gait disturbance.

3. **Vancomycin-resistant gram-positive bacteria.** Vancomycin-resistant isolates of *Enterococcus* (VRE) have become common. Additionally, vancomycin-resistant strains of *Staphylococcus aureus* have also emerged.

C. Linezolid, an oxazolidinone, is bacteriostatic and acts by inhibiting bacterial protein synthesis. Of note, there is equivalent bioavailability with intravenous and oral administration.

1. **Spectrum.** Linezolid is active against highly resistant gram-positive bacteria including MRSA, penicillin-resistant *Streptococcus pneumoniae,* and VRE.

2. **Adverse reactions** to linezolid include headache, diarrhea, tongue discoloration, thrombocytopenia, mild reversible anemia, leucopenia, peripheral neuropathy, optic neuropathy, and lactic acidosis. Because linezolid reversibly inhibits monoamine oxidase, there is potential for interaction with adrenergic and serotonergic agents. **Serotonin syndrome** has been reported in patients who are treated concomitantly with linezolid and agents that increase serotonin levels, such as various classes of antidepressants, and several analgesics.

D. Quinupristin/dalfopristin (Synercid) is a mixture of streptogramin A and B antibiotics that act by inhibiting bacterial protein synthesis.

1. **Spectrum.** Synercid is active against MRSA, methicillin-resistant coagulase-negative staphylococci, *Streptococcus pneumoniae,* and most strains of *Enterococcus faecium. Enterococcus faecalis* may be resistant.

2. **Adverse reactions** include discomfort or swelling at the infusion site, nausea, vomiting, diarrhea, rash, myalgias, arthralgias, increased bilirubin, increased gamma-glutamyl transferase, and rarely increased serum creatinine, thrombocytopenia, and anemia.

3. Synercid has multiple drug interactions including those with cyclosporine, carbamazepine, calcium channel blockers, diazepam, midazolam, disopyramide, lidocaine, methylprednisolone, astemizole, cisapride, and statins.

E. Daptomycin is a bactericidal cyclic lipopeptide.

1. **Spectrum.** Daptomycin is active against MRSA, MRSE, and VRE.

2. **Adverse reactions** include nausea, diarrhea, constipation, and elevated creatine phosphokinases.

3. Daptomycin is used for treatment of complicated skin and skin structure infections, and *Staphylococcus aureus* bloodstream infections and

right-sided endocarditis. Efficacy has not yet been established in left-sided endocarditis. Daptomycin should not used for the treatment of pneumonia.

4. Daptomycin is cleared by the kidneys. Thus, dosage reduction is recommended in patients with a creatinine clearance <30 mL/min.

F. **Aminoglycosides** are bactericidal agents that interfere with bacterial protein synthesis. The most commonly used aminoglycosides in the ICU are gentamicin, tobramycin, and amikacin. Aminoglycosides are available in parenteral and nebulized formulations.

1. **Spectrum.** Aminoglycosides are active against gram-negative organisms and are synergistic with the cell wall active agents (β-lactams, vancomycin) against *Enterococcus* spp, *Staphylococcus* spp, and *Streptococcus viridans*. Most enteric gram-negative bacteria are sensitive to aminoglycosides. Resistance occurs regularly among nonenteric gram-negative bacteria such as *B. cepacia* and *S. maltophilia*. Tobramycin is used preferentially over gentamicin for infections with *P. aeruginosa*.

2. **Environmental considerations** and **penetration into tissues and fluids.** Aminoglycosides are not effective under acidic or anaerobic conditions such as with ascites or within abscesses. Tissue concentrations are variable. For example, there is poor penetration of systemic aminoglycosides into tracheobronchial secretions, bile, the prostate, and into the CNS.

3. **Adverse reactions** include nephrotoxicity, ototoxicity, weakness, and potentiation of neuromuscular blockade. Nephrotoxicity is generally mild, nonoliguric, and reversible. Risk factors for nephrotoxicity include advanced age, overall debilitation, baseline renal dysfunction, hypotension, hypovolemia, and concomitant administration of other nephrotoxins. In extreme circumstances such as *Enterococcus* or *Pseudomonas* endocarditis, aminoglycoside administration is indicated despite the potential for renal toxicity.

4. **Dosing and drug level monitoring considerations.**
   a. Monitoring of aminoglycoside levels is often utilized to guide therapy. Peak levels can verify that bactericidal concentrations have been achieved and trough levels can confirm adequate clearance and thus aid in avoiding toxicity.
   b. **Renal dysfunction** requires dosage adjustments of parenteral aminoglycosides. Specific adjustments are based on the degree of renal function impairment, and the type of renal replacement therapy (RRT) if RRT is in progress.
   c. **Once-daily administration** may have some advantages including less renal toxicity, maximization of concentration-dependent bactericidal activity, and a "postantibiotic effect" whereby bacterial growth is suppressed even after the serum level drops below the minimal inhibitory concentration. Animal studies have demonstrated a trend toward decreased nephrotoxicity with daily dosing.

G. **Fluoroquinolones (levofloxacin, ciprofloxacin, ofloxacin)** are bactericidal agents that act by inhibiting DNA synthesis. Enteral absorption of fluoroquinolones is excellent, but is decreased by concomitant administration of iron, zinc, antacids, sucralfate, and enteral tube feedings. Fluoroquinolones are concentrated in the urine, prostate, kidney, bowel, and lung.

1. **Spectrum. Ciprofloxacin, ofloxacin,** and **levofloxacin** are primarily active against aerobic gram-negative bacilli, including *P. aeruginosa*. Levofloxacin is active against some gram-positive bacteria including penicillin-resistant *Streptococcus pneumoniae*, but are not consistently

active against anaerobes. **Levofloxacin** is often used in combination with agents that cover gram-positives and anaerobes, such as clindamycin. Levofloxacin is also active against atypical bacteria such as *Legionella* spp, *Chlamydia* spp, and some *Mycobacterial* spp. They are potentially useful for many conditions including bone and joint infections, complicated urinary tract infections, bacterial gastroenteritis, and intra-abdominal infections.

2. **Adverse reactions** include GI upset, neurologic dysfunction (headache, dizziness, confusion, hallucinations, seizures), and hypersensitivity reactions.

3. **Drug interactions** are often a result of the fact that fluoroquinolones are metabolized via the hepatic P-450 enzyme system. Administration of ciprofloxacin to patients taking theophylline can result in theophylline toxicity.

4. **Fluoroquinolones and enteral feedings.** Studies indicate that continuous enteral feeding may significantly reduce absorption of fluoroquinolones. Thus, it is often recommended that enteral tube feeds be off for 2 hours prior to and for up to 4 hours after enteral administration of fluoroquinolones.

H. **Metronidazole** is bactericidal and acts by cleaving bacterial DNA. It is well absorbed from the GI tract and is metabolized in the liver.

1. **Spectrum.** Metronidazole is only active against anaerobes. It is the treatment of choice for pseudomembranous colitis due to *Clostridium difficile* colitis. It may be used in combination with other agents for the treatment of peritoneal or thoracic infections arising from the GI tract and for aspiration pneumonia.

2. **Adverse reactions**, although uncommon, can include GI symptoms such as metallic taste, anorexia, and nausea, as well as neurologic dysfunction, including peripheral neuropathy, seizures, ataxia, and vertigo.

I. **Clindamycin** is bacteriostatic and inhibits bacterial protein synthesis. It is well absorbed from the GI tract and is metabolized in the liver.

1. **Spectrum.** Clindamycin is active against most anaerobes and gram-positive aerobes. Resistant organisms include gram-negative aerobes and facultative anaerobes, *Enterococcus* spp, and some isolates of *B. fragilis*. Clindamycin may be used alone or with other agents for the treatment of aspiration pneumonia or for thoracic or abdominal infections originating from the upper GI tract.

2. **Adverse reactions** include GI upset, rash, and elevated liver enzymes. Clindamycin is the antibiotic that is most commonly associated with the development of *C. difficile* colitis.

J. **Macrolides** including erythromycin, clarithromycin, and azithromycin are bacteriostatic and work by inhibiting bacterial protein synthesis. They are well absorbed from the GI tract and undergo hepatic metabolism and biliary excretion.

1. **Spectrum.** Erythromycin is active against many gram-positives (especially *Streptococcus* spp), *Legionella* spp, *L. monocytogenes*, *Chlamydia pneumoniae*, and *Mycoplasma pneumoniae*. The main indication for erythromycin in critically ill patients is atypical pneumonia. **Azithromycin** and **clarithromycin** have a similar spectrum of activity as erythromycin but have increased activity against *H. influenzae* and are much better tolerated due to fewer GI side effects versus erythromycin.

2. **Adverse reactions** include GI upset with enteral administration, thrombophlebitis with intravenous administration, tinnitus, and rarely, transient deafness.

K. **Chloramphenicol** inhibits protein synthesis.
   1. **Spectrum.** Chloramphenicol is active against a wide range of gram-positive and gram-negative aerobic and anaerobic organisms. It is indicated for the treatment of meningitis or endocarditis due to VRE.
   2. The major **adverse reaction** which greatly limits the use of chloramphenicol is aplastic anemia. Adverse hematologic effects range from dose-dependent but reversible bone marrow depression to fatal aplastic anemia (approximately 1 per 25,000–50,000). Other adverse reactions include GI upset, hypersensitivity reactions, and optic neuritis.

III. **Antifungal agents**
   A. **Amphotericin B** acts by creating pores in the cell membrane. It is administered via intravenous or intrathecal routes or by local instillation into the bladder.
      1. **Spectrum.** Amphotericin B is broadly active against most *Candida* spp, including non–*albicans Candida* (*glabrata* and *krusei*) and many isolates of *Aspergillus*.
      2. **Adverse reactions** are multiple. Fever and rigors are common. Hypotension and hypoxemia can also occur. The incidence and severity of the above side effects can be decreased by pretreatment with acetaminophen, antihistamines, low-dose corticosteroids, and meperidine. Occasionally, the daily dose must be decreased to enable continued treatment. Some degree of renal dysfunction occurs in most patients treated with amphotericin B. Risk factors for **severe renal failure** include simultaneous administration of other nephrotoxic drugs, pre-existing renal disease or renal transplantation, and severely ill patients who are hypotensive and/or hypovolemic. Alternate-day dosing and administration of saline (1 L/d in excess of baseline fluid requirements) may be of benefit in preventing or blunting renal toxicity.
      3. **Lipid formulations** of amphotericin B are now commonly used instead of standard formulations to reduce the renal complications.
   B. **Triazoles**, including **fluconazole** and **voriconazole**, act by inhibiting fungal membrane sterol synthesis. Enteral absorption of fluconazole is excellent (≥90%) in patients who are tolerating enteral feedings. CNS penetration is reasonably good. Voriconazole also has excellent enteral bioavailability.
      1. **Spectrum.** Triazoles are active against many *Candida* spp (*albicans, parapsilosis*, and *tropicalis*) and *Cryptococcus neoformans*. *Candida krusei* and *Candida glabrata* are frequently resistant. Voriconazole has a broader spectrum of activity which includes molds such as *Aspergillus*. Potential uses of fluconazole include prophylaxis against invasive fungal infections in immunocompromised hosts, treatment of candidemia, and treatment of invasive fungal infections in stable patients due to *Candida* spp, excluding some isolates of *krusei* and *glabrata*. Fluconazole can be used to treat *C. krusei* and *C. glabrata* if the isolates are documented to be fluconazole sensitive by the microbiology laboratory.
      2. **Adverse reactions** include GI upset, rash, headaches, increased hepatocellular enzyme levels, and rarely exfoliative dermatitis and severe hepatotoxicity.
      3. Significant **drug interactions** include potentiation of Coumadin, phenytoin and cyclosporine effects, increased fluconazole levels with rifampin administration, and QT prolongation or polymorphic ventricular tachycardia when administered with cisapride.
   C. **5-Fluorocytosine** is an antimetabolite that inhibits fungal protein and DNA synthesis. It is synergistic with amphotericin B in the treatment of severe

systemic candidiasis or cryptococcal meningitis. Toxicity (primarily hematologic) correlates with high serum levels.

D. Echinocandins such as **caspofungin** and **micafungin** inhibit the synthesis of β-(1,3)-D-glucan, a component of fungal cell walls.

    1. Spectrum. Caspofungin and micafungin are active against *Candida* spp, including those that are resistant to fluconazole. Echinocandins are indicated in the treatment of candidal infections in patients who are intolerant to or are not responding to traditional agents, or who have a high risk of developing renal failure during treatment with amphotericin B. Caspofungin is also active against *Aspergillus*, and may be considered for treating critically ill patients who are infected with *Aspergillus* and are either not responding to or who are at high risk of developing renal failure with conventional therapy. The efficacy of micafungin against *Aspergillus* has not yet been established.

    2. Adverse effects are rare and include increases in transaminases and pruritus at the infusion site.

IV. Antiviral agents

    A. Acyclovir inhibits viral DNA replication. It is available in enteral and parenteral formulations.

        1. Spectrum. Acyclovir is active against herpes simplex virus (HSV) and varicella-zoster virus (VZV). Oral acyclovir is indicated in the treatment of mucocutaneous HSV. Parenteral treatment is indicated for serious infections such as varicella pneumonia or herpes encephalitis.

        2. Adverse reactions include renal dysfunction, especially in hypovolemic patients, and those with pre-existing renal disease as well as neurotoxicity, such as confusion, tremulousness, and seizures.

    B. Famciclovir and valacyclovir are antivirals with spectra similar to acyclovir. They are only available in enteral formulations.

    C. Ganciclovir

        1. Spectrum. Ganciclovir is active against HSV, VZV, and cytomegalovirus (CMV). It is used for treatment of CMV infections including retinitis, colitis, and pneumonitis in immunocompromised patients. It can also be used as prophylaxis against CMV infections in transplant recipients.

        2. Adverse reactions include myelosuppression and nephrotoxicity.

V. Infections in immunocompromised hosts. Immunocompromised hosts are at increased risk of community-acquired, nosocomial, and opportunistic infections. Prompt intervention is required to successfully treat these infections, but their diagnosis is often difficult because of the lack of clear localizing signs. A thorough search for the source of the infection is imperative and should include cultures of blood, urine, and sputum and a chest radiograph. There are many etiologies of immunocompromise including immunosuppressive therapy, burns, malignancy, HIV infection, chemotherapy, corticosteroids, and severe malnutrition. While infectious disease complications are variable, the most common site of infection in the immunocompromised patient is the lung.

    A. Infections in neutropenic patients

        1. Neutropenia is defined as an **absolute neutrophil count [ANC] <500 cells/mm³ or <1,000 cells/mm³ with anticipated decrease of >500 cells/mm³ within 48 hours; severe neutropenia** is often defined as an **ANC <100/μL.** Neutropenia most often results from leukemia, chemotherapy, or bone marrow transplantation. Occasionally, neutropenia is due to drug reactions or aplastic anemia. Bacteria, particularly enteric and nonenteric gram-negative bacteria and gram-positive bacteria, and fungi

(*Candida* spp, *Aspergillus* spp) characteristically cause infection in neutropenic patients. Severe viral infections (HSV, CMV, and Epstein-Barr virus) may also occur.

2. **Fever** in patients with neutropenia should always be assumed to be due to infection.

3. **Treatment of neutropenic fever**

   a. **Initial treatment** involves **broad-spectrum** antibacterial agents directed against gram-positive and gram-negative bacteria, including *Pseudomonas* spp. Antibiotics should be continued for a minimum of 10 days or until the ANC rises above $500/\mu L$. In patients who are critically ill, **combination therapy** should be administered. Empiric treatment involves using agents that are likely to treat nosocomial antibiotic-resistant organisms and organisms such as *Enterobacter* spp and *Citrobacter* spp that rapidly become resistant to β-lactams. Potential combinations include a third- or fourth-generation cephalosporin, a carbapenem, or an antipseudomonal penicillin/β-lactamase combination as well as an aminoglycoside or a fluoroquinolone. Vancomycin should be added if there is suspicion of infection due to resistant gram-positive bacteria. In patients who are not critically ill, **monotherapy** may be appropriate. In such cases, a third- or fourth-generation cephalosporin, a carbapenem, or an antipseudomonal penicillin/β-lactamase combination may be employed.

   b. **Subsequent treatment** may involve **antifungal agents** such as amphotericin or an echinocandin if fever is ongoing for 4 to 7 days despite broad-spectrum antibacterial therapy.

B. **Infections in transplant recipients.** Transplant recipients are most susceptible to life-threatening infections during the first 6 months after organ transplantation. During this time, they are maximally immunosuppressed, they are exposed to many nosocomial organisms, and they may be experiencing **allograft rejection** or **graft-versus-host disease (GVHD)**. Infections can be caused by bacteria, fungi, viruses, protozoa, parasites, and mycobacteria. Bacterial infections are caused by aerobic gram-positive and gram-negative bacteria. Fungal infections are most commonly caused by *Candida* and *Aspergillus* spp. Some infections, such as CMV, can be transmitted from the organ to the recipient, or via transfused blood products. Fever in the absence of localized findings is often the first manifestation of infection. Short courses of parenteral antibiotics are generally given before and after solid-organ transplantation. Patient and environmental factors dictate antibiotic choices. Some antibiotics have significant interactions with immunosuppressive agents. Metabolism of cyclosporine (CSA) by the cytochrome P-450 system can be increased or decreased by administration of fluoroquinolones, macrolides, fluconazole, rifampin, and isoniazid. Aminoglycosides, amphotericin B, vancomycin, pentamidine, and high-dose trimethoprim/sulfamethoxazole enhance the nephrotoxicity of CSA. CSA levels should be monitored in patients receiving these agents.

   1. **Solid-organ transplantation**

      a. **In the first month** post transplantation, infections are usually caused by the same bacteria and fungi that cause infections in immunocompetent postsurgical patients. Early post-transplant infections are usually nosocomial, occurring at the surgical site, or as a result of indwelling catheters or prolonged endotracheal intubation.

      b. **Between 1 and 6 months**, viral and opportunistic infections, such as *Pneumocystis carinii* pneumonia and aspergillosis predominate.

      c. **After 6 months**, infections depend on the degree of immunosuppression and environmental exposures. Patients on minimal immunosuppressive therapy develop similar infections as immunocompetent hosts. High doses of immunosuppressive agents predispose patients to infections with opportunistic pathogens such as *P. carinii, L. monocytogenes, Aspergillus fumigatus,* and *C. neoformans.* Pre-existing viral infections may progress and cause damage to infected organs. CMV infection can cause isolated fever, hepatitis, pneumonitis, hypotension, enterocolitis, and glomerulonephritis. Manifestations of CNS infections (generally caused by *L. monocytogenes* or opportunistic pathogens) can be atypical. CT of the head and lumber puncture are necessary for transplant patients with unexplained fever or headache. Chest CT may be useful in evaluating transplant patients with pulmonary symptoms because the typical radiographic signs of inflammation are often attenuated.

2. **Bone marrow transplantation.** Allogeneic and autologous bone marrow transplants are performed for the treatment of acute and chronic leukemias, lymphoma, solid tumors, multiple myeloma, and severe aplastic anemia. There are three phases of infectious disease complications after bone marrow transplantation:

   a. **The first month** is characterized by ongoing neutropenia from prior chemotherapy. Bacterial, fungal, and viral infections occur. Bacterial infections are caused by gram-positive aerobes, including coagulase-negative *Staphylococcus, Streptococcus viridans, Staphylococcus aureus,* and *Corynebacterium* spp, and enteric and nonenteric gram-negative aerobes and facultative anaerobes. Reactivation of HSV can also occur. **Empiric antibiotic therapy** for febrile neutropenic bone marrow transplant patients should include agents that cover gram-negative and gram-positive bacteria. Antipseudomonal coverage should be included. Empiric coverage is often undertaken using a combination of β-lactams (one antipseudomonal cephalosporin and one antipseudomonal penicillin such as piperacillin or mezlocillin) or an antipseudomonal β-lactam plus vancomycin, or a carbapenem (imipenem or meropenem) plus vancomycin. **Antifungal coverage** should be considered if fevers persist despite broad antibacterial coverage.

   b. **From 1 to 3 months,** patients are prone to viral infections (CMV), opportunistic infections, and gram-positive and gram-negative bacterial infections.

   c. **Late infections,** occurring after 3 months, often involve the respiratory tract and are caused by respiratory viruses and encapsulated organisms such as *Streptococcus pneumoniae* and *H. influenzae.* Mucocutaneous damage due to GVHD also predisposes these patients to infections with skin flora.

C. **Human immunodeficiency virus (HIV).** Progress in antiretroviral therapy and prophylaxis against opportunistic infections has resulted in longer survival of patients infected with HIV and in improved survival of HIV-infected patients in the ICU. The **T4-helper (CD4)** count is an accurate predictor of sites and organisms involved in infection in HIV patients, as indicated in **Table 12-4.** Infection with HIV predisposes patients to opportunistic infections and increases susceptibility to infection with encapsulated bacteria, including *Streptococcus pneumoniae* and *H. influenzae.*

   1. **Pulmonary infections** in HIV patients are caused by a variety of microorganisms. In patients with normal CD4 counts, pneumonia may be due to community-acquired organisms. As the CD4 count drops, the likelihood that pulmonary infection is due to opportunistic infections, particularly *P. carinii* and CMV, increases. Evaluation for the etiology of

TABLE 12-4	Relationship of CD4 Count to Infection in HIV Patients

CD4 Count (per µL)	Microbiologic Predisposition
>800	Community-acquired organisms
<800	*Mycobacterium tuberculosis* (pulmonary)
<500	*Candida* species, *Cryptococcus neoformans, Histoplasma capsulatum, Coccidioides* species
<300	*Pneumocystis carinii*
<100	*Mycobacterium avium intracellulare, Mycobacterium tuberculosis* (disseminated), *Cryptosporidium,* cytomegalovirus

pneumonitis should be prompt, and should include induced sputum examination, deep aspiration, or bronchoscopy with bronchoalveolar lavage. Empiric antibiotic therapy should cover most likely pathogens based on the CD4 count and geographic location. Above a CD4 count of roughly 200 to 300/µL, antibiotics should cover community-acquired organisms. Below a CD4 count of 200, treatment also should cover *P. carinii.*

2. **CNS infections** such as brain abscess, meningitis, and encephalitis can be caused by a variety of organisms, including bacteria, fungi, viruses, and parasites in patients with HIV. Evaluation for CNS infections, including CT scans or magnetic resonance imaging of the brain and lumbar puncture, should be performed if CNS infection is suspected, and empiric antibiotics should be administered while awaiting the results.

Selected References

Bochud PY et al. Antimicrobial therapy for patients with severe sepsis and septic shock: an evidence-based review. *Crit Care Med* 2004;32:S495.

Cohen J, Powderly WG. *Infectious diseases.* 2nd ed. New York: Elsevier, 2004.

Cunha BA. Sepsis and septic shock: selection of empiric antimicrobial therapy. *Crit Care Clin* 2008;24:313–334.

David N, Gilbert RC, Moellering GM, et al. *The Sanford guide to antimicrobial therapy.* 38th ed. Vienna, VA: Antimicrobial Therapy, 2008.

Dellinger RP, Levy MM, Carlet JM, et al. Surviving Sepsis Campaign: International guidelines for management of severe sepsis and septic shock: 2008. *Crit Care Med* 2008;36:296–327.

Endo S, Aikawa N, Fujishima S, et al. Usefulness of procalcitonin serum level for the discrimination of severe sepsis from sepsis: a multicenter prospective study. *J Infect Chemother* 2008;14:244–249.

Fishman JA. Infection in solid-organ transplant recipients. *N Engl J Med* 2007;357(25): 2601–2614.

Kumar A, Roberts D, Wood KE, et al. Duration of hypotension before initiation of effective antimicrobial therapy is the critical determinant of survival in human septic shock. *Crit Care Med* 2006;34:1589.

Lawrence KR, Adra M, Gillman PK. Serotonin toxicity associated with the use of linezolid: a review of postmarketing data. *Clin Infect Dis* 2006;42(11):1578–1583.

Mehrotra R, De Gaudio R, Palazzo M. Antibiotic pharmacokinetic and pharmacodynamic considerations in critical illness. *Intensive Care Med* 2004;30:2145–2156.

Rivers E, Nguyen B, Havstad S, et al. Early goal-directed therapy in the treatment of severe sepsis and septic shock. *N Engl J Med* 2001;345:1368–1377.

Schuetz P, Christ-Crain M, Müller B. Biomarkers to improve diagnostic and prognostic accuracy in systemic infections. *Curr Opin Crit Care* 2007;13:578–585.

13
Quality Improvement and Prophylaxis
Karsten Bartels and Ulrich Schmidt

I. **Quality improvement and patient safety**
   A. **Improving patient care.** Patients in the United States receive only approximately 50% of the recommended care. Initiatives to improve the quality of care have been launched in various institutions and on a national level. Measuring and improving quality of care will become essential for all health care providers. The federal Deficit Reduction Act of 2005 authorized the Centers for Medicare and Medicaid to implement a value-based purchasing plan by the year 2009. Value-based purchasing links payment to the quality of care provided by measuring and rewarding high-quality and efficient clinical care.
   B. **Measuring quality of care.** Quality measures used for public reporting should be both feasible to measure and scientifically supported. This constitutes an ongoing conundrum. Especially in the ICU, there is often only limited amount of data to guide a clinical decision. Evidence for the beneficial effects of certain interventions is subject to constant reanalysis and change. For example, perioperative administration of β-blockers had been included in several pay-for-performance initiatives before further evidence that contradicted the initial recommendations became available.
   C. **Design and implementation of institutional protocols.** To develop, implement, and adapt quality improvement and patient safety measures, institutions should develop their own protocols. Imperative for any successful quality improvement measure is the creation of a multidisciplinary team to guide the improvement process and to ensure support by all stakeholders. The following outline exemplifies this strategy for a common area of quality improvement: hand hygiene.
      1. Identifying the problem: *Lack of hand hygiene results in avoidable hospital-acquired infections. Obtain baseline measurements of current adherence to hand hygiene guidelines.*
      2. Selecting areas of performance improvement: *Hand hygiene practiced by medical staff in the ICU, assessed by rates of disinfection/washing of hands before and after every patient contact.*
      3. Test the strategy for change: *Education of staff, ensuring easy access to disinfectant solutions, staff bonus pay tied to adherence rates.*
      4. Assess data to see if performance is improved: *Monitor rates of appropriate hand hygiene before and after performance improvement measure was implemented.*
      5. Create plans to implement improvement throughout the system: *Build institutional task force to develop plan to implement similar processes across entire system.*
      6. Continue to monitor effectiveness and make changes as needed: *Assess impact of hand hygiene improvements on rates of hospital-acquired infections.*

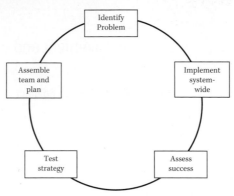

FIGURE 13-1 Strategy for initiating performance improvement measures in the ICU (counterclock wise, starting from 'Identify Problem').

A strategy for initiating performance improvement measures in the ICU is summarized in **Fig. 13-1**.

II. **Infection control in the ICU.** ICU patients have an increased risk for nosocomial infection. Pneumonia, urinary tract infection, and bloodstream infection are the most common. Both host and environmental factors are important in the development of nosocomial infections. Elderly patients and immunosuppressed patients are at increased risk of acquiring infections. Chronic diseases increase the risk of site-specific infections. Patients with underlying lung disease are more likely to develop pneumonia, and patients with chronic renal disease and diabetes are prone to develop urinary tract infections. Environmental factors impair host defenses. Antibiotics shift the endogenous colonizing flora. Instrumentation of the airway for the delivery of mechanical ventilation constitutes a port of entry for nosocomial pathogens and compromises clearing of bronchial secretions. Invasive monitors break the skin and mucosal barriers. These impaired host defenses facilitate transmission of microorganisms to patients by personnel, equipment, or ventilation systems.

   A. **General infection control.** Microorganisms are transmitted in hospitals by contact, droplets, airborne particles, and contaminated items.

      1. **Contact.** Spread of microorganisms can occur by direct and indirect contact. Transmission by hand to body surface is much more common than indirect contact to a contaminated surface. For example, almost all cases of methicillin-resistant *Staphylococcus aureus* are transmitted by hand contamination of health care providers.

      2. **Droplets** are particles larger than 5 μm in diameter. Droplets can only be transmitted over a short distance—less than 3 ft. They are transmitted through coughing and sneezing. Droplets transmit microorganisms including *Neisseria meningitidis, Haemophilus influenzae, Mycoplasma pneumoniae,* adenovirus, and rubella virus.

      3. **Airborne particles** are smaller (<5 μm) than droplets and can remain in the air for a long period of time. **Tuberculosis (TB), measles, varicella,** and **disseminated varicella-zoster** virus are spread by airborne particles.

      4. **Contaminated items.** Infection by contaminated items is rare. However, improper sterilization of bronchoscopes and endoscopes has led to

TABLE 13-1	Precaution for Transmission of Infectious Diseases	
Standard precautions	All hospitalized patients	Hand washing and disinfection. Gloves, gowns, eye protection. Safe disposal of sharps, safe disposal of contaminated material
Airborne precautions	Tuberculosis, measles, varicella, varicella-zoster virus	Isolation room Special mask
Droplet precautions	*Neisseria meningitidis, Haemophilus influenzae, Rubella Mycoplasma,* adenovirus, severe acute respiratory syndrome	Private room Face mask for contact
Contact precautions	Multidrug-resistant bacteria	Nonsterile gloves and gowns. Hand washing

infection with microorganisms such as *Pseudomonas aeruginosa* and *Serratia marcescens.*

B. **Specific infection control measures** decrease the risk of nosocomial infection and prevent transmission of pathogens from ICU staff to patients and vice versa. Aggressive surveillance strategies might help to reduce nosocomial infections. The **Center for Disease Control and Prevention (CDC)** has implemented a system based on standard precautions and transmission-based precautions (**Table 13-1**).

1. **Standard precautions** are intended for all patients. They decrease the risk of infections for patients and health care workers. They include

a. **Hand hygiene** has been identified as a major factor for transmission of infectious disease in the hospital setting. Disinfection of the hands should take place **prior and following every patient contact**. Hand washing with soap and water should take place if hands are visibly soiled or if *Clostridium difficile* is suspected. Interestingly, an inverse correlation between level of professional education and compliance with hand washing has been reported.

b. **Gloves, gowns,** and **protective eyewear** are recommended for working with all ICU patients.

c. **Safe disposal of sharps** in specially designed, safe containers is warranted. According to the Occupational Safety and Health Administration (OSHA), 385,000 needle injuries from needles and other sharps occur annually in hospitals throughout the United States. The most important pathogens transmitted include human immunodeficiency virus (**HIV**), hepatitis B virus (**HBV**), and hepatitis C virus (**HCV**). OSHA requires all health care facilities to implement plans to decrease the transmission of **blood-borne pathogens**. These include the following measures:

(1) Annual education for health care workers regarding the minimization of transmission of blood-borne pathogens.

(2) Standard precautions for working with all patients.

(3) Hepatitis B immunization as pre-exposure prophylaxis.

(4) Decreasing the use of sharps (e.g., use of prefilled syringes, safety and closed blood collection systems) and engineering tools to reduce the risk of injury with sharps (self-containing needle systems, special containers, etc).

d. Following exposure to blood, tissue, or other body fluids, wounds should be cleaned thoroughly with soap and water. The health care worker should undergo an immediate evaluation by a physician with expertise in occupational health and infectious disease. This evaluation includes documentation of the incidence. After obtaining consent, blood from both the health care worker and from the source should be tested for HBV, HBC, and HIV. For details of post-exposure prophylaxis, refer to regularly updated CDC guidelines: http://www.cdc.gov/ncidod/dhqp/wrkrProtect_bp.html

e. Soiled material should be placed in special bags. Feces and urine should be discarded in sanitary toilets.

2. Airborne precautions are used in patients with suspected or confirmed infection with *Mycobacterium tuberculosis, Varicella*, and disseminated *Varicella zoster* virus. A single, negative-pressure isolation room is required for patients with airborne precautions.

a. Special considerations for TB

(1) Negative-pressure rooms should have 12 or more air exchanges per hour, should be exhausted to the exterior, and should have anterooms to effectively separate them from the rest of the ward.

(2) Respiratory protection masks (N-95) are designed to filter inhaled air. They filter small particles (<1 μm) with at least 95% efficiency. These masks should be fitted to each person's face in advance to ensure optimal fit and limit leakage. Persons in contact with patients at risk should wear respiratory protection masks. In contrast, the patient should wear a surgical mask when leaving the isolation room. Surgical masks are designed to prevent secretions from entering the environment.

(3) Discontinuation of TB isolation. The patient can be transferred to a regular room when TB is ruled out or when the patient is felt to have been treated effectively. Treated patients must show clinical signs of improvement and have three consecutive sputum samples that are negative for acid-fast bacilli.

3. Droplet precautions are used to limit the spread of infectious agents that are transmitted over a short distance by coughing and sneezing. Patients should be placed in a single room. Personnel and visitors who come in close proximity to patients on droplet precautions must wear a surgical mask.

4. Contact precautions minimize spread of microorganisms from direct contact or indirect contact with environmental surfaces.

a. They are used for patients colonized or infected with antibiotic-resistant bacteria.

b. Patients should be placed in private rooms.

c. Health care providers must wear gloves and gowns to minimize direct contact with patients and surfaces.

d. Disinfection of hands must occur before and after every patient contact.

e. After a patient is brought to a new environment, all surface areas need to be cleaned.

C. Prevention of intravascular catheter-related infections. The average rate of intravascular **central venous catheter (CVC)**–related bloodstream infections in the United States is 5.3 per 1,000 catheter days. This results in approximately 80,000 infections per year, and morbidity has been reported to increase by up to 35% when controlled for severity of illness. The annual cost attributed to CVC-related bloodstream infections has been estimated at US $2.3 billion. Hence, line infections have become a focal point of concern for hospital administrations and regulating agencies. Recent evidence demonstrated that by using protocolized efforts CVC-related infections could be largely eliminated. Measures recommended include

1. **Education** of clinicians about best practices to control infection is pivotal to implementing a successful program for decreasing CVC-related bloodstream infections.
2. **A central line cart** with all necessary supplies should be provided.
3. **Catheter site selection:** Central lines are placed mainly in internal jugular, subclavian, and femoral veins. Subclavian vein catheters have the lowest risk of infection. If possible, the femoral vein should be avoided in adult patients.
4. **Aseptic technique** is recommended for the insertion of CVCs. The importance of infection control practices should be included in the training of health care providers. Operators should disinfect their hands. Sterile gloves, gowns, caps, and surgical masks should be worn for insertion of central lines. Complete sterile barrier drapes should be used.
5. **Skin preparation with 2% aqueous chlorhexidine** has been shown to decrease the number of central line infections.
6. During the insertion of a line, one team member should run a **checklist** to ensure adherence to infection-control practices and be empowered to hold the procedure (in nonemergency situations) if these practices are not being followed. The checklist used at our institution is depicted in **Fig. 13-2**.
7. The need for central venous access should be re-evaluated at daily rounds, and catheters should be removed as early as possible. Other strategies include
   a. **Selection of catheters.** The material and coating of catheters influence the incidence of line infections.
      (1) **Material.** Bacterial adherence is decreased in catheters made from polyurethane, Teflon, and silicone elastomers. It is therefore recommended to use catheters made from one of these materials.
      (2) **Coating**
         i. Heparin sodium bonding decreases the incidence of catheter-related thrombus as a possible source of infection. Heparin-bonded catheters reduce the incidence of catheter infection.
         ii. **Chlorhexidine-/silver sulfazidine**–impregnated catheters lead to a significant reduction in catheter colonization and catheter-related bacteremia.
         iii. **Minocycline-/rifampin-**impregnated catheters decrease the rate of line infections. The impregnation does not cause changes in antibiotic resistance.
      (3) **Number of catheter lumens.** Multilumen catheters have a higher number of infections. When possible, it is recommended to insert catheters with a lower number of lumens.
   b. **Feedback** regarding the number and rates of catheter-related bloodstream infections should be provided to the care team regularly.
   c. **Change of central lines.** Routine change of central lines either by new stick or guide wire change does not seem to decrease the incidence of line infection. Instead of scheduled line changes, it is recommended to evaluate the patient for line infection on a continuous basis.

Central Line Infection Prevention Checklist   MASSACHUSETTS
GENERAL HOSPITAL

Goal	To decrease patient harm from catheter-related blood stream infections
Who	An operator & a monitor
What	Assure compliance with and documentation of checklist elements
Where	At the site of the procedure
When	During all central venous line insertions or rewires
How	The monitor verifies that the steps have occurred, immediately informs the operator/supervisor of deviations, & completes the checklist *Patient label*

Roles:
Operator: the clinician placing the central line
Supervisor: an experienced operator that is involved in training the operator in central line placement
Monitor: an individual that is qualified to observe the procedure and watch for breaks in sterile technique. If a break in sterile technique is observed, the monitor asks the operator to repeat a portion of the procedure after correcting the observed break. Please identify a monitor for this line placement prior to the time out.

Procedure Planning					
Line Insertion Site:	❑ Subclavian	❑ Internal Jugular	❑ Femoral ❑ PICC	❑ Other (specify)	

	Yes	No	Comments/Reason
Emergent placement	❑	❑	
Timeout documented separately	❑	❑	
Consent documented separately	❑	❑	

If there is a deviation in any of the critical steps, immediately notify the operator and stop the procedure until corrected. If the step is completed properly, check the "Yes" box. If the step is not completed properly, check the "No" box and note the issue in the "Comments/Reason" section. Contact the Attending if any item on the checklist is not adhered to or with any concerns.

Critical Step for Line Insertion	Yes	No	Comments/Reason
Before the procedure, the operator will:			
Confirm hand sanitizing (Cal Stat) or antimicrobial soap immediately prior	❑	❑	
Disinfect procedure site (chlorhexidine) using a back & forth friction scrub for 30 seconds. In patients < 2 months of age, use povidone iodine instead of chlorhexidine.	❑	❑	
Allow site to dry for 30 seconds	❑	❑	
Operator(s): hat, mask, sterile gown/gloves, eye protection	❑	❑	
Assistant/Monitor: hat, mask & standard precautions (if at risk for entering sterile field use sterile gown/gloves)	❑	❑	
Use sterile technique to drape from head to toe; Pediatrics use judgment to determine extent of draping.	❑	❑	
During the procedure, the operator will:			
Maintain a sterile field	❑	❑	
Flush and cap line before removal of drapes	❑	❑	
After the procedure, the operator will:			
Remove blood with antiseptic agent (chlorhexidine), if present, before placement of sterile dressing	❑	❑	
Apply appropriate (green = all "yes", red = 1 or more "no") dated sticker on patient's line	❑	❑	
Date & Time:		Unit:	
Operator:	MD/RN	Monitor:	Credentials

FIGURE 13-2 Central line insertion checklist.

    d. Percutaneously inserted central catheters (PICC) are inserted centrally via peripheral arm veins, generally at the antecubital fossa. Maintenance and follow-up are important, since the line infection risk in the hospital setting is comparable or even higher compared to central lines.

D. Prevention of catheter-associated urinary tract infections. Urinary tract infections affect approximately 600,000 patients per year in acute care hospitals. Approximately 1% of these patients develop severe gram-negative sepsis with often multiresistant bacteria. Similar to line infections, UTIs may be regarded as preventable complications with implications on payment in the future.

    1. Catheter placement: Indwelling urinary catheters should be placed only in patients for whom frequent measurement of urinary output is beneficial. Alternatives to indwelling devices such as condom catheters or intermittent catheterization should be considered. Indwelling urinary catheters

TABLE 13-2	Prevention of Ventilator-Associated Pneumonia (VAP)	
Approach		**Recommendation**
Nonpharmacologic		
Positioning	Semirecumbent position	$++$
	Kinetic beds	$+$
Airway	Short intubation	$++$
	Oral intubation and use of orogastric tubes	$+$
	Drainage of subglottic secretions	$+$
	Infrequent change of humidifier and no change of ventilatory circuit	$+$
Other	Noninvasive mechanical ventilation for patients with COPD and cardiogenic pulmonary edema	$+$
	Standardized protocols for weaning and enteral feedings	$++$
Pharmacologic	No stress ulcer prophylaxis in low-risk patients	$+$
	Restriction of antibiotics	$+$
	Oral decontamination with chlorhexidine	$++$
	DVT prophylaxis	$+$

COPD, chronic obstructive pulmonary disease; DVT, deep vein thrombosis.
Note: $++$, strong evidence, $+$, some evidence supporting the recommendation.

must be placed under strict aseptic technique by trained personnel. For most adult patients, 14 to 18 French catheters are an appropriate size. Smaller catheters are preferable in terms of infection prevention.

2. **Catheter maintenance and removal:** Clinicians should wash their hands and wear gloves prior to handling the indwelling catheter or drainage tubing. Closed drainage systems should be utilized. The incidence of urinary tract infection increases with breaks in the drainage system. Catheters should be secured to the patient's leg to prevent movement or traction of the catheter. Catheters should not be changed unless there is frequent occlusion of the catheter that requires repeated irrigation. Routine irrigation should be avoided. The most often cited strategies for avoiding catheter-associated urinary tract infections are the following:
   a. Removal of the urinary catheter as soon as possible. The need for the catheter should be re-evaluated at daily rounds.
   b. Use of closed drainage systems.

E. **Prevention of ventilator-associated pneumonia (VAP).** VAP (**Chapter 29**) is one of the most common nosocomial infections within the ICU, resulting in increased length of stay, cost of care, and mortality. Prevention strategies are aimed at minimizing aspiration and prevention of colonization of the airway and the gastrointestinal (GI) tract with pathogens. The incidence of VAP resembles a possible target for implementation of pay-for-performance policies; however this is a subject of ongoing debate. Commonly used pharmacologic and nonpharmacologic approaches and their efficacy are summarized in **Table 13-2**.

1. **Positioning**
   a. **Semirecumbent position** decreases the incidence of aspiration and VAP. It is therefore recommended to keep the head of the bed elevated at greater than 30 degrees whenever possible.

   b. **Kinetic therapy.** Altering a patient's position has been shown to enhance mobilization of secretions and decrease atelectasis. Evidence
   is limited, and due to high costs we recommend restricting the use
   of these beds to patients who are difficult to mobilize.
2. **Airway management**
   a. **Duration of intubation.** Intubation of the airway is a prerequisite for
   developing VAP. Noninvasive ventilation (**Chapter 5**) has emerged as
   a successful alternative to intubation especially in patients with
   congestive heart failure and chronic obstructive pulmonary disease
   (COPD). Development of VAP increases with the duration of
   mechanical ventilation. Strategies to shorten time on the ventilator
   have the potential to decrease VAP.
   b. **Route of intubation.** The oral route for tracheal intubation is recommended. The presence of a nasotracheal or a nasogastric tube promotes sinusitis and VAP.
   c. **Coating of endotracheal tube.** Silver coating of the endotracheal tube
   has been recently shown to decrease VAP. However, the absence of a
   difference in mortality and the high costs of the endotracheal tubes
   may limit the widespread use of these tubes to high-risk populations.
   d. **Subglottic suctioning.** Most intubated patients have secretions in the
   upper airways that tend to pool above the balloon of the endotracheal tube. Constant microaspiration occurs. Strategies for
   decreasing these secretions may aid in preventing VAP. Special
   endotracheal tubes with a separate dorsal hole allowing continuous
   suction have been developed. Use of these tubes has decreased the
   incidence of VAP in patients intubated for >48 hours. In patients
   where these tubes are not placed, intermittent suctioning of the
   back of the throat is recommended.
3. **Stress ulcer prophylaxis.** Decreasing intragastric acidity by histamine-2
   blockers or proton pump inhibitors may increase the incidence of VAP.
   However, intubated patients are at increased risk of developing GI
   bleeding, and transfusion is a risk factor for VAP. It is therefore recommended that prophylaxis for GI bleeding be continued in these patients.
4. **Prevention of colonization of GI tract.** Colonization of the oropharynx is
   a major pathophysiologic factor in the development of VAP.
   a. **Oral decontamination** is effective for decreasing the incidence of VAP.
   Topical treatment of the oral cavity with chlorhexidine in patients
   intubated for more than 24 hours showed reduction in the development of VAP, and is therefore recommended. Although topical oral
   antibiotics have also been shown to decrease the incidence of VAP,
   their use has been associated with emergence of antibiotic resistance and can therefore not be universally recommended.
   b. **Selective decontamination** of the digestive tract (SDD) uses a combination of topical and nonabsorbable antibiotics to eradicate pathogenic
   organisms from the GI tract. It has been shown to decrease nosocomial pneumonia and ICU mortality. However, there is concern that
   SDD may promote the emergence of antibiotic resistance. Because of
   these concerns, SDD is not widely used in the United States.
5. **Antibiotics.** The use of antibiotics in general is associated with the emergence of antibiotic-resistant bacteria. This is associated with an increase
   of antibiotic-resistant VAP. The following strategies have been shown to
   decrease the incidence of pneumonia by antibiotic-resistant bacteria.
   a. **Prophylactic antibiotics.** Prolonged use of prophylactic antibiotics
   is associated with an increased incidence of VAP; therefore, it is

recommended to limit the duration of prophylactic antibiotics to 24 hours or less.

b. **Antibiotic rotation.** Cycling antibiotic therapy has been shown to decrease the incidence of VAP. This strategy should be part of a wider strategy to limit the emergence of antibiotic-resistant infections.

c. **Shortening the course of empiric antibiotic** therapy has been shown to decrease the emergence of resistant bacteria. This approach may help to reduce the incidence of subsequent infections including VAP.

III. **Prophylaxis of GI bleeding.** The majority of patients admitted to the ICU develop mucosal damage of the GI tract. Clinically significant GI bleeding develops in approximately 2% to 15% of critically ill patients, and carries a high mortality. Mechanical ventilation of more than 48 hours and coagulopathy have been identified as risk factors for GI bleeding. These patients are most likely to benefit from prophylaxis. In nonintubated noncoagulopathic patients, GI prophylaxis might not be necessary. The following strategies are used to decrease the incidence of GI bleeding.

A. **Histamine-2 (H-2) receptor antagonists** decrease the stimulatory effects of histamine on acid production. H-2 blockers decrease the incidence of GI bleeding in the ICU. They can be given in enteral and intravenous (IV) form. Continuous infusion has the best control over gastric pH. The use of H-2 blockers is limited by the development of tolerance. It is unclear whether H-2 blockers increase the risk of VAP.

B. **Proton pump inhibitors (PPIs)** inactivate the hydrogen–potassium ATPase pump and thereby decrease gastric pH. PPIs are effective in decreasing GI bleeding. In contrast to H-2 blockers, there is no tolerance development against PPIs. To date, no trials prove the superiority of PPIs over ranitidine in the prevention of GI bleeding.

C. **Enteral feeding** may decrease the incidence of GI bleeding in critically ill patients. The mechanism is unknown. In patients with risk for GI bleeding, it is recommended to combine enteral feeding with pharmacotherapy.

D. **Antacids** decrease gastric acidity by direct neutralization of stomach acid. The efficacy of these drugs in critically ill patients is questionable. In addition, these drugs have to be given in large volume (30–60 mL) every 1 to 2 hours. In general, antacids are not recommended in the ICU population.

E. **Cytoprotection.** Sucralfate is a polysaccharide that provides protection of gastric mucosa by coating the surface. In mechanically ventilated patients, sucralfate was less effective than ranitidine in preventing clinically important GI bleeding. However, sucralfate is less expensive and has not been associated with an increase in VAP. Prostaglandin analogues have also been shown to be cytoprotective. There are not enough data to support their widespread use in critically ill patients.

IV. **Prophylaxis of deep vein thrombosis (DVT) and pulmonary embolism (PE).** DVT occurs in 13% to 31% of patients admitted to critical care unit, and is associated with significant morbidity. It has been reported that among patients who died in the ICU, PE was present in 7% to 27% of the cases.

A. **High-risk** patients include those immobilized or at bed rest and who have severe head injury (Glasgow Coma Score ≤8), severe blunt chest or abdominal injury, pelvic fractures, severe lower extremity injuries, and selected burns, especially electrical burns.

B. **Relatively immobile patients** should receive prophylaxis, if possible, if they have additional risk factors such as previous history of DVT or PE, obesity,

age more than 60 years, presence of femoral venous catheter, pregnancy, cancer, and marginal cardiopulmonary reserve.
  C. **Critically ill patients.** All critically ill patients require prophylaxis.
  D. **Prophylaxis** includes nonpharmacologic and pharmacologic measures.
    1. **Elastic stockings** and **sequential compression boots** are used routinely, but their efficacy appears to be marginal. Increasing patient mobility reduces venous stasis and the formation of DVT. These measures should usually be supplemented by pharmacologic prophylaxis, especially in critically ill patients, though the efficacy of combined therapy has not been evaluated. Critically ill patients at high risk of bleeding should receive sequential compression boots.
    2. If a mild to moderate risk of bleeding exists, **subcutaneous unfractionated heparin (UFH)** (in the adult, 5,000 Units every 12 hours, or every 8 hours for patients who are high risk or weigh >100 kg), alternatively, **low-molecular-weight heparin (LMWH)** can be administered. Both UFH and LMWH reduce the incidence of PE and DVT.
    3. **If anticoagulation is contraindicated**, periodic systematic screening for deep venous thrombosis with venous ultrasound should be conducted. In high-risk patients, this is usually performed twice per week.
    4. If surveillance cannot be adequately performed, prophylactic placement of an **inferior vena cava filter** can be considered in high-risk patients.
    5. For patients who present with thrombocytopenia associated with HIT, **lepirudin, argatroban,** and **fondaparinux** can be used for prophylaxis. Because argatroban is metabolized by the liver, it should be avoided in patients with severe hepatic dysfunction. Lepirudin is cleared by the kidney and should not be used in patients with renal impairment. Fondaparinux is a synthetic pentasaccharide, which binds to antithrombin, thereby indirectly selectively inhibiting factor Xa. Fondaparinux can be used for the prevention and treatment of venous thromboembolism in patients with HIT. Its half-life elimination is increased in renal impairment.

Selected References

Bouza E, Pérez MJ, Muñoz P, Rincón C, Barrio JM, Hortal J. Continuous aspiration of subglottic secretions in the prevention of ventilator-associated pneumonia in the postoperative period of major heart surgery. *Chest* 2008;134(5):938–946.

Craven DE. Preventing ventilator-associated pneumonia in adults: sowing seeds of change. *Chest* 2006;130(1):251–260.

Kantorova I, Svoboda P, Scheer P, et al. Stress ulcer prophylaxis in critically ill patients: a randomized controlled trial. *Hepatogastroenterology* 2004;51(57):757–761.

Kollef M. SMART approaches for reducing nosocomial infections in the ICU. *Chest* 2008;134(2):447–456.

Kollef MH, Afessa B, Anzueto A, et al; NASCENT Investigation Group. Silver-coated endotracheal tubes and incidence of ventilator-associated pneumonia: the NASCENT randomized trial. *JAMA* 2008;300(7):805–813.

Limpus A, Chaboyer W, McDonald E, Thalib L. Mechanical thromboprophylaxis in critically ill patients: a systematic review and meta-analysis. *Am J Crit Care* 2006;15(4):402–410.

McGlynn EA, Asch SM, Adams J, et al. The quality of health care delivered to adults in the United States. *N Engl J Med* 2003;348(26):2635–2645.

Proceedings of the National Sharps Injury Prevention Meeting, September 12, 2005 Crown Plaza Atlanta Airport Hotel, Atlanta GA. Accessed at: http://www.cdc.gov/sharpssafety/pdf/proceedings.pdf.

Pronovost P, Needham D, Berenholtz S, et al. An intervention to decrease catheter-related bloodstream infections in the ICU. *N Engl J Med* 2006;355:2725.

Pronovost PJ, Berenholtz SM, Goeschel CA. Improving the quality of measurement and evaluation in quality improvement efforts. *Am J Med Qual* 2008;23(2):143–146.

14

Ethical and Legal Issues
in ICU Practice
Rae Allain and Sharon Brackett

I. **Introduction.** Care of the critically ill patient necessarily involves acknowledg-
ment that some patients will die despite best medical therapy. Mortality rates
in ICUs vary widely, depending on practice type and patient population, but
a minimum 10% mortality rate is typical. Approximately one in five deaths in
the United States today occurs during or after ICU admission, and **most
deaths in ICUs are preceded by decisions to withhold or withdraw some form of
therapy.** Thus, imminent death is usually a predictable event that has been
discussed among the critical care team, patient's family, and patient, if possible. In this setting, ethical and end-of-life issues come to the forefront and
sometimes provoke conflict. This chapter explores the ethical and legal
issues that frequently arise in the ICU and offers suggestions for avoiding and
resolving conflicts. Customs, laws, ethical beliefs, and religious practices differ considerably in different cultures and societies. This chapter describes
the prevailing practice at the Massachusetts General Hospital and is meant
to be thoughtful rather than definitive.

II. **Treatment decisions**
  A. Our society highly values patient **autonomy** (i.e., respect for an individual's
    preferences) as a guiding ethical principle in medicine. Competent adults
    can and may choose to accept or refuse medical therapies offered. If a
    patient's competence is questionable, a psychiatrist should evaluate the
    patient to determine whether he/she has **decision-making capacity.** This
    requires an ability to receive and understand medical information, to dis-
    cern the various options presented, and to choose a course based on the
    information offered and one's values.
  B. **Informed consent** is the process where permission is freely obtained from the
    patient for treatments rendered. The process consists of a dialogue between
    the patient and care provider with a description of the risks and benefits of
    each treatment as applied to the individual's situation and is a means of pre-
    serving autonomy. Ideally, informed consent should be obtained for
    1. **Procedures** (e.g., endotracheal intubation, mechanical ventilation, cen-
      tral venous cannulation, flexible fiberoptic bronchoscopy).
    2. **Therapies** (e.g., vasopressors, blood transfusions, chemotherapy).
    3. **Research.** The challenges to obtaining informed consent for research in-
      volving critically ill patients are formidable. Many patients lack decision-
      making capacity due to the gravity of their illness or due to sedative/
      analgesic medications employed to diminish suffering. Often, surro-
      gate decision-makers are unavailable until after enrollment in a
      research study must be decided, especially if the study is of emergent
      therapies. While a practical solution to this problem is a waiver of con-
      sent, the U.S. Code of Federal Regulations for the Protection of Human
      Subjects restricts waivers to specific situations, including the require-
      ment that research participation potentially provides "direct benefit"
      to the subject. Researchers who plan enrollment of critically ill

patients in study protocols are referred to their local institutional review board for further guidance.

C. Patients **lacking decision-making capacity** are common in the critical care unit (see above) and provide challenges to pursuing care congruent with patient autonomy.

1. An **advance directive** is a statement specifying the patient's health care wishes should he/she become unable to communicate for himself/herself and is very useful in this circumstance. The exact form of advance directives honored varies by U.S. state.

   a. A **health care proxy** or **durable power of attorney for health care** is a legal document prepared by the patient in advance of an incapacitated state. It delineates the person **(Health Care Agent)** whom he/she would wish to make health care decisions under those circumstances. These documents frequently provide an alternate agent if the primary is unable or unwilling to fulfill the role. Ideally, the patient has shared his or her wishes regarding treatments and life values with the proxy such that the agent can accurately render the substituted judgment (see **Section II.D.6.d**) of the patient.

   b. A **living will** is a document describing the therapies or interventions that a patient would wish to receive or refuse under specific circumstances. These documents can elucidate a patient's prior expressed wishes and should be considered as part of the decision-making process, but U.S. states vary as to whether they are legally binding. These documents range from very general to extraordinarily detailed, depending upon the individual. Since it is usually impossible for patients to predict exactly what health circumstances may arise, some living wills are only marginally helpful in the modern critical care environment. For example, many documents specify that a patient would not wish to be sustained by life support in the event of a persistent vegetative state (PVS) or agreement by physicians of no hope for meaningful recovery. However, PVS is a rare outcome of neurologic injury, and "no hope for meaningful recovery" requires an absolute prognosis as well as subjective interpretation of what "meaningful recovery" means to the individual patient. The intensivist may not be able to provide this information. Interpretation of living wills is best supplemented by communication with people closest to the patient (see **Section II.D**).

   c. Increasingly, the judicial system is recognizing that **advance directives may be verbal in nature,** and what a patient stated to family, close friends, or health care providers regarding treatment preferences can provide an acceptable framework for care decisions in the absence of written documents.

2. Options for decision-making in the absence of an advance directive include

   a. A de facto **surrogate,** usually the next of kin, or in some circumstances, a trusted friend. This individual should be reminded to offer **substituted judgment** for the patient, providing decisions that the patient would make if competent.

   b. A court-appointed legal **guardian,** who may be the last resort when no family member or friend exists or is able to make decisions in the best interest of the patient. One recent study suggests that up to 25% of deaths in the ICU may occur in this patient population, although the average was 5%. In an attempt to determine who this vulnerable population would wish to be in charge of life-determining decisions for them if the need arose, a survey of homeless persons without family indicated a preference for their physician as opposed to a court-appointed guardian. There is no medical consensus about who should make decisions in this circumstance—a wide range of recommendations from various professional medical organizations exist. Some recommend judicial review while others counsel against this, instead suggesting that the clinicians caring for the patient are in the best position to make decisions. The critical care team ought to be familiar with hospital policy and state law when confronted with an incapacitated patient who lacks advance directive, designated surrogate, or available family or friends. This situation may be an indication for the institutional ethics committee involvement (see **Section II.F**).

D. Family involvement

1. **Discussions** with family members regarding treatment of a patient who lacks capacity are vital to appropriate care and are best conducted in a quiet, private **environment** in an unhurried fashion. If the patient has capacity, he/she should be included in the discussion whenever possible. Physicians should refrain from such discussions in the ICU or in hospital corridors because real or apparent distractions and breaches of confidentiality will threaten to destroy the family's confidence in the critical care team, in addition to risking legal infraction under the **Health Insurance Portability and Protection Act (HIPPA)**. The patient's private ICU room may be used for patients able to participate; otherwise, a comfortable conference room near the ICU is the ideal setting.

2. **Attendants** to the family meeting should include the following:

   a. The patient's close family, including the **health care agent** or person who will serve as surrogate.

   b. The patient's **primary care physician** or alternate physician with whom the patient has had a long-term, trusting relationship.

   c. The **ICU attending physician and ICU nurse**. Occasionally, it may be helpful to have adjuvant team members (e.g., respiratory therapist, physical therapist, or occupational therapist) present.

   d. **Consulting specialists**, if needed, to present information regarding the patient's condition, therapeutic options, or prognosis.

   e. Ancillary support staff, including **social worker** and **chaplain**.

3. **Cultural differences** in the approach to serious illness and end-of-life care should be anticipated and respected by the ICU team.

4. **Disclosure of errors** in the ICU or hospital course may be revealed during family discussions. This trend toward transparency in the U.S. medical system is in part an ongoing departure from a prior era of paternalistic care as well as recognition of the high chance of some error occurring during hospitalization, especially in the critically ill. Estimates suggest that up to one-third of ICU patients are subject to a drug error during their course. The complex care involved in the ICU, including procedures with significant risk, vast amount of data collected per patient, and involvement of multiple caregivers as part of the team, invites potential error. When error occurs, most experts agree that disclosure be considered if (1) harm occurred and (2) an alternate action would have been undertaken by a similarly trained person who would have recognized the error. **The intent of disclosure is to apologize, to be honest,** and to **express empathy for the patient's (and family's) situation.** Observational data suggest that this type of approach to medical errors may, despite physicians' fears, reduce risk for

malpractice claims. Physicians are advised to seek expert consultation at their specific institutions in preparation for a disclosure meeting. Formal training in communication, akin to the concept of "how to deliver bad news" may aid all members of the team in this endeavor.

5. **Family presence at codes** (resuscitation) is a controversial topic that is gaining support amongst some practitioners and professional organizations. Part of the movement toward "family-centered care," which seeks to continue treatment of the critically ill patient in the context of the social environment where he/she usually lives, the presence of family during resuscitation may offer such advantages as tangible family support to the patient during life/death experience, improved handling of grief by the family, and a strengthened family bond to the caregiver team. Counterarguments to family presence include potential detriment to code team performance, physical impediment to resuscitation efforts, and worsened trauma to the family who witness the gruesome nature of some resuscitations. Keys to success of family presence include buy-in of all members of the care team, advance preparation via role playing or simulation, careful screening and support of the family member before and during presence, and debriefing after an actual event. Studies suggest that nurses are more supportive of family presence during resuscitation than their physician counterparts, and that there may be regional variation in the United States in health care provider acceptance of this new concept.

6. **The goals of ICU therapy** should be confirmed with the family. For many patients, the obvious goals will include preventing imminent death, curing the acute disease, preventing and relieving pain and suffering, and eventually returning the patient to his or her premorbid level of function. Some patients may only hope to delay the disease process sufficiently to gain a few more months or years of meaningful living. Occasionally, ICU care is requested to prolong a patient's life long enough for close relatives to arrive to pay last respects or consent to organ donation.

   a. **The prognosis** of the patient is very important to setting realistic therapeutic goals. It is important for the health care team to discuss the patient's prognosis and arrive at a consensus before meeting with the family.

      (1) **Consistency** in the message is important. Variant opinions about a patient's prognosis only serve to confuse the family, often resulting in delayed decisions, additional anguish, and sometimes hostility toward the care team. If opinions of consulting specialists differ, the intensivist or trusted primary physician should assume responsibility for summarizing the patient's overall condition for the family.

      (2) **Patience** is required during family discussions. Presenting a poor prognosis can be devastating; care should be taken to express compassion and empathy. Adequate time must be allowed for the family to contemplate what has been said and to ask questions. Often the first response is denial of the loved one's condition. The intensivist should gently reaffirm what has been presented and allow family members to express their grief. Acceptance of a poor prognosis may require several discussions over days or even a few weeks.

      (3) **Time-limited trials** of therapies may be suggested. For example, a short-term (e.g., 7 days) trial of renal replacement therapy may be initiated in the patient suffering from acute renal failure

where the prognosis for recovery is unclear. It is important that at the conclusion of such a trial, the care team reconvenes with the family to discuss the response (or lack thereof) of treatment and to determine further plans of action.

b. **Values** of the patient should be elicited and emphasized during discussions of goals. This requires listening on the part of the care team. Open-ended questions such as "What makes life most worth living for you (your father, your sister, etc)?" should be posed. If the prognosis is poor and death is expected, asking "Have you witnessed a relative or friend's death, and if so, what went well or poorly?" may help glean insight into the family's past experiences with death and address concerns.

c. Once the prognosis has been discussed, the family may request or the physician may suggest a **limitation of life-sustaining treatment** status for the patient, also defined as **"do not resuscitate" (DNR)**. The DNR status seeks to clarify what therapies will be offered to the patient in case of acute, life-threatening instability that requires immediate treatment to prevent death. **Clear instructions** should be given and documented in the chart regarding preferences for specific interventions such as cardiopulmonary resuscitation, endotracheal intubation, electrical therapy, and medical therapy in case of sudden cardiac or respiratory failure. The simple phrase "DNR" in the physician's orders is insufficient because the meaning will vary to different caregivers. When discussing limitations to treatment with the family, physicians should use their best clinical judgment to describe each therapy, including the potential risks and benefits and the expected outcome or prognosis for recovery. Physicians should also guide the family to internal consistency in decision-making—for example, a decision to pursue aggressive surgical therapy of disease without acceptance of perioperative endotracheal intubation and mechanical ventilation may indicate a lack of understanding on the part of the family and may require a more lengthy discussion regarding treatment options and expected consequences. It must also be emphasized to the family that any agreed limitation of treatment status does not signify that a patient's condition is hopeless or that therapies other than those specifically discussed will be withheld. In this sense, the term DNR has been inappropriately associated by patients and caregivers with a general withdrawal of care and often carries an ominous implication. Families may need to be reassured that current therapies intended to improve the patient's health will be continued unless a further decision to withdraw or withhold therapy has been made (see later discussion).

d. Eventually, a decision to **withdraw** or **withhold** therapies may be made. The majority of critically ill patients are incompetent to make this decision, and, thus, a **surrogate** is involved. As in deciding the possible limitations of care, the patient's surrogate should approach this decision using substituted judgment or determining what type of care **the patient would have wanted for himself/herself.** The surrogate should refer to written indications of the patient's preferences or to past conversations concerning end-of-life wishes. Surrogates should refrain from incorporating their own preferences or values into decision-making. If the patient's wishes regarding end-of-life care are unknown, the principle of relative **benefit versus burden** may be used. In this process, the potential helpful versus harmful effects of each therapy are weighed, resulting in a choice to accept or reject each therapy. Thus, a surrogate may choose, for example, to accept antibiotics for the patient in the hopes of curing pneumonia, but to reject a lung biopsy because of the pain associated with the procedure. Neither an ethical nor a legal distinction exists between withdrawing and withholding therapies, including hydration and nutrition, but some families may see a psychological advantage to withholding rather than withdrawing life-sustaining measures.

e. The point at which the family decides to withdraw or withhold therapy may be the opportune time to address questions about wishes after death. For example, either the family or the care team may have an interest in a **postmortem examination** to determine or confirm the cause of death. Queries about the patient's or family's desires regarding **organ donation** (see **Section VI**) may also be aired. Although discussion may be viewed as awkward while the patient still lives, most families appreciate honest attempts by the care team to prepare them for what lies ahead. In addition, it is often easier to have such discussions in advance, separate from the often intense grief which occurs at the time of death.

7. If the ICU team determines that ongoing care is **futile** (i.e., only serves to prolong the dying process), the team may advise that therapies be withdrawn to reduce the suffering of the dying patient. Determining futility may be problematic because technology can prolong the survival of patients with multiorgan failure and because few physicians are able to judge with unequivocal certainty that a patient will die in the ICU. All members of the ICU team should agree that further treatment of the patient is futile before meeting with the family. Again, patience and compassion are paramount to the family's acceptance of this determination. If conflict arises, the input of the institutional ethics committee (see **Section II.F**) is advisable.

E. **The pediatric patient** deserves special consideration. Legally, end-of-life decisions are deferred to the parents. Ethically, however, the child may participate in these decisions depending on his or her developmental level and decision-making capacity. If the child is too immature to participate in decisions, parents are relied on to make decisions in the child's best interest by weighing the benefit versus burden of each therapy. Pediatric intensivists must be sensitive to individual family dynamics and parenting styles when approaching end-of-life discussions for the pediatric ICU patient.

F. The **institutional ethics committee** is generally made up of a group of health care professionals trained in medical ethics.

1. **The purpose** of the ethics committee is to educate and advise clinicians regarding ethical dilemmas and to enable resolution of ethical **conflicts**. The ethics committee offers an objective analysis of the patient's case and may draw on basic ethical principles to guide the patient, clinicians, and family to a consensus about the therapeutic course. The ethics committee should

a. Be **accessible** to all members of the health care team and to the patient and family. This diminishes inequalities of power present in the hospital environment and promotes a climate of respect for all viewpoints.

b. Be presented with a **specific question** to be answered. The patient's condition and prognosis should be documented.

c. **Not be a substitute** for communication with the family regarding end-of-life issues.

2. Hospital or institutional policy may **mandate** input of the ethics committee in certain circumstances. For example, withdrawal of care decisions in traditionally "vulnerable" populations such as children or those lacking any surrogate decision-maker may be assisted by ethics consultation.

3. Ethics committees may be involved with formulating and implementing the institutional **conflict-resolution policy.** This policy is useful in those rare situations where irreconcilable differences exist between the physician and the patient and/or family and where the usual mechanisms for decision-making (e.g., informal discussions, team/family meetings, assistance of social workers, clergy, or ethics consultants) have proven ineffective. The policy should describe a specific, stepwise process toward achieving accord or, if none can be achieved, may describe the process whereby the patient's care may be transferred to another accepting physician, care team, or institution.

III. Guidelines for withdrawing life-sustaining therapies
A. **Goals** for withdrawal of life-sustaining therapies include the following:
1. Promoting comfort and respecting the wishes of the patient.
2. Promoting comfort of the family.
3. Maintaining or achieving the patient's ability to communicate.
4. Withdrawing burdensome therapies.
5. Allowing death to occur.
B. All physician orders should be reexamined with a goal toward **palliative** and **comfort care**. A **palliative care consult** may be requested, particularly if care of the patient will continue outside the ICU. Therapies that increase patient comfort or relieve pain, anxiety, or agitation should be continued or added (**Table 14-1**). Therapies directed toward supporting physiologic homeostasis or treating the underlying disease process is no longer indicated and may be discontinued. These include many of the "routine" procedures and interventions associated with being an ICU patient (**Table 14-2**). The benefit-to-burden ratio of each intervention should be used to determine which interventions should be eliminated. The precise order of discontinuation is often determined by patient's or family's preference or the patient's situation. Most commonly, a stepwise approach is followed, with mechanical ventilation discontinued only after the withdrawal of vasopressors, antibiotics, or enteral feedings. There can be no substitute for the continual presence of a concerned and caring medical staff, especially

TABLE 14-1	Examples of Comfort and Palliative Measures

Clearance of oral secretions
Continuation of general nursing care and cleanliness
Offering of food/water to alert patients
Antiseizure or antiepileptic regimens
Narcotics
Sedatives
Antipyretics
Nonsteroidal anti-inflammatory drugs
Prophylaxis for gastrointestinal bleeding
Antiemetics
Humidified air

TABLE 14-2	Examples of Routine Measures that may be Withdrawn During the Process of Withdrawing Life-sustaining Therapy

Frequent phlebotomy for laboratory tests
Frequent vital sign determinations
Placement of intravenous and central lines
Radiographic examinations
Aggressive chest physiotherapy and endotracheal suctioning
Debridement of wounds

including the experienced physician, at the bedside. Clear plans for monitoring the patient's level of discomfort and intervening with additional medications should be made and shared with the family in attendance. The decision to withdraw life-sustaining treatment should be accompanied by an increase of vigilance and bedside attention, not withdrawal of the medical staff.

C. A large variability of **individual situations** should be anticipated. Each situation is unique. Paramount during the process is the wishes of the patient or the patient's surrogate. Patient autonomy must be respected. Immediately secondary to this is assurance of patient comfort and the comfort of the patient's family. Cultural practices and beliefs of the patient and the family should be identified and respected. In each situation, the process of withdrawal should be clearly explained and the family educated in what to expect. For example, it is helpful to describe changes in skin color that occur with cyanosis, noises due to retained secretions from respiratory impairment, and the irregular breathing pattern preceding death. Practical wishes of the patient and family concerning the desirability of extubation can usually be easily accommodated. The anticipated rapidity of the dying process or realities of the patient's medical condition, however, may dictate specific choices concerning therapies to be withdrawn, the rate of withdrawal, and the ability to accommodate the requests of families. When a rapid death is anticipated, it may be impossible to accommodate requests to extubate and communicate with the patient or hold prolonged vigils.

D. Specific life-sustaining therapies that may be withdrawn include the following:

1. **Vasopressor** and **inotropic** medications. Continuous chemical circulatory support can be discontinued without weaning. The gradual withdrawal of circulatory support appears to offer no benefit for patient comfort.

2. **Extracorporeal support** therapies are usually considered quite invasive by the patient and the family. These therapies require maintenance of vascular cannulae and the presence of additional equipment and personnel at the bedside. Intermittent extracorporeal support (e.g., intermittent hemodialysis) may simply not be restarted. Continuous renal support (e.g., continuous venovenous hemofiltration) can be discontinued. **Death is usually not immediate following the discontinuation of dialysis,** often occurring more than 1 week following discontinuation. Continuous circulatory support (e.g., ventricular assist, extracorporeal membrane oxygenation, intraaortic balloon pump) can be discontinued and death anticipated soon after termination of support. Decisions regarding removal of vascular access devices should reflect patient comfort, family preference, but also may take into account the risk of excessive bleeding due to uncorrectable coagulopathy.

3. **Antibiotics** and other curative pharmacotherapy. Once the decision to terminate life-sustaining treatments is made, it is no longer consistent to consider therapies directed toward curing the patient. Such therapies include cancer chemotherapy, radiation therapy, steroids, and antibiotics. It is reasonable, however, to continue treatments such as topical antifungal agents used for oral hygiene or antibiotics aimed at treating painful lesions.

4. **Supplemental oxygen.** Because the avoidance of hypoxemia is no longer a therapeutic goal, supplemental oxygen may be discontinued and the patient returned to breathing room air. This is reasonable even if it is decided that mechanical ventilation will be continued. If the patient is removed from the ventilator but continues to have an artificial airway in place (e.g., endotracheal tube or tracheostomy), **humidified air** can be administered to avoid the irritation of drying of the airway and tracheal secretions.

5. **Mechanical ventilation.** Several studies have suggested that mechanical ventilation is the most common therapy withdrawn when life-sustaining therapies are discontinued. Some physicians, however, prefer to withdraw therapies other than mechanical ventilation (such as vasopressors) with the expectation that the patient will die while still receiving mechanical ventilation. Similarly, during a prolonged illness, patients' families may have become comfortable with the surroundings of the ICU, the monitors, the artificial airway, and the mechanical ventilator. They may voice fears that the patient may suffer if mechanical ventilation or airway support is withdrawn. In such cases, it is reasonable to continue mechanical ventilation and airway support while discontinuing other life-sustaining therapies. Nevertheless, mechanical ventilation does not differ morally or legally from other life-sustaining treatments such as dialysis, and can be discontinued if the patient or his or her proxy believes that it represents unwanted therapy.

   a. **Mechanical ventilation may be gradually withdrawn** by decreasing the inspired oxygen to room air, decreasing positive end-expiratory pressure, and then slowly decreasing ventilatory rate. The rate of decrease is quite variable among practitioners. A relatively slow weaning process may prolong the dying process and may provide the family with a misleading hope for survival.

   b. **Mechanical ventilation may be discontinued** entirely and humidified air administered via T-piece, or the patient can simply be removed from the ventilator and the trachea extubated. Extubation may more quickly result in death compared with gradually decreasing the intensity of mechanical ventilation. It is important that extubation not appear to be objectively associated with greater discomfort or with the administration of greater doses of opioids. Each technique is applicable in certain situations. The ability of the patient to maintain a patent airway, the presence of secretions, the perceptions of the patient and family, and the confounding presence of anesthetic drugs and neuromuscular blocking agents all may dictate a particular method of discontinuing mechanical ventilation. Invasive monitoring and analysis of arterial blood gas tensions or oxygen saturation are unnecessary during withdrawal of mechanical ventilation.

   c. The **timing of death** after the withdrawal of mechanical ventilation is uncertain and depends on the etiology and severity of respiratory failure. Usually death occurs within a few hours to one day. In some studies, however, a small proportion of patients with chronic lung disease did well and were discharged alive from the hospital after deciding to forgo mechanical ventilation.

6. **Nutrition** (enteral or parenteral), fluid resuscitation, blood replacement, and intravenous (IV) hydration are all therapies that have the goal of returning the patient to health and may be discontinued. Nasogastric and orogastric tubes may be discontinued. Case reports and controlled studies suggest that **little, if any, discomfort accompanies the withdrawal of enteral nutrition and IV hydration.**

E. **Indications for pharmacologic intervention**

1. Presumption for **comfort measures.** Clinicians should not withhold comfort measures for fear of hastening death. Patients who are given large doses of opioids to treat discomfort during the withdrawal of life-sustaining treatments on average live as long as patients not given opioids, suggesting that it is the underlying disease process, not the use of palliative medications, that usually determines the time of death.

2. **Standard of care.** The administration of sedatives and analgesics during the withholding or withdrawal of life-sustaining treatments is consistent with the standard of care for critically ill patients. The majority of ICU patients do receive these medications during the withholding or withdrawal of support. Certainly, competent patients may refuse pharmacologic intervention to preserve lucidness. Drugs may not be indicated for patients who will gain no benefit (e.g., comatose patients).

F. **Specific indications**

1. **Pain.** The patient's report of pain or discomfort is certainly the best guide of treatment. Frequently, the patient is unable to communicate effectively. Other signs and symptoms of pain such as vocalizations, diaphoresis, agitation, tachypnea, and tachycardia may be valuable.

2. **Air hunger/dyspnea.** Especially with the withdrawal of supplemental oxygen and mechanical ventilatory support, discomfort should be expected and anticipatory doses of anxiolytics and opioids should be administered. Additional doses should be immediately available and opioids continued as a continuous infusion. Clinicians must be immediately and continuously available to assess the patient's level of comfort and provide additional medication as necessary.

3. **Death rattle.** Noisy, gargling breathing may occur in patients who are close to death, particularly in extubated patients. Although these sounds may be accompanied by dyspneic symptoms in the patient, they are usually more distressing to family members who are present. Treatment can include repositioning, gentle oropharyngeal suctioning, anticholinergics, and preparation and reassurance of the family.

4. **Anxiety.** Alert patients may display varying levels of anxiety at the prospect of termination of life support. Although nonpharmacologic means of allaying anxiety can be extremely effective, sometimes patients request to be deeply sedated or unconscious prior to the discontinuation of life-sustaining therapies such as mechanical ventilation. Although death may be hastened by deep sedation, such requests should be honored.

5. **Agitation or excessive motor activity.** Nonspecific motor activity may occur in some patients. Such activity is often interpreted as discomfort or distress by those attending the patient. It is reasonable that the level of sedation be increased in such situations. Neuromuscular blockade is never indicated because it does not treat the presumed underlying distress of the patient.

6. **Avoidance of drug withdrawal.** Often, patients are already receiving high doses of opioids or sedatives during the course of their illness. The patient's individual dose ranges can be used as a guide to provide increased amounts of opioids and sedatives during the discontinuation of support. Certainly, there appears to be little reason to decrease therapeutic doses of sedatives or opioids prior to the discontinuation of support for fear that the patient will not breathe adequately once the ventilator is discontinued.

IV. **Pharmacologic choices (see also Chapter 7 and Appendix)**
   A. **Opioids** are the first line of treatment for pain, dyspnea, or tachypnea during the discontinuation of life-sustaining measures. It is imperative that the route, dose, and schedule be individualized. IV administration is by far the most common route of administration with bolus administration providing the fastest pain relief, followed by a continuous infusion and additional bolus doses available as needed. For patients lacking adequate IV access, subcutaneous, oral, or transdermal routes of administration are options. Commonly used opioids and their doses are summarized in **Table 14-3**. Opioid doses for **children** are not as well established as for adults. For babies and infants, continuous morphine infusions (10–25 μg/kg/h) can be administered after an initial bolus (0.1–0.2 mg/kg IV as a starting point). Sometimes very large doses may be necessary to ensure the absence of discomfort.
   B. **Benzodiazepines** are the drugs of choice for the treatment of anxiety. **Lorazepam** is a common choice because of its pharmacodynamic predictability in both IV and oral forms.
   C. **Haloperidol** may be indicated in the presence of delirium (acute confusional states) or agitation not controlled with benzodiazepines and opioids. In one survey of practitioners, haloperidol was used at least occasionally as an adjunct to the discontinuation of life-sustaining measures by almost one-fourth of physicians. Haloperidol does not affect the respiratory drive.
   D. **Propofol** is a potent hypnotic agent that can be used for sedation or for rapid induction of unconsciousness. This may be helpful for procedures and to rapidly reach a desired level of sedation. Dose-dependent decreases of arterial blood pressure and ventilatory drive should be expected.
   E. **Barbiturates,** such as thiopental, are potent hypnotics that rapidly produce unconsciousness. Their pharmacodynamic effects are similar to those of propofol, but their pharmacokinetic profile is much less favorable. Hence, propofol has essentially substituted for the short-acting barbiturates in most ICUs.

TABLE 14-3	Examples of Initial Opioid Doses	
Generic Name	**Bolus Dose**	**Infusion**
Hydromorphone	0.015–0.05 mg/kg	0.25–2 mg/h
Fentanyl	0.5–1.5 μg/kg	2–4 μg/kg/h
Methadone	0.1 mg/kg	—
Meperidine	0.5–1.0 mg/kg	0.5 mg/kg/h
Morphine	0.05–0.1 mg/kg	0.1–0.5 mg/kg/h

These represent typical initial doses for a patient without tolerance. Doses should be titrated to effect without regard to a maximal dose.

F. **Anticholinergic medications,** such as **atropine, ipratropium bromide,** and **glycopyrrolate,** may be used to diminish copious oral and respiratory secretions that can produce death rattle. In general, atropine should be avoided because of its potential central nervous system side effects. Glycopyrrolate is a potent antisialogogue that may be administered intravenously or nebulized (5–10 μg/kg every 4 hours via either route). Scopolamine offers the advantage of availability in a transdermal formulation.

G. **Neuromuscular blocking agents** are sometimes administered in the ICU to facilitate mechanical ventilation in patients with severe acute respiratory failure (**Chapter 7**). **The indication for the use of neuromuscular blocking agents is lost** once the decision to forgo life-sustaining treatments is made. Neuromuscular blocking agents do not contribute to comfort of the patient and have no analgesic or sedative properties. Paralyzed patients are unable to express discomfort by attempting to communicate, move, or become tachypneic. The precise doses of opioids and anxiolytics necessary to avoid discomfort are then difficult to determine. Although it may be preferable to permit reversal of neuromuscular blockade prior to the withdrawal of mechanical ventilation, sometimes a prolonged drug effect that precludes adequate reversal or profound weakness is present. Many clinicians are uncomfortable with extubating a patient with no capability of maintaining spontaneous ventilation or a patent airway. In such cases, physicians may decide to forgo the withdrawal of mechanical ventilation or proceed only after administering high doses of sedatives and opioids to ensure the absence of patient awareness.

H. **Euthanasia** is illegal in United States (see **Section VIII**). Drugs should not be administered with the sole and express purpose of causing death. Such interventions include the administration of neuromuscular blocking agents to produce apnea or the administration of potassium chloride to produce asystole.

V. **Brain death**
A. **Brain death** means that death has been determined via evaluation of brain function, and as such is distinct from cardiac death. Ethically and legally, brain death is equivalent to death, even when other organs, such as the heart, may still be functioning. Occasionally, this concept presents difficulties in patients and families from cultures and religions that do not consider the concept of brain death as outlined here. Because these patients are dead, clinicians are obligated to end care, even though this may be stressful to the family. In our experience at MGH, families understand this concept, even though it may require the additional efforts of social workers and chaplains who are part of the same culture or religion and are trusted by the family. Practically, the diagnosis of brain death means that a patient can potentially become an organ donor if the conditions of consent (premortem by the patient or postmortem by the family) and medical acceptability are met.

B. **Locally accepted guidelines** are used to establish the diagnosis of brain death. Our guidelines are outlined in **Chapter 36.**

VI. **Organ donation.** Traditionally, the majority of organ procurements derive from **heart-beating patients who have been declared brain dead.** Recently, however, a renewed interest in **donation after cardiac death (DCD)** has occurred because of the dramatic mismatch between the number of organs available for transplant and the number of patients on the waitlist. Often, critically ill patients are unable to become organ donors due to the nature of illness (e.g., sepsis) or due to failure of the vital organs, but because some are eligible and a significant number die in the ICU, the critical care unit is a natural environment to discuss the issue.

A. **Early contact** with the organ procurement organization (OPO) is important. In an effort to increase the number of potential organ donors in the United States, the Centers for Medicare and Medicaid Services (CMS) has mandated that hospitals notify their local OPO about all deaths, including imminent deaths. Additionally, the local OPO must be involved in collaboration with clinicians when families are approached regarding organ donation, because it has been demonstrated that consent for donation is more likely to be obtained if presented by an experienced requester. OPO preferences regarding medications (such as vasopressors, diuretics), mechanical ventilator settings, and laboratory blood work after death should be known to the ICU team. The United Network for Organ Sharing publishes a convenient checklist for organ donors (both heart-beating and DCD) that can be easily accessed at the following URL: http://www.unos.org/resources/donorManagement.asp?index=2.

B. **Approaching the family** regarding organ donation must be done tactfully and in consultation with trained professionals from the OPO. In the case of DCD, ethical treatment of the patient mandates that discussion about organ donation occurs after the health care agent or family has agreed on withdrawing life-sustaining therapies. Ideally, the discussion should be overseen by a physician with whom the family has developed a rapport. The topic may be introduced by asking the family whether the patient had ever expressed an opinion regarding use of his or her organs after death. Many families are consoled by the thought that their loved one's body parts may be life-saving to another individual and may in some sense carry on the life that has been lost.

C. **Care of the patient** for organ donation is challenging. Physiologic problems frequently include hypotension, dysrhythmias, hypoxemia, and diabetes insipidus. If a successful donation is to occur, the vigilant attendance of the ICU team, in concert with direction from the organ procurement agency, is necessary. In the case of DCD, compassionate care aimed at ensuring patient comfort, including the use of opioids and amnestic agents, supersedes the goals of organ preservation. DCD requires thoughtful consideration by the institution and is best guided by a written protocol which clearly stipulates the following:

1. The nonoverlapping roles of caregivers to the donor and the recipient, to avoid a conflict of interest.

2. The physician responsible for pronouncing cardiac death.

3. The time interval after asystole at which death is declared; currently at MGH, this is **5 minutes.**

4. The process for obtaining consent and administering medications/treatments necessary for organ procurement (e.g., heparin).

5. The process for enabling family presence at the time of death (either in the ICU or operating room).

6. The time interval after which organ procurement will not be attempted in the case of unexpected patient survival following withdrawal of life-sustaining therapies; currently this is **2 hours** at MGH.

D. If the institutional transplant team will participate in procuring or transplanting organs, it is prudent to establish contact with the team and immediately apprise them of any change in the donor's condition that might warrant an expedited approach.

VII. Supporting survivors

A. Support of the patient's survivors during the dying process and following death begins with honest, frequent, and compassionate communication from physicians and nurses in the ICU. Families appreciate the guidance of experienced practitioners to prepare them for what to expect during the dying process, especially when life-sustaining therapies have been withdrawn. Reassurance should be given that measures will be taken to ensure the patient's comfort and that some sights (e.g., gasps) and sounds (e.g., gurgling) are normal during dying and may not be completely obliterated. The environment where death occurs should accommodate the wishes of the patient and family as much as possible.

1. **Privacy** is important for a dignified death. This may be achieved by closing ICU cubicles and shielding the dying patient and family from the routine commotion of a busy ICU. Alternatively, the patient or family may request to be moved to a private room on a hospital ward or to an in-hospital hospice unit to die. If the condition of the patient allows transfer before death will occur, these requests should be granted.

2. **Cultural background and individual values** will affect who is at the bedside of a dying patient. For some patients, one or two close family members may attend; for others, a vigil is maintained by a large extended family. The ICU staff should strive for flexibility when presented with each situation.

   a. The medical social worker may be an important source for understanding the family's religious and cultural background and for communicating the family's wishes to the medical care team.

   b. Many patients and families find solace in the presence of clergy at death. If so, arrangements can be made for the patient's religious representative or a hospital-based chaplain to attend.

B. Support of the caring team is also important. Members of the team (particularly trainees and junior staff) are often distressed by the process of allowing a patient to die. Very little is formally taught in medical schools about end-of-life situations, and doctors and nurses learn by experience. **Debriefings** (**Chapter 38**) with the whole team and the addition of senior staff and hospital ethicists are very helpful.

VIII. Legal considerations.

Physicians who follow the preceding process regarding honest, open communication with patients and their families about ethics and end-of-life care should rarely find themselves resolving such issues in a court of law. Federal rulings have outlined general principles regarding end-of-life care, but specific details may be contained in state statutes. For this reason, clinicians are advised to familiarize themselves with their specific state's laws surrounding end-of-life. Following is a general outline of legal principles and their implications that may prove useful to the clinician when confronted with ethical and end-of-life issues.

A. Patient autonomy is primary in decision-making. That patients may refuse life-sustaining or other therapies has been repeatedly affirmed.

B. Advance directives provide the best source of information for guidance with medical decisions for patients lacking capacity. As such, most states recognize advance directives from another state or executed in nonstandard form. Oral communications regarding preferences may be utilized as advance directives. The role of a surrogate in providing substituted judgment has been supported.

C. Human life has qualification beyond mere biologic existence. Thus, a surrogate's decision to withdraw care may be based on the potential for meaningful existence **(quality of life)**.

D. **Care once rendered may be withdrawn.** The idea that a life-sustaining therapy that has been implemented can never be stopped is not valid.

E. **End-of-life decisions** are best addressed by the physician and the patient and/or family with help from institutional facilitators (e.g., ethics committee) as needed. Judicial intervention should, in the vast majority of circumstance, be unnecessary and only sought when state law mandates or hospital policy requires. The latter circumstance usually applies to situations where serious irresolvable conflicts occur regarding patients who lack capacity to make treatment decisions.

F. **Withdrawal of hydration or nutrition is not legally different** from withdrawal of other life support. In addition to legal decisions, this stance has been supported by numerous medical societies, including the American Medical Association and the American Academy of Neurology. Most recently, the judicial action in the 2005 Terri Schiavo case supported this dictum, despite attempts at intervention by the Congress.

G. **Physicians are not bound to provide care that they deem futile.** Although still somewhat controversial, this was supported by a jury decision involving a patient at the Massachusetts General Hospital from whom ventilatory support was withdrawn despite the objection of one family member. It is advisable for a physician, however, to pursue every avenue of conflict resolution (see **Section II.F.3**), including removing oneself from the care of a patient, before exercising this dictum against a family's wishes.

H. Provision of medications intended to treat pain or suffering but which result in the unintended consequence of hastening death (principle of **"double effect"**) do not place the prescribing physician at risk of criminal prosecution. For patients with intractable pain or suffering when death is imminent, terminal sedation may be legally offered.

I. **Physician-assisted suicide** is currently legal only in Oregon.

J. **Euthanasia** is currently not legal in the United States.

K. **Hospital risk managers** need not be consulted before termination of life-sustaining therapies. Some institutions may suggest or require this course, but there is no legal precedence. Physicians should be aware, too, that hospital risk managers are tasked with protecting the institution's interest, and do not necessarily represent best ethical or clinical practice for the patient.

L. **For unusual or questionable cases,** it is appropriate to seek the advice of both the institutional ethics committee and legal counsel before acting on decisions.

Selected References

Annas GJ. "Culture of life" politics at the bedside—the case of Terri Schiavo. *N Engl J Med* 2005;352:1710–1715.

Bigatello LM, George E, Hurford WE. Ethical considerations for research in critically ill patients. *Crit Care Med* 2003;31:3(suppl):S178–S181.

Bloche MG. Managing conflict at the end of life. *N Engl J Med* 2005;352:2371–2373.

Boyle D, O'Connell D, Platt FW, et al. Disclosing errors and adverse events in the intensive care unit. *Crit Care Med* 2006;34:1532–1537.

McClenathan BM, Torrington KG, Uyehara CFT. Family member presence during cardiopulmonary resuscitation. *Chest* 2002;122:2204–2211.

Meisel A, Snyder L, Quill T. Seven legal barriers to end-of-life care: myths, realities, and grains of truth. *JAMA* 2000;284:2495–2501.

Quill TE. Initiating end-of-life discussions with seriously ill patients: addressing the "elephant in the room." *JAMA* 2000;284:2502–2507.

Sharma BR. Withholding and withdrawing of life support: a medicolegal dilemma. *Am J Forensic Med Pathol* 2004;25:150–155.

Truog RD, Campbell ML, Curtis JR, et al. Recommendations for end-of-life care in the intensive care unit: a consensus statement by the American Academy of Critical Care Medicine. *Crit Care Med* 2008;953–963.

White DB, Curtis JR, Wolf LE, et al. Life support for patients without surrogate decision maker: who decides? *Ann Int Med* 2007;147:34–40.

15

Evidence-Based Practice and Basic Statistics in Critical Care

Ala Nozari, H. Thomas Stelfox, and Edward Bittner

I. **Evidence-based medicine** (EBM) is defined as the conscientious, explicit, and judicious use of current best evidence in making decisions about the care of individual patients. It requires the integration of the best research evidence with clinical expertise and the unique values and circumstances of the patient. By encouraging physicians to explicitly explain their medical decision-making processes, including the evidence on which their decisions are based, we may enhance the opportunity for optimal clinical outcomes. Scientific evidence will never be available to guide all medical decisions, but a clear understanding of the benefits and boundaries of EBM will help to optimize patient care. The practice of EBM can be organized in four steps (**Fig. 15-1**).

  A. **Asking an answerable clinical question.** The more precisely the question is framed, the more likely it is the physician will find an appropriate answer in the literature. Each question should specify

    1. A patient or a problem.

    2. An intervention or a diagnostic test (if relevant).

    3. A comparison group (if relevant).

    4. An outcome.

  B. **Searching for the best evidence** that will provide an answer. Two excellent databases for clinical medicine include **Medline** *(www.pubmed.gov)* and the **Cochrane Library** *(www.cochrane.org)*.

  C. **Evaluating the evidence,** by asking two simple questions:

    1. Is the evidence valid?

    2. Are the results important?

    For systematic reviews, as an example, you should determine if a strenuous effort has been made to locate all original reports on the topic of interest, if the reports have been critically evaluated, and whether conclusions have been drawn based on a synthesis of the studies which meet preset quality criteria. The review should include **confidence intervals (see Section II.A)** of all results, both of individual studies and the meta-analysis.

  D. Once it has been established that the evidence is valid, we need to ask whether the **results will help in caring for patients**. Evaluating and applying a specific piece of evidence can be guided by asking additional questions depending on the exact nature of the evidence (**Table 15-1**).

    1. **Diagnostic studies.** Rarely does any symptom, sign, laboratory test, or any combination of them completely distinguish between those patients with and those without a disease. Instead, disease is generally defined using a gold standard, and formal approaches to studies evaluating diagnostic instruments are essential to solidifying the foundation for diagnostic decision making.

    2. **Prognostic studies.** Prognosis is a prediction of the outcome of a disease process. It describes the duration, the timing, and the nature of the disease as it progresses along its clinical course.

Ask a clinically relevant question

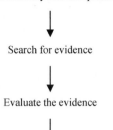

Search for evidence

Evaluate the evidence

Apply the evidence

FIGURE 15-1 An approach to evidence-based medicine.

3. **Treatment or prevention studies.** The course of disease may be greatly affected by the choice of treatment options. Not all therapies are equally effective, and in fact some may be deleterious.
4. **Systematic reviews, overviews, and meta-analyses.** The terms systematic review and overview are used for any summary of the medical literature, and meta-analysis is used for reviews that use quantitative methods to summarize results.
5. **Clinical decision analyses.** Decision making is the choosing of a course of action after weighing the benefits and harms of the alternatives. Clinical decision analysis is the application of quantitative methods to decision making under conditions of uncertainty.
6. **Economic analyses** compare alternative clinical strategies with respect to both outcomes and resource utilization.
7. **Clinical practice guidelines** are published recommendations that employ subject experts to synthesize the medical literature into practical recommendations for guiding clinical practice.

II. **Study design and measurement of the validity and importance of the evidence**
   A. **Definitions**
      1. **Bias** is systematic error or deviation from the truth. We are generally concerned with two forms of bias in clinical studies, selection bias and information bias. Selection bias pertains to noncomparability in how subjects are selected. Information bias pertains to noncomparability in how information is obtained or reported.
      2. **Confounding** is a mixing of effects between the study variable, the outcome, and a third factor that is associated with the study variable and independently affects the risk of developing the outcome. The extraneous factor is called a confounding variable.
      3. **Effect modification** is a change in the magnitude of an effect according to the value of some third variable.
      4. **Cointervention** is an intervention made in the intervention group, the control group, or both that is outside of the study protocol and that might contribute to a study's outcome.
      5. **Efficacy** is the extent to which medical interventions achieve health improvements under ideal circumstances (e.g., clinical trials).
      6. **Effectiveness** is the extent to which medical interventions achieve health improvements in real, practical settings.

TABLE
15-1

A Basic Guide for Systematically Evaluating and Applying Evidence-Based Medicine

Study	Is the Evidence Valid?	What Are the Results?	Will the Results Help Me Care for My Patients?
Diagnostic	Was there an independent, blind comparison with a gold standard? Did the patient sample include an appropriate spectrum of patients? Was the gold standard applied to all patients?	Are likelihood ratios presented?	Will the test results be reproducible and applicable to patients in my clinical setting? Will the test results change my management?
Prognostic	Did the patient sample include a well-defined, appropriate spectrum of patients at a similar disease stage? Was there adequate follow-up? Were the outcome criteria objective? Were important prognostic factors measured and accounted for?	How large and precise (95% confidence interval) are the estimates of the likelihood of the outcome in a period of time?	Were the study patients similar to my own? Will the results change my management? Can I use the results to counsel my patients?
Treatment and prevention	Were patients assigned to treatments using randomization? Were all patients accounted for at the conclusion of the study? Were patients analyzed in the groups to which they were randomized (intention-to-treat analysis)? Were patients, health workers, and study personnel blind to treatment? Were the study groups similar at the start of the study? Were the groups treated equally except for the assigned treatment?	How large and precise (95% confidence interval) are the estimates of the treatment effect?	Were the study patients similar to my own? Were all clinically important outcomes (positive and negative) considered? Are the benefits worth the harms and costs?
Systematic reviews	Was a focused clinical question asked? Were appropriate criteria used to select the individual articles?	How large and precise (95% confidence interval) are the results?	Were the study patients similar to my own? Were all clinically important outcomes considered? Are the benefits worth the harms and costs?

(continued)

227

TABLE 15-1 A Basic Guide for Systematically Evaluating and Applying Evidence-Based Medicine *(continued)*

Study	Is the Evidence Valid?	What Are the Results?	Will the Results Help Me Care for My Patients?
	Is it likely that important studies were missed? Was the validity of the selected studies appraised? Were similar results found across the different studies?		
Clinical decision analyses	Were all important clinical strategies and outcomes examined? Was an explicit and reasonable process used to assign probabilities? Was an explicit and reasonable process used to assign utilities? Were sensitivity analyses performed to determine the potential impact of any uncertainty in the evidence?	Does one strategy result in a clinically important difference? How strong is the evidence used in the analysis? How much does allowance for uncertainty change the results?	Do the probability estimates approximate my patients' clinical features? Do the utilities reflect my patients' values?
Economic analyses	Was a full economic comparison of different strategies provided? Were all costs and outcomes properly measured? Were allowances made for uncertainties? Are the costs and outcomes related to the baseline risk in the treatment population?	What were the incremental costs and outcomes of each strategy? Could the uncertainty in the evidence change the results?	Could my patients expect similar health outcomes and costs? Are the benefits worth the harms and costs?
Clinical practice guidelines	Were all important options and outcomes clearly specified? Was an explicit and reasonable approach used to identify, select, and combine evidence? Is the guideline reasonably up to date? Has the guideline been subject to peer review?	Are the recommendations practical and clinically relevant? What is the impact of uncertainty and of any value judgments?	Is the primary objective of the guidelines consistent with my goals? Are the recommendations applicable to my patients?

Adapted from Guyatt G, Rennie D. *User's guide to the medical literature: essentials of evidence-based clinical practice.* Chicago: American Medical Association, 2001.

7. **The *p* value** is the probability of obtaining a value at least as extreme as the one that was actually observed, given that the null hypothesis is true. In other words, it is the probability of observing a particular result or one that is more extreme due solely to chance. It reflects the sample size and the magnitude of the association. By convention, $p \leq 0.05$ is considered statistically significant.

8. The **confidence interval** is the estimated range of values within which the true magnitude of effect lies with a certain degree of probability or confidence. Confidence intervals provide information about statistical significance (**a 95% confidence interval is the complement of $p = 0.05$**) and data variability.

9. **A Type I error** is committed when the null hypothesis is rejected when it is actually true. The probability of making a Type I error is designated by α.

10. **A Type II error** is committed when one fails to reject the null hypothesis when it is in fact false. The probability of making a Type II error is designated by β. A study's power is calculated by subtracting the probability of a Type II error from a Type I error (Power $= 1 - \beta$).

11. **Internal validity** is the extent to which an observed association between an exposure and outcome is valid.

12. **External validity** is the extent to which one can generalize the study conclusions to populations and settings outside the study.

B. **Epidemiologic studies** can be broadly divided in two groups, descriptive studies and analytic studies. **Descriptive studies** are designed to generate hypotheses, while analytic studies are designed to test hypotheses. Descriptive studies include case series, correlational series, and cross-sectional studies. **Analytic studies** can be subdivided into observational studies (case-control studies and cohort studies) and experimental studies (intervention studies or clinical trials as they are generally called in medicine).

1. **Case reports and case series** document unusual medical occurrences and may represent the first clues in the identification of new diseases, adverse effects of exposures, or presence of an epidemic.
    a. Strength
        (1) Very useful for hypothesis generation. If the outcome is unusual and dramatic enough, such case reports or series will generate a hypothesis.
    b. Limitations
        (1) Interpretation is limited by the lack of a comparison group.
        (2) Cannot be used to test for a valid statistical association.
        (3) Based on the experiences of a single individual or small group of individuals.

2. **Correlational studies** describe a variable of interest in relation to an outcome in an entire population.
    a. Strengths
        (1) Can often be performed quickly with minimal resources because the information is often already available.
        (2) May allow for geographic comparisons.
    b. Limitations
        (1) Inability to link exposure and outcome in individuals because the data are aggregated at a higher level (e.g., city, county, state).
        (2) Inability to control for confounding.

3. **Cross-sectional studies (prevalence studies)** assess both the exposure and outcome status of individuals at a specific point in time.

  a. Strength
  (1) Both exposure and outcome data are obtained from individuals.
  b. Limitations
  (1) Inability to establish temporal sequence between exposure and outcome.
  (2) Prevalent outcomes are assessed, so any association between the exposure and the outcome may reflect determinants of survival.

4. Case-control studies are observational studies where study individuals are selected on the basis of whether they do (cases) or do not (controls) have a particular outcome. The groups are then examined for a history of an exposure or a particular characteristic.
  a. Strengths
  (1) Good for studying rare outcomes.
  (2) Can evaluate multiple exposures.
  (3) Efficient from both a time and economic perspective.
  (4) Particularly well suited to studying diseases with long latent periods.
  b. Limitations
  (1) Do not allow a direct estimate of outcome rates.
  (2) Inefficient for evaluating rare exposures.
  (3) Susceptible to selection and information bias.
  (4) Temporal sequence of exposure and outcome may be difficult to establish.

5. Cohort studies are observational studies where disease-free individuals are selected and classified based on the presence or absence of exposure and then followed over time (retrospectively or prospectively) for the development of the outcome of interest.
  a. Strengths
  (1) Establish a temporal relationship between the exposure and outcome.
  (2) Allow a direct estimate of the incidence rate for the outcome.
  (3) Good for evaluating rare exposures.
  (4) Allow multiple outcomes to be evaluated.
  (5) Minimize bias in exposure assessment.
  b. Limitations
  (1) Prospective cohort studies have numerous feasibility considerations including the availability of participants, the ability to ensure complete follow-up, and the extensive time and cost required.
  (2) Retrospective cohort studies require access to sufficient numbers of adequate quality records.
  (3) Not efficient for examining rare outcomes.

6. Clinical trials are generally considered the gold standard of clinical research because the investigator assigns exposure status. In most clinical trials, participants are allocated to exposure groups at random.
  a. Strength
  (1) Provide the strongest causal evidence.
  b. Limitations
  (1) Ethical considerations make it difficult for many interventions to be evaluated in a clinical trial.
  (2) It may be difficult to find a sufficiently large population of individuals willing to forego an intervention that is believed to be beneficial even if there is no evidence to support this view.

(3) Clinical trials generally have numerous feasibility considerations including being very resource intensive.

(4) Findings may reflect the relationship between an exposure and an outcome in a clinical trial setting (efficacy), but not necessarily in the real-world setting (effectiveness).

C. Quantitative measures

1. **The selection and interpretation of diagnostic tests** is a sequential process whose goal is to reduce uncertainty about a patient's diagnosis until either the threshold for treating or for not treating the patient is reached. A test result is best interpreted considering the probability of disease before the diagnostic result was obtained. When the **pretest probability** of disease is high, a positive test result confirms the presence of disease, but a negative test result is insufficient to rule out disease. When the pretest probability of disease is low, a negative test result excludes the presence of disease, but a positive test is insufficient to consider disease **(Table 15-2)**.

   a. **Sensitivity** is the proportion of patients with the disease who have a positive test result:

   $$A/(A + C)$$

   b. **Specificity** is the proportion of patients without the disease who have a negative test result:

   $$D/(B + D)$$

   c. **Positive predictive value** is the proportion of patients with a positive test result who have the disease:

   $$A/(A + B)$$

   d. **Negative predictive value** is the proportion of patients with a negative test result who do not have the disease:

   $$D/(C + D)$$

   e. **Likelihood ratio for a positive test result** is the relative odds of having the disease given a positive test result:

   $$[A/(A + C)]/[B/(B + D)]$$

   f. **Likelihood ratio for a negative test result** is the relative odds of having the disease given a negative test result:

   $$[C/(A + C)]/[D/(B + D)]$$

   g. **Pretest odds** are the odds that the patient has the disease before the test is carried out:

   (Probability of disease present) = (1 − Probability of disease absent)

TABLE
15-2   Two-by-Two Table for Evaluating a Diagnostic Test

	Disease	
Test Result	**Present**	**Absent**
Disease present	True positive (A)	False positive (B)
Disease absent	False negative (C)	True negative (D)

	Outcome	
Exposure	Yes	No
Yes	A	B
No	C	D

TABLE 15-3 Data Presented in Two-by-Two Tables for The Calculation of Measures of Association

  h. **Posttest odds** are the odds that the patient has the disease after the test is carried out:

  (Pretest odds) $\times$ (Likelihood ratio for the test result)

  i. **Posttest probability** is the proportion of patients with a particular test result who have the disease:

  (Posttest odds)/(Posttest odds + 1)

2. **Measures of association** are descriptive statistics used to determine the degree to which one variable changes in relation to another, for example, the association between an exposure and an outcome. They generally involve either calculating the ratio or the absolute difference of the measures of outcome for two groups, which indicates on a relative or an absolute scale, respectively, how much more likely one group is to develop the outcome than the other (**Table 15-3**).

  a. **Relative risk** is the likelihood of developing the outcome in one group (e.g., treated or exposed patients) relative to another group (e.g., untreated or unexposed patients):

  $$[A/(A + B)]/[C/(C + D)]$$

  b. **Relative risk reduction** is the proportional reduction in event rates between two groups:

  (1 − Relative risk)

  c. **Absolute risk reduction** is the absolute difference in event rates:

  $$[A + (A + B)] − [C/(C + D)]$$

  d. **Number needed to treat** is the number of patients who need to be treated to prevent one additional event:

  1/(Absolute risk reduction)

  e. **Odds ratio** is the ratio of the odds of exposure or outcome (depending on study design) between two study groups:

  (A/B)/(C/D)

  f. When the outcome is undesirable, a relative risk or odds ratio of less than 1.0 represents a beneficial treatment.

3. **Levels of evidence.** Many different systems exist for grading the strength of a body of scientific evidence. Although there is no universal agreement on the best approach, there is general agreement that certain research methodologies are less likely to be subject to bias and are consequently apt to provide stronger levels of scientific evidence (**Table 15-4**). The Agency for Health Care Research and Quality has

TABLE 15-4	Levels of Evidence

Increasing strength of evidence ⬆

Randomized controlled trials
All-or-none case series[a]
Cohort studies
Case-control studies
Case series
Expert opinion

Systemic reviews can be used to aggregate evidence when more than one study is available and can be particularly valuable if the studies included are of high quality and demonstrate consistent findings.
[a]All-or-none case series refer to clinical scenarios where rigorous scientific evaluation of new interventions was difficult because either all patients died before the treatment became available and some now survive or some patients died before the treatment became available but now none die (e.g., penicillin).

identified three important elements for any system used to grade the strength of scientific evidence:

   a. **Quality** is an aggregate measure of quality ratings for the individual studies based on the extent to which they minimize bias.
   b. **Quantity** is an aggregate measure of the magnitude of the overall effect based on the numbers of studies, the total sample size, or the overall power.
   c. **Consistency** is the extent to which similar findings are reported in different studies employing various methodologies.
 D. **Grading of practice guidelines and recommendations**
   1. A variety of systems have been employed to evaluate the quality of clinical practice guidelines and recommendations. Differences in criteria between systems can lead to substantial differences in recommendations depending on the system applied. A systematic approach to making judgments about the quality of evidence and the strength of recommendations is, hence, desirable to reduce errors, improve the communication of this information, and support well-informed choices in clinical practice.
   2. The **Grades of Recommendation, Assessment, Development and Evaluation (GRADE)** system is an evidence-based methodology for assessing and rating the quality of evidence and strength of recommendations for clinical guidelines. The GRADE methodology is based on a sequential assessment of quality of evidence, followed by assessment of the balance between benefits versus risks, burden and cost, and, based on the preceding, development and grading of recommendations. A crucial feature of the GRADE system is to keep the rating of "quality of evidence" separate from "strength of recommendation."
     a. **Quality of evidence** is classified as high (grade A), moderate (grade B), low (grade C), or very low (grade D). Quality of evidence is based on four key elements:
       (1) **Study design:** Basic study design, broadly categorized as randomized or observational.
       (2) **Study quality:** Detailed study methods and execution, such as the adequacy of allocation concealment, blinding, and follow-up.
       (3) **Consistency:** The similarity of estimates of effects across studies. The direction, size, and significance of the differences determine the importance of the inconsistency.

(4) **Directness:** The extent to which the subjects, interventions, and outcome measures are similar to that of the population or intervention of interest.
b. **Randomized trials** begin as high-quality evidence but may be downgraded due to limitations in implementation, inconsistency or imprecision of the results, indirectness of the evidence, and possible reporting bias.
c. **Observational studies** begin as low-quality evidence, but may be upgraded on the basis of large magnitude of effect. Any other evidence is graded very low.
d. **Recommendations** are classified as strong (grade 1) or weak (grade 2).
(1) A strong recommendation in favor of an intervention reflects that the desirable effects of adherence to a recommendation will clearly outweigh the undesirable effects (net benefit).
(2) A weak recommendation indicates that the desirable effects of adherence to a recommendation probably will outweigh the undesirable effects (tradeoff between benefits and harm), but the benefit of this tradeoff is uncertain.

III. **Evidence-based medicine in the intensive care unit**
A. **Severity-of-illness scoring systems** use elements of the history, physical examination, and diagnostic tests to objectively gauge illness severity and determine prognosis. There are four main applications for these scoring systems: clinical research, performance assessment, resource allocation, and guidance in individual patient decisions. The most commonly used scoring systems for adult critical care medicine are the **Acute Physiology and Chronic Health Evaluation (APACHE)** system, the **Simplified Acute Physiology Score (SAPS),** and the **Mortality Probability Model (MPM).** In addition, several organ dysfunction scores have been developed for use in the critically ill. Although these scores have been developed primarily to describe organ dysfunction, there is clearly a relationship between organ failure and patient outcomes.
1. **APACHE (I–IV)** is based on the premise that severity of illness on ICU admission is based on a patient's physiologic reserve (age and the presence of comorbidities) and the extent of any acute common physiologic abnormalities (worst abnormalities within 24 hours of admission) including body temperature, arterial blood pressure, heart rate, an index of arterial oxygenation, and so on. APACHE II scores can be calculated by signing on to easily accessible Web sites, such as http://www.sfar.org/scores2/apache22.html. The APACHE II system was developed due to the complexity of the original model, and was further refined to perform better with regard to discrimination and outcome prediction in its subsequent models (APACHE III and IV). APACHE IV also includes a separate scoring system for coronary bypass patients.
2. **SAPS (I–III)** was initially developed as a simplification of the APACHE I classification system. SAPS II uses 17 variables and performs similarly to APACHE II. In SAPS III, three subscores (patient characteristics before admission, circumstances of admission, and acute physiology) are summed up to avoid serious shortcomings that are inherent in the exclusively physiology-based scoring systems.
3. **MPM (I and II)** is a statistical modeling system that uses patient clinical variables to predict the probability of hospital mortality rather than to measure severity of illness. The strength lies in its simplicity of scoring

and the possibility of sequential assessment of mortality risk throughout the ICU stay.

4. **Trauma and Revised Injury Severity Score (TRISS)** is a severity-of-injury scoring system for trauma patients, but is not specific to ICU trauma admissions.

5. **Multiple Organ Dysfunction Score (MODS)** is an organ dysfunction score that is calculated based on a patient's respiratory, renal, hepatic, cardiovascular, hematologic, and neurologic functions.

6. **Sequential Organ Failure Assessment (SOFA)** is an organ dysfunction score that mainly differs from MODS in that it includes therapeutic interventions in its assessment of a patient's cardiovascular function. It also takes into consideration the changing severity over time of the process of organ dysfunction.

B. **Outcomes of special interest in the intensive care unit**

1. **In-hospital mortality** is the incidence of death in a particular population during the period of the hospitalization.

2. The **28-day mortality** is the incidence of death in a particular population during a specific period of time (28 days is commonly used).

3. **Hospital length of stay** is frequently assessed to examine the length of a patient's acute illness. It may be subdivided into length of stay in the intensive care unit, in the hospital, as well as in any subsequent rehabilitation facilities.

4. **Ventilator-free days** is a measure of the number of days that patients spend in the intensive care unit alive but not on a ventilator in a specified time period (e.g., 28 days). It is a commonly used measure because of the frequency of respiratory failure in most intensive care units.

Selected References

Boyd CR, Tolson MA, Copes WS. Evaluating trauma care: the TRISS methodology. *J Trauma* 1987;27:370–378.

GRADE Working Group. Grading quality of evidence and strength of recommendations. *BMJ* 2004;328:1490–1498.

Guyatt G, Rennie D. *User's guide to the medical literature: essentials of evidence-based clinical practice.* Chicago: American Medical Association, 2001.

Knaus WA, Draper EA, Wagner DP, et al. APACHE II: a severity of disease classification system. *Crit Care Med* 1985;13:818–829.

Le Gall JR, Lemeshow S, Saulnier F. A new simplified acute physiology score (SAPS II) based on European/North American multicenter study. *JAMA* 1993;270:2957.

Lemeshow S, Teres D, Klar J, et al. Mortality probability models (MPM II) based on an international cohort of intensive care unit patients. *JAMA* 1993;270:2478.

Marshall JC, Cook DJ, Christou NV, et al. Multiple Organ Dysfunction Score: a reliable descriptor of a complex clinical outcome. *Crit Care Med* 1995;23:1638–1652.

Sackett DL, Strauss SE, Richardson WS, et al. *Evidence-based medicine: how to practice and teach EBM.* 2nd ed. Edinburgh: Churchill Livingstone, 2000.

Strand K, Flaatten H. Severity scoring in the ICU: a review. *Acta Anaesthesiol Scand* 2008;52:467–478.

Vincent JL, Moreno R, Takala J, et al. The SOFA (Sepsis-related Organ Failure Assessment) score to describe organ dysfunction/failure. *Intensive Care Med* 1996;22:707–710.

16

Transport of the ICU Patient

Emily Apsell and Michael Fitzsimons

I. Increasingly ill patients are requiring transport within the hospital for diagnostic and therapeutic procedures as well as between hospitals to receive a higher level of care. Critical care clinicians are expected to be familiar with the indications, complications, technical aspects, and published guidelines for patient transfer, in their roles as leaders of intensive care units, operating rooms, and direct care providers.

A. **Intrahospital transport** refers to the movement of a patient to various sites throughout that same hospital for diagnostic or therapeutic procedures that cannot be performed safely or with a high degree of safety at their primary location. For example, patients considered too ill for care in the operating room may be transferred to endoscopy or radiology for an alternative procedure. **Interhospital transport** refers to the transportation of a patient from one hospital to another for a patient to receive a higher level of care. Often the destination is a "referral center" whose staff has a higher level of training, offers a wider range of services, or has expertise in a particular area.

B. **Indications** for transport are either patient specific or, in the case of interhospital transport, institution specific. The risks must always be balanced with the potential benefit to the patient.

1. Intrahospital transport commonly occurs to diagnostic or therapeutic locations. **A "travel" out of the intensive care unit results in a change in patient management up to 40% of the time.** The radiography suite remains the most common destination. Angiography and abdominal computed tomography most commonly result in a diagnosis leading to a change in patient management.

2. Studies have demonstrated a morbidity and mortality benefit to patients when they are transported to centers of excellence in certain medical and surgical specialties. This is referred to as "regionalization." Benefits are observed in neonatal and perinatal medicine, trauma, burn management, and spinal injury. A higher level of physician training, broader range of consultative services, and clinical research may be available. Other specialized care only provided in certain medical centers may include hyperbaric medicine and mechanical cardiac assist.

a. **Pregnant patients** may be transported for either maternal or neonatal reasons. Neonatal outcomes are improved when the mother is transported to a tertiary care center prior to delivery, as opposed to transporting a distressed neonate. Transport of the pregnant patient requires equipment and technical ability to respond to premature labor, premature rupture of membranes, pre-eclampsia, eclampsia, bleeding, and delivery. Often it may be difficult to maintain access to both the maternal airway and pelvis simultaneously during transport. Therefore, optimal positioning for transport must be determined on a case-by-case basis. During transport of pregnant patients, left uterine displacement must be maintained to ensure adequate maternal venous return.

Potential Causes of Hemodynamic Instability During Transport	
Patient Specific	**Technical**
Anxiety	Interruption of infusions
Pain	Mechanical ventilation
Sedation level	Care provider unfamiliar with infusion systems
Fluid redistribution	
Bleeding	
Worsening illness	
Interruption of monitoring	
Emergence from anesthesia	
Neuraxial anesthesia	

  b. **Spinal injuries.** The early transfer to a center of excellence of spinal cord injury patients is of proven benefit, especially if completed within 12 hours. It is of critical importance to minimize any additional movement of the spine to avoid exacerbating cord injury.

  c. **Critically ill children** and those with congenital disease benefit from treatment at specialized centers. Furthermore, transport by specially trained pediatric transport teams improves the outcome once the child arrives at the center.

 C. The **risks of patient transfer** must always be balanced with perceived benefits. The risks include seemingly minor complications such as a decrease in blood pressure to major mishaps resulting in death. Hemodynamic and respiratory changes may occur in as high as 70% of patients. Patients who require transport out of the ICU ultimately have a higher rate of death but this is likely related to their severity of illness as opposed to transport alone.

 D. **Physiologic changes** and complications related to transfer occur in nearly every organ system.

  1. **Hemodynamic instability** (hypertension or hypotension) is likely the most common adverse event occurring during transport and may be seen in 25% to 50% of movements. Arrhythmias occur in up to half of transports. The causes of hemodynamic changes may be patient-specific or due to technical factors (**Table 16-1**).

  2. **Respiratory compromise** such as hypoxemia may occur in up to 86% of intubated patients requiring transport (**Table 16-2**). Patients requiring positive end-expiratory pressure (PEEP) or high inspired concentration of oxygen (FiO_2) prior to transport appear to have a higher risk of hypoxemia. Secondary respiratory complications must be considered

Possible Respiratory Complications During Transport
Hypercarbia with respiratory acidosis
Hypocarbia with respiratory alkalosis
Drying of secretions
Dislodgement of the endotracheal tube
Hypoxemia
Aspiration of gastric contents

including the effects of hypercarbia on intracranial hypertension, pulmonary hypertension, or existing acidosis. **Accidental extubation** is unfortunately common in the critically ill patient, and transport is a risk factor for this. Finally, dynamic hyperinflation and auto-PEEP (**Chapter 2**) as a result of overly aggressive manual ventilation may impair venous return and result in hypotension.

3. **Hypothermia** may result when a patient is moved from the warmth of an intensive care unit to an isolated site such as radiology, which is often unprepared to deal with temperature maintenance. Worsening of pulmonary vasoconstriction, coagulopathy, arrhythmias, and depression of mental status may result. The highest risk may be in children and the elderly.

4. **Other injuries** may result when the care provider responsible for the patient is occupied with monitoring and maintaining stability. Dislodgement of central lines may result in cessation of the delivery of critical medications and acute hemodynamic instability. Dislodgment of a chest tube may convert a simple pneumothorax into a tension pneumothorax. Movement of unstable spinal injuries and fractures (see **Chapter 36**) may exacerbate injury.

E. **Complications** during transport may be both **equipment-related** and **staff/patient management-related.** The Australian Incident Monitoring Study in Intensive Care revealed that 39% of incidents were equipment-related and 61% due to patient/staff management issues. Most complications occur at the destination of the transfer and likely relate to different monitors, drug infusion systems, need to disconnect patient from ventilation, and limited battery life of transport systems. In order to minimize equipment-related complications, certain minimum requirements should be met: Alarms that indicate a disconnected ventilator, low oxygen delivery, and low pressure should be activated; batteries should be fully charged; back-up supplies of life-sustaining medications (i.e., vasopressors) should be readily available, and airway management tools should accompany the patient.

F. **Patient assessment and planning** prior to transport is critical to ensure safe and beneficial care. Even the sickest patients can be safely transported, including those on extracorporeal circulation and ventricular assist devices. The level of care and monitoring delivered must be maintained at all times. **Nine principles of safe patient transfer** have been outlined (**Table 16-3**). Studies that have looked at injury scores demonstrate that the greater a patient's severity of illness, the more likely they are to have an adverse event during transport. Others studies looking at laboratory analysis and support have

TABLE 16-3	Principles of Safe Patient Transfer

1. Experienced staff
2. Appropriate equipment
3. Full assessment and investigation
4. Extensive monitoring
5. Careful stabilization of patient
6. Reassessment
7. Continuing care during transfer
8. Direct handoff
9. Documentation and audit

failed to demonstrate a consistent predictor of risk. Each organ system must be assessed and specific plans made for transport and potential complications that may be encountered.

1. **Airway.** The stability of the patient's airway must be assessed prior to any movement. The position, function, and stability of an ETT must be confirmed prior to any movement. Studies show that intubation can be safely accomplished during transport; however, certain patients may benefit from elective intubation prior to transport (**Table 16-4**).

2. Adequate **breathing and ventilation** must be confirmed and documented before movement. Increases in $PaCO_2$ and respiratory acidosis may indicate inadequate ventilation while a decrease in PaO_2 or hypoxemia may require PEEP, an increase in FiO_2, change in ventilator settings, or diuresis. The presence of a simple pneumothorax may require placement of a chest tube, especially if interhospital transport is to be accomplished by air. The benefits of mechanical ventilation versus manual ventilation are unclear. Respiratory therapists, anesthesiologists, and trained nurses can perform safe and effective manual ventilation when the settings and parameters are known prior to transport. Transport of patients on specialized modes of ventilation or those subject to long-distance transport would be more likely to benefit from maintenance of mechanical ventilation.

3. Patients on **cardiovascular** support prior to transport are likely to experience some instability during transport. Current dosages of vasopressors and inotropic drugs should be noted. Appropriate function of transport monitors including display, sufficient battery life, and a system of backup must be confirmed. Personnel responsible for providing care during transport must be familiar with use of the equipment and troubleshooting. The appropriate level of hemodynamic monitoring for the patient's illness and treatments must be determined and provided. Noninvasive blood pressure monitors may be subject to error and unreliable readings with the movement associated with air or ground transport.

4. The **neurologic status, level of sedation,** and **adequacy of pain management** must be assessed prior to any movement. Complications during transport such as hypercarbia, hypocarbia, hypoxemia, and hypotension can worsen neurologic outcome by compromising cerebral perfusion. A

TABLE 16-4	Indications for Pretransport Tracheal Intubation

Glasgow Coma Score less than 9
Respiratory acidosis and impending failure
Status asthmaticus
Shock (septic, hemorrhagic, cardiogenic, neurogenic)
Multitrauma
Recurrent seizures or status epilepticus
Facial or extensive burns
Acute epiglottitis
Angioedema
Anaphylaxis
Laryngeal–tracheal trauma
Combative patients

plan must be made to address increases in intracranial pressure including ventilation, raising the head of the bed, spinal fluid drainage, or mannitol. Often patients with elevated intracranial pressure have an intracranial pressure monitoring device in place. Care must be maintained to avoid dislodgment and appropriate zero reference established. Appropriate pain control and sedation is necessary to ensure patient well-being as increased levels of epinephrine and norepinephrine have been demonstrated in volunteers subject to transport. Short-acting agents such as midazolam and fentanyl may be used to control agitation and discomfort with acceptable risk.

5. **Consent** and disclosure of risks for transport is commonly implied when a patient is moved for a procedure within the same hospital. The risks to the patient associated with the transport itself are separate from the procedure and should be explained to the patient or family member. Current guidelines suggest that a competent patient or legally authorized representative give informed consent when a patient is transferred to another facility. **Transfer that is simply financially motivated is illegal** under the Emergency Medical treatment and Active Labor Law (EMTALA, 1986).

6. **Communication between providers** when a patient is transferred to another hospital or within a hospital but to different sites is imperative. Verbal communication between care providers is a necessity when a patient's care is to be shifted to another provider, even if only temporary. This should happen at both a physician-to-physician level as well as a nurse-to-nurse level. There are substantial data on nurse-to-nurse handovers, but little data on physician-to-physician, or physician-to-nurse handovers. There is no standardized formula, but our hospital uses certain guidelines to govern a safe handoff. A proper transfer of care mandates that the following information be communicated: patient identification; primary condition and reason for transfer; past medical history; current medications or infusions and pertinent medications that the patient may be taking at home; allergies; important physical findings and vital signs; significant laboratory values, procedures performed and their results; access devices such as peripheral IVs, arterial lines, central lines, endotracheal tubes, chest tubes, and so on, and any difficulty encountered in their placement; fluids or blood products given (and lost, if significant;) code status; and plan for management en route. The provider receiving the information must be given the opportunity to clarify details and ask questions. They may request that additional access be obtained prior to transport. When a patient is moved to another facility, copies of all relevant records and studies must accompany the patient along with a complete summary of the hospital course to that point. When a patient is moved within the hospital, even for a brief study, the chart should accompany them.

G. **Equipment** and **monitoring.** No specific standards exist to define what type of equipment should accompany a patient during transport. At a minimum, heart rate and rhythm, noninvasive blood pressure, pulse oximetry, and respiratory rate should be monitored. As a general rule, equipment should be small, portable, and designed to function in the setting of movement. Displays should be bright, alarms easy to identify, and adjustment buttons protected from accidental change.

1. Equipment for **airway management** (**Chapter 4**) including supplies for urgent intubation should accompany all transports. Equipment should include laryngoscopes and a variety of blades, various size

endotracheal tubes, oral and nasal airways, and rescue devices such as a bougie or laryngeal mask airway (LMA). The LMA has been used successfully to manage failed intubation cases in transport. A recently placed tracheostomy that becomes displaced may prove to be a significant challenge and plans must be made to address this situation.

2. **Breathing** and **adequate oxygenation** must be assured. Capnography (**Chapter 2**) ensures correct position of the endotracheal tube and the presence of ventilation. It may prove valuable in transport of the head-injured patient. Capnography may be less subject to errors caused by movement than pulse oximetry is, but pulse oximetry should be monitored on all patients transported from an intensive care setting. Portable ventilators have the advantage of hands-free operation and less variability of respiratory parameters (for prolonged transport), but have the risk of mechanical dysfunction and are expensive.

3. Continuous monitoring of **circulatory status** is also required. Intra-arterial pressure monitoring is more accurate (**Chapter 1**) than noninvasive methods during transport. All invasive hemodynamic monitors should have their "zero" recalculated after the patient is placed on the transport system and when they are positioned at the receiving destination. The accidental dislodgement of invasive monitors may lead to improper clinical decisions, cessation of medication delivery, neurovascular compromise, and hemorrhage.

H. **Transport personnel.** No clear standards define which individual should accompany a patient during movement. Two individuals should accompany all critical care transports at a minimum. One of these individuals must be a nurse, an advanced medical technician, or a physician, and skilled in airway management, intravenous therapy, arrhythmia interpretation, hemodynamic monitoring, treatment, and familiar with all monitors. Studies have shown that specially trained ICU transport teams have fewer adverse outcomes. It is recommended that a physician accompany all unstable patients. Patients subject to the highest level of hemodynamic support such as extracorporeal circulation, ventricular assist, and intra-aortic balloon counterpulsation should only be transported with an individual highly trained in management of these devices.

I. **Ground transport** is safe for the vast majority of patients requiring movement to another hospital. The advantages include lower cost, better monitoring, and rapid mobilization. The transferring physician should be aware of the scope of practice of the transporting personnel. Ground transport is probably faster than air transport for distances less than 10 miles.

J. **Transportation by air** may be accomplished by fixed wing or rotor wing (helicopter). Rotor wing transport is generally more efficient than ground transport for distances more than 45 miles while fixed wing transport is best utilized for distances more than 250 miles. The primary advantages of air transport are efficiency for long distance movement and in the case of fixed wing, less vibration and more space for care providers to operate. Rotor wing can be more rapidly mobilized and land at or near a hospital. Patients are subject to certain physiologic changes with air transport that a care provider must understand.

1. The FiO_2 in air remains at 21% at altitude (5,000–8,000 ft above sea level) but the drop in barometric pressure places the patient at risk for **hypoxemia**. Supplemental oxygen is required for all patients transported by either rotor or fixed wing. For patients with high O_2 requirements, increases in PEEP may be more effective than increasing FiO_2. Fixed wing aircraft may fly at lower altitude to increase O_2 availability

TABLE 16-5	Medical Conditions Potentially Worsened by Altitude

Pneumothorax
Pneumopericardium
Subcutaneous emphysema
Gas gangrene
Decompression sickness
Systemic air emboli
Gastric distention
Pneumocephalus

but with the risk of increased turbulence, slower speed, and poorer fuel efficiency.

2. The **decrease in ambient pressure** may allow the expansion of gases in a closed cavity placing a patient at risk for multiple complications (**Table 16-5**). Decompression drainage tubes should be placed prior to takeoff.

3. Temperature and humidity decrease at altitude, potentially contributing to hypothermia, drying of secretions and dehydration.

4. **Acceleration, deceleration,** and **vibration** contribute to patient pain and anxiety, while potentially interfering with appropriate equipment function.

K. **Transport critical incident review** is imperative to maintaining and improving transportation outcomes within a system. Critical incident review allows a root cause analysis of problems with a goal of improving patient care without establishing blame. This will result in better training, guideline development, and ongoing modification of practices.

Selected References

Andrews PJ, Piper IR, Dearden NM, Miller JD. Secondary insults during intrahospital transport of head injured patients. *Lancet* 1990;335:327–330.

Austin PN, Campbell RS, Johanningman JA, et al. Transport ventilators. *Respir Care Clin* 2002;8:119–150.

Beckmann U, Gillies DM, Berenholtz SM, et al. Incidents relating to the intrahospital transfer of critically ill patients. Analysis of the reports submitted to the Australian Incident Monitoring Study in Intensive Care. *Intensive Care Med* 2004;30:1579–1585.

Chang DM. Intensive care air transport: the sky is the limit; or is it? *Crit Care Med* 2001;29:2227–2230.

Diaz MA, Hendey GW, Bivins HG. When is the helicopter faster? A comparison of helicopter and ground ambulance transport times. *J Trauma* 2005;58:148–153.

Fitzsimons M, Sims N. Transport and monitoring of the critically ill patient. In: Longnecker D, Brown D, Newman M, Zapol W, eds. *Principles and practice of anesthesiology.* McGraw-Hill, 2008:1811–1827.

Indek M, Peterson S, Smith J, Brotman S. Risk, cost, and benefit of transporting ICU patients for special studies. *J Trauma* 1988;28:1020–1025.

Insel J, Weissman C, Kemper M, et al. Cardiovascular changes during transport of critically ill and postoperative patients. *Crit Care Med* 1986;14:539–542.

Kanter RK, Tomkins JM. Adverse events during interhospital transport: physiologic deterioration associated with pretransport severity of illness. *Pediatrics* 1989;84:43–48.

Low RB, Martin D, Brown C. Emergency air transport of pregnant patients: the national experience. *J Emerg Med* 1988;41–48.

Sheldon P, Day MW. Sedation issues in transportation of acutely and critically ill patients. *Crit Care Nurs Clin N Am* 2005;205–210.

Smith AF, Pope C, Goodwin D, Mort M. Interprofessional handover and patient safety in anaesthesia: observational study of handovers in the recovery room. *Br J Anaesth* 2008:101:332–337.

Smith I, Fleming S, Cernaianu A. Mishaps during transport from the intensive care unit. *Crit Care Med* 1990;18:278–281.

Szem JW, Hydo LJ, Fischer E, et al. High-risk intrahospital transport of critically ill patients: safety and outcome of the necessary "road trip." *Crit Care Med* 1995;23:1660–1666.

Warren J, Fromm RE, Orr RA, et al. Guidelines for the inter- and intrahospital transport of critically ill patients. *Crit Care Med* 2004;32:256–262.

Waydhas C. Intrahospital transport of critically ill patients. *Crit Care* 1999;3:R83–R89.

Woodward GA, Insoft RM, Pearson-Shaver AL, et al. The state of pediatric interfacility transport: consensus of the second National Pediatric and Neonatal Interfacility Transport Leadership Conference. *Ped Emerg Care* 2002;18:38–43.

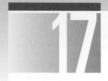

Coronary Artery Disease

Corry "Jeb" Kucik and Michael Fitzsimons

I. **Introduction.** Coronary artery disease (CAD) is the leading cause of adult morbidity and mortality in the United States. More than 64 million Americans have some form of cardiovascular disease such as CAD, heart failure (HF), hypertension (HTN), peripheral vascular disease, and stroke. Nearly 39% of all U.S. deaths stem from these causes. While about a third of patients with acute myocardial infarction (MI) die immediately, most deaths are due to early prehospital dysrhythmias. Medical treatment focuses on identifying at-risk patients and preventing sequelae through risk modification. The major **risk factors** of CAD are HTN, diabetes mellitus (DM), smoking, dyslipidemia (high LDL or low HDL), age over 45 (for men), age over 55 (for women), obesity, elevated homocysteine levels, physical inactivity, and a family history of CAD. African American, Mexican American, and Native American patients also tend to have higher incidences of CAD.

A. **Definitions**

1. **Angina pectoris** is retrosternal tightness, pressure, or pain that occurs at rest or with physical or emotional stress, lasting up to 10 minutes. It can radiate to the back, jaw, arm, or shoulder, usually on the left. Angina usually reflects compromise of at least one epicardial artery and implies ischemia, but not necessarily myocardial necrosis. Symptoms also include nausea, vomiting, diaphoresis, and shortness of breath. Angina may present in valvular heart disease, hypertrophic cardiomyopathy, or uncontrolled HTN. The Canadian Cardiovascular Society Classification System grades angina from Class I (ordinary physical exertion does not cause angina) to Class IV (angina with minimal exertion or at rest).

    a. **Stable angina** demonstrates a pattern that has not changed in frequency, duration, or ease of relief for several months. Predictable symptoms present with exertion and abate with rest. A fixed coronary atheroma with a fibrous cap is generally to blame.

    b. **Variant (Prinzmetal's) angina** occurs at rest, is often worse in the morning, lasts several minutes, and is accompanied by transient ST-segment elevation and/or ventricular dysrhythmias. It can be induced by exercise, stemming from vasospasm in a coronary artery that may not have significant atheromatous disease. Smoking is a major risk factor. Hyperventilation, hypocalcemia, cocaine, pseudoephedrine, and ephedrine have also been implicated.

2. **Acute coronary syndromes (ACS)** are three conditions associated with acute myocardial ischemia secondary to poor myocardial blood

supply: unstable angina, non–ST-segment elevation myocardial infarction **(NSTEMI)**, and ST-segment elevation myocardial infarction **(STEMI)**.

   a. Unstable angina has a recent onset (2 months), increasing frequency and intensity, and recurs at progressively lower levels of stress, even at rest. The prognosis is poor, as 10% of patients have significant disease of the left main coronary artery, and approximately 20% of patients will suffer an acute MI within 3 months. Plaque rupture, platelet aggregation, thrombosis, and vasospasm are the underlying causes.

   b. NSTEMI indicates myocardial ischemia. In the setting of suggestive angina, NSTEMI presents with ST-segment depressions or prominent T waves and may be associated with a rise in cardiac biomarkers. The management of NSTEMI focuses on improving oxygen (O_2) supply and reducing demand in at-risk myocardium, thus preventing progression of damage. It must always be borne in mind that **a nondiagnostic ECG does not rule out MI.**

   c. STEMI reflects severe, possibly irreversible damage to the myocardium, with the appearance of a new ST-segment elevation at the J-point in two contiguous leads ($\geq$0.2 mV in men or $\geq$0.15 mV in women in leads V2–V3 and/or $\geq$0.1 mV in other leads). Left bundle branch block, left ventricular hypertrophy, hyperkalemia, pericarditis, early repolarization, or paced rhythms complicate the diagnosis. Treatment focuses on timely reperfusion.

3. Noncardiac chest pain is not related to coronary ischemia, but may be life threatening. Aortic dissection, pulmonary embolism, and pneumothorax must be ruled out immediately.

4. Perioperative MI is one of the most significant threats in major noncardiac surgery. Patients who suffer MI after surgery have a 15% to 25% risk of in-hospital death and a significant increase in 6-month morbidity and mortality. While there is controversy over accepted definitions of perioperative MI, its incidence may be up to 6% in patients with CAD. While a MI is normally diagnosed on the basis of three criteria (chest pain, biomarker levels, ECG changes), a perioperative MI may be obscured by pain or pain-control techniques to the point of being "silent." A high index of suspicion is critical, and increased consideration should be given to the ECG and cardiac enzymes.

B. Pathophysiology

1. Myocardial O_2 supply–demand balance. Even at rest, the myocardium extracts O_2 maximally. During exertion, O_2 delivery must increase to meet demand. Myocardial ischemia and infarction occur when O_2 demand exceeds delivery.

   a. Myocardial O_2 supply is determined by

     (1) Coronary blood flow is determined by the aortic root pressure at the beginning of diastole minus the resistance of transmural pressure. As transmural resistance is low in diastole, myocardial blood flow is higher during this period. Tachycardia, which minimizes diastolic time, can thus induce ischemia. Normal coronaries compensate by dilating to increase blood flow four- to fivefold during exercise or stress. However, stenoses can reduce the coronaries' ability to dilate and thus limit O_2 supply downstream. Polycythemia, hyperviscosity, and sickle cell disease may further compromise coronary flow.

     (2) O_2 content is dependent on hemoglobin (Hgb) concentration and its saturation with O_2 (SaO_2), and to a lesser extent on dissolved O_2 concentration **(Chapter 2)**. An ideal Hgb level is not known, but compensation through increased cardiac output (CO) occurs with anemia.

   b. **Myocardial O_2 demand** is influenced by

      (1) **Ventricular wall tension (T),** which according to Laplace's law is

$$T = PR/2h$$

where P is transmural pressure, R is ventricular radius, and h is wall thickness. Increase in pressure or radius will increase O_2 demand.

      (2) **Heart rate (HR),** which increases O_2 demand by increasing contractility. Tachycardia shortens diastole and maximal coronary perfusion in atherosclerotic vessels, also limiting O_2 supply. Hyperthyroidism, sympathomimetics (e.g., cocaine), or anxiety can increase HR and O_2 demand.

      (3) **Contractility,** which is the intrinsic property of the myocyte to contract against a load, is proportional to O_2 demand. Positive inotropes (e.g., digoxin, norepinephrine) increase O_2 demands of myocardium that may already be at risk.

   2. **Etiologies of myocardial O_2 demand imbalance.** More than 90% of myocardial ischemia and infarction result from atherosclerosis. Accordingly, most perioperative MIs stem from abrupt, unpredictable partial or complete occlusion secondary to acute atherosclerotic plaque rupture. Other causes include coronary vasospasm or thromboembolism, vasculitis, trauma, valvular heart disease (e.g., aortic stenosis), hypertrophic or dilated cardiomyopathies, and thyrotoxicosis.

II. Angina

   A. **History** should ascertain whether risk factors (DM, smoking, HTN, family history of early coronary disease) exist. Pain is characterized by character, location, duration, radiation, and exacerbating (emotional stress, eating, cold weather) or alleviating (rest, medications) factors. Pain is often a "pressure," "heavy," or "grip-like," with radiation to the arm or jaw. An unstable, changing constellation of symptoms must be differentiated from a stable anginal pattern. Severe angina of recent onset; angina at rest; or angina of increasing duration, frequency, or intensity is classified as unstable and considered a part of the spectrum of ACS.

   B. **Physical examination** may be nonspecific. Findings of distress, anxiety, tachycardia, HTN, an S_4 gallop, pulmonary rales, xanthomas, or peripheral atherosclerosis may be evident. Pulmonary edema, a new or worsening murmur of mitral regurgitation, and angina with hypotension are associated with a high risk of progression to nonfatal MI or death.

   C. **Noninvasive studies**

   1. The **resting ECG** is normal in many patients with ischemia. ECG changes indicative of myocardial ischemia that may progress to MI include new ST-segment elevations at the J-point in two or more contiguous leads that are ≥ 0.2 mV in leads V_1 to V_3 and >0.1 mV in all other leads. Ischemia from coronary vasospasm may present with ST-segment elevation. ST depression or T-wave abnormalities may also signal risk for MI. However, isolated J-point elevation may occur as a normal variant in young, healthy adults. Significant Q waves are suggestive of a prior MI. A bundle branch block (BBB) or artificial pacer may complicate detection of ST-segment or T-wave abnormalities. Serial ECGs in 15- to 20-minute intervals can determine whether ischemia is evolving. In general, reversibility of ECG changes after therapeutic interventions is

TABLE 17-1	Location of Ischemia or Infarct by Electrocardiographic Criteria	
Region	**Leads**	**Vessel**
Anterior	V_2–V_5	Left anterior descending
Anteroseptal	V_1–V_2	Left anterior descending
Apical	V_5–V_6	Left anterior descending
Lateral	I, aVL	Circumflex
Inferior	II, III, aVF	Right coronary artery
Posterior (inferolateral)	Large R wave in V_1, V_2, or V_3 with ST depression	Right coronary artery[a]
Right ventricular	V_3R, V_4R	Right coronary artery

[a]The posterior and inferolateral designate the same segment of the left ventricle. A posterior myocardial infarction may be the result compromise of the right coronary artery or an obtuse marginal branch of the circumflex.

highly suggestive of ischemia **Table 17-1** outlines the ECG changes associated with specific regions of ischemic myocardium.

2. **Exercise ECG.** Exercise stress testing involves monitoring blood pressure (BP) and ECG while the patient exercises on a treadmill or a bicycle. Indications for exercise testing include diagnosis of obstructive CAD, risk assessment and prognosis in suspected or known CAD, asymptomatic patients with multiple risk factors, and certain post-revascularization situations. Each level of exercise reflects increased O_2 uptake or metabolic equivalents (METs). A single MET is 3.5 cm^3 O_2/kg/min. The test is discontinued when a patient reaches 85% to 90% of maximal predicted HR; the patient requests its termination; or when angina, serious arrhythmias, CNS symptoms, decreased BP, or evidence of poor peripheral perfusion occurs. A **positive test** (i.e., one which demonstrates ST-segment elevation or depression, a fall in BP with exercise, development of serious arrhythmias, or the development of anginal chest pain with exercise) indicates a high likelihood of significant CAD. Sensitivity for obstructive CAD increases with the severity of stenotic disease. For CAD involving the left main coronary or for three-vessel disease, sensitivity is 86% and specificity is 53%. Positive tests should prompt consideration of cardiac catheterization and revascularization. Absolute contraindications to exercise stress testing include a recent MI (within 2 days), severe aortic stenosis, symptomatic HF, arrhythmia causing hemodynamic compromise, acute pulmonary embolus, and aortic dissection. Relative contraindications include uncontrolled HTN (systolic BP higher than 200 mm Hg or diastolic BP higher than 110 mm Hg), tachy- or bradyarrhythmias, hypertrophic cardiomyopathy, high-grade atrioventricular block, and a physical or mental limitation to exercise. ECG changes occurring at lower workloads are generally more significant than those at higher workloads.

3. **Myocardial injury enzymes.** Biomarker analysis is undertaken immediately to help determine whether angina is stable or unstable. Negative results within 6 hours of symptom onset necessitate further testing at 6- to 8-hour intervals if ACS is suspected. When damaged (e.g., by trauma or infarction), cardiac myocytes release various proteins such as **creatine kinase-MB fraction** (CK-MB), **troponin,** and myoglobin into the blood. Myocardial troponin is considered the most accurate marker. Troponin levels may be especially valuable in the perioperative

period where CK-MB may be elevated for other reasons and may not reflect myocardial necrosis.

4. **Radionuclide perfusion imaging** assesses both myocardial perfusion and function in a patient with stable angina.

   a. **Exercise myocardial perfusion imaging.** Thallium[201] is a radioactive potassium analog that is avidly extracted by viable myocardium in proportion to regional myocardial blood flow during exercise. Regions of decreased uptake correlate with the severity of coronary stenosis supplying the regions. Imaging after rest may show a "fixed defect" that takes up no tracer at all, which represents an area of prior infarct, while a "reversible defect," a region that regains uptake, is considered to be myocardium at risk of ischemia. This test has a sensitivity of 85% and a specificity of 90% for detecting myocardium at risk of ischemia.

   b. **Exercise radionuclide ventriculography.** Intravenous technetium[99m] sestamibi accumulates in myocardium in proportion to blood flow, and multiple ventricular images that are synchronized to the cardiac cycle are acquired at rest and during exercise. Ischemia is suggested by regional wall motion abnormalities and the inability to increase left ventricular ejection fraction (LVEF) during exercise.

   c. **Pharmacologic stress perfusion imaging.** Adenosine and dipyridamole are coronary vasodilators commonly used in stress imaging. Adenosine increases blood flow in disease-free coronary vessels. Dipyridamole inhibits cellular uptake and degradation of adenosine, indirectly increasing coronary flow in nonstenotic vessels. Because stenotic areas are already maximally dilated, the dilation of disease-free vessels creates differential flow patterns upon coronary imaging. Both drugs may cause angina, headache, or bronchospasm, and must be used with caution in patients with obstructive pulmonary disease. Dobutamine, an inotrope, increases HR, systolic BP, and contractility, causing increased blood flow secondarily. Imaging after dobutamine administration may show heterogeneous flow due to nondilating stenotic areas.

D. **Invasive studies. Coronary angiography** remains the gold standard for quantifying the extent of CAD and guiding percutaneous coronary intervention (PCI; e.g., angioplasty, stenting, atherectomy) or coronary artery bypass grafting (CABG). Coronary angiography will reveal hemodynamic parameters, cardiac and coronary anatomy, and wall motion abnormalities. A coronary obstruction is clinically significant when more than 70% of the luminal diameter is narrowed. Coronary angiography is not without risk; the mortality rate is approximately 0.5%.

E. **Medical management.** Once it has been determined that angina is stable, appropriate management should be initiated.

   1. **Smoking cessation.**

   2. **BP control** to a goal of 140/90 mm Hg.

   3. **Dietary modification.**

   4. **Medically supervised physical activity and weight reduction.**

   5. **Aspirin (ASA)** inhibits platelets by irreversibly acetylating cyclooxygenase and decreasing thromboxane levels. If no contraindications exist, it should be started at 81 to 325 mg/d.

   6. **Angiotensin-converting enzyme (ACE) inhibitors** reduce sympathetic tone and have a survival benefit in HF. They should be started in all patients with no contraindications and an ejection fraction of less than 40%, especially if HTN, DM, or renal disease coexists.

	Contradictions to β-blockers in the ACS

Marked first-degree AV block
Any form of second or third-degree block
History of asthma
Evidence of left ventricle dysfunction
High risk for shock (e.g., time delay to presentation, lower blood pressure)

   7. β-Blockers should be initiated in all patients with a history of MI or ACS unless contraindicated (**Table 17-2**).
   8. HMG-CoA reductase inhibitors ("statins") improve lipid profiles, limiting progression of atherosclerotic disease and coronary calcium deposition while stabilizing existing plaques.
   F. Invasive management for unstable angina includes **percutaneous coronary intervention (PCI)**. Occasionally, **CABG** may be urgently indicated.

III. Acute coronary syndromes. Regardless of whether ACS is due to unstable angina, NSTEMI, or STEMI, the goal is to minimize ischemic time and, when appropriate, initiate reperfusion therapy with thrombolysis, PCI, or CABG.
   A. The **history** should attempt to differentiate between UA from MI. Symptoms are often indistinguishable (see **Section II.A**).
   B. The **physical examination** is unlikely to distinguish UA from an acute MI (see **Section II.B**).
   C. As for angina, noninvasive studies include the ECG and cardiac enzymes.
      1. A **12-lead ECG** should be obtained as soon as possible to determine whether a STEMI is occurring and immediate revascularization is needed. Transient ST-segment elevations ($\geq$0.05 mV) that resolve with rest likely indicates true ischemia and severe underlying CAD. Elevation of less than 0.05 mV, ST-segment depression, or T-wave inversion is more often associated with NSTEMI or UA. A normal ECG does **not** rule out MI, as up to 6% of patients later confirmed to have had MIs may present as such. Serial ECGs are more accurate than an isolated study.
      2. The best **biomarker** confirmation is a rise in cardiac troponin I or T (>99th percentile). If clinical suspicion for MI is high, troponins should be drawn at 0, 6 to 9, and 12 to 24 hours. Cardiac troponins I and T are highly specific for myocardial damage but do not indicate the mechanism of damage. CK-MB is less sensitive, but may be substituted if troponin measurement is not available.
      3. The **chest x-ray** can detect MI complications such as pulmonary venous congestion, and can rule out aortic dissection, pneumonia, pleural effusion, and pneumothorax.
      4. Transthoracic echocardiography (TTE) is not an initial diagnostic study in most presentations of ACS. If biomarkers and ECG analysis are equivocal, TTE may elucidate complications of ischemia or MI such as regional wall motion abnormalities, thromboembolic events, valve morphologies, and changes in global ventricular function. If TTE is available and the echocardiographer is experienced, this modality offers a convenient method by which a more complete clinical picture can be gained while awaiting the return of biomarker labs.
   D. Management of acute MI
      1. The **general approach** to acute MI focuses on minimizing total ischemic time (onset of symptoms to start off reperfusion). Ideally, this

time should be <90 minutes. Initiation of thrombolysis in <30 minutes is the system goal for STEMI when PCI is not available.

2. **Supportive measures.** Supplemental O_2, IV access, routine vitals, and continuous ECG should be begun. Unless HF or hypoxemia (SpO_2 <90%) occurs, supplemental O_2 is generally required only for 2 to 3 hours after uncomplicated MI. Patients with severe HF or cardiogenic shock may need intubation and mechanical ventilation. Laboratory studies include electrolytes with magnesium, lipid profile, and complete blood count to detect anemia. Continuous pulse oximetry is critical to evaluate oxygenation, especially in patients with HF or cardiogenic shock.

3. **Treatments.** See **Appendix** for additional pharmacologic information. Unless contraindicated, a β-blocker, ASA, anticoagulation, a glycoprotein IIb/IIIa inhibitor, and a thienopyridine should be administered.

   a. β-Blockade appears to reduce myocardial O_2 consumption by slowing the HR and reducing cardiac contractility. However, there is evidence that β-blockers may be detrimental in patients with acute HF (**Table 17-2**). If no contraindications exist, β-blockers should be initiated. Initially, **metoprolol** 5 mg IV every 5 minutes to a total of 15 mg may be given. If tolerated, metoprolol 25 to 50 mg orally every 6 hours can be administered for 2 days and then increased up to 100 mg orally twice daily. **Carvedilol** 6.25 mg administered orally twice a day, titrated up to a maximum of 25 mg twice a day, may reduce mortality in patients with an acute MI and LV dysfunction.

   b. The benefit of **calcium channel blockers** in ACS is related to symptom reduction in patients already receiving β-blockers and nitrates or who cannot tolerate these agents. **Nifedipine** 30 to 90 mg orally can be administered. If tolerated, a longer-acting agent such as Diltiazem (slow release) 120 to 360 mg once daily or Verapamil (slow release) 120 to 480 mg by mouth once a day may be initiated.

   c. **Nitrates** increase venous capacitance, thus decreasing preload and cardiac work. Nitrates dilate epicardial coronary arteries and collateral circulation, and also inhibit platelet function. Evidence does not support routine long-term nitrate therapy in MI unless pain persists. IV nitroglycerin (NTG) is started at 10 μg/min and titrated until symptom relief or BP response. Patients with acute MI or HF, large anterior infarcts, persistent ischemia, or HTN may benefit from IV NTG for the first 24 to 48 hours. Those with continuing pulmonary edema or recurrent ischemia or angina may benefit from even more prolonged use of NTG. Ideally, IV NTG should be changed to an oral route within 24 hours; for instance, **isosorbide dinitrate** 5 to 80 mg orally 2 to 3 times per day. NTG is generally not indicated in hypotension or persistent bradycardia.

   d. **ACE inhibitors** are of benefit in diabetic patients with a recent MI associated with LV dysfunction.

   e. **Analgesia.** Morphine sulfate (1–5 mg IV) for analgesia and anxiolysis are reasonable unless contraindicated by hypotension or history of morphine intolerance. Modest reductions in HR and BP decrease O_2 consumption. Side effects include hypotension, respiratory depression, bradycardia, or nausea.

   f. **Antiplatelet therapy** should be considered in any patient presenting with ACS. Agents are chosen based on whether the proposed management will be conservative or invasive (e.g., CABG or PCI, which yield an increased risk of hemorrhage).

(1) **ASA** 325 mg by mouth should be given to all patients, unless contraindicated by hypersensitivity or a history of major GI bleeding. By irreversibly inhibiting cyclooxygenase-1 in platelets, ASA prevents formation of thromboxane A2 and decreases platelet aggregation.

(2) If a contraindication to using ASA exists, a 300-mg oral loading dose of **clopidogrel** followed by 75 mg once a day can be started. Clopidogrel and ASA are given together if invasive management is planned.

(3) **Glycoprotein IIb/IIIa inhibitors** may be added pending the decision about a conservative or invasive protocol.

g. Further **anticoagulation** depends upon whether conservative or invasive management is pursued. Unfractionated heparin **(UFH)**, low-molecular-weight heparin **(LMWH)**, a direct thrombin inhibitor (bivalirudin), or a factor Xa inhibitor (fondaparinux) may be chosen.

(1) **UFH** has the advantage of common use but the disadvantage of a risk of heparin-induced thrombocytopenia (HIT). Initial dosing is to target an APTT of 1.5 to 2 × normal. A normal dose is 60 U/kg as a bolus followed by 12 U/kg/h.

(2) **LMWH** has a lower risk of HIT and is easier to administer. Concerns about the ability to monitor the effectiveness of LMWH compared to UFH and less effective reversal with protamine have limited its use when PCI is planned.

(3) **Direct thrombin inhibitors** have no risk of HIT and are associated with more bleeding complications and an inability to reverse effects with protamine or FFP. **Bivalirudin** is a direct-acting synthetic antithrombin that acts against clot-bound thrombin with a very short half-life (25 minutes). Its major advantages may be a lower rate of bleeding when compared to UFH plus a GP IIb/IIIa inhibitor.

(4) **Fondaparinux** is a **factor Xa inhibitor** that confers a lower risk of bleeding when compared to UFH and GP IIb/IIIa inhibitors.

h. **Magnesium** dilates coronary arteries, inhibits platelet activity, suppresses automaticity, and may protect against reperfusion injury. Supplemental magnesium in indicated for hypomagnesemia and *torsades de pointes*. Hypomagnesemia is corrected with magnesium sulfate 2 g IV over 30 to 60 minutes, while torsades de pointes is treated with 1 to 2 g IV over 5 minutes. Since most magnesium in the body is intracellular, hypomagnesemic patients may require multiple replacement doses to achieve normal levels. Prophylactic administration in acute MI is not indicated.

i. An **insulin** infusion should maintain a glucose homeostasis in patients presenting with ACS, generally aiming for a goal of 110 to 150 mg/dL.

j. Pharmacologic or mechanical **reperfusion therapy** reduces infarct size and mortality and improves function, even after a prolonged period. Temporary myocardial impairment ("stunned myocardium") may exist after the injury is reversed. In general, PCI is preferred if performed less than 1 hour from presentation. If the anticipated time is greater than 1 hour, thrombolysis is preferred. Reperfusion is assessed noninvasively through relief of symptoms, restoration of hemodynamic or respiratory stability, or a 50% or better reduction in initial ST-segment elevation.

(1) **Thrombolysis** is only indicated in the presence of ST-segment elevation >0.1 mV in at least two contiguous leads. Thrombolysis

TABLE 17-3	Comparison of Thrombolytic Drugs		
	tPA	**Streptokinase**	**APSAC**
Half-life	6 min	20 min	100 min
Dosage	100 mg[a]	1.5 million units	30 units
Administration	90 min	60 min	5 min
Fibrin-selective	Yes	No	Partial
Artery patency rate[b]	79%	40%	63%
ICH	0.6%	0.3%	0.6%
Lives saved/1,000 treated	35	25	25
Antigenic	No	Yes	Yes
Hypotension	No	Yes	Yes
Heparin required	Yes	No	No

tPA, tissue plasminogen activator; APSAC, anisoylated plasminogen streptokinase activator complex; ICH, intracranial hemorrhage.
[a]15 mg bolus, then 0.75 mg/kg over 30 minutes (maximum 50 mg), then 0.5 mg/kg over 60 minutes (maximum 35 mg) to provide total of 100 mg over 90 minutes.
[b]Artery patency rate at 90 minutes after treatment.

yields the greatest benefit when initiated within 6 hours of symptom onset, although definite benefit exists even at 12 hours. Patients presenting within 12 to 24 hours but with continuing symptoms may also benefit. Response to therapy results in improvement in ST-segment elevation and resolution of chest discomfort. Persistent symptoms and ST-segment elevation 60 to 90 minutes after thrombolysis are indications for urgent angiography and possible PCI. Thrombolysis offers no benefit in patients without ST-segment elevation or new BBB, or in those with MI complicated by HF or cardiogenic shock. **Table 17-3** shows a comparison of the commonly used thrombolytic agents. **Absolute contraindications** are any prior intracranial hemorrhage, a cerebral vascular malformation or neoplasm, suspected aortic dissection, active bleeding, or significant head trauma or ischemic stroke within 3 months (does not include an acute CVA within 3 hours). **Relative contraindications** include known bleeding diathesis, concurrent anticoagulation, recent trauma (2–4 weeks), prolonged cardiopulmonary resuscitation (>10 minutes), recent major surgery (<3 weeks), recent internal bleeding (2–4 weeks), severe HTN (systolic BP >180/110 mm Hg), other intracranial pathology, noncompressible vascular puncture sites, pregnancy, active peptic ulcer disease, or prior exposure (5 days to 2 years) to streptokinase or anisoylated plasminogen streptokinase activator complex (APSAC). **Patients requiring retreatment**, having failed streptokinase or APSAC, should receive tissue plasminogen activator. Those with contraindications to thrombolysis should be considered for PCI.

   i. **Streptokinase** is a bacterial protein produced by α-hemolytic streptococci. It induces activation of free and clot-associated plasminogen, eliciting a nonspecific systemic fibrinolytic state. It may decrease mortality by 18%. Side effects are hypotension and allergic-type reactions.

ii. **Tissue plasminogen activator (t-PA)** is a recombinant natural protein. By increasing plasmin binding to fibrin, it provides relative clot-selective fibrinolysis without inducing a systemic lytic state. When given with heparin, its early reperfusion rate is slightly better than other agents. Compared to streptokinase, it is less likely to cause hemorrhage requiring transfusion, and has greater survival benefit (10 additional lives in 1,000 treated).

iii. **Anisoylated plasminogen streptokinase activator complex (APSAC)** (Eminase or anistreplase) has clinical characteristics between those of t-PA and streptokinase (**Table 17-3**).

(2) **PCI and stenting** has replaced percutaneous transluminal coronary angioplasty as atherectomy and stenting have improved patency rates above that of angioplasty alone. In addition to the absence of a thoracotomy and associated complications, there are fewer neurological sequelae with PCI compared to CABG. The primary constraint of PCI is the availability of personnel and support facilities that are only available in approximately 20% of hospitals in the United States. Adjuncts to PCI that reduce coronary reocclusion include **IV heparin, ASA, ticlopidine, and GP IIb/IIIa inhibitors.** The benefit of LMWH compared to UFH in PCI is unclear at this time. A glycoprotein IIb/IIIa inhibitor (e.g., abciximab) may decrease mortality, MI recurrence, and the need for urgent revascularization.

(3) **Acute surgical reperfusion** may be emergently indicated for patients with operable coronary anatomy who have failed medical management but are not candidates for PCI; have failed PCI; have persistent ischemia, hemodynamic instability, or cardiogenic shock; have surgically correctable complications of MI (e.g., severe mitral regurgitation or ventricular septal defect); or have life-threatening arrhythmias in the presence of severe left main or three-vessel disease. Mortality from emergent CABG is high.

k. **Intra-aortic balloon counterpulsation** with an intra-aortic balloon pump (**IABP**) may be indicated in patients awaiting PCI or CABG who have low CO unresponsive to inotropic support or who demonstrate refractory pulmonary congestion. The effects of IAB counterpulsation include diastolic BP augmentation—thus increasing coronary perfusion, and systolic BP reduction—thus decreasing impedance to ejection.

IV. Complications of myocardial infarction

A. **Recurrent ischemia and infarction.** Common causes of chest pain after MI are pericarditis, ischemia, and reinfarction. Up to 58% of patients show early recurrent angina after reperfusion. Reinfarction occurs in approximately 3% to 4% of patients within 10 days of thrombolysis and ASA. Patients with reinfarction are at risk of cardiogenic shock and fatal dysrhythmias. The initial approach optimizes medical therapies and may include repeat thrombolysis or PCI. Emergency CABG may benefit those who have failed or are not candidates for medical treatment or PCI. Patients with active ischemia unresponsive to medical therapy may receive an IABP while awaiting angiography.

B. **Mechanical complications**

1. **Mitral regurgitation (MR)** can occur from papillary muscle rupture, often presenting 3 to 5 days post-infarct, and is commonly associated with an

inferoposterior MI. Findings may include pulmonary edema, hypotension, cardiogenic shock, and a new apical systolic murmur. A pulmonary artery occlusion pressure waveform may exhibit large V waves. A ruptured papillary muscle and mitral regurgitation may be evident on echocardiography. Treatment includes afterload reduction, inotropes, and IABP while awaiting emergent surgical repair. Medical management alone yields a mortality of roughly 75% in the first 24 hours.

2. **Ventricular septal defect (VSD)** most commonly occurs between 3 and 5 days after an anterior MI. Clinical signs include a new holosystolic murmur with systolic thrill and cardiogenic shock. A septal defect will be seen on echocardiography. An increased SaO_2 between blood sampled from the right atrium and right ventricle can confirm an interventricular shunt. Treatment includes afterload reduction, inotropy, and IABP. Hemodynamically stable patients may not require immediate surgical repair, but mortality in patients with cardiogenic shock is up to 90% without surgical intervention.

3. **Ventricular free wall rupture** accounts for approximately 10% of peri-infarct death. Risk factors include sustained HTN after MI, a large transmural MI, late thrombolysis, female sex, advanced age, and exposure to steroids or nonsteroidal anti-inflammatory agents. It is most common in the first 2 weeks after MI, with peak incidence 3 to 6 days post-infarct. Recurrent chest pain, acute HF, and cardiovascular collapse suggest free wall rupture. Death can occur rapidly and overall mortality is high. Diagnosis is by echocardiography. Volume expansion, tamponade decompression, and IABP temporize prior to emergent surgical repair.

4. **Ventricular aneurysm** is usually due to thinning of the infarcted ventricular wall. It is characterized by a protrusion of scar tissue in association with HF, malignant dysrhythmias, and systemic embolism. Persistent ST-segment elevation may be evident, while echocardiography confirms. Anticoagulation is required, especially in patients with documented mural thrombus. Surgical correction of ventricular geometry may be necessary.

5. **Pericarditis,** due to extension of myocardial necrosis to the epicardium, occurs in approximately 25% of patients within weeks of MI. Pleuritic chest pain or positional discomfort, radiation to the left shoulder, a pericardial rub, diffuse J-point elevation, concave ST-segment elevation, reciprocal PR depression, and pericardial effusion on echocardiography may be evident. Treatment includes **ASA** 162 to 325 mg daily, increased to 650 mg every 4 to 6 hours if necessary. Indomethacin, ibuprofen, and corticosteroids are avoided, as wall thinning in the zone of myocardial necrosis may predispose to ventricular wall rupture.

C. **Dysrhythmias,** including premature ventricular contractions, bradycardia, atrial fibrillation, atrioventricular blocks, ventricular fibrillation, ventricular tachycardia, and idioventricular rhythms, are common in the setting of MI. Multiple etiologies may include HF, ischemia, re-entrant rhythms, reperfusion, acidosis, electrolyte derangements (e.g., hypokalemia, hypomagnesemia, intracellular hypercalcemia), hypoxemia, hypotension, drug effects, and heightened reflex sympathoadrenal and vagal activity. Treatment of any precipitating cause should be undertaken immediately. **Chapter 19** discusses these dysrhythmias and their treatments in detail.

D. **Heart failure and cardiogenic shock.** The incidence of cardiogenic shock after MI is approximately 7.5%. Mortality is extremely high. Contractility of approximately 40% of the ventricular myocardium must be lost for cardiogenic shock to develop. Causes include VSD, acute MR, tamponade, and right ventricular failure. Management includes hemodynamic support with pressors, IABP, or immediate revascularization.

E. **Hypertension** increases myocardial O_2 demand and may worsen ischemia. Causes of HTN after MI include premorbid HTN, HF, and elevated catecholamines due to pain and anxiety. Treatment includes adequate antianginal therapy, analgesia, anxiolysis, IV NTG, β-blockade, and ACE inhibitors. Calcium channel blockers (verapamil or diltiazem) may be indicated in patients who have contraindications to other agents. Nitroprusside may be required if HTN is severe.

V. **Perioperative myocardial ischemia and infarction**

A. **Definition, incidence, and implications.** As medical and surgical therapy for cardiovascular disease continues to improve, more patients with these conditions are living longer, healthier lives. However, as a result, more patients with CAD or related risk factors (advanced age, HTN, DM, HF, decreased exercise tolerance, and renal disease) are presenting for cardiac and noncardiac surgery than ever before, and this number is only expected to rise. Normal risks of surgery and anesthesia (pain, tachycardia, HTN, increased sympathetic tone, coronary vasoconstriction, hypoxemia, anemia, shivering, hypercoagulability) place this population at increased risk for ischemia and perioperative MI. Of more than 27 million patients undergoing noncardiac surgery each year, approximately 1 million suffer some form of perioperative cardiac complication, contributing to more than $20 billion of added health care costs. In patients with pre-existing CAD, roughly 6% will experience a perioperative MI. Patients who suffer MI after surgery have a 15% to 25% risk of in-hospital death and a significant increase in 6-month morbidity and mortality.

B. **Perioperative monitoring and diagnosis.** Under normal conditions, MI is diagnosed on the basis of history (see **Sections I.A.1, II.A**), increased biomarkers (see **Section III.C.2**), and characteristic ECG changes (see **Section III.C.1**). However, postoperative pain and pain-control techniques may render a perioperative MI "silent." As perioperative MI occurs most often on the day of surgery or postoperative day 1, increased diagnostic weight must be given to ECG changes and cardiac enzymes early in the postoperative course. A high index of suspicion, especially in a population likely to have pre-existing ECG abnormalities (e.g., arrhythmias, bundle branch blocks, left ventricular hypertrophy, pacemakers), should be maintained. Comparison of a daily ECG to baseline is a cost-effective monitoring plan. Biomarkers should be obtained for confirmation rather than for surveillance, bearing in mind that these enzymes may be elevated as a direct result of surgery (e.g., in CABG). Transthoracic and transesophageal echocardiography **(Chapter 3)** are excellent investigative modalities when an adverse cardiac event is suspected, as regional wall motion abnormalities will precede both ECG changes and biomarker increases.

C. **Preventive strategies.** Surgical stress and anesthesia provoke myriad physiologic and biochemical changes that can be influenced to the betterment of postoperative care.

1. **β-Blockade.** There is evidence supporting the use of perioperative β-blockade to decrease cardiovascular complications in patients at risk, including those older than age 65, or those with CAD, HTN, DM, tobacco use, hypercholesterolemia, or a family history of CAD. Prescribed β-blockade should be continued up to and including the

morning of surgery. Patients not on a regimen can be treated with **metoprolol** 5 mg IV unless HR is <60 beats per min or systolic BP is <110 mm Hg. Metoprolol may also be given in the operating or recovery room to maintain an HR of 50 to 80 beats per min. Upon completion of surgery, chronic β-blockade should be resumed and patients at risk may be started on metoprolol 25 mg by mouth twice a day for at least 2 weeks. Contraindications include bronchospasm, symptomatic HF, third-degree heart block, or prior adverse reaction to β-blockers.

2. **Pain control.** The patient may have postoperative or ischemic pain, but due to sedation, intubation, or pain control modalities may not be able to report it. Surgical pain may cause tachycardia, HTN, sympathetic discharge, and coronary vasoconstriction, all of which can raise myocardial O_2 consumption while compromising supply. Adequate **sedation and analgesia** (using opioids, benzodiazepines, propofol, or regional anesthesia) are mainstays of postoperative care that may contribute to improved cardiac outcomes. Nonsteroidal anti-inflammatory drugs (NSAIDs), such as **ketorolac,** have both analgesic and antiplatelet effects. **Clonidine,** an α-2 agonist, inhibits presynaptic norepinephrine release and produces beneficial effects on HR, BP, and thrombosis.

3. **O_2 carrying capacity.** A true or dilutional anemia may result from excessive intra- or postoperative blood loss or from aggressive IV hydration, respectively. Either etiology may limit O_2 delivery to myocardium at risk. Treatment should be individualized to patient and procedure and should consider the risk of complications of impaired oxygenation. While absolute transfusion "triggers" should be avoided, judicious fluid resuscitation and transfusion practice should maintain a hematocrit between 25% and 30%.

4. **Temperature regulation.** Postanesthesia homeothermic derangement may cause shivering and an augmented O_2 demand. Low temperatures may also compromise postsurgical hemostasis. Unless contraindicated, patients should be kept normothermic by means of limiting unnecessary exposure, forced air warmers, and warmed IV fluids and blood products. In an intubated, ventilated patient, a non-depolarizing muscle blocker can prevent shivering.

5. **Glucose homeostasis.** Surgical stress can exacerbate pre-existing DM or impaired glucose tolerance. High glucose levels can worsen to endothelial dysfunction. An insulin infusion or sliding scale should maintain a goal of 110 to 150 mg/dL.

6. **Coagulation.** Surgery can induce a protective hemostatic state that may be detrimental to the patient with CAD. Decreased fibrinolysis, increased platelet count and function, and increased fibrinogen and coagulation factor levels may cause intracoronary thrombosis. ASA, NSAIDs, and α-2 agonists have a role in preventing untoward thrombotic complications.

D. Management

1. **Consultation** with a cardiologist, the primary surgical team, and when indicated, a cardiac surgeon should begin the moment a perioperative MI is suspected, as emergent reperfusion by PCI or CABG may be warranted (see **Section III.D.3.j**). Because of the patient's recent surgery, thrombolysis will likely be contraindicated.

2. **Supportive measures** include continued ECG, biomarker, and invasive monitoring as appropriate, as well as intervention in all parameters listed under "Preventive Strategies" (see **Section V.C**) can contribute to improved outcomes after a cardiac complication.

3. Current **medications** (as discussed in **Sections II.E, III.D.3, and V.C**) should be reviewed in light of the change in clinical status. If not begun already, ASA, β-blockade, ACE inhibitors, and statins should be started if no contraindications exist. Again, thrombolysis may not be an option due to the patient's recent surgery.

4. As mentioned earlier, **invasive management** strategies such as PCI or CABG should be considered. An IABP may be useful for improving coronary blood flow, though device placement may be complicated in vasculopathic patients.

Selected References

Antman EM, Anbe DT, Armstrong bates ER, et al. ACC/AHA guidelines for the management of patients with ST-elevation myocardial infarction—executive summary: a report of the American College of Cardiology/American Heart Association Task Force on Practice Guidelines (Writing Committee to Revise the 1999 Guidelines for the Management of Patients with Acute Myocardial Infarction). *Circulation* 2004;110;588–636.

Antman EM, Hand M, Armstrong PW, Bates ER, et al. 2007 Focused update of the ACC/AHA 2004 guidelines for the management of patients with ST-elevation myocardial infarction. A report of the American College of Cardiology/American Heart Association Task Force on Practice Guidelines. *Circulation* 2008;117:296–329.

Auerbach AD, Goldman L. β-blockers and reduction of cardiac events in noncardiac surgery scientific review. *JAMA* 2002;287:1435–1444.

Butterworth J, Furberg CD. Improving cardiac outcomes after noncardiac surgery. *Anesth Analg* 2003;97:613–615.

Devereaux PJ, Goldman L, Yusuf S, et al. Surveillance and prevention of major perioperative ischemic cardiac vents in patients undergoing noncardiac surgery: a review. *CMAJ* 2005;173:779–788.

Eagle KA, Guyton RA, Davidoff R, et al. ACC/AHA 2004 guideline update for coronary artery bypass graft surgery: a report of the American College of Cardiology/American Heart Association Task Force on Practice Guidelines (Committee to Update the 1999 Guidelines for Coronary Artery Bypass Graft Surgery). *Circulation* 2004;110:340–437.

Fraker TD, Fihn SD, Gibbons RJ, Abrams J, et al. 2007 Chronic angina focused update of the ACC/AHA 2002 guidelines for the management of patients with chronic stable angina. *J Am Coll Cardiol* 2007;50:2264–2276.

Landesberg G. The pathophysiology of perioperative myocardial ischemia: facts and perspectives. *J Cardiothorac Vasc Anesth* 2003;17:90–100.

Lubbrook GL, Webb RK, Currie M, Watterson LM. Crisis management during anaesthesia: myocardial ischaemia and infarction. *Qual Saf Health Care* 2005;14:e13.

Podgoreanu MV, White WD, Morris RW, Mathew JP, et al. Inflammatory gene polymorphisms and risk of perioperative myocardial infarction after cardiac surgery. *Circulation* 2006;114:I275–I281.

Priebe HJ. Perioperative myocardial infarction—aetiology and prevention. *Br J Anaesth* 2005;95:3–19.

Thygesen K, Alpert JS, White HD. Universal definition of myocardial infarction. *Circulation* 2007;116:2634–2653.

18

Valvular Heart Disease

Jonathan Bloom and Theodore Alston

Each of the cardiac valves is subject to malfunction. Advances in portable echocardiography permit quantitative assessment of valvular function as an aid to management of critically ill patients.

I. **Aortic stenosis (AS)** is usually **valvular** but can be **supravalvular** or **subvalvular**. Rheumatic heart disease, congenital bicuspid valve, and senile degeneration are the primary causes of valvular AS.

   A. **Pathophysiology**

   1. As the valve orifice decreases, the heart maintains stroke volume through increased pressure generation. This results in **concentric hypertrophy** of the left ventricle (LV). Critical AS eventually results in LV dysfunction with pulmonary edema, myocardial ischemia, or sudden lethal dysrhythmias.

   2. There are a number of causes of morbidity in the patient with AS:

      a. Elevated intracavitary pressures can compress the subendocardium and impair perfusion. Ischemia may be difficult to treat. **Though afterload is increased, a high aortic pressure may be required to maintain adequate coronary perfusion.**

      b. Increased LV systolic and diastolic pressures increase wall tension and so increase myocardial oxygen demand.

      c. Tachycardia or supraventricular dysrhythmias may decrease stroke volume and cause ischemia. Atrial contraction normally contributes 20% to 25% of the total stroke volume. In severe AS, the atrial contribution increases to 30% to 40%. Thus, normal atrial contraction is essential for optimal cardiac function in patients with AS.

      d. Reduction in systemic vascular resistance (SVR) can result in hypotension that can be difficult to treat in view of the inability of the heart to compensate through a fixed stenotic valve and the onset of ischemia. Yet, perhaps counterintuitively, carefully titrated nitroprusside sometimes improves cardiac output.

   B. **Signs, symptoms, and diagnosis**

   1. AS may be asymptomatic for years. Onset of symptoms indicates severe disease. The triad of angina pectoris, syncope, and congestive heart failure (CHF) indicates a life expectancy of less than 5 years in untreated AS.

   2. **Angina** can result from coexisting atherosclerotic coronary artery disease or from AS in isolation.

   3. **Physical findings** indicative of AS include the following:

      a. A loud systolic murmur that is best heard at the base of the heart and radiates to the neck.

      b. A strong apical impulse.

      c. A slow-rising carotid upstroke.

   4. The **degree of AS** is measured by echocardiography or by cardiac catheterization (**Fig. 18-1**). **Stenosis** is graded as trace, mild, moderate,

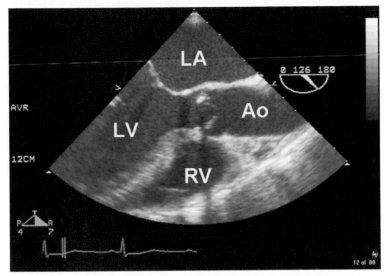

FIGURE 18-1 Transesophageal echo image of a stenotic aortic valve. Right ventricle (RV), left atrium (LA), left ventricle (LV), and aorta (Ao) are labeled. Courtesy of Mark S. Adams RDCS.

or severe. The **normal adult aortic valve area** (AVA) is 2.5 to 3.5 cm^2. Severe stenosis occurs when the AVA is less then 0.7 cm^2 or the mean systolic pressure gradient is more than 50 mm Hg.

C. Hemodynamic changes

  1. The **systemic arterial pressure wave** typically shows a slow upstroke. The anacrotic notch occurs low in the pressure wave, and the dicrotic notch is often absent.

  2. The **pulmonary artery occlusion pressure (PAOP)** is increased in AS because of the elevated left ventricular end-diastolic pressure. As the disease progresses, atrial hypertrophy ensues and the mitral valve annulus widens, resulting in a prominent v-wave of mitral regurgitation (MR).

D. Management

  1. **Hypotension** must be treated promptly. Ischemia resulting from aortic root pressure falling below the subendocardial pressure may initiate a downward spiral of further ischemia, dysrhythmias, and hemodynamic instability. Cardiopulmonary resuscitation efforts may prove ineffective because of thickened myocardium and small valvular area.

  2. **Dysrhythmias** can quickly result in unstable hemodynamics that may be refractory to pharmacologic treatment. The hypertrophic LV is highly dependent on atrial kick for adequate filling. Both **tachycardia and bradycardia** are poorly tolerated. Tachycardia may not allow enough time for proper diastolic filling. Bradycardia may overdistend the heart or inhibit adequate perfusion. Cardiac depressants (β-blockers, calcium channel blockers) and cardiac stimulants (atropine, dopamine) should be used with caution. **Nodal rhythms** are poorly tolerated. Atropine (0.4 mg) may convert a slow nodal rhythm into a normal sinus rhythm. Atrial pacing may be needed.

3. **Nitroglycerin,** if needed, should be administered cautiously because high venous pressure may be required to maintain stroke volume.

4. **Pulmonary artery catheters** (PACs) can help to guide fluid balance and monitor cardiac performance. Insertion of a PAC may precipitate dysrhythmias. A catheter with **pacing** capabilities can prove useful.

5. **Inotropic support** may be needed in severe AS. **Norepinephrine** can be helpful because of its combined inotropic and vasoconstrictive effects. Milrinone and dobutamine may be useful, but they decrease SVR and may decrease the aortic root pressure more than is desired. β-Agonists carry a risk of tachydysrhythmias.

E. **Postoperative care after aortic valve replacement or commissurotomy.** Although stroke volume increases and LV end-diastolic pressure decreases following aortic valve replacement or repair, the LV remains **hypertrophied** for months. Maintaining adequate coronary artery perfusion is essential, along with maintenance of sinus rhythm. After the hypertrophied myocardium has returned to a near-normal state, increased subendocardial pressures are less problematic.

F. **Hypertrophic obstructive cardiomyopathy (HOCM).** Unlike valvular AS, HOCM causes a dynamic obstruction to the forward flow of blood from the LV. The large muscle mass of the subaortic region causes obstruction of the LV outflow tract. The dynamic obstruction of the outflow tract is worsened by tachycardia, β-agonism, and by low filling volumes. Management includes maintenance of a slow heart rate to allow for longer diastolic filling, adequate intravascular volume repletion, and maintenance of adequate aortic root pressure (often with phenylephrine). Patients with HOCM are prone to lethal ventricular dysrhythmias.

II. **Aortic regurgitation (AR)** can be acute or chronic. Causes include rheumatic fever, syphilitic aortitis, bacterial endocarditis, aortic dissection, trauma (often blunt chest trauma), and congenital abnormalities.

A. **Pathophysiology**

1. The compensatory response to AR is increased sympathetic tone, resulting in tachycardia and increased inotropy. If this response is inadequate, CHF ensues. In acute AR, the LV has not had time to remodel through eccentric hypertrophy (an increase in the size of the ventricular cavity and the thickness of the myocardium). Both LV end-diastolic pressure and LV end-diastolic volume (LVEDP and LVEDV) increase acutely. In addition, a reduction in systemic arterial diastolic pressure can decrease coronary perfusion pressure and so result in ischemia.

2. In **chronic AR**, elevated LVEDV results in an eccentric myocardial hypertrophy. Although the LVEDV increases, there is little change in LVEDP because of compensatory changes in LV size and muscle mass. Thus, the heart may function normally for years. In general, function remains near normal if the regurgitant fraction remains less then 40%. Symptoms often result when the regurgitant fraction exceeds 60%. An LVEDP of greater then 20 mm Hg is a sign of poor compensation.

B. **Signs, symptoms, and diagnosis**

1. **Acute AR** often presents with CHF, angina, and tachycardia. **Chronic AR** may be asymptomatic for years. When symptoms (shortness of breath, palpitations, fatigue, or angina) develop, average survival without valve replacement is approximately 5 years.

2. **Physical findings** that are indicative of AR include the following:
   a. Widened arterial pulse pressure.
   b. Bounding peripheral pulses.

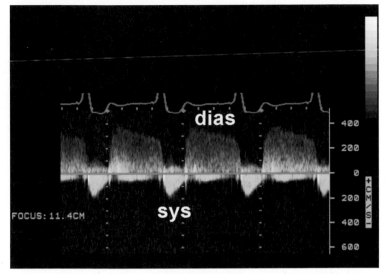

FIGURE 18-2 Doppler recording of diastolic (dias) flow reversal in aortic regurgitation. Blood velocity is shown as a function of time. Anterograde flows are depicted downward. The retrograde regurgitant jet (positive deflection) is of higher velocity than the forward systolic (sys) flow (negative deflection). Courtesy of Mark S. Adams, RDCS.

    c. Quincke's pulses (visible capillary pulsations with compression of the nail bed).

    d. Decrescendo diastolic murmur along the left sternal border.

    e. Austin–Flint murmur (an apical diastolic rumble caused by regurgitant flow impinging on the anterior mitral leaflet).

    f. Maximal cardiac impulse shifted downward and to the left.

  3. The **degree of AR** depends upon the hemodynamic state (i.e., afterload, heart rate, inotropy). The echocardiographic grading system distinguishes severe, moderate, mild, and trace categories, depending on the width and height of the regurgitant jet (**Fig. 18-2**). Jets of fluid passing through a narrow orifice exhibit a hydraulic constriction occurring just past the orifice. The width of this constriction, termed the **vena contracta** by Newton, is more than 6 mm in severe AR. In severe AR, Doppler examination shows holodiastolic flow reversal in the descending aorta.

C. Hemodynamic changes

  1. The systemic arterial pulse pressure often is widened, with a very rapid upstroke due to the large stroke volume.

  2. A rapid descent of the arterial pressure waveform results from the rapid flow of blood back into the LV.

  3. The PAOP may exhibit prominent *v*-waves because of LV volume overload and accompanying MR. The PAOP may underestimate the LVEDP because the aortic regurgitant jet causes premature closure of the mitral valve.

D. Management

  1. **Afterload reduction,** an **increased heart rate** (to decrease filling time and thus decrease LVEDV), and **inotropic support** are keys to acute management. Urgent surgical intervention may be necessary.

2. Echocardiography can be useful in guiding therapy. Echo imaging reveals dynamic changes in the regurgitant jet, inotropic state, and LV filling.

3. **Dobutamine** often is the inotrope of choice for patients with AR. It increases contractility, reduces peripheral resistance, and maintains a relatively rapid heart rate. Milrinone also provides inotropic support and afterload reduction, but with less increase in heart rate.

E. **Postoperative care after aortic valve repair or replacement for AR**

1. Because of persistent cardiomegaly in patients with longstanding AR, adequate ventricular filling remains essential for good cardiac function.

2. Inotropic support may be required postoperatively.

3. An intra-aortic balloon pump (IABP) is contraindicated in patients with AR prior to valve replacement. The IABP augments aortic diastolic pressure and therefore worsens the regurgitation. However, the device may provide support after valve replacement.

III. **Mitral stenosis (MS)**

A. **Pathophysiology. Rheumatic fever** results in scarring and calcification of the edges of the valve leaflets, with eventual fibrosis of the commissures. Patients with rheumatic heart disease can remain asymptomatic for years. When symptoms appear, there is a 20% chance of death within the first year. **Senile calcification** is another mechanism of MS and may begin with calcification of the valvular annulus.

B. **Signs, symptoms, and diagnosis**

1. **Symptoms** usually first present during exercise or other high-output states. Inactive patients may present upon the onset of atrial fibrillation or flutter caused by atrial distention.

2. Patients complain of dyspnea, palpitations, fatigue, chest pain, and paroxysmal nocturnal dyspnea. Some patients develop hoarseness due to the compression of the left recurrent laryngeal nerve by the dilated left pulmonary artery or left atrium. Patients can also present with hemoptysis because of high pulmonary venous pressures.

3. **Atrial fibrillation** may trigger CHF because of decreased diastolic filling time and increased left arterial pressure (LAP).

4. An **echocardiogram** confirms the diagnosis of MS (**Fig. 18-3**). The mitral valve area (MVA) is inversely proportional to the pressure half-time (PHT), where PHT is the time for the Doppler peak velocity across the valve to decline by 30%. MVA (cm^2) equals 220 divided by PHT (ms). A PHT longer than 220 ms indicates severe stenosis (MVA <1 cm^2).

5. **Physical findings** that are indicative of MS include the following:
   a. A loud S_1 heart sound on auscultation.
   b. A presystolic or mid-diastolic rumble.
   c. A prominent jugular a-wave.

C. The **degree of MS** can be assessed by echocardiography or angiography.

1. The area of the normal mitral valve is 4 to 6 cm^2.

2. Patients with **moderate MS** (1.5–2.5 cm^2) often show symptoms only with increased cardiac demand. Symptoms (dyspnea, fatigue) are related to increased LAP.

3. **Critical MS** is defined as a valve area of less than 1 cm^2. Patients with critical MS are often asymptomatic at rest but tolerate exercise poorly. Increased pulmonary vascular pressures can precipitate pulmonary edema.

D. **Hemodynamic changes**

1. The PAOP is increased and may not accurately reflect LVEDP.

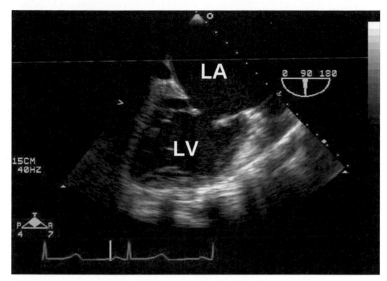

FIGURE 18-3 Transesophageal echo image of a stenotic mitral valve. Left atrium (LA) and left ventricle (LV) are labeled. Courtesy of Mark S. Adams, RDCS.

2. The PAOP waveform can exhibit a large *a*-wave if normal sinus rhythm is present. Because MS often is associated with some degree of MR, large *v*-waves may also be present.

3. **Pulmonary hypertension** is common. Because of the increased PA pressures and decreased PA compliance, there is increased risk of PA rupture with inflation of the balloon of a PAC. Severe pulmonary hypertension can lead to RV failure (cor pulmonale).

E. Management

1. **Adequate preload** is essential for good cardiac function. Flow across the mitral valve is dependent on elevated left atrial pressures. This requirement must be balanced with the propensity of patients with MS to develop CHF. No specific PAOP is universally correct. Parameters used to gauge optimum preload for a given patient include signs and symptoms of organ perfusion, oxygenation, and CHF.

2. A **slow heart rate** facilitates LV filling. Because blood flow across the MV occurs during diastole, a heart rate that is too fast does not allow enough time for proper filling. This consideration must be balanced with the fact that too slow a heart rate will reduce cardiac output. The goal is a heart rate that maintains adequate organ perfusion in the absence of CHF.

3. If AV pacing is required, a long PR interval (0.2 seconds) will allow more time for blood to flow across the mitral valve.

4. Patients with MS may need **inotropic support**. Digoxin is commonly used in these patients because it has both negative chronotropic and positive inotropic effects. If more aggressive inotropic support is needed, drugs without positive chronotropy (such as milrinone) may be useful.

5. **Supraventricular dysrhythmias** that are hemodynamically significant (i.e., cause a decrease in blood pressure) must be treated aggressively, usually with electrocardioversion. Many clinicians suggest starting

with high energy (i.e., 200 J monophasic or equivalent biphasic). Cardiopulmonary resuscitation is often ineffective in the setting of a stenotic mitral valve.

6. **Percutaneous balloon valvuloplasty** can greatly relieve stenosis without need for postoperative anticoagulation. The best candidates have no left atrial thrombus, mild or no MR, and low echocardiographic scores for leaflet immobility, valvular thickening, subvalvular thickening, and valvular calcification. MR is not improved, and there is a risk of severe MR after balloon valvuloplasty.

F. **Postoperative care after mitral valve replacement or commissurotomy**

1. **Preload augmentation** is often needed in the postoperative period. Stroke volume, PAOP, and TEE can guide proper fluid replacement.

2. **Afterload reduction** can improve hemodynamics postoperatively, although preoperatively it has little effect due to the fixed stenosis.

3. **Inotropic support** may be required following valve repair or replacement because of an underlying decrease in LV function caused by chronic underfilling of the ventricle.

4. **Chronic atrial fibrillation** is common in patients with long-standing MS. The use of amiodarone or overdrive pacing may be beneficial.

5. If there is a sudden decrease in blood pressure following MV repair or replacement, one should consider the very rare possibilities of atrioventricular disruption or (in the case of valve replacement) a valve that is caught in the closed position. Both processes are emergencies that often require surgery at the bedside.

IV. **Mitral regurgitation (MR)**

A. **Pathophysiology.** The etiology of MR can be rheumatic or nonrheumatic.

1. **Rheumatic MR** often occurs concomitantly with MS. Like MS, the asymptomatic period can last for years.

2. **Nonrheumatic MR** can be caused by papillary muscle dysfunction (often seen in patients with posterior septal or anterior septal ischemia or infarction), bacterial endocarditis, or ruptured cordae tendinea.

3. **Acute MR** occurs when there is a sudden backflow of blood across the mitral valve into the left atrium. This results in a sudden volume overload of the atrium, causing increased pulmonary vascular pressures and often CHF. The compensatory response of increased sympathetic output results in tachycardia and increased inotropy. The increased LV volume can lead to annular dilation of the MV and worsen the amount of regurgitation. **Myocardial ischemia** may occur because of increased myocardial oxygen demand (from increased sympathetic output) and increased LVEDP.

4. **Chronic MR** differs from acute MR in that there is time for the LV to compensate for the increased volume load. Adaptations include eccentric hypertrophy of the LV, which causes the heart to dilate and allows a relatively constant LVEDP despite a greatly increased LVEDV. The left atrium enlarges and may maintain a normal pressure. In the late stage of the compensatory process, the dilation of the LV may lead to dilation of the mitral annulus and thus increased MR. The LV ejection fraction often remains normal, but forward flow may decrease. When the regurgitant fraction exceeds 60%, the likelihood of CHF increases dramatically. A decreasing ejection fraction (<50%) indicates failing LV function. In the final stages of chronic MR, the increased pulmonary pressures can precipitate right ventricular (RV) failure (cor pulmonale).

B. Signs, symptoms, and diagnosis

1. **Acute MR** often presents as sudden dyspnea, fatigue, or acute CHF. Patients may suffer palpitations because of atrial fibrillation. Some develop chest pain. **Chronic MR** may remain asymptomatic for years, but the onset of symptoms usually indicates a rapid downward course. Patients may present with dyspnea, fatigue, CHF, or atrial fibrillation.

2. The **physical examination** can aid in the diagnosis of MR. Physical findings that are indicative of MR include the following:
   a. A hyperdynamic apex with or without an apical lift or thrill.
   b. A holosystolic murmur best heard at the apex (that may radiate to the left axilla).
   c. Rarely, a mid-systolic rumble.

3. The grade of MR depends on the hemodynamic state (i.e., afterload, heart rate, and inotropy). When evaluating MR with echocardiography, many physicians use the grading system of severe, moderate, mild, and trace, depending on the width and height of the regurgitant jet (**Fig. 18-4**).

4. **Echocardiography**. Two-dimensional echocardiography may visualize flail leaflet or ruptured papillary muscle. In severe MR, Doppler can reveal systolic flow reversal in pulmonary veins. The flow reversal may not be observed if the jet of MR is not directed toward the pulmonary vein under examination. A color jet reaching the posterior wall of the left atrium or comprising more than 40% of the LA indicates severe MR. The narrow portion of the base of the jet is the vena contracta. A

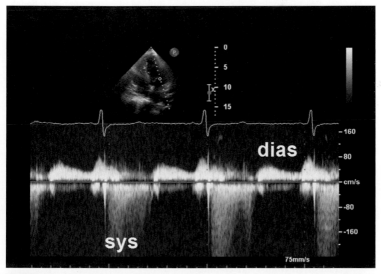

FIGURE 18-4 Doppler recording of systolic (sys) flow reversal in mitral regurgitation. Blood velocity is shown as a function of time. Anterograde flows are depicted upward (toward the probe at the apex of the sector seen as an inset). The retrograde regurgitant jet (negative deflection) is of higher velocity than the forward diastolic (dias) flow (positive deflection). Courtesy of Mark S. Adams, RDCS.

vena contracta width of more than 6.5 mm indicates severe regurgitation. The LA may be enlarged to a diameter of more than 5.5 cm.

C. Hemodynamic changes

1. The PAOP waveform is characterized by giant *v*-waves. The size of the *v*-wave depends on the compliance of the LA and pulmonary vasculature and may not reflect the amount of regurgitation.

2. The giant *v*-waves can make the PAOP difficult to differentiate from the PAP waveform. A helpful sign is that the peak of the pressure waveform shifts to the right, compared to the systemic arterial waveform, when the PA balloon is inflated and a PAOP tracing is obtained.

D. Management

1. The **heart rate** should be kept in a normal to high-normal range. A slow heart rate can cause volume overload of the LV.

2. **Maintenance of adequate LV preload** must be weighed against the possibility that excess LV volume may dilate the mitral annulus and make the severity of the regurgitation worse.

3. **Afterload reduction** is often necessary. A decreased peripheral resistance increases the forward ejection of the stroke volume. In patients with coronary artery disease and MR, nitroglycerin may be a reasonable intervention, achieving coronary vasodilation and some afterload reduction. Calcium channel blockers have also been used.

4. **Inotropic agents** can increase forward flow. Dobutamine and milrinone increase contractility and can beneficially decrease afterload.

5. **Pulmonary hypertension** develops in severe cases of MR and can lead to right heart failure. In fragile patients, it is prudent to avoid further increasing PA pressures (i.e., avoid hypoxia, hypercarbia, and acidosis). Prostaglandin E_1, prostacyclin, or inhaled nitric oxide may be beneficial in patients with right heart failure. Intra-aortic balloon counterpulsation may be life saving.

E. Postoperative care after mitral valve repair or replacement for MR

1. After repair of MR, the entire stroke volume is ejected into the aorta. The LV may fail because of the increased afterload.

2. **Inotropic support** is often needed. In severe cases, intra-aortic balloon counterpulsation may be necessary to augment forward flow and coronary perfusion.

3. **Atrial fibrillation** is not well tolerated postoperatively. Every attempt should be made to maintain normal sinus rhythm. Antidysrhythmics (such as amiodarone) or overdrive atrial pacing may be necessary.

4. **Transesophageal echocardiography** can be useful for determining valvular function and LV performance.

V. Tricuspid stenosis (TS)

A. Pathophysiology. The occurrence of TS is rare compared to the previously mentioned valvular lesions. Patients with TS often have associated MS. Tricuspid stenosis is most often caused by rheumatic fever, carcinoid syndrome, systemic lupus erythematosus, or endomyocardial fibroelastosis. There is generally a long asymptomatic period. As TS worsens, flow across the valve decreases, and right atrial size and pressures increase. Atrial tachydysrhythmias are common.

B. Signs, symptoms, and diagnosis

1. TS can cause peripheral edema, jugular venous distention, ascites, hepatomegaly, and hepatic dysfunction, all secondary to elevated right atrial pressures. As is the case with MS and AS, symptoms of fatigue with exercise may be the presenting complaint. In addition, patients

may first present with palpitations caused by supraventricular dysrhythmias.
2. Physical findings indicative of TS include the following:
    a. A holosystolic murmur that is best heard at the left sternal border.
       The murmur often becomes louder during inspiration.
    b. A right ventricular heave.
    c. Associated murmurs of other valvular abnormalities.
    d. Hepatic pulsations, ascites, and peripheral cyanosis in severe cases.
3. The normal area of the tricuspid valve is 7 to 9 cm^2. Tricuspid stenosis
   is considered significant when the valve area decreases to 1.5 cm^2. The
   normal tricuspid gradient is 1 mm Hg. A gradient as small as 3 mm Hg
   indicates a moderate stenosis, whereas a gradient of 5 mm Hg is
   severe.
C. **Hemodynamic changes**
   1. A large a-wave is evident on the central venous pressure (CVP) wave-
      form. This corresponds to the right atrium contracting against a high-
      resistance orifice.
   2. CVP may be increased because of systemic volume overload.
D. **Management**
   1. A **slow normal heart rate** is essential to allow sufficient diastolic filling
      of the RV.
   2. **Tachydysrhythmias** can decrease cardiac output and increase CVP.
   3. **Adequate preload** is essential for forward flow. However, care must be
      taken not to overfill the right atrium because this will stretch the right
      atrium and predispose to supraventricular tachydysrhythmias.
   4. Although reducing RV afterload and increasing contractility will not
      directly affect the degree of TS, these maneuvers may help to maintain
      cardiac output.
E. **Postoperative care after tricuspid valve replacement or repair for stenosis**
   1. The patient may have right-sided dysfunction because of the chroni-
      cally underfilled RV. Afterload reduction and inotropic support may be
      needed.
   2. Avoiding increased pulmonary artery pressures is essential.
      Prostacyclin, prostaglandin E_1, or inhaled nitric oxide may reduce PA
      pressure, thereby reducing RV afterload.
   3. **Tachydysrhythmias** should be avoided. Antidysrhythmics such as amio-
      darone may be necessary.
   4. Because of the prosthetic valve, the patients are often managed with-
      out a PA line. If a PAC is deemed necessary, then it must be placed sur-
      gically when a nontissue prosthesis is implanted. Alternatively, a sur-
      gically placed LA line may be used.

VI. **Tricuspid regurgitation (TR)**
   A. **Pathophysiology**
      1. TR usually accompanies other valvular lesions such as MS or AS.
         Rarely, isolated TR may be caused by endocarditis, chest trauma, or
         carcinoid syndrome.
      2. TR results in volume overload of the atrium and increased pressure
         within the systemic venous system. Isolated TR can be well tolerated.
         When TR is due to pulmonary hypertension from valvular abnormali-
         ties or LV dysfunction, the ability to compensate is poor.
   B. **Signs, symptoms, and diagnosis**
      1. The increased volume load in the RA can distend the atrium and cause
         atrial fibrillation.

2. **Physical findings** that are indicative of TR include the following:
   a. An S_3 gallop (accentuated by inspiration).
   b. A systolic murmur that increases during inspiration.
   c. An accentuated P_2 heart sound.
3. Doppler evidence of systolic flow reversal in hepatic veins is evidence of severe TR. Echocardiography may reveal an annulus diameter of more than 4 cm or a regurgitant jet covering more than 30% of the right atrial area.

C. **Hemodynamic changes**
   1. The **CVP** may be normal or increased in TR.
   2. The CVP waveform may exhibit giant **v-waves,** corresponding to the large regurgitant jet during right ventricular systole. The size of the *v*-wave depends in part on the compliance of the right atrium and does not simply correspond to the size of the regurgitant volume.

D. **Management**
   1. **A high heart rate** helps to minimize peripheral congestion and RV volume overload while increasing forward flow from the RV.
   2. **Atrial fibrillation** is common. Hemodynamic parameters nearly always improve if a sinus rhythm can be achieved.
   3. **Adequate preload** is essential for forward flow. Decreased RV filling can severely limit cardiac output.
   4. **Minimizing pulmonary vascular resistance** (i.e., avoiding hypoxemia, hypertension, and acidosis) will aid forward flow.
   5. **Inotropic support** of the failing RV can be useful in TR. Dobutamine and milrinone are examples of drugs that provide increased inotropy but do not greatly increase PA pressures. Agents that decrease PA pressures (e.g., prostaglandin E_1, prostacyclin, and inhaled nitric oxide) may be helpful when used in conjunction with inotropic medications.

E. **Postoperative care after tricuspid valve replacement or repair of TR**
   1. Because the TR is no longer present to provide a "pop off" and limit RV pressure, the pressure load of the RV can be acutely increased after tricuspid valve repair. RV dysfunction may occur, and inotropic support may be necessary.

VII. Pulmonic valve disease

A. Congenital pulmonic stenosis presents as right heart failure. Acquired pulmonic stenosis is rare.

B. **Pulmonic regurgitation** is well tolerated as long as right ventricular function is adequate. Acquired pulmonic regurgitation can result from infective endocarditis or rheumatic heart disease. Operative intervention in pulmonic regurgitation due to endocarditis generally consists in excision of the affected valve without replacement by a prosthetic device.

VIII. Endocarditis.
Bacteremia can seed both native and prosthetic valves. Bacterial endocarditis induces metaplasia of the endothelial cells, which then lose contact with each other. Collagen fibers are removed, resulting in large cavities. Localized hyperplasia results in the development of valvular vegetations that can often be visualized by echocardiography. The vegetations may result in regurgitant valvular pathology. Endocarditis can lead to papillary muscle rupture, the result of which is abrupt severe mitral valve incompetence. The microbiology, manifestations, complications, diagnosis, and management of infective endocarditis are reviewed in detail in **Chapter 29.**

IX. Antibiotic prophylaxis against bacterial endocarditis.
Transient bacteremia following invasive procedures, surgery, and dental procedures can lead to valvular

endocarditis. Blood-borne bacteria lodge on damaged or abnormal tissues. Because of a lack of data demonstrating efficacy for prophylaxis, recent recommendations have grown more conservative since 2005. In 2007, the American Heart Association published their new guidelines, recommending prophylaxis only in high-risk patients (previous infective endocarditis, prosthetic valve, unrepaired or incompletely repaired cyanotic congenital heart disease, congenital heart disease repaired with prosthetic material less than 6 months prior, and valve disease in cardiac transplant patients) who are undergoing dental procedures involving manipulation of gingival tissues, the periapical region of teeth, perforation of the oral mucosa, invasive procedures of the respiratory tract needing incision, or biopsy of the respiratory mucosa. Prophylaxis is not recommended for either an increased lifetime risk of acquisition of infective endocarditis, or in patients who undergo a genitourinary or gastrointestinal tract procedure. Transesophageal echo studies are not associated with bacteremia. Depending on allergy and available route of administration, antibiotic regimens for applicable dental procedures include ampicillin, amoxicillin, ceftriaxone, cephalexin, clindamycin, azithromycin, or clarithromycin.

Selected References

Abaci A, Oguzhan A, Unal S, et al. Application of the vena contracta method for the calculation of the mitral valve area in mitral stenosis. *Cardiology* 2002;98:50–59.

Buffington CW, Nystrom EUM. Neither the accuracy nor the precision of thermal dilution cardiac output measurements is altered by acute tricuspid regurgitation in pigs. *Anesth Analg* 2004;98:884–890.

Khot UN, Novaro GM, Popovic GC, et al. Nitroprusside in critically ill patients with left ventricular dysfunction and aortic stenosis. *N Engl J Med* 2003;348:1756–1763.

Krishnagopalan S, Kumar A, Parrillo JE, et al. Myocardial dysfunction in the patient with sepsis. *Curr Opin Crit Care* 2002;8:376–388.

Levine RA, Vlahakes GJ, Lefebvre X, et al. Papillary muscle displacement causes systolic anterior motion of the mitral valve. Experimental validation and insights into the mechanism of subaortic obstruction. *Circulation* 1995;91:1189–1195.

Oh JK, Seward JB, Tajik AJ. *The echo manual.* 2nd ed. Philadelphia: Lippincott Williams & Wilkins, 1999.

Palacios IF, Sanchez PL, Harrell LC, et al. Which patients benefit from percutaneous mitral balloon valvuloplasty? Prevalvuloplasty and postvalvuloplasty variables that predict long-term outcome. *Circulation* 2002;105:1465–1471.

Quere JP, Tribouilloy C, Enriquez-Sarano M. Vena contracta width measurement: theoretic basis and usefulness in the assessment of valvular regurgitation severity. *Curr Cardiol Rep* 2003;5:110–115.

Wison W et al. Prevention of infective endocarditis: guidelines from the American Heart Association: a guideline from the American Heart Association Rheumatic Fever, Endocarditis, and Kawasaki Disease Committee, Council on Cardiovascular Disease in the Young, and the Council on clinical Cardiology, Council on Cardiovascular Surgery and Anesthesia, and the Quality of Care and Outcomes Research Interdisciplinary Working Group. *Circulation* 2007;116(15):1736–1754.

Yoerger DM, Weyman AE. Hypertrophic obstructive cardiomyopathy: mechanism of obstruction and response to therapy. *Rev Cardiovasc Med* 2003;4:199–215.

19

Cardiac Dysrhythmias

Cosmin Gauran and Jagmeet Singh

I. **Epidemiology**
   A. Dysrhythmias of both supraventricular and ventricular origin are common in critically ill patients. Of the two, supraventricular dysrhythmias occur more frequently.
   B. Of all perioperative dysrhythmias, postoperative **atrial fibrillation (AF)** is the most intensely studied, given its high incidence (10%–65%) and associated morbidity.

II. **Clinical significance.** Perioperative dysrhythmias are associated with increased mortality, cardiac and noncardiac morbidity (primarily neurologic and pulmonary), and utilization of resources in terms of increased ICU days, ICU readmissions, and hospital length of stay.

III. **Classification.** Types of dysrhythmia can be essentially divided into **stable** and **unstable**.
   A. **Unstable dysrhythmias** are defined by the presence of hemodynamic instability (hypotension, myocardial ischemia, congestive failure, etc) or cerebral hypoperfusion (syncope, altered mental status) in conjunction with dysrhythmia.
   B. **Stable dysrhythmias** can be subclassified by considering the following factors:
      1. Rate (bradydysrhythmias vs. tachydysrhythmias).
      2. Presence or absence of P waves.
      3. Relationship of P waves to the QRS complex.
      4. Width of the QRS complex (narrow vs. wide).
      5. Regularity of the QRS complex (regular vs. irregular).

IV. **Bradydysrhythmias**
   A. **Classification**
      1. **Sinus node dysfunction**
         a. Describes a host of bradycardic dysrhythmias involving the sinus node, including sinus bradycardia, sinus pauses, and the tachycardia–bradycardia syndrome.
         b. Risk factors include advanced age and structural heart disease.
         c. Frequently associated with a malignant course involving progressive nodal dysfunction.
         d. One of the most common causes of permanent pacemaker placement in the United States.
      2. **Atrioventricular (AV)** nodal dysfunction
         a. **First-degree AV block**
            (1) Characterized by a PR interval exceeding 200 ms (normal 120–200 ms).
            (2) Typically a benign condition, unless associated with another form of conduction disease or problems with AV synchrony.

b. **Second-degree AV block**
   (1) **Mobitz type 1 (Wenckebach)**
      i. Characterized by a progressive widening of the PR interval with a subsequently nonconducted P wave (i.e., nonconducted atrial contraction).
      ii. Disease is typically high in the AV node.
   (2) **Mobitz type 2**
      i. Characterized by a fixed, normal PR interval with episodic nonconducted P waves.
      ii. Disease is typically lower in the AV node or bundle of His.
   (3) Differentiation between Mobitz types 1 and 2 cannot be made if AV block is 2:1. This is important because the risk of proceeding to a complete heart block is higher with a Mobitz type 2 block.
c. **Third-degree AV block** (complete heart block)
   (1) No conductance of P waves across the AV node and **complete AV dissociation.**
   (2) Can be associated with a junctional or ventricular escape.
   (3) Presence of a junctional escape (typical rate 40–50 beats per minute [bpm]) suggests disease high up in the AV node. Presence of a ventricular escape (typical rate 30–40 bpm) suggests disease is lower down in the conduction pathway.
d. **Fascicular blocks**
   (1) The conduction system is comprised of the **sinoatrial (SA) node,** the AV node, the bundle of His, and the left and right bundle branches. The left bundle branch divides into the anterior and posterior fascicles.
   (2) A bifascicular block is defined as a **right bundle-branch block (RBBB)** in conjunction with either a left anterior or a left posterior hemiblock.
   (3) A trifascicular block is defined as a bifascicular block in conjunction with a first-degree AV block.
B. **Etiopathogenesis** of bradydysrhythmias can be divided into intrinsic and extrinsic causes.
   1. **Common intrinsic causes** seen in the critically ill patient include degenerative sinus node dysfunction and ischemia/infarction.
      a. The SA node and AV node are predominantly supplied by the right coronary circulation.
      b. The His-Purkinje system is predominantly supplied by the left coronary circulation.
      c. Therefore, right coronary disease is more commonly associated with SA or AV nodal aberrancies, whereas left coronary disease is more commonly associated with bundle-branch blocks.
   2. **Common extrinsic causes** seen in critically ill patients include neurocardiogenic causes (e.g., vagal response to intubation or tracheal suctioning, imbalance of sympathetic/parasympathetic tone postoperatively or related to sepsis, or the systemic inflammatory response), medications, hypothermia, electrolyte imbalances, infection (endocarditis/myocarditis), and trauma (e.g., iatrogenic due to valvular surgery or central venous catheter placement). The incidence of causing an RBBB while placing a pulmonary artery catheter has been estimated at 3%. Therefore, it is recommended that backup ventricular pacing be available when placing a pulmonary artery catheter in a patient with a pre-existing **left bundle-branch block (LBBB).**

C. **Treatment options** include
   1. Correction of an underlying disorder.
   2. Observation, if the patient is "stable."
   3. Temporary or permanent pacing.
      a. **Pacing modalities** include epicardial, transvenous (directly or through a pulmonary artery catheter), transesophageal, and transcutaneous. Transvenous approaches are preferred and most practical.
      b. Transesophageal pacing typically enables only atrial capture. Therefore, this modality should not be used in patients with AV conduction aberrancies.
      c. Transcutaneous pacing enables ventricular capture. Loss of AV synchrony can be associated with hypotension. This modality is also associated with significant discomfort in an awake patient.
      d. Thresholds can be affected by multiple factors in the critically ill including myocardial ischemia or infarction, hypothermia, electrolyte imbalances, medications, and defibrillation/cardioversion events.
      e. **Dual chamber (physiologic AV) pacing** is preferable in patients who are hemodynamically tenuous and may have depressed ventricular function. The most recent evidence suggests that physiologic pacing is superior by lowering risk of progression to AF, reducing hospital admissions for congestive failure, and improving quality-of-life scores.

V. **Tachydysrhythmias**
   A. **Etiopathogenesis** is related to a complex interaction between pre-existing pathology (ischemia, scar, etc), triggering factors (premature beats, high sympathetic tone, etc), and aggravating factors (atrial stretch, trauma, etc).
   B. **Classification**
      1. **Narrow QRS complex, regular rhythm**
         a. Sinus tachycardia.
         b. Sinus nodal reentry
            (1) P-wave morphology is similar to sinus origin with heart rates usually not greater than 160 bpm.
            (2) Can be differentiated from sinus tachycardia by abrupt onset and termination, suggestive of a reentrant circuit. It is frequently set off by atrial extra stimuli.
            (3) Responsive to calcium channel blockers.
         c. Ectopic atrial tachycardia (AT)
            (1) Consequence of an ectopic atrial focus with enhanced automaticity that overdrives the sinus node. The atrial rate is regular and typically is between 100 and 200 bpm. The ventricular rate may vary depending on the presence of a concomitant AV nodal block.
            (2) P-wave morphology is dependent on the origin of the ectopic focus. The PR interval is dependent on the rate, and the QRS morphology is dictated by normal conduction or aberrancy.
            (3) Common causes of atrial tachycardia include increased sympathetic tone, pulmonary disease, coronary artery disease, hypoxia, and electrolyte imbalances. One of the most common causes of paroxysmal atrial tachycardia with block is **digoxin toxicity.**
            (4) **Treatment is** directed at the etiology. **Heart rate controlling agents** such as **β-blockers** and **calcium channel antagonists** may be used to slow the ventricular rate. **Digoxin** is typically less efficacious in

settings associated with high sympathetic tone as frequently seen in the critically ill. Alternate agents such as **procainamide, sotalol,** and **amiodarone** may be used for resistant tachycardias. Catheter ablation can be employed in situations where medical treatment is ineffective, contraindicated, or refused. It is important to distinguish sinus tachycardia from ectopic atrial tachycardia. The primary etiology needs addressing in sinus tachycardia rather than an antiarrhythmic strategy, while the latter is more useful in patients with an ectopic atrial arrhythmia.

d. Atrial flutter
   (1) The most common form is classified as type I atrial flutter and involves a reentrant loop within the right atrium, moving in a counterclockwise direction.
   (2) It is classically associated with an atrial rate of 300 bpm with 2:1 AV block, producing a ventricular rate of 150 bpm. A saw-toothed pattern is characteristic of typical atrial flutter (see **Fig. 19-1**).
   (3) Therapy is similar to that for AF **(Section V.B.b)**. Direct current (DC) cardioversion should be attempted in the setting of clinical instability.
      i. A clear role for anticoagulation with atrial flutter is not established. However, given the frequent coexistence of AF, anticoagulation should be considered.
      ii. In certain circumstances (e.g., in patients with implanted pacemakers), overdrive pace termination may be attempted. Radiofrequency catheter ablation can also be attempted as a definitive cure for both typical and atypical forms of atrial flutter.

e. AV nodal reentrant tachycardia (AVNRT)
   (1) Typical
      i. Associated with conduction down a slow anterograde limb and up the fast retrograde limb (**Fig. 19-2**).
      ii. Resulting atrial and ventricular activation times are such that P waves are typically buried within the QRS complex (**Fig. 19-3**). Often the retrograde P waves can produce a "pseudo R-wave" pattern in lead V_1.
   (2) Atypical
      i. Associated with conduction down the fast anterograde limb and up the slow retrograde limb.
      ii. Resulting atrial and ventricular activation times are such that P waves typically precede each QRS complex. However, because the atria are depolarized from the AV node upward (as opposed to the normal SA node downward), atypical AVNRT is associated with inverted P waves in the inferior leads.

f. Orthodromic AV reentrant rhythm (AVRT)
   (1) Associated with a reentrant loop involving the AV node and an accessory pathway in the ventricular wall (**Fig. 19-2**).
   (2) Results in a narrow complex rhythm because the anterograde limb of the reentrant loop involves the AV node and His-Purkinje system (as opposed to an *antidromic* AVRT described in **Section V.B.3.b**).
   (3) Abrupt onset is usually suggestive of AVNRT or AVRT.
   (4) The Valsalva maneuver or carotid massage can be used to diagnose (and/or treat) AV nodal-dependent tachycardias.

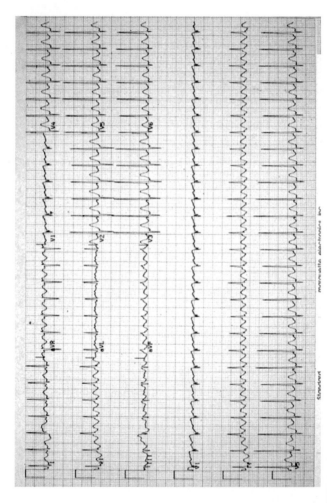

FIGURE 19-1 Twelve-lead electrocardiogram of typical atrial flutter. Saw-toothed P waves, with a ventricular rate of 150 beats per minute.

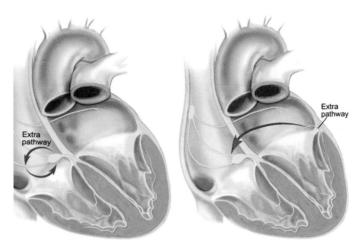

FIGURE 19-2 Schematic representation of atrioventricular nodal reentrant tachycardia (AVNRT, left panel) and atrioventricular reentrant tachycardia (AVRT, right panel). The left panel shows the presence of an accessory pathway along the left lateral wall. From Wang PJ, Estes M. Supraventricular tachycardia. *Circulation* 2002;106:e206–e208, with permission.

g. **Wolff-Parkinson-White (WPW)** syndrome
   (1) Evidence of preexcitation (shortened PR interval and delta wave) on the electrocardiogram (ECG) may indicate the presence of an accessory pathway (**Fig. 19-4**).
   (2) AV nodal blockade with WPW may facilitate rapid conduction down the accessory pathway and precipitate ventricular tachycardia/fibrillation. Therefore, cardioversion/defibrillation capability should be available whenever a nodal agent is used in the treatment of a tachycardia with a possible preexcitation syndrome.

h. **AV junctional tachycardia**
   (1) Occurs from increased automaticity of the AV node, and is characterized by heart rates of 60 to 120 bpm.
   (2) Inciting factors include digoxin toxicity, increased catecholamine levels, myocarditis, electrolyte imbalances, and trauma (postcardiac surgery).
   (3) The characteristic ECG shows retrograde P waves in the inferior leads. The QRS complex, although typically narrow, may occasionally be wide from concomitant aberrancy.
   (4) In certain circumstances, as with the isorhythmic AV dissociation seen with inhalation anesthesia, a junctional tachycardia may coexist with AV dissociation from competitive activation of both SA and AV nodes. Here the relationship between the P waves and the QRS complex may vary.
   (5) Typically, AV junctional tachycardias are benign and self-limited. Therapy involves treatment of triggering factors and/or withdrawal of offending agents. **Atrial overdrive** pacing may suppress a junctional focus, and allow the sinus node to regain

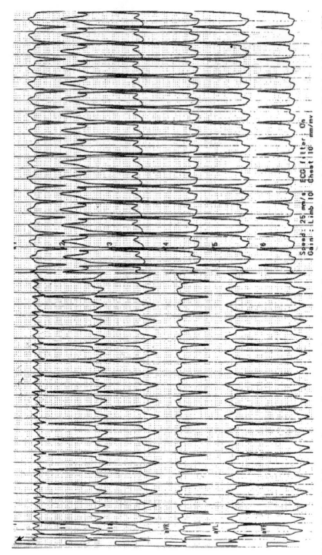

FIGURE 19-3 Twelve-lead electrocardiogram of narrow complex tachycardia. P waves are not well appreciated and are most likely buried in the QRS complex.

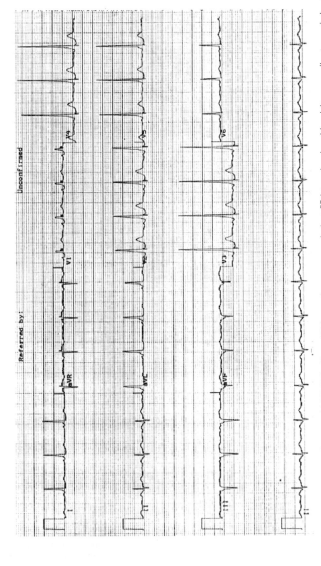

FIGURE 19-4 Twelve-lead electrocardiogram with Wolff-Parkinson-White syndrome pattern. A short PR interval and positive delta waves (best seen in leads V2–V5) are appreciated. Negative delta waves are seen in leads 3 and aVF.

control of conduction and normalize AV synchrony. **Phenytoin, lidocaine,** and β-**adrenergic antagonists** may also be of benefit.

    i. Incidence. Among supraventricular tachycardias in the general population, the incidence of AVNRT (50%–60%) is higher than that of AVRT (30%–40%) and atrial tachycardia (10%). Atrial tachycardia is relatively more common in the critically ill.

2. Narrow QRS complex, irregular rhythm

  a. Multifocal atrial tachycardia (MAT)

    (1) Narrow complex, irregular tachycardia exhibiting at least three separate P waveforms and associated PR intervals.

    (2) A similar rhythm with heart rate less than 100 bpm is termed a **wandering atrial pacemaker.**

    (3) Commonly seen in patients with chronic obstructive pulmonary disease or congestive failure.

    (4) Treatment is similar to that for ectopic atrial tachycardia **(Section V.B.1.c).**

  b. AF

    (1) The reported incidence of postoperative AF varies between 10% and 65%, with a recent large meta-analysis describing an incidence of 26.5%.

    (2) Risk factors include male sex, old age, history of prior AF, structural heart disease, hypertension, chronic obstructive lung disease, obesity, type of surgery (i.e., surgery involving cardiac valves, coronary bypass surgery, thoracic surgery, etc), withdrawal of medications (β-blockers, angiotensin-converting enzyme inhibitors, nonsteroidal anti-inflammatory agents), and prolonged mechanical ventilation.

    (3) Postoperative AF (see also **Chapter 40**) can result from alteration in the atrial myocyte conduction velocity or refractory period due to atrial trauma, stretch, or ischemia. Hypoxia, electrolyte imbalances, or increased sympathetic nervous system activity may trigger AF.

    (4) Recent evidence also supports the activation of foci within the distal pulmonary veins or, less commonly, in the right atrium as playing a pivotal role in the genesis of AF.

    (5) Regardless, the final common pathway in the pathogenesis of AF is the formation of multicircuit reentrant loops within the atria.

    (6) Significant (50%–75%) reductions in the rate of postoperative AF have been demonstrated by using β-blockers, sotalol, and oral or parenteral amiodarone during the perioperative period.

    (7) Classification

      i. Lone AF is AF without structural heart disease or hypertension. In patients age less than 60 years, lone AF is associated with a benign prognosis.

      ii. Recurrent or paroxysmal AF.

      iii. Persistent AF is characterized as AF persisting for more than 1 week.

    (8) More than 50% of AF episodes will spontaneously convert to sinus rhythm within 24 hours. After 24 hours, the incidence of spontaneous conversion to sinus rhythm declines precipitously. The rate of spontaneous conversion of persistent AF is negligible.

(9) Treatment options include electrical or pharmacologic therapy.
 i. Electrical
   (a) Synchronized cardioversion is indicated if a patient is unstable.
   (b) Cardioversion can begin at 50 J and escalate as needed (150 J with current biphasic devices or 360 J with the older, monophasic devices). The lowest possible energy is preferred to minimize myocardial injury.
   (c) Risk factors for poor response to cardioversion include presence of high sympathetic tone, critical illness, a large left atrium, and history of chronic dysrhythmia.
 ii. Pharmacologic therapy specific to AF can be divided into three components.
   (a) Anticoagulation.
   (b) Heart rate control.
   (c) Rhythm control.
 iii. Cardioversion without anticoagulation for rhythm control can be performed in a stable patient if the duration of AF is less than 48 hours.
 iv. Cardioversion without anticoagulation for AF exceeding 48 hours is associated with an increased risk of thromboembolic complications.
 v. If elective cardioversion is planned in a patient with AF of unknown or greater than 48-hour duration, evidence supports either
   (a) Ruling out the presence of atrial thromboses by transesophageal echocardiography, systemic heparin therapy with target **activated partial thromboplastin time (aPTT)** 1.5 to 2.5 times control, and postcardioversion warfarin therapy with target **international normalized ratio (INR)** 2 to 3 for 3 to 4 weeks.
   (b) Precardioversion warfarin therapy with target INR 2 to 3 for 3 to 4 weeks followed by postcardioversion warfarin therapy with similar INR target for 3 to 4 weeks.
 vi. Controversy exists regarding the relative benefit or rhythm control over heart rate control in specific populations.
   (a) Rate control appears to *not be inferior* to rhythm control in elderly patients with recurrent or persistent AF. Recent controlled trials suggest that rate control may be superior to rhythm control in elderly patients with recurrent or paroxysmal AF. New-onset AF in the critical care setting is often secondary to a trigger, and the approach to treatment should be individualized. The need for rate or rhythm control in this situation is often decided based on the underlying clinical scenario and cardiac substrate. For example, rhythm control may be a preferred option if there is a contraindication for anticoagulation and/or the patient is hypotensive and thereby intolerant to nodal agents.
 vii. Current evidence indicates that **cerebral thromboembolic complications** occur in patients with persistent or recurrent AF in the presence of inadequate (INR <2) or discontinued anticoagulation. Most of the embolic strokes originate in the left atrial appendage. Currently there are clinical trials

involving devices that obstruct the left appendage and if proven useful could circumvent the need for anticoagulation in patients with contraindications.

viii. Heart rate control can be attempted using nodal agents that decrease AV conduction. Commonly used agents include **β-blockers, calcium channel blockers,** and **digoxin** (**Table 19-1**).

ix. Acute pharmacologic conversion:

    (a) Timing of chemical conversion with respect to thromboembolic risk is similar to that with electrical cardioversion.

    (b) Pharmacologic agents from most classes of antiarrhythmics can be used for acute conversion where electrical conversion is not warranted. With most antiarrhythmics, patients should be closely monitored for QT-interval prolongation and drug-induced arrhythmia such as torsades de pointes. Most antiarrhythmic agents also have a negative inotropic effect, and, thus, monitoring for hypotension and heart failure is warranted.

x. Drugs commonly used include the following:

    (a) **Amiodarone.** Intravenous (IV) loading dose of 150 mg over 10 minutes, followed by a 1 mg/min infusion for 6 hours and then 0.5 mg/min for another 18 hours. A repeat load of 150 mg can be considered for recurrent dysrhythmias. **Droneradone,** a new drug with significantly fewer side effects than amiodarone has recently been shown to be a useful oral agent in the treatment of AF.

    (b) **Procainamide.** Dose 15 mg/kg IV at a rate less than 50 mg/min. Alternatively, 500 to 750 mg enterally, followed by a four-time daily regimen.

    (c) **Ibutilide.** Dose 1 mg IV over 10 minutes, repeated once if necessary. Pretreatment with magnesium sulfate is recommended.

TABLE 19-1	Common Agents Used for Rate Control in Atrial Fibrillation

Agent	Class	Dose
Metoprolol	β-blocker	5 mg IV over 2 min; may repeat as necessary
Propranolol	β-blocker	1 mg IV over 2 min; may repeat as necessary
Verapamil	Calcium channel blocker	5–10 mg over 2 min; may repeat in 30 min
Diltiazem	Calcium channel blocker	Bolus: 0.25 mg/kg (or 20 mg) IV over 2 min; may repeat after 15 min, with 0.35 mg/kg (25 mg) Continuous infusion: 5–10 mg/h; increase in 5 mg/h increments up to 15 mg/h maintained for up to 24 h
Digoxin	NaK-ATPase pump inhibitor	0.5 mg IV, then may give 0.25 mg every 6 h for two doses to a maximum of 1 mg as initial load

(d) **Flecainide.** Loading dose of 300 mg enterally, followed by a twice-daily regimen of 50 to 150 mg. Contraindicated in patients with coronary disease.

(e) **Propafenone:** Loading dose of 600 mg enterally, followed by a thrice-daily regimen of 150 to 300 mg.

(f) **Sotalol:** Enteral dose of 80 to 240 mg twice daily.

(g) **Dofetilide:** Enteral dose of 125 to 500 μg twice daily depending on QT-interval duration and renal function.

(h) **Vernakalant hydrochloride:** This is a new intravenous agent that may soon become available for the acute conversion of AF. It is an atrial selective agent with a low risk for ventricular arrhythmias.

(i) **Drug combinations:** Although combining drugs (e.g., propafenone and ibutilide) may increase the likelihood for pharmacological conversion, there is an increased risk for ventricular proarrhythmia, providing no added benefit over electrical cardioversion.

xi. Long-term treatment

(a) Rate control may be attempted using calcium channel blockers, β-blockers, or digoxin and needs to be combined with long-term anticoagulation.

(b) Rhythm control may be attempted using one of the agents discussed previously.

3. Wide complex, regular rhythm

a. **Ventricular tachycardia (VT)**

(1) VT is defined as three or more consecutive complexes of ventricular origin with a rate greater than 110 bpm.

(2) VT may be nonsustained (< 30- seconds' duration) or sustained (> 30- seconds' duration). Morphologically, VT is classified as monomorphic when the QRS morphology is uniform and polymorphic when the QRS morphology is variable. In general, polymorphic VT is more ominous than monomorphic VT. In the structurally normal heart, monomorphic VT, originating from the right or left ventricular outflow tract (**Fig. 19-5**), is usually well tolerated, and often may be treated conservatively.

(3) Hemodynamic consequences are related to the underlying cardiac function, comorbidities, the chamber of origin, and rate of the VT.

(4) Risk factors include coronary artery disease with previous scar, acute ischemia, nonischemic cardiomyopathy, myocarditis, drug-induced proarrhythmias, infiltrative disorders, electrolyte abnormalities, and myocardial toxins.

(5) **Treatment**

i. Unstable VT should be immediately treated with synchronized DC cardioversion (**Chapter 34**).

ii. Stable forms can be treated pharmacologically.

(a) The choice of the antiarrhythmic agent should be determined by the underlying left ventricular function.

(b) Patients with preserved function may be treated with lidocaine, procainamide, or amiodarone (doses as in **Section V.B.2.c**). **Lidocaine** may be initially administered as a bolus of 50 to 100 mg followed by a maintenance drip at 1 to 4 mg/min.

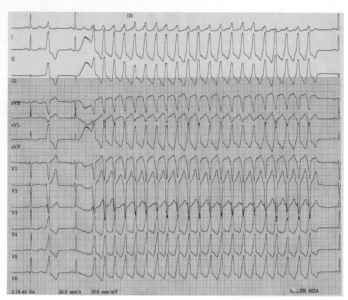

FIGURE 19-5 Twelve-lead electrocardiogram showing a monomorphic ventricular tachycardia originating from the right ventricular outflow tract. Classic features are a left bundle-branch–like morphology, evidence of atrioventricular dissociation, and inferior axis in the inferior leads (2, 3, and aVF).

    (c) Patients with compromised ventricular function may be treated with lidocaine and **amiodarone**. Alternately, urgent cardioversion can be attempted.

    (d) In some patients with recurrent VT (MMVT, see **Fig. 19-4**), autonomic blockade using incremental doses of β-blockers can be attempted. Intravenous esmolol is often times a useful agent in the ICU setting, since it enables careful titration. Refractory cases may require a more definitive approach such as catheter ablation (**Table 19-2**).

   iii. Long-term strategies and selection of antiarrhythmic agents depend on the cardiac substrate (ischemic vs. nonischemic), precipitating factors, renal function, exercise testing, cardiac function, and ambulatory ECG monitoring.

b. Antidromic AV reentrant tachycardia (AVRT)

   (1) Involves a reentrant pathway with an anterograde limb involving a ventricular accessory pathway and a retrograde limb involving the His-Purkinje system (contrast with an orthodromic AVRT described in **Section V.B.1.f**).

   (2) Typically occurs with an underlying preexcitation syndrome such as WPW.

   (3) Caution must be exercised in the use of AV nodal agents to treat AF in patients with preexcitation with AV nodal agents. AV nodal blockade may paradoxically increase ventricular rate by promoting conduction down the accessory pathway.

Arrhythmia	Success (%)
WPW or AVRT	90+
Atrioventicular node reentry	95+
Atrial fibrillation	
Atrioventricular node ablation	95+
Pulmonary vein isolation	75
Typical atrial flutter	90
Atrial tachycardia	80
Ventricular tachycardia	
Normal heart	95
Structural heart disease	70

WPW, Wolff-Parkinson-White syndrome; AVRT, atrioventricular reentrant tachycardia.

c. Accelerated idioventricular rhythm (AIVR)

(1) AIVR is an abnormal automatic rhythm originating from the terminal His-Purkinje system.

(2) Risk factors include acute ischemia, digitalis toxicity, and myocarditis.

(3) There is a monomorphic, wide-complex rhythm with a heart rate between 60 and 110 bpm on ECG. Retrograde P waves with AV dissociation and sinus capture beats can be seen.

(4) Typically a benign, self-limited rhythm except when patients are dependent on AV synchrony for adequate cardiac output. In symptomatic patients, therapy (atrial overdrive pacing, isoproterenol or atropine) is directed at increasing the sinus nodal rate to overdrive and suppress the ectopic ventricular focus.

d. SVT with aberrancy

(1) A pre-existing bundle-branch block or rate-dependent aberrancy can cause confusion regarding whether a wide-complex tachycardia is supraventricular or ventricular in origin.

(2) The presence of VT is favored by
   i. History of structural heart disease.
   ii. Old ECG without evidence of conduction disease.
   iii. Evidence of AV dissociation: canon *a*-waves on a central venous pressure tracing, fusion beats or capture beats on ECG, evidence of organized yet dissociated atrial activity on an esophageal ECG.
   iv. Other electrocardiographic evidence of ventricular tachycardia includes the following:
      (a) Positive concordance of the QRS complex across the precordial leads.
      (b) LBBB with right-axis deviation, QRS axis less than -90 or more than 180 degrees.
      (c) QRS duration greater than 140 ms with an RBBB or QRS duration greater than 160 ms with an LBBB.

(3) In the critically ill patient, when in doubt, it is typically more prudent to treat a wide-complex tachycardia as if it were ventricular in origin.

4. Wide-complex, irregular rhythm
   a. **Ventricular fibrillation (VF,** see also **Chapter 34)**
      (1) INITIATE BLS!
      (2) Pharmacologic treatment
         i. **Epinephrine** 1 mg boluses remain the mainstay of pharmacologic therapy. Current evidence does not support the use of high-dose epinephrine therapy.
         ii. **vasopressin** 40 U IV can be used as a single dose either as a first line of therapy or following the administration of epinephrine.
         iii. Data from out-of-hospital arrest trials support a single bolus dose of **amiodarone** 300 mg IV.
         iv. Current evidence and recommendations do not support routine use of lidocaine.
      (3) Electrical treatment
         i. **Defibrillation:** Single 150 J biphasic current defibrillation every 5 BLS cycles (or alternatively 300, 360, 360 J defibrillations series with the older devices)
         ii. **Automated implantable cardiac defibrillators (AICD)**
            (a) Current evidence supports use of AICDs for both primary and secondary prevention of sudden death in patients with ischemic cardiomyopathy (left ventricular ejection fraction <35%–40%).
            (b) Patients with hypertrophic obstructive cardiomyopathy at risk for sudden death may benefit from placement of AICDs.
            (c) Recent evidence supports prophylactic use of AICD with nonischemic dilated cardiomyopathy and heart failure.
   b. *Torsades de pointes* **(TDP)**
      (1) Classically associated with a prolonged QT interval (see **Fig. 7-4**)
         i. Although an absolute threshold for TDP is not defined, almost all cases of TDP are reported with a **corrected QT value exceeding 500 ms.**
         ii. QT prolongation can be produced by a number of medications (**Table 19-3**), electrolyte imbalances (hypomagnesemia, hypokalemia, hypocalcemia), and associated conditions (myocardial ischemia, hypothyroidism, anorexia/starvation, HIV infection, intracranial pathology, hypothermia).
         iii. Onset of TDP is typically associated with short-long-short sequences of the ventricular cycle length (measured by the RR interval).
         iv. Occasionally, TDP can develop in patients without marked prolongation of the QT interval. It is the relative change in the QT interval, rather than the absolute duration of the QT interval in these patients that predicts the occurrence of the arrhythmia.
      (2) Characteristic appearance on ECG, where the undulating peaks of sequential QRS complexes and T waves give it an appearance of twisting about an axis (**Fig. 19-6**).
      (3) Treatment
         i. Cardioversion/defibrillation.
         ii. Treatment of any concurrent precipitating factor discontinuing medications that are know to prolong the QT interval (**Table 19-3**).

TABLE 19-3	Drugs Causing QT-Interval Prolongation and/or Torsades de Pointes

Antiarrhythmic drugs	
— Class III (TdP reported in all)	Sotalol
	Amiodarone
	Ibutilide
	Amakalant
— Non-class III	
Sodium channel blockers	Quinidine
	Disopyramide
	Procainamide
	Encainide, flecanide
Other cardiovascular, diuretics	Dobutamine
	Oxprenolol
	Amiloride
Noncardiovascular drugs	
Neuroleptics	Chlorpromazine, perphenazine
	Haloperidol, droperidol
	Risperidone
	Thioridazine
	Olanzapine
Antidepressants	Amitriptyline
	Citalopram
	Fluoxetine
	Imipramine
H1-antihistamines	Terfenadine
	Diphenhydramine
	Promethazine
	Hydroxyzine
Antimalarials	Chloroquine
Antimicrobials	Erythromycin
	Clarithromycin
	Ketoconazole
	Levofloxacin
	Amantidine
	Pentamidine
Serotonin (5-HT) antagonists	Ketanserin
Anticancer drugs	Tacrolimus
	Adriamycin
	Tamoxifen
	5-Fluorouracil

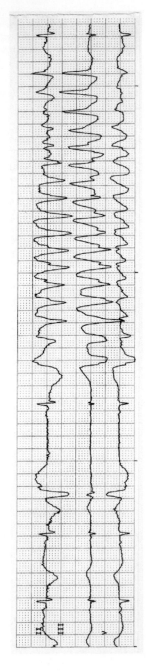

FIGURE 19-6 Rhythm strip of a patient with hypokalemia-induced prolonged QT interval and torsades de pointes.

    iii. Magnesium sulfate 1 to 2 g IV in setting of hypomagnesemia.
    iv. Overdrive pacing using either temporary pacing or isopro-
    terenol infusion that acts to shorten the QT interval and
    decrease the likelihood of short-long-short sequences.
    v. Patients at increased risk for recurrences without clearly
    reversible causes may benefit from prophylactic AICD
    implantation.

VI. Radiofrequency ablation (RFA)
    A. RFA is an elective and definitive strategy for most supraventricular and
    ventricular arrhythmias.
    B. In many situations, RFA has become the first line of therapy for supraven-
    tricular arrhythmias inclusive of AVNRT, AVRT, atrial flutter, and focal
    atrial tachycardias. It still constitutes the second line of therapy for AF and
    ventricular tachycardias.
    C. RFA is performed under conscious sedation with local anesthesia. Three
    to five transvenous catheters are placed, with occasional need for arterial
    or transseptal catheter approach. A diagnostic evaluation is performed,
    including induction of arrhythmia, determination of the potential mecha-
    nism, and assessment of the activation map. Therapeutic intervention
    immediately follows using current delivered through a catheter electrode
    to ablate the target. To conclude the procedure, a reassessment for pres-
    ence of arrhythmia is performed.
    D. Success rates for RFA are shown in **Table 19-2**.

Suggested Reading

American College of Cardiologists, American Heart Association, European Society of cardiologists (ACC/AHAESC) 2006 guidelines for the management of the patients with atrial fibrillation. *Circulation* 2006;114:e257–e354.[c4]

Amar D. Perioperative atrial tachyarrhythmias. *Anesthesiology* 2002;97:1618–1623.

Bakhtiary F et al. Impact of high thoracic epidural anesthesia on incidence of perioperative
atrial fibrillation in off-pump coronary bypass grafting: a prospective randomised study. *J
Thorac Cardiovasc Surg* 2007;134:460–464.

Dimarco JP. Implantable cardioverter-defibrillators. *N Engl J Med* 2003;349:1836–1847.

Lamas GA et al. Ventricular pacing or dual-chamber pacing for sinus-node dysfunction. *N
Engl J Med* 2002;346:1854–1862.

Mangrum JM, Dimarco JP. The evaluation and management of bradycardia. *N Engl J Med*
2000;342:703–709.

Opolski A et al. Rate control vs rhythm control in patients with nonvalvular persistent atrial
fibrillation: the results of the Polish How to Treat Chronic Atrial Fibrillation (HOT CAFE)
Study. *Chest* 2004;126:476–486.

Scott NB et al. A prospective randomized study of the potential benefits of thoracic epidural
anesthesia and analgesia in patients undergoing coronary bypass artery grafting. *Anesth
Analg* 2001;93:528–535.

Sick P et al. Initial worldwide experience with the WATCHMAN left appendage system for
stroke prevention in atrial fibrillation. *J Am Coll Cardiol* 2007;49;13:1490–1495.

Singh B et al. Dronedarone for maintenance of sinus rhythm in atrial fibrillation or flutter. *N
Engl J Med* 2007;357:987–989.

Stone KR, McPherson CA. Assessment and management of patients with pacemakers and
implantable cardioverter defibrillators. *Crit Care Med* 2004;(4 suppl):S155–S165.

The AFFIRM Trial Investigators. A comparison of rate control and rhythm control in patients
with atrial fibrillation. *N Engl J Med* 2002;347:1825–1833.

Zebis L et al. Practical regimen for amiodarone use in preventing postoperative atrial fibrillation. *Ann Thorac Surg* 2007;83:1326–1331.

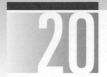

The Acute Respiratory Distress Syndrome

Kathrin Allen and Luca Bigatello

I. Although great progress has been made in understanding the pathophysiology of **acute lung injury (ALI)** and **acute respiratory distress syndrome (ARDS)**, treatment remains largely supportive. However, recent randomized trials have provided evidence the proper administration of mechanical ventilation may avoid additional damage to the lungs of patients with ALI/ARDS and may increase their survival.

II. Epidemiology

A. **Definition (Table 20-1)**. ARDS defines a syndrome of acute respiratory failure of diverse etiology, characterized by noncardiogenic pulmonary edema, hypoxemia, and diffuse lung parenchymal consolidations. ALI defines an early clinical stage of the same syndrome, with a milder degree of hypoxemia. The reason we identify an early stage of the syndrome is so we can apply and test therapeutic measures in a larger patient population before substantial damage to the lung has occurred.

B. **Etiology. Table 20-2** lists common causes of ALI/ARDS. Infectious pneumonia, aspiration pneumonitis, and lung contusion are frequent **pulmonary** etiologies. Abdominal sepsis, acute pancreatitis, and multiple trauma are **extrapulmonary** etiologies. Regardless of the anatomic origin, the lung is the target organ, but the radiographic pattern of injury may be quite variable. **Figure 20-1** shows representative computed tomography (CT) scans of two different patients. ARDS secondary to acute pancreatitis (**Fig. 20-1A**) shows a diffuse, almost homogeneous pattern of consolidation. ARDS secondary to bronchopneumonia (**Fig. 20-1B**) shows dense consolidations localized preferentially to the lower lung fields. Although there is no evidence that these are two separate syndromes from a pathophysiologic standpoint, they present different mechanical characteristics that may affect the choice of therapeutic strategies (see **Sections VI.B** and **VI.C**).

C. **Incidence.** A recent cohort study of a county served by 21 hospitals indicated that ALI/ARDS has a greater incidence than previously believed and

TABLE 20-1	Definition of Acute Lung Injury (ALI) and Acute Respiratory Distress Syndrome (ARDS)

Acute onset of respiratory distress
Hypoxemia
    ALI: $Pao_2/Fio_2 \leq 300$ mm Hg
    ARDS: $Pao_2/Fio_2 \leq 200$ mm Hg
Bilateral consolidation of chest radiograph
Absence of clinical findings of cardiogenic pulmonary edema

American-European Consensus Conference on ARDS. Bernard GR, Artigas A, Brigham KL, et al. Am J Respir Crit Care Med 1994;149:818–824

TABLE 20-2	Common Etiologies of the Acute Respiratory Distress Syndrome
Direct lung injury	Aspiration and other chemical pneumonitis
	Infectious pneumonia
	Lung contusion, penetrating chest injury
Distant injury	Inflammation, necrosis, ischemia–reperfusion injury
	Sepsis: intra-abdominal, bacteremia, fungemia, meningitis
	Multiple trauma, burns
	Shock
	Acute pancreatitis

carries a substantial impact on the United States health care. ALI occurs with an incidence of 79 per 100,000 person-years, and ARDS with an incidence 59 per 100,000 person-years. The impact on health care occurs not only because of the high mortality rate, but also because the survivors of ARDS have complex morbidity, and prolonged times of rehabilitation and away from the workplace.

D. Survival from ARDS depends on a number of factors, both acute (type and severity of the original cause, coexisting injuries, and additional organ failures) and pre-existing (age and comorbidity). Overall, the mortality rate of patients with ALI/ARDS seems to have improved over the past 5 to 10 years, and it averages between 30% and 40%. Factors that are unequivocally associated with a poor prognosis are old age and sepsis. On the other hand, trauma carries consistently a better outcome, and it is a category of ARDS patients in whom the most prolonged and intense treatments may be justified because of the realistic possibility of survival.

E. Recovery. The same categories of patients who enjoy higher survival rates, young patients with low comorbidity, also have the fastest recovery from ARDS. Over the first 3 to 6 months following discharge from the ICU, lung function steadily improves, reaching a level of approximately 70% of normal, allowing these patients to lead a productive life. However, consequences of ARDS are not limited to the respiratory system. Patients who undergo extended periods of mechanical ventilation in the ICU are susceptible to prolonged muscle wasting and weakness; a lower health-related quality of life; and some degree of impairment of memory, cognition, and ability to concentrate.

III. Pathogenesis

A. Regardless of the site of origin, the original insult triggers a systemic inflammatory response that injures the lungs as well as other organs. It is possible that the lung itself is a site where the inflammatory response is amplified by a combination of factors, included the mechanical stress induced by positive-pressure ventilation (**ventilator-induced lung injury (VILI)**, see below). Activated leukocytes release mediators that further amplify local and systemic injuries and may contribute to the onset of multiple organ system failures.

B. VILI refers to direct injury of the lungs by mechanical ventilation, and can be induced by several mechanisms.

  1. Trauma at end-inspiration occurs when an excess volume or pressure delivered results in alveolar overdistension. This excess transalveolar pressure may cause macroscopic (pneumothorax, pneumomediastinum,

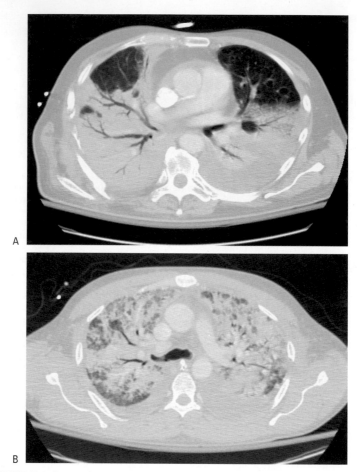

FIGURE 20-1 Computed tomography (CT) scans of two patients. **A.** ARDS secondary to bronchopneumonia shows dense consolidations localized preferentially to the lower lung fields. **B.** ARDS secondary to acute pancreatitis shows a diffuse, almost homogeneous pattern of consolidation.

pneumoperitoneum) or cellular damage, leading to worsening inflammation and disease process. In an ARDS patient, the normally aerated portion of the lung is reduced and therefore delivering a "normal" tidal volume can induce VILI.

2. **Trauma at end-expiration** refers to the cyclic opening and closing of alveoli throughout the respiratory cycle. Repetitive opening of the alveoli leads to epithelial damage through shear stress. **Positive end-expiratory pressure (PEEP)** has been shown to keep the alveoli open and reduce the trauma at end-expiration.

3. **Oxygen toxicity.** Elevated Fio_2 leads to formation of cytotoxic free radicals that may damage epithelial cells. Absorption atelectasis may also

result from a high Fio_2. Although a "safe" level of Fio_2 is not known, it seems reasonable to try to keep it, when possible, at 60% or less.

IV. The lung tends to respond to acute, nonneoplastic injuries in a reproducible manner, generating an anatomic picture known as **diffuse alveolar damage (DAD)**, whose main characteristics include

  A. Acute alveolar injury. The initial injury involves both the **endothelial** and the **epithelial** sides of the alveolocapillary membrane. This is important in order to understand the evolution of ARDS as a syndrome of both airways and vasculature. The degree of initial epithelial damage may affect the ultimate evolution of the syndrome. Of particular importance is the injury of the metabolically active type II alveolar cells, which are responsible for the production of surfactant, clearance of edema by fluid transport, and differentiation into the flat, parietal type I cells. Damage to type II cells fosters systemic amplification of the inflammatory response and affects the degree of subsequent high-grade fibroproliferative response.

  B. Exudative phase. Interstitial and alveolar edemas of DAD develop from endothelial damage rather than from hydrostatic forces. The exudate contains plasma proteins, white and red blood cells, platelets, and coagulation factors, and eventually lines the alveolar walls with hyaline membranes. Inactivation of the existent surfactant and production of abnormal surfactant may occur. Alveolar edema, consolidation, and collapse produce hypoxemia and reduce lung compliance.

  C. Vascular lesions. Tissue injury and activation of the coagulation cascade may result in alveolar hemorrhage and in thrombosis of small arteries. Remodeling may later obliterate sections of the pulmonary vasculature. Loss of vascular cross-sectional area, vasoconstrictive mediators, and **hypoxic pulmonary vasoconstriction (HPV)** may contribute to the onset of moderate pulmonary artery hypertension, which fosters the formation of pulmonary edema.

  D. Fibroproliferative phase. Within approximately 7 to 10 days, the inflammatory infiltrate acquires chronic characteristics, with a predominance of macrophages, monocytes, and eventually fibroblasts. The initial lesions heal by collagen deposition, leading to obliteration of air spaces and interstitial fibrosis. The intensity of fibroproliferative phenomena is variable and may be related to the severity of the initial injury (see **Section IV.A.**).

V. Physiology. Hypoxemia and low lung compliance are the physiological hallmarks of ARDS.

  A. Hypoxemia in ALI/ARDS is caused by alveolar edema, consolidation, and collapse. As ventilation decreases or completely ceases in different areas of the lung, partially or fully desaturated blood mixes with oxygenated blood. When true shunt (i.e., no ventilation) rather than ventilation/perfusion mismatch (i.e., low ventilation) is the main determinant of hypoxemia, as it is in ARDS, the Pao_2 can be increased only through the recruitment of nonventilated alveoli. Hypoxemia in ARDS is in part attenuated by the physiologic response of HPV, which diverts pulmonary blood flow away from hypoventilated alveoli. **HPV** may be inhibited by local production of vasodilator substances such as prostanoids and nitric oxide (NO) during inflammation. It may also be blunted by the administration of vasodilators such as nitroglycerin and sodium nitroprusside.

  B. Decreased pulmonary blood flow, vascular occlusion, airways overdistention, and hypovolemia may create areas of high ventilation/perfusion and true **dead space** (i.e., no perfusion). An increased ratio of dead space to tidal volume hinders CO_2 elimination and leads to **hypercapnia** and respiratory acidosis. A high dead space ventilation fraction early in the course of ALI/ARDS has been associated with a high mortality rate.

C. Low lung compliance. In the early phase of ARDS, lung compliance decreases because of diffuse alveolar edema, consolidation, and collapse. Because this injury is not homogeneous, the low compliance of early ARDS is really the average of the various mechanical characteristics of individual lung regions. The two CT scans in **Fig. 20-1** illustrate how a certain value of compliance measured in patients with ALI/ARDS may be determined by very different distributions of the lesions, which have implications in the choice of ventilatory management **(Section VI)**.

D. The chest wall is comprised of the rib cage and the abdomen. Low chest wall compliance may occur as a result of skeletal deformity, morbid obesity, ascites, abdominal compartment syndrome, massive trunk edema, circumferential burns, and tight chest bandages. **Abdominal distention** is frequent in surgical patients. It is important to recognize that a decrease in chest wall compliance will also decrease the transpulmonary pressure (i.e., the distending pressure of the alveoli), and these patients will require higher plateau pressures to achieve adequate change in lung volume. Intrathoracic pressure can be estimated by means of an **esophageal balloon;** making it possible to separate the mechanics of the lung and the chest wall. **Measuring respiratory compliance** is useful for following the evolution of the syndrome and testing the effect of changes of ventilatory settings. Bedside methods to assess respiratory compliance are described in **Chapter 3**.

VI. Treatment of ARDS

A. General measures. ALI/ARDS must be viewed as part of a systemic inflammatory injury that has a specific etiology and is commonly associated with the failure of other vital organs.

1. **Diagnosis and treatment** of the underlying condition must be sought, even when respiratory failure dominates the clinical picture. Important early interventions in surgical patients include the drainage of abscesses, debridement of devitalized tissue, fixation of fractures, and grafting of burned tissue.

2. **Hemodynamic management.** Judicious **fluid restriction** limits the formation of pulmonary edema, improves gas exchange and respiratory mechanics. In a recent study of the ARDS Network ([ARDS-Net] a federally funded consortium of academic centers performing clinical trials aimed at increasing survival of ALI/ARDS patients), a conservative fluid management improved lung function and decreased the duration mechanical ventilation and ICU stay.

3. **Treatment of infections.** Antimicrobial therapy should be targeted to cultured organisms whenever possible. The appeal of broad-spectrum antibiotic prophylaxis and coverage must be weighed against the potential for toxicity and selection of resistant microbial flora (see **Chapters 12, 13,** and **29**). **Nosocomial pneumonia** is frequent in patients with acute respiratory failure and is associated with a high mortality. Skillful airway management and measures for reducing the risks of aspiration (infection control measures, head-up position, oral hygiene, gastric decompression) decrease the incidence of nosocomial pneumonia.

4. **Nutrition** should be started early because a prolonged ICU course is likely. Enteral feeding is generally preferred **(Chapter 11)**.

5. **Support of other organ system functions** is an integral part of the treatment of ALI/ARDS. Hemodynamic instability, acute renal failure,

gastrointestinal hemorrhage, coagulation abnormalities, and neuro-muscular changes may complicate the course of these critically ill patients. We refer to the relevant specific chapters for their management.

B. Mechanical ventilation of ALI/ARDS patients

  1. The current approach to mechanical ventilation of patients with ALI/ARDS is based on the delivery of **small tidal volumes (V_T)** and a **moderate level of PEEP.**

    a. Large V_T and high alveolar pressure damage the lung. This injury **(VILI, Section III.B)** compounds the original alveolar injury and may adversely affect the outcome of patients with ALI/ARDS. **Figure 20-2** shows the portable chest radiogram (panel A) and the CT scan (panel B) of a patient who developed VILI in our ICU. However, in most cases, the damage of VILI is not visible by x-ray or CT scans, and the occurrence of pneumothorax, pneumomediastinum, and other classical signs of lung trauma from mechanical ventilation are rare.

    b. A multicenter clinical trial (ARDS-*Net*) showed that ventilating ALI/ARDS patients with a **lung-protective strategy** of low V_T (6 mL/kg of ideal body weight) and low airway pressure (inspiratory plateau pressure <30 cm H_2O) might improve survival.

    c. A number of subsequent studies in smaller patient populations have confirmed the above finding.

  3. Based on the current evidence, we suggest to

    a. Limit the size of the V_T, ideally to 6 mL/kg. You may allow for a slightly higher V_T if the **end-inspiratory plateau airway pressure** measured in a relaxed patient (see **Chapter 3**) is lower than 25 to 30 cm H_2O, if the patient is dyssynchronous with the ventilator, or if the patient is acidemic. If the use of low V_T causes significant acidemia, you may first increase the respiratory rate, aiming at an arterial pH value (admittedly arbitrary) close to 7.30 (see also **Section VI.B.3.d**).

    b. Apply a level of PEEP aimed at optimizing respiratory mechanics, that is, at preventing alveolar collapse at end-expiration (**Section III.B.2**) and recruitment of alveoli leading to a decrease in intrapulmonary shunting. The ideal level of PEEP is not precisely set, as the amount of recruitable lung is highly variable. In two recent studies of ALI/ARDS comparing low versus moderate PEEP levels, the strategies aimed at improving recruitment with a moderate PEEP level resulted in better lung function, reduced duration of mechanical ventilation, and a reduced rate of deaths from hypoxemia. A simple and practical way to test the effect of a change in PEEP on lung volume at the bedside is to apply a stepwise increase in PEEP while maintaining a set level of pressure above PEEP **("PEEP trial"),** during fully controlled ventilation. If the V_T increases or stays the same, this is an indication that the new level of PEEP has recruited lung tissue and has not overdistended a significant portion of previously recruited lung.

    c. Further recruitment of the lung. The pressure necessary to open collapsed alveoli may be several times higher than the levels of PEEP commonly used. Furthermore, ventilating with a low V_T tends to promote alveolar collapse. Therefore, lung-protective strategies of low V_T and airway pressure tend to include additional means to recruit the lung **(recruitment maneuvers)** by applying higher pressures at the airway for limited periods of time. Recruitment maneuvers are of two main varieties:

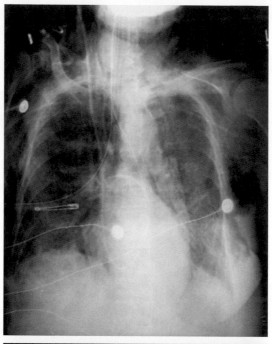

A

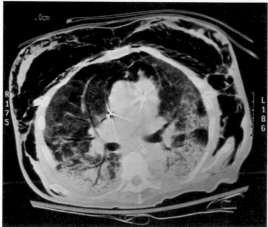

B

FIGURE 20-2 Portable chest radiogram **(A)** and chest computed tomography (CT) **(B)** of a patient with early acute respiratory distress syndrome and ventilator-induced lung injury. Note the striking difference in the morphologic information provided by the two techniques. In the CT image, one can distinguish inhomogeneous areas of consolidation, preferentially located in the dependent regions of the lungs, the massive subcutaneous emphysema, the peribronchial and pericardial air, and the subpleural loculated pneumothoraces.

(1) **A sustained inflation** of 30 to 60 seconds at a pressure higher than the inflating pressure, for example, 40 to 60 cm H_2O, increases the Pao_2 in the majority of patients with ALI/ARDS. Its effect is transient, but can be enhanced by increase the level of PEEP. However, sustained inflations may cause **hemodynamic instability** and **lung damage.** Hence, they should be carried out by experienced clinicians, with **continuous monitoring** of the arterial blood pressure, and only in patients whose hypoxemia is suspected to be due to alveolar collapse.

(2) A **sigh** is a large breath interspersed among the breaths of a set V_T or pressure. Although not a new concept, current ventilators may provide higher versatility to set the parameters of a sigh. A simple way to deliver a sigh is to have the patient breathe on pressure-support ventilation and add a single pressure-control breath of the desired pressure and duration.

(3) Despite their apparent immediate benefits, recruitment maneuvers have not been proven beneficial beyond their transient effect on gas exchange. While patients who have recruitable lungs may benefit from these maneuvers, others may be harmed by alveolar overdistension and hemodynamic instability. We recommend careful risk analysis of these maneuvers and considering that the ARDS lung may not need to be fully recruited at all times.

d. **$Paco_2$ control.** Low V_T may cause hypoventilation. Acute acidemia is best avoided by increasing the respiratory rate and/or by temporarily administering a buffer such as sodium bicarbonate or tromethamine for pH <7.20. A slow rise of the $Paco_2$, on the other hand, may not be harmful as long as pH compensation is allowed to occur. This approach, called **permissive hypercapnia,** has been advocated as a way to limit ventilator-associated acute lung injury. Experimental studies have suggested a possible protective benefit to hypercapnic acidosis against volutrauma. Considering the current data, it seems that allowing hypercapnia to avoid VILI is a safe practice; however, each patient must be evaluated on an individual basis. Contraindications to permissive hypercapnia include increased intracranial pressure, right ventricular failure, and ongoing acidemia.

4. **Modes of ventilation.** The basic concepts of mechanical ventilation, as well as the principles of the most common modes of mechanical ventilation, are discussed in **Chapter 5.** Here we will briefly review them in the context of the ALI/ARDS patient.

a. **Pressure** versus **volume-control ventilation.** Potential advantages of **pressure-control** ventilation include a **high and variable inspiratory flow rate,** which may enhance synchrony during patient-triggered breaths, and the ability to reach **the set airway pressure early in inspiration,** providing a higher mean airway pressure than an equivalent setting in the volume-control mode. The higher mean airway pressure may promote alveolar recruitment and increase the Pao_2. However, current mechanical ventilators can deliver **volume-control ventilation** with airflow patterns similar to what we just described for pressure control. In addition, volume control always **ensures the set minute ventilation,** which may be desirable in some patients. Hence, the choice between pressure and volume ventilation when using a modern ventilator is not a factor that affects patient outcome, but rather an individual preference.

   b. **Mandatory versus spontaneous ventilation**
      (1) **Mandatory ventilation** makes it possible to deliver high levels of alveolar pressure with complex and often "unphysiologic" flow waveforms that may improve gas exchange. For example, a prolonged inspiratory time may recruit alveoli and improve Pa_{O_2}, but is not generally tolerated by a spontaneously breathing patient. Hence, ventilation with high levels of support may require heavy sedation and neuromuscular blockade (see **Section VI.B.5.a**).
      (2) Conversely, maintaining some degree of **spontaneous breathing** activity may have beneficial effects. It may improve gas exchange due to the prevailing role of the diaphragm during spontaneous breathing, which applies inflating pressure to the lung bases, a larger and less expanded lung field. In addition, the maintenance of respiratory muscle activity may reduce the degree of weakness and atrophy of the respiratory muscles that is common after a prolonged course of acute respiratory failure (see **Section II.E**).
   c. **"Bilevel" modes** include those ventilatory modes that deliver two levels of airway pressure, and allow various combinations of spontaneous breathing. **Airway pressure release ventilation (APRV)** is a bilevel mode where the high level of pressure is held for several seconds, then briefly released to allow exhalation. Spontaneous breaths can occur at both pressure levels, but mostly at the higher level, because of its longer duration. These spontaneous breaths add to the minute ventilation without increasing the high level of pressure at the airway. Ventilation/perfusion mismatching may be improved by the spontaneous breathing activity. The ultimate benefits of APRV in ALI/ARDS are still under investigation.
   d. **High-frequency ventilation (HFV)** and **high-frequency oscillation (HFO)** deliver very small V_T at high rates and a set mean airway pressure. They provide gas exchange at low measurable airway pressures, presumably limiting VILI. However, expiratory flow limitation may cause high levels of auto-PEEP that are not reflected in the measured airway pressures. The use of HFV and HFO in adults is limited while waiting for the results of ongoing clinical trials.
   e. **Pressure control inverse ratio ventilation (PCIRV)** increases mean airway pressures by prolonging the inspiratory time (increased I:E ratio). Hence, Pa_{O_2} is increased at lower alveolar pressures. Common adverse consequences of PCIRV include auto-PEEP, decreased cardiac output, and the increased need for sedation.
5. **Additional strategies**
   a. **Sedation and neuromuscular blockade** may improve gas exchange by enhancing patient–ventilator synchrony and allowing the delivery of high levels of ventilatory support. Most clinicians limit the use of neuromuscular blockade to the most difficult cases to ventilate and oxygenate (see **Chapter 7**). The use of neuromuscular blocking agents, particularly of the steroid group, has been associated with prolonged weakness and polyneuropathy of critical illness (see **Chapter 32**).
   b. **Prone ventilation.** A significant increase in Pa_{O_2} occurs in more than half of ARDS patients who are turned prone, tends to last throughout the period of prone ventilation, and fades at variable rates as the supine position is resumed. Patients can be kept prone for

several hours at a time and turned supine for nursing care, physical examination, and relief of skin pressure. Complications of prone ventilation are rare in experienced hands, and are mostly related to the loss of lines, tubes (endotracheal tube!), and monitoring devices during the turning procedure. Rarely, skin pressure sores and nerve damage from incorrect positioning may occur. Transient hemodynamic instability may also occur, which makes proning a **high-risk maneuver in unstable patients.** We prefer to fully sedate patients who are ventilated prone, and often use neuromuscular blockade to facilitate this practice. The **mechanism** of the effect of prone ventilation on gas exchange in ARDS is not fully understood. Although gravitational factors redistribute ventilation to the previously collapsed dorsal areas of the lung, they do not explain the persistence of the effect of the prone position over time. It is also possible that changes in the geometry and mechanical properties of the chest wall may redirect airflow away from inflated ventral lung areas to previously collapsed dorsal areas. If this last concept is correct, simply compressing the anterior portion of the chest with **sand bags** during supine ventilation should improve gas exchange. Occasionally, the effects of using sand bags on gas exchange are obvious and reproducible. We use two sand bags of 2.5 lb each placed on each hemithorax particularly in patients who are deemed at increased risk for prone ventilation (see prior discussion).

C. **Additional therapeutic options**
   1. **Inhaled nitric oxide** (NO) reduces pulmonary hypertension and increases PaO_2 in the majority of patients with ARDS. Unfortunately, this beneficial effect is transient, and most of the time it does not result in an appreciable change in ventilatory management. Currently, the best indication for inhaled NO in ARDS seems to be as a **bridge to more complex therapies** during the initial stabilization of severely hypoxemic patients.
   2. **Extracorporeal membrane oxygenation (ECMO)** provides a temporary substitute for transpulmonary respiration while severely injured lungs are allowed to rest and recover. Extracorporeal gas exchange techniques in adults are confined to a few, highly specialized centers for limited indications.
   3. **Corticosteroids.** Because the disease process of ARDS includes persistent inflammation and parenchymal cell proliferation, the hope had been that corticosteroids may alter this disease process. Initially, small, single-institution studies suggested a benefit of treating late-phase ARDS with substantial doses of corticosteroids. However, a recent multicenter study failed to show any improvement beyond the known, physiological benefit of increasing PaO_2 and possibly lung compliance. Methylprednisolone failed to show an overall survival benefit and indicated an increased risk when treatment was initiated more than 13 days after ARDS onset. Based on this study, the routine use of corticosteroids for ARDS cannot be supported.

Selected References

ARDS Clinical Trials Network (ARDS-Net, National Heart, Lung and Blood Institute). Ventilation with lower tidal volumes as compared with traditional tidal volumes for acute lung injury and the acute respiratory distress syndrome. "ARMA Trial". *N Engl J Med* 2000;342: 1301–1308.

ARDS-Net. Comparison of two fluid-management strategies in acute lung injury. *N Engl J Med* 2006;354:2564.

ARDS-Net. Efficacy and safety of corticosteroids for persistent acute respiratory distress syndrome. *N Engl J Med* 2006;354:1671.

Artigas A, Bernard G, Claret J, et al. The American-European consensus conference on ARDS, Part 2. *Am J Respir Crit Care Med* 1998;157:1332–1347.

Bernard GR, Artigas A, Brigham KL, et al. The American-European consensus conference on ARDS, Part 1. *Am J Respir Crit Care Med* 1994;149:818–824.

Dreyfuss D, Saumon G. Ventilator-induced lung injury. *Am J Respir Crit Care Med* 1998;157:294–323.

Gattinoni L, Caironi P, Massimo C, et al. Lung recruitment in patients with acute respiratory distress syndrome. *N Engl J Med* 2006;354:1775.

Herridge MS, Cheung AM, Tansey CM, et al. One-year outcomes of survivors of the acute respiratory distress syndrome. *N Engl J Med* 2003;348:683–693.

Hess D, Bigatello LM. The chest wall in acute lung injury/acute respiratory distress syndrome. *Curr Opin Crit Care* 2008;14:94.

Meade M, Cook D, Guyatt G, et al. Ventilation strategy using low tidal volumes, recruitment maneuvers, and high positive end-expiratory pressure for acute lung injury and acute respiratory distress syndrome. *JAMA* 2008;299(6):637.

Mercat A, Richard J, Vielle B, et al. Positive end-expiratory pressure setting in adults with acute lung injury and acute respiratory distress syndrome. *JAMA* 2008;299(6):646.

Rubenfeld GD, Caldwell E, Peabody E, et al. Incidence and outcomes of acute lung injury. *N Engl J Med* 2005;353:1685.

Stapleton RD, Wang BM, Hudson LD, et al. Causes and timing of death in patients with ARDS. *Chest* 2005;128:525–532.

Ware LB, Matthay MA. The acute respiratory distress syndrome. *N Engl J Med* 2000;342:1334–1349.

21

Chronic Obstructive Pulmonary Disease and Asthma

Robert Owens and Fiona Gibbons

I. **Introduction.** Patients with an exacerbation of chronic obstructive pulmonary disease (COPD) or asthma present with a wide spectrum of disease severity. This chapter provides a guide to the care of patients with moderate to severe stable or unstable obstructive lung disease requiring care in an ICU.

  A. The following **definitions** consider each disease as an isolated entity. Although relatively pure forms of these diseases occur, there is overlap. Thus, many of the clinical findings and treatment modalities are similar. Nonetheless, COPD and asthma differ sufficiently in certain respects (e.g., cellular response, inflammatory mediators, degree of reversibility) to warrant individual discussion.

    1. **COPD** is a preventable and treatable disease characterized by **airflow limitation** that is not fully reversible. The airflow limitation is usually progressive and is associated with an abnormal inflammatory response of the lungs to noxious gases or particles. The airflow limitation in COPD is caused by both small airway disease (**obstructive bronchiolitis**) and parenchymal destruction (**emphysema**). The degree of obstructive bronchiolitis and emphysema varies among individuals.

      a. **Emphysema** is anatomically defined as permanent, destructive enlargement of the air spaces (alveoli) distal to the terminal bronchioles with accompanying destruction of the air space walls.

      b. **Chronic bronchitis** is a term that has been included in previous definitions of COPD, but is not part of the current definition. Chronic bronchitis, defined as the presence of cough and sputum for at least 3 months in each of 2 consecutive years, is a clinically useful term, but it does not reflect the major impact of airflow limitation on morbidity and mortality in COPD patients. While cough and sputum may precede the development of airflow limitation, some patients develop airflow limitation without chronic cough and sputum.

    2. **Asthma** is a chronic inflammatory disorder of the airways caused by inflammatory cell infiltration including neutrophils, eosinophils, lymphocytes, mast cells, and their mediators. This chronic inflammation is associated with airway hyperresponsiveness leading to recurrent episodes of wheezing, breathlessness, chest tightness, and coughing. These episodes are associated with widespread but variable airflow obstruction that is often spontaneously reversible or reversible with treatment. In some patients, the chronic inflammation leads to persistent changes in airway structure, such as subbasement membrane fibrosis, mucus hypersecretion, epithelial cell injury, smooth muscle hypertrophy, and angiogenesis.

    3. **Airflow obstruction** is a characteristic of both asthma and COPD. For asthma, airflow limitation is usually intermittent and reversible, whereas for COPD there is progressive airflow obstruction. However, individuals with asthma exposed to noxious agents such as cigarette smoke may also develop fixed airway obstruction. In addition,

longstanding asthma alone can lead to fixed airflow limitation. Airway obstruction usually improves with bronchodilators and corticosteroids in patients with asthma, whereas in patients with COPD there is a smaller response. For asthma, the cellular inflammation is mainly characterized by CD4$^+$ lymphocytes and eosinophils. For COPD, CD8$^+$ cells, macrophages, and neutrophils play a larger role. However, some patients with severe asthma display neutrophilic infiltration of the airways, and some patients with COPD may have features of asthma such as mast cell and eosinophilic airway infiltration.

B. Epidemiology

1. COPD is a leading cause of morbidity and mortality worldwide, affecting an estimated 210 million people. The disease affects men and women almost equally. The World Health Organization (WHO) reports that more than 3 million people died of COPD in 2005, which represents 5% of all deaths globally that year. Almost 90% of COPD deaths occur in low- and middle-income countries. Total deaths from COPD are projected to increase by more than 30% in the next 10 years without interventions to cut risks such as exposure to tobacco smoke. In the year 2000, the *MMWR* reported 726,000 hospitalizations and 119,000 deaths for COPD.

2. Asthma affects an estimated 300 million people worldwide and 20 million people in the United States. It is the most common chronic disease among children. It occurs in all countries regardless of level of development, but most asthma-related deaths occur in low- and middle-income countries. In 2004, the estimated number of hospital discharges where asthma was listed as the primary diagnosis was 497,100. The number of deaths attributed to asthma that year was 3,816.

II. ICU Evaluation

A. History.
The interview with the acutely ill patient with obstructive lung disease attempts to identify those at risk for mechanical ventilation, intubation, and/or death.

1. In asthma, **risk factors** identified for **death** during an exacerbation are
   - Previous severe exacerbation (e.g., intubation or ICU admission for asthma)
   - Two or more hospitalizations for asthma in the past year
   - Three or more emergency department visits for asthma in the past year
   - Hospitalization or emergency department visit for asthma in the past month
   - Use of more than two canisters of short-acting β-agonist (SABA) per month
   - Difficulty perceiving asthma symptoms or severity of exacerbations
   a. A subgroup of patients with **asthma with sudden onset of symptoms** (<6 hours) may also have a higher risk of intubation and/or death.

2. A history of intubation, a hospitalization of asthma within the last 5 years, and the physical examination finding of pulsus paradoxus have also been validated as **predictors of length of stay**, and thus may also be markers for severity of disease. Unfortunately, the lack of any of these risk factors does not preclude the possibility of a life-threatening illness.

3. Medications that have previously precipitated wheezing or asthma exacerbations such as aspirin, nonsteroidal anti-inflammatory drugs, or β-blockers should be reviewed.

4. Patients with COPD tend to be older and suffer from more comorbidities than those with asthma. **Predictors of mortality in COPD** exacerbations are
   - Increased age
   - Lower baseline FEV_1
   - Presence of cardiac disease
   - Higher APACHE II score

   Of those admitted to the ICU, in-hospital mortality has been predicted by previous intubation, chronic steroid use, and was inversely related to serum albumin.

   a. Review of the patient's record may also reveal chronic CO_2 retention (chronic respiratory acidosis), and can be useful in interpreting arterial blood gases.

   b. If obtainable, a prior history of difficult intubation may allow time to gather needed resources.

5. In patients with asthma or COPD exacerbation, a history of infectious symptoms (fever, cough, changes in sputum, sick contacts) will help guide management. In patients with COPD, a lack of these common symptoms or any other evidence of infection might suggest pulmonary embolism as the cause of the exacerbation.

B. **Physical examination.** Similar to the history, the physical examination focuses on markers of impending respiratory failure and the need for mechanical ventilation.

1. Many of the physical findings in patients with asthma or COPD become progressively more disordered with increasing respiratory distress, but **may normalize as respiratory arrest becomes imminent** (**Table 21-1**). For example, wheezing typically increases with increasing respiratory distress, but its absence may signal lack of air movement due to progressive obstruction or respiratory muscle fatigue. There is a typical sequence of events leading to respiratory acidemia following muscle fatigue: increased respiratory rate, followed by alternation between abdominal and rib cage breathing (respiratory *alternans*), paradoxical inward abdominal motion during inspiration (abdominal paradox), and finally an increase in $Paco_2$ associated with a fall in minute ventilation and respiratory rate, and worsening of respiratory acidemia.

2. Auscultation of the chest may reveal other causes of respiratory distress, such as pneumonia or pneumothorax, and may help guide management. **Wheeze is the expected finding in patients with asthma or COPD**, as a result of airway obstruction and/or bronchospasm. Absence of wheeze may be an ominous sign. Rhonchi in the spontaneously breathing patient suggest large airway secretions. Crackles may suggest a cardiac cause of wheeze. Inspiratory stridor suggests the presence of upper airway obstruction.

3. If time permits, a survey of the head and the neck, especially with regard to anatomy, may be helpful prior to intubation. Findings might include nasal polyps (suggestive of sensitivity to aspirin and other nonsteroidal medications, which could hinder nasotracheal intubation) or prior tracheotomy scars.

C. **Labs and imaging**

1. Arterial blood gas and pH measurement can be useful. However, the results must be interpreted with caution.

   a. In asthma exacerbations, initial respiratory distress may cause hyperventilation. As the exacerbation worsens, or the patient tires,

TABLE 21-1 Symptoms and Examination Findings During Asthma Attack

	Mild	Moderate	Severe	Subset: Respiratory Arrest Imminent
Symptoms				
Breathlessness	While walking can lie down	While at rest (infant—softer, shorter cry, difficulty feeding) Prefers sitting	While at rest (infant— Sits upright stops feeding)	
Talks in	Sentences	Phrases	Words	
Alertness	May be agitated	Usually agitated	Usually agitated	Drowsy or confused
Signs				
Respiratory rate	Increased	Increased often >30/min. Guide to rates of breathing in awake children: Age <2 mo 2–12 mo 1–5 years 6–8 years	Normal Rate <60/min <50/min <40/min <30/min	
Use of accessory muscles; suprasternal retractions	Usually not	Commonly	Usually	Paradoxical thoracoabdominal movement
Wheeze	Moderate, often only end expiratory	Loud; throughout exhalation	Usually loud; throughout inhalation and exhalation	Absence of wheeze

Pulse/minute	<100	100–120	>120 Guide to normal pulse rates in children: Age 2–12 mo <160/min 1–2 years <120/min 2–8 years <110/min	Bradycardia
Pulsus paradoxus	Absent <10 mm Hg	May be present 10–25 mm Hg	Often present >25 mm Hg (adult) 20–40 mm Hg (child)	Absence suggests respiratory muscle fatigue
Functional assessment				
PEF percent predicted or percent personal best	≥70%	Approx. 40%–69% or response lasts <2 h	<40%	<25% Note: PEF testing may not be needed in very severe attacks
Pa_{O_2} (on air) and/or Pc_{O_2}	Normal (test not usually necessary) <42 mm Hg (test not usually necessary)	≥60 mm Hg (test not usually necessary) <42 mm Hg (test not usually necessary)	<60 mm Hg: possible cyanosis ≥42 mm Hg: possible respiratory failure (see pages 393–394, 399)	
Sa_{O_2} percent (on air) at sea level	>95% (test not usually necessary)	90%–95% (test not usually necessary)	<90% Hypercapnia (hypoventilation) develops more readily in young children than in adults and adolescents.	

Pa_{O_2}, arterial oxygen pressure; Pc_{O_2}, partial pressure of carbon dioxide; PEF, peak expiratory flow; Sa_{O_2}, oxygen saturation.

Notes: The presence of several parameters, but not necessarily all, indicates the general classification of the exacerbation. Many of these parameters have not been systematically studied, especially as they correlate with each other. Thus, they serve only as general guides.

From *Expert Panel Report 3: Guidelines for the Diagnosis and Management of Asthma*, National Heart Lung and Blood Institute, National Asthma Education and Prevention Program, 2007. Available from: www.nhlbi.nih.gov/guidelines/asthma/asthgdln.htm.

Pa_{CO_2} increases. **Thus, a Pa_{CO_2} of 40 mm Hg may indicate severe obstruction and impending respiratory failure.**

   b. In patients with COPD, Pa_{CO_2} may be **chronically elevated**, such that this should not drive clinical decision-making. Instead, **change in pH** is a more useful measurement of acute respiratory acidosis. Alternatively, the Pa_{CO_2} can be followed over time.

   c. **Venous pH** often correlates with arterial pH. However, venous and arterial P_{CO_2} differ. A venous P_{CO_2} >45 mm Hg is a sensitive cutoff suggesting arterial hypercarbia.

2. In addition to standard laboratory tests, measurement of **theophylline** level is appropriate in patients using this medication.

3. The **chest radiography** may aid in diagnosis of pneumonia or complications such as pneumothorax, and can also reveal other causes of wheezing such as congestive heart failure.

4. The **electrocardiogram (ECG)** may show right axis deviation, poor R-wave progression, and right heart strain with hyperinflation. The ECG may also be useful in older patients in assessment for supraventricular tachycardia, either as a result of respiratory distress or bronchodilators and steroids used in treatment.

   a. **Multifocal atrial tachycardia (MAT)** is associated with COPD, and treatment typically focuses on reversing the respiratory distress. It may also portend a poor outcome. If necessary, β-blockade, calcium channel blockers, amiodarone, and magnesium can all be used to help control heart rate and rhythm. Cardioversion and digoxin do not have a role in management.

5. **Peak expiratory flow (PEF)** can be used in the acute setting to assess severity of an asthma flare, and provides information about response to treatment.

III. **ICU Management.** Despite differences in pathophysiology, the ICU management of asthma and COPD are often similar.

   A. Patients with obstructive lung disease are generally treated with **supplemental oxygen.**

   1. Concern is often expressed about treating patients with emphysema who have a chronic respiratory acidosis with supplemental oxygen. The fear is that supplemental oxygen will abolish the hypoxemic respiratory drive, decrease minute ventilation, and lead to hypercarbic respiratory failure. In general, suppression of the drive to breathe likely plays a minor role, and studies have found either small or no change in minute ventilation with application of supplemental oxygen.

   a. Supplemental oxygen does reverse the normal protective hypoxic vasoconstriction of the pulmonary vessels in poorly ventilated areas of the lungs. With supplemental oxygen, the vasoconstriction is reversed and blood flow increases through poorly ventilated areas, causing $\dot{V}/\dot{Q}$ **mismatch.**

   b. Supplemental oxygen may also cause hypercarbia via the **Haldane effect**, which describes the decrease in hemoglobin–CO_2 binding, which occurs with increasing hemoglobin oxygen saturation. As Pa_{O_2} increases, hemoglobin will bind oxygen preferentially and offload carbon dioxide. Although total CO_2 content will not change, the partial pressure of Pa_{CO_2} increases.

   2. To minimize the effects of supplemental oxygen, only an amount sufficient to maintain **arterial oxygen tension 55 to 60 mm Hg (oxygen saturation of 88%–92%)** should be provided.

B. **Heliox** is a combination of helium and oxygen (usually in a 80:20 or 70:30 ratio) that is less dense than oxygen or air.
   1. With turbulent flow, a less dense gas will have a higher flow rate. Decreased density favors laminar flow, which is more efficient than turbulent flow.
   2. Heliox has been advocated in obstructive lung disease to increase gas flow, decrease hyperinflation, and decrease work of breathing. Despite these claims, high-level evidence is lacking. While small studies generally purport small advantages, most meta-analyses fail to support routine use, either for asthma or COPD. Nevertheless, heliox is sometimes used in an effort to avoid intubation.
C. **Chest physiotherapy** is usually not indicated in patients with an exacerbation of asthma or COPD.
D. **Noninvasive positive pressure ventilation (NPPV)**. A growing body of evidence supports the use of NPPV in appropriately selected patients. NPPV can increase alveolar ventilation and decrease work of breathing. Two important contraindications are the patient's inability to clear secretions and to protect the airway.
   1. **In COPD patients with acute respiratory failure and $Paco_2$ of >45 mm Hg, NPPV has been shown to reduce intubation and death by almost 50%.**
   2. NIV is not as well studied in patients with acute asthma exacerbation. A meta-analysis of NPPV in asthma was unable to demonstrate consistent benefit. Nevertheless, several small studies suggest that NPPV in acute asthma may have benefit.
   3. Patients receiving NPPV must be monitored closely. A concern is that NPPV may delay endotracheal intubation. **Patients should be assessed for improvement or deterioration after 30 to 60 minutes of NPPV .**
E. **Intubation** and mechanical ventilation are required for respiratory failure and loss of consciousness. **The timing of intubation is often a clinical decision**, based on the clinical perception of increased work of breathing, patient fatigue, altering mental status, failure of NPPV , hemodynamic instability, hypercapnia, or hypoxemia.
   1. **Postintubation hypotension** is common in these patients for a number of reasons:
      ■ Dehydration from increased respiratory losses
      ■ Preload dependence in patients with cor pulmonale
      ■ Worsening hypercapnia
      ■ Auto-PEEP, causing a decrease in systemic venous return, especially during preoxygenation
      Hypotension can be minimized with fluid administration prior to intubation, and vasopressors, if necessary.
F. The aim of **mechanical ventilation** is to achieve adequate oxygenation (SpO_2, 88%–92%) and ventilation. Management of the ventilator is a compromise between an appropriate $Paco_2$ and avoidance of hyperinflation. Increased airway resistance and auto-PEEP (intrinsic positive end expiratory pressure) are the principal considerations during mechanical ventilation of patients with obstructive lung disease.
   1. **Auto-PEEP** can be assessed for qualitatively, or measured quantitatively:
      ■ Inspiratory efforts by the patient that do not trigger the ventilator.
      ■ Expiratory **flow** does not return to 0 before initiation of the next breath.
      ■ Esophageal manometry or an **end-expiratory pause** can be used to measure auto-PEEP quantitatively.
   2. Auto-PEEP can contribute to patient–ventilator dyssynchrony, $\dot{V}/\dot{Q}$ mismatch, hemodynamic instability, and barotrauma.

3. Strategies to decrease auto-PEEP

a. Treatment of underlying airflow obstruction (steroids, bronchodilators).

b. **Shorten the inspiratory time** (which increases the expiratory time) may decrease auto-PEEP without significantly altering the minute ventilation.

c. **Decrease the minute ventilation.** Decreasing the respiratory rate or the tidal volume will decrease the minute ventilation. These changes may also lead to **"permissive hypercapnia"** or "controlled hypoventilation." The recommended respiratory rate is 10 to 15 breaths/min and tidal volumes of 6 to 8 mL/kg of ideal body weight.

d. CO_2 production can be minimized through sedation, analgesia, and antipyretics, which decreases the required minute ventilation.

e. **Deep sedation** to decrease or eliminate the patient's respiratory drive may also be necessary.

   (1) **Propofol** is often favored as it also acts as a bronchodilator. Benzodiazepines and opioids are also added as needed to reduce respiratory drive.

   (2) **Neuromuscular blockade**, in the setting of steroid use, raises concern for myopathy, and should be avoided if possible. Because myopathy has been demonstrated to occur in a dose-dependent fashion, neuromuscular blockade, if needed, should be given as intravenous boluses, rather than as a continuous infusion.

f. **Counterbalancing auto-PEEP with PEEP set** on the ventilator may improve patient–ventilator synchrony. In some cases, there is a decrease in hyperinflation with increasing PEEP set on the ventilator. When PEEP is used to counterbalance auto-PEEP, care must be taken to avoid additional hyperinflation, which would result in increased inspiratory plateau pressures.

4. Initial ventilator settings (Fig. 21-1)

a. **Pressure-controlled ventilation** versus **volume-controlled ventilation.** No data favor either pressure-controlled ventilation or volume-controlled ventilation.

   (1) Pressure-controlled ventilation has the advantage of limiting hyperinflation, but it can result in low tidal volumes and hypoventilation if auto-PEEP worsens.

   (2) Volume-controlled ventilation maintains minute ventilation, but may contribute to hyperinflation with worsening auto-PEEP.

b. **Tidal volume** of 6 to 8 mL/kg of ideal body weight is recommended.

c. A low **respiratory rate** of 10 to 15 breaths/min is set to allow for a long expiratory time.

d. The inspiratory **flow** should be constant, rather than descending ramp, and set high to decrease inspiratory time and maximize expiratory time.

e. **PEEP is selected to counterbalance auto-PEEP,** but avoid increasing hyperinflation by monitoring plateau pressure and auto-PEEP.

IV. Pharmacologic treatment

A. **Bronchodilators.** Patients with COPD and asthma may experience significant benefit from small improvements in airway resistance. For this reason, bronchodilators are the mainstay of therapy during acute exacerbations of these diseases.

1. **Anticholinergics** have direct bronchodilating effects. Because the site of bronchospasm in COPD is often in central airways that have parasym-

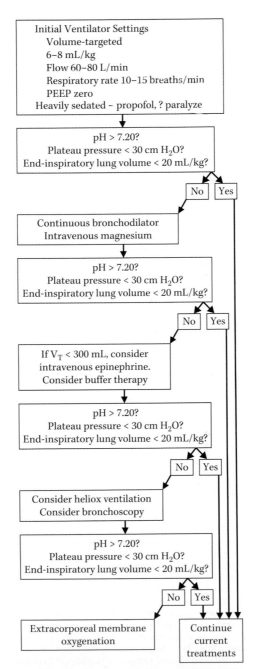

FIGURE 21-1 Initial ventilator settings and suggested management algorithm. Note that mild-moderate acidosis is allowed. From Medoff BD. *Respir Care* 2008.

TABLE 21-2	Common Inhaled Anticholinergic Drugs			
Drug	**Brand Name**	**Administration**	**Initial Adult Dose**	**Interval (h)**
Ipratropium bromide	Atrovent	MDI (21 μg) Nebulizer (0.2 mg/mL)	2 puffs 2.5 mL (500 μg)	4–6 6–8
Albuterol/ ipratropium	Combivent	120 μg albuterol/ 21 μg ipratropium	1–2 puffs	4 times daily
Albuterol/ ipratropium	DuoNeb	3 mg albuterol/ 0.5 mg ipratropium in 3 mL	3 mL	4
Tiotropium	Spiriva	DPI (18 μg/capsule)	1 capsule	24

Initial adult doses are for spontaneously breathing adults. Increased doses may be required for patients who are tracheally intubated. MDI, metered-dose inhaler; DPI, dry-powder inhaler.

pathetic innervation, these drugs, which are administered by inhalation, are often effective in patients with COPD. Short-acting agents include **ipratropium bromide** and **glycopyrrolate** (**Table 21-2**).

  a. Ipratropium produces rapid bronchodilation (within 15 minutes), most likely by competitive inhibition of cholinergic receptors in bronchial smooth muscles (antagonizing the action of acetylcholine at its membrane-bound receptor site), thereby blocking the bronchoconstrictor action of vagal efferent impulses.

  b. While SABAs are the drugs of choice in asthma exacerbations, ipratropium is an alternative agent for patients with significant side effects from β-agonists or with severe coronary disease to avoid deleterious increases in heart rate.

  c. A recent meta-analysis showed a statistically significant **improvement in pulmonary function** and a **reduction in the rate of hospital admissions when ipratropium was added** to β-agonist therapy. This effect is most pronounced in those patients with severe obstruction. However, the addition of ipratropium to albuterol has not been shown to provide further benefit once the patient is hospitalized.

  2. Sympathomimetics: β_2-adrenergic receptor agonists cause bronchodilation via cyclic adenosine monophosphate (cAMP)–mediated relaxation of bronchial smooth muscle.

  a. Short-acting agents such as **albuterol** are indicated in the acute setting (**Table 21-3**).

  b. β-agonists are usually administered by inhalation, but can be given intravenously.

  c. A meta-analysis comparing the use of continuous versus intermittent β-agonists for acute asthma revealed a reduction in hospital admissions and a small but statistically significant improvement in pulmonary function with continuous β-agonist use. Patients with severe airway obstruction seem to benefit the most from this intervention.

  d. **Epinephrine** (by continuous infusion, nebulization, subcutaneous, or intramuscular injection) is used when other measures have failed (**Table 21-3**). Intravenous epinephrine can be used safely, but the clinician should recognize the higher likelihood of dysrhyth-

TABLE 21-3	Common β_2-Adrenergic Drugs			
Drug	**Brand Name**	**Administration**	**Initial Adult Dose**	**Interval (h)**
Albuterol	Proventil HFA	MDI (108 μg)	2 puffs	4–6
	Proair HFA	MDI (108 μg)	2 puffs	4–6
	Ventolin HFA	MDI (108 μg)	2 puffs	4–6
	AccuNeb	0.083% 3 mL	2.5 mg (1 vial)	4–6
	Generic	5 mg/mL (0.5%) 20 mL	2.5 mg (0.5 mL)	4–6; 10–15 mg/h continuous
Levalbuterol	Xopenex	MDI (45 μg)	2 puffs	4–6
		0.31, 0.63, 1.25 mg in 3 mL	0.63–1.25 mg	6–8
Formoterol	Foradil	DPI (12 μg capsule)	1 capsule	12
	Perforomist	20 μg in 2 mL	20 μg	12
Arformoterol	Brovana	15 μg in 2 mL	15 μg	12
Pirbuterol	Maxair (breath-actuated)	MDI (200 μg)	2 puffs	4–6
Racemic epinephrine	VapoNefrin	Nebulizer (2.25%)	0.25–0.5 mL	3–4
Epinephrine	Adrenalin	1:1,000 solution	0.1–0.5 mg subcutaneous	20 min–4 h
		0.25–2 μg/min IV		Continuous Infusion
Terbutaline	Generic		0.25–0.5 mg subcutaneous	15–30 min × 2

Initial adult doses are for spontaneously breathing adults. Increased doses may be required for patients who are tracheally intubated. MDI, metered-dose inhaler; DPI, dry-powder inhaler.

mias and other undesirable side effects in older patients. Furthermore, there is no proven advantage of systemic therapy with epinephrine over aerosol therapy.

3. **Long-acting bronchodilators**

   a. The long-acting anticholinergic agent **tiotropium** is useful for management of stable COPD, but has not been studied in the setting of acute exacerbations of COPD. It has not been studied in the long-term management of asthma, and is not FDA approved for treatment of asthma.

   b. Long-acting β-agonists (e.g., **salmeterol** and **formoterol**) are never indicated for acute bronchospasm due to their slow onset of action (30 minutes), but are useful in the management of chronic asthma and COPD.

4. **Nebulizer versus inhaler:** The use of a nebulizer or an inhaler for the delivery of aerosolized medications is controversial.

   a. In mild or moderate exacerbations, adequate bronchodilation can be achieved either by the use of a metered-dose inhaler (MDI) with

	TABLE 21-4	Inhaled steroids		

Drug	Brand Name	Administration	Initial Adult Dose	Interval (h)
Beclomethasone	QVAR	40 μg 80 μg	40–320 μg	12
Fluticasone	Flovent	HFA (44, 110, 220 μg) Diskus (50 μg)	88–880 μg 100–1000 μg	12
Mometasone furoate	Asmanex	DPI (220 μg)	220–880 μg	Daily or 12
Salmeterol/ fluticasone	Advair	DPI (50 μg salmeterol + 100, 250, or 500 μg fluticasone) MDI (21 μg salmeterol + 45, 115, or 230 μg fluticasone)	1 inhalation 2 puffs	12 12
Budesonide/ formoterol	Symbicort	MDI (4.5 μg formoterol + 80 μg or 160 μg budesonide)	2 puffs	12
Triamcinolone	Azmacort	MDI (75 μg)	2 puffs 4 puffs	6–8 12
Flunisolide	Aerobid	MDI (250 μg)	2–4 puffs	12
Budesonide	Pulmicort	DPI (90, 180 μg) Respules (0.25, 0.5, 1.0 mg/2 mL)	360–720 μg	12

Initial adult doses are for spontaneously breathing adults. Increased doses may be required for patients who are tracheally intubated. MDI, metered-dose inhaler; DPI, dry-powder inhaler.

a valved holding chamber, under the supervision of trained personnel, or by nebulizer.

   b. The use of a holding chamber improves the performance of the MDI in patients with poor hand–breath coordination. The holding chamber also decreases pharyngeal deposition, which is important with inhaled steroids.

   c. During exacerbations, many patients have difficulty using the MDI correctly. Therefore, a nebulizer may be preferred in patients who are unable to use the MDI effectively due to age, agitation, or the severity of the exacerbation.

   d. Dry-powder inhalers (DPI) are increasingly becoming available. As with the MDI, patients must be instructed in the proper technique for use of a DPI (**Table 21-4**).

B. Methylxanthines are weak bronchodilators.

   1. Specific agents include **theophylline** and **aminophylline** (80% theophylline by weight) (**Table 21-5**).

   2. These agents may improve respiratory drive and muscle function, but this is controversial and their effect is small.

   3. The mechanisms of action for these agents are complex, multiple, and incompletely understood. These include nonspecific inhibition of

TABLE 21-5	Methylxanthines		
Drug	**Administration**	**Initial Adult Dose**	**Interval**
Theophylline	4.6 mg/kg IBW/30 min loading dose IV	0.4 mg/kg/h IV Max 900 mg/d	Continuous infusion
Aminophylline	5.7 mg/kg IBW/30 min loading dose IV	0.5 mg/kg/h Max dose 1125 mg/day	Continuous infusion

Doses above are for theophylline naïve patients who are nonsmokers between the ages of 16 and 60. Dose adjustments are indicated for patients who have receive theophylline in last 24 hours or who are older than 60.

phosphodiesterase to increase intracellular cAMP, blockade of adenosine, direct activation of histone deacetylases, and release of endogenous catecholamines.

4. These agents are not recommended for treatment of asthma attacks.
5. Use of these agents in the treatment of COPD exacerbations is controversial. When used for COPD, methylxanthines are administered intravenously (with or without a loading bolus) in the ICU and have a half-life of 3 to 4 hours, which is prolonged unpredictably in patients with right heart failure and with certain concomitant drugs.
6. Methylxanthines can cause gastrointestinal symptoms such as nausea and more serious toxic reactions such as dysrhythmias and seizures.
7. Methylxanthines have limited use. When they are used, clinical findings and serum levels should be followed closely with dose adjusted accordingly, keeping serum theophylline levels <20 μg/dL. They are currently considered second-line therapy when there is an inadequate or insufficient response to short-acting bronchodilators.

C. **Corticosteroids.** These drugs act via complex and incompletely understood mechanisms to reduce airway inflammation, airway responsiveness, mucus secretions, and edema. Steroids enhance β-adrenergic responsiveness and relax bronchial smooth muscle.
1. In exacerbations of asthma, systemic administration of corticosteroids is often necessary.
   a. In patients with moderate (dyspnea interfering with or limiting usual activity, PEF 40%–69% predicted or personal best) and severe exacerbations (dyspnea at rest and with speaking, PEF $<$40% predicted or personal best), oral systemic corticosteroids are indicated. Oral administration of prednisone has been shown to have effects equivalent to those of intravenous methylprednisolone, provided gastrointestinal transit time or absorption is not impaired.
   b. In patients with life-threatening asthma who are too dyspneic to speak with PEF $<$25% predicted or personal best, intravenous corticosteroids are usually administered. The **early use (within 1 hour of arrival)** of systemic corticosteroids in patients with acute asthma presenting to the emergency room has been shown to significantly reduce admission rates. This effect is most pronounced in those patients not receiving systemic steroids prior to ED presentation and in those with more severe asthma.
   c. Doses of prednisone or **methylprednisolone of 40 to 80 mg/d** in one or two divided doses is recommended until PEF reaches 70% of predicted or personal best. There is no known advantage for higher doses of corticosteroids in severe asthma exacerbations.

2. Oral or intravenous steroids have been shown to reduce treatment failure, improve lung function, hypoxemia, and dyspnea in the first 72 hours of a COPD exacerbation.

   a. The exact recommended dose is not known. High doses are associated with significant risk of side effects such as hyperglycemia. Usually, 30 to 40 mg of oral prednisolone daily for 7 to 10 days is effective and safe.

D. Antibiotics: Both viral and bacterial infections can be a factor in a COPD exacerbation. The most common pathogens include *Hemophilus influenzae*, *Streptococcus pneumoniae*, and *Mor catarrhalis*.

1. Antibiotics should be administered to patients with COPD exacerbations who present with increased dyspnea, increased sputum volume, and increased sputum purulence, as well as patients with severe exacerbations requiring invasive or noninvasive mechanical ventilation.

2. Antibiotics are *not* generally recommended for the treatment of acute asthma exacerbations unless the patient presents with fever, purulent sputum, or evidence of bacterial sinusitis or pneumonia.

E. Mucolytics such as nebulized acetylcysteine or hypertonic saline are generally not recommended in treating asthma or COPD exacerbations. Because they induce bronchospasm, they should be administered with caution and in combination with inhaled β_2-adrenergic agonists.

F. Leukotriene receptor antagonists (zafirlukast and montelukast) and synthesis inhibitors (zileuton) are often used for maintenance treatment of chronic asthma. They may have potential benefit in the treatment of acute asthma as they have a relatively rapid onset of action after oral administration.

1. One study examined administration of intravenous montelukast versus placebo in addition to standard therapy in patients who presented to the emergency room with moderate to severe acute asthma. Those who received montelukast had an improved FEV_1 for up to 2 hours compared with placebo, less β-agonist use, and fewer treatment failures.

2. Although some studies suggest efficacy, presently there are insufficient data to make recommendations about these drugs as an adjunctive therapy for acute asthma or COPD.

G. Magnesium sulfate is a calcium channel blocker that has been shown to cause smooth muscle relaxation in vitro and in vivo, leading to an interest in magnesium as an adjunctive therapy for acute asthma in the emergency room.

1. In patients with severe acute asthma, magnesium sulphate PEF improves PEF, FEV_1, and is associated with a reduced rate of admissions.

2. Inhaled magnesium sulfate in addition to β-agonists may improve lung function in severe asthmatics, but further investigation is required.

3. Intravenous magnesium sulfate should be considered in patients with life-threatening exacerbations and in those whose exacerbations remain in the severe category after 1 hour of intensive conventional treatment (**Table 21-6**).

TABLE 21-6	Magnesium	
Drug	**Initial Adult Dose**	**Interval (h)**
Magnesium sulfate	2 g IV over 20 min	×1

Selected References

Aubier M, Murciano D, Milic-Emili J, et al. Effects of the administration of O_2 on ventilation and blood gases in patients with chronic obstructive pulmonary disease during acute respiratory failure. *Am Rev Respir Dis* 1980;122:747–754.

Behbehani NA, Al-Mane F, D'yachkova Y. Myopathy following mechanical ventilation for acute severe asthma: the role of muscle relaxants and corticosteroids. *Chest* 1999;115: 1627–1631.

Caramez MP, Borges JB, Tucci MR, et al. Paradoxical responses to positive end-expiratory pressure in patients with airway obstruction during controlled ventilation. *Crit Care Med* 2005;33:1519–1528.

Carmargo CA Jr, Spooner CH, Rowe BH. Continuous verus intermittent beta-agonists for acute asthma. *Cochrane Database Syst Rev* 2003;(4):Art. No.:CD001115. DOI:10.1002/14651858.CD001115.

Carmargo Jr CA, Smithline HA, Malice MP, et al. A randomized controlled trial of intravenous montelukast in acute asthma. *Am J Respir Crit Care Med* 2003;167:528–533.

Colebourn CL, Barber V, Young JD. Use of helium-oxygen mixture in adult patients presenting with exacerbations of asthma and chronic obstructive pulmonary disease: a systematic review. *Anaesthesia* 2007;62:34–42.

Expert Panel Report 3. Guidelines for the Diagnosis and Management of Asthma, National Heart Lung and Blood Institute, National Asthma Education and Prevention Program, 2007. Available from: www.nhlbi.nih.gov/guidelines/asthma/asthgdln.htm.

Global Strategy for Asthma Management and Prevention, Global Initiative for Asthma (GINA) 2007. Available from: http://www.ginasthma.org.

Global Strategy for the Diagnosis, Management and Prevention of COPD, Global Initiative for Chronic Obstructive Lung Disease (GOLD) 2007. Available from: http://www.goldcopd.org.

Medoff BD. Invasive and noninvasive ventilation in patients with asthma. *Respir Care* 2008;53:740–750.

Oddo M, Feihl F, Schaller MD, Perret C. Management of mechanical ventilation in acute severe asthma: practical aspects. *Intensive Care Med* 2006;32:501–510.

Ram FS, Picot J, Lightowler J, Wedzicha JA. Non-invasive positive pressure ventilation for treatment of respiratory failure due to exacerbations of chronic obstructive pulmonary disease. *Cochrane Database Syst Rev* 200;(3).

Rodrigo G, Rodrigo C, et al. A meta-analysis of the effects of ipratropium bromide in adults with acute asthma. *Am J Med* 1999;107:363–370.

Rowe BH, Bretzlaff JA, Bourdon C, et al. Magnesium sulfate for treating exacerbations of acute asthma in the emergency department. *Cochrane Database Syst Rev* 2000;(2):CD001490.

Soroksky A, Stav D, Shpirer I. A pilot prospective, randomized, placebo-controlled trial of bilevel positive airway pressure in acute asthmatic attack. *Chest* 2003;123:1018–1025.

22

Pulmonary Embolism and Deep Venous Thrombosis

B. Taylor Thompson

I. **Overview.** Embolization of thrombus from the deep venous system to the pulmonary vascular bed results in a nonspecific clinical presentation that is frequently unrecognized. The estimated annual incidence of pulmonary embolism in the United States is 500,000, and the prevalence for nonfatal pulmonary embolism approaches 20 per 1,000 inpatients. Treatment with anticoagulants reduces mortality from between 30% and 40% to between 2% and 8%, primarily by preventing further emboli. Pulmonary embolism and deep venous thrombosis (DVT) have been less well studied in critically ill patients, but studies indicate that approximately 13% of critically ill patients may develop DVT even with prophylaxis.

II. **Natural history**
   A. **Deep venous thrombosis (DVT)** usually begins in the lower extremities, although occasional thrombi form in pelvic veins, renal veins, upper extremity veins, and the right heart. Most thrombi originate in the soleal veins of the calf near valve cusps or bifurcations. Calf thrombi may resolve spontaneously, and embolization to the lung is uncommon. Approximately, 20% to 30% of clots propagate to the popliteal, femoral, or iliac veins (so-called proximal DVT), and an additional 10% to 20% of all DVT begin in the thigh without prior calf involvement.
   B. **Pulmonary emboli (PE).** Once in the pulmonary circulation, large emboli may lodge at the bifurcation of the pulmonary and lobar arteries, causing acute right ventricular (RV) dilation and dysfunction leading to reduced left ventricular filling and hypotension. Smaller emboli continue distally into small arteries or arterioles. The lower lobes are more often involved than the upper lobes, and multiple emboli are usually present at the time of diagnosis. Only 10% to 20% of emboli cause infarction, usually in patients with pre-existing cardiopulmonary disease.

III. **Risk factors for DVT and PE**
   A. Prior venous thromboembolism.
   B. Factors promoting stasis such as more than 48 hours of immobility, congestive heart failure, or surgery with general anesthesia.
   C. Endothelial damage such as lower extremity surgery or trauma.
   D. Hypercoagulable states such as inherited thrombophilias (e.g., factor V Leiden or the prothrombin gene mutation) or acquired thrombophilias (e.g., lupus anticoagulant and antiphospholipid antibody).
   E. Malignancy. Approximately 15% of patients with venous thromboembolic disease who have no known risk factors for DVT or PE will have an occult malignancy diagnosed within 2 years.
   F. Spinal cord injury. DVT occurs in 38% of these patients within 3 months of paralysis, with a corresponding frequency of PE of approximately 5%.
   G. **Heparin-induced thrombocytopenia (HIT).** In patients who develop HIT and have heparin therapy discontinued, 38% to 76% subsequently develop DVT and/or PE.

H. Pregnancy or oral contraceptives, especially when combined with an inherited thrombophilia.

IV. Clinical manifestations
A. Symptoms and signs
1. **DVT.** Many lower extremity venous thrombi are asymptomatic, probably because they remain nonocclusive or because of the development of collaterals. Symptomatic thrombi produce calf pain, edema, venous distention, and pain on passive dorsiflexion of the foot (Homan's sign). These symptoms and signs are nonspecific. Prospective studies of outpatients with symptoms suggestive of DVT actually find DVT by objective testing in only one-third of patients. In patients with leg symptoms suggesting DVT but in whom venography is normal, musculoskeletal injuries, Baker's cysts, and chronic lymphatic or venous insufficiency are the usual explanations.
2. **PE.** Autopsy series suggest that many PE are silent. When clinically apparent, symptoms and signs depend on the size of the embolus. Symptoms of small to medium emboli include dyspnea, chest pain, and cough. Tachypnea and tachycardia are present in the majority of patients. Mild fever less than 39°C is common, and wheezing occurs in less than 5% of patients. If infarction occurs, hemoptysis, pleuritic pain, and pleural rub are present. Massive emboli often produce near-syncope, tachycardia, and hypotension along with signs of RV dysfunction such as an RV heave, an RV S_3, or a murmur of tricuspid regurgitation. If massive PE is the only explanation for hypotension, the central venous pressure will be elevated.

B. **Hemodynamic findings.** After PE, cardiac output is usually normal, but in hypotensive patients with massive PE the stroke volume is reduced and compensatory tachycardia is usually insufficient to maintain cardiac output. In this setting, RV diastolic and right atrial mean pressures are always elevated. Pulmonary artery pressure tends to be increased but correlates poorly with the size of the embolus and may be normal even in massive PE.

C. **Differential diagnosis.** Smaller PE may mimic pneumothorax, hyperventilation, asthma, myocardial infarction, congestive heart failure, pleurodynia, or serositis. If infarction is present, clinical findings may resemble pneumonia, bronchial obstruction by mucus or tumor, or pleural effusion. The differential diagnosis for massive PE includes RV infarction, pericardial tamponade, and venous air embolism.

V. Diagnosis
A. **The electrocardiogram (ECG)** is often abnormal in small to medium PE, but findings are nonspecific. The ECG is normal in 23% of patients with submassive embolism and in 6% of patients with massive PE.
B. **Chest radiography.** Even without infarction, radiographic abnormalities occur in the majority of patients with PE and include elevation of a hemidiaphragm, atelectasis, and effusion. An infarct appears as a pleural-based infiltrate with a convex margin directed toward the hilum.
C. **Noninvasive studies** for DVT. **Color-flow Doppler** with compression ultrasound (referred to as **venous ultrasound**) has high sensitivity (89%–100%) and specificity (89%–100%) in comparison with venography for the detection of proximal DVT and slightly less sensitivity and specificity for calf vein thrombi. Venous ultrasound is also useful for the detection of a Baker's cyst. Sensitivity falls dramatically when venous ultrasonography is used for asymptomatic, high-risk patients (33%). **Impedance plethysmography (IPG)**

also offers high sensitivity, slightly less specificity, and lower cost in comparison to venous ultrasound. IPG is not accurate for the detection of calf vein thrombi.

D. **D-Dimers** are usually present in the serum of patients with PE, but are nondiagnostic. However, a level less than 500 ng/mL by quantitative ELISA or semiquantitative latex agglutination has a high negative predictive value and is sufficient to exclude pulmonary embolism with low or moderate pretest probability of PE. However, D-dimer levels less than 500 ng/mL are uncommon in critically ill patients due to fibrin turnover during critical illness, thus limiting the value of D-dimer testing to exclude PE from diagnostic consideration.

E. **HIT antibodies.** HIT testing should be performed in all patients being treated with any form of heparin treatment when there is a platelet count decrease of more than 50% from baseline or to less than 100,000/μL. Heparin should be discontinued while awaiting results of HIT testing.

F. **Lung scintigraphy.** Perfusion lung scans are performed by injection of radiolabeled albumin macroaggregates or microspheres. Scans are sensitive; a negative perfusion scan virtually excludes PE. Results are also nonspecific. Because pulmonary arterioles constrict in response to hypoxia, perfusion defects, especially if nonsegmental, these may be secondary to a ventilatory abnormality and not to obstruction of flow by an embolism. Perfusion scans may be abnormal in atelectasis, asthma, chronic airway obstruction, and other causes of regional hypoventilation. The value of lung scintigraphy in intubated patients or unconscious patients is limited due to poor image quality, and this modality has largely been replaced by spiral CT angiography.

G. **Spiral CT angiography (Fig. 22-1).** Spiral (or helical) CT scanning with intravenous contrast has high sensitivity for the detection of segmental or greater thrombi. An additional benefit is the ability to detect alternative pulmonary pathologies that may explain the patient's clinical presentation. Considerable reader expertise is needed to interpret spiral CT scans, especially if the timing of the contrast injection and image acquisition is not perfect, which in critically ill patients is not uncommon. The largest study to systematically examine the diagnostic accuracy of CT scanning for PE diagnosis was PIOPED II; 83% of patients with PE had a positive spiral CT (i.e., sensitivity) and 96% of patients without PE had a negative spiral CT (i.e., specificity). Addition of CT venography (imaging of the veins during the venous-phase of the contrast circulation) improved the sensitivity to 90%. Specificity was also high (95%). If there is a low clinical risk of PE and the spiral CT is negative, no further testing is needed. However, if the spiral CT results are discordant with clinical suspicion, additional testing should be performed.

H. **Pulmonary angiography.** Despite the advantages of noninvasive techniques, a significant proportion of patients require angiography to confirm or exclude pulmonary embolism with certainty. Mortality of the procedure is less than 0.5%. Morbidity occurs in approximately 5%, usually related to catheter insertion and contrast reactions.

I. **Magnetic resonance angiography (MRA)** has high sensitivity and specificity. Emergency availability of MRA and the appropriate monitoring of unstable patients in the scanner are potential limitations.

VI. Treatment

A. **Resuscitation.** PE causes hypoxemia early in the course by altering ventilation/perfusion balance. Supplemental oxygen usually restores arterial oxygen tension during this phase. However, massive PR may result in intracardiac

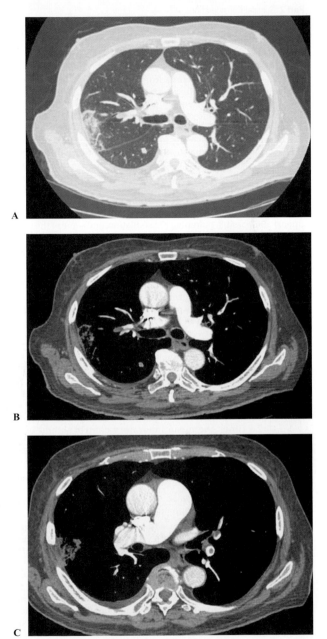

FIGURE 22-1 Computed tomography of the chest of a patient with acute thromboembolism. Panel A (lung windows) shows a right upper lobe infarct. Panel B shows an acute thromboembolus of the right upper lobe and right lower lobe segmental arteries. Panel C shows an acute thromboembolus of the left lower lobe and lingual arteries. Courtesy of Dr. Jo- Anne Shepard.

shunting in patients with a patent foramen ovale or atrial septal defect and refractory hypoxemia following PE should alert clinicians to this possibility and the potential for paradoxical arterial embolization. Later in the course of PE (24–48 hours), atelectasis from surfactant dysfunction, or less commonly pulmonary infarction or hemorrhage, produces intrapulmonary shunting and more refractory hypoxemia. Patients with hypotension require cautious volume resuscitation as increased RV volumes with fluid resuscitation will increase RV wall tension and RV oxygen consumption at a time when aortic diastolic pressure and right coronary blood flow are jeopardized. The net effect may be RV ischemia and worsening shock. It is recommended that volumes of isotonic crystalloid more than 500 to 1,000 mL be administered with caution. Hypotension refractory to volume resuscitation requires intravenous vasopressor therapy. No randomized trials are available. Initial treatment with norepinephrine is rationale. The addition of dobutamine can be tried for refractory hypotension for additional inotropic support and possible pulmonary vasodilation, and some of the elevated pulmonary vascular resistance following PE appears to be due to vasoconstriction in addition to physical obstruction of the vascular bed by thrombi. Inhaled NO may also improve hemodynamics in this setting while suitable patients are prepared for embolectomy.

B. **Unfractionated heparin.** Anticoagulation with an unfractionated heparin or low-molecular-weight heparin (LMWH) should be considered as soon as pulmonary embolism is suspected in patients without contraindications. LMWH is the treatment of choice for most patients with hemodynamically stable PE. However, patients with massive PE and critically ill patients with PE in the ICU requiring numerous procedures or surgeries and those with renal failure are best treated initially with unfractionated heparin, barring contraindications to anticoagulation.

   1. **Dose.** The constant intravenous infusion of unfractionated heparin is the current standard of care for most patients with DVT or PE. A bolus of 75 u/kg should be followed by approximately 18 u/kg/h in most patients. An activated partial thromboplastin time (aPTT) of 1.5 to 2.5 times the mean laboratory control should be achieved within 24 hours, and this should correspond to a heparin level of 0.2 to 0.4 u/mL in plasma. Fatal recurrences on anticoagulant therapy usually occur within the first week after diagnosis, and failure to reach a therapeutic aPTT increases the risk for recurrence or extension of DVT 10-fold.

   2. **The duration** of heparin therapy for massive PE should be at least 5 to 7 days, with 5 days of overlap with **Coumadin.**

   3. **Complications.** Hemorrhage is the major complication of heparin therapy, occurring in approximately 1% of patients per day after the first day. Heparin may also cause thrombocytopenia (3%–4%) with or without thrombosis.

   4. **Contraindications.** Absolute contraindications to heparin are intracranial bleed or tumor, active gastrointestinal (GI bleeding), retroperitoneal hemorrhage, proliferative retinopathy with hemorrhage, heparin-associated thrombocytopenia, and malignant pericarditis. A known bleeding diathesis and recent surgery are relative contraindications.

C. **LMWH** are typically administered by subcutaneous injection, have more predictable dose–response characteristics than unfractionated heparin, and can be given without the need for monitoring of an anticoagulant effect. They are equally effective and possibly safer than unfractionated heparins.

It is important to note that **spinal or epidural hematomas** have been associated with spinal or epidural anesthesia and lumbar punctures in patients receiving LMWH or heparinoids. The risk of epidural hematoma formation is increased in patients who have indwelling epidural catheters or are also receiving other drugs that may adversely affect hemostasis.

D. Direct thrombin inhibitors. Lepirudin and **argatroban** are direct thrombin inhibitors that can be used for treatment of thrombosis associated with HIT. Argatroban is given at 0.5 μg/kg/min intravenously and adjusted until steady-state aPTT is 1.5 to 3 times the initial baseline value (not to exceed 100 seconds). Because argatroban artificially elevates the international normalized ratio (INR), when starting warfarin, discontinue argatroban when INR reaches 4.0. Recheck INR in 4 hours to confirm therapeutic range has been achieved with warfarin. Lepirudin is given intravenously with a loading dose of 0.4 mg/kg followed by 0.15 mg/kg/h until steady-state aPTT is 1.5 to 3 times the initial baseline value. Lepirudin does not artificially elevate the INR.

E. Oral anticoagulants

1. **Onset of action.** Because the antithrombotic effect of Coumadin is due to prothrombin (factor II) depletion, and because it takes roughly 5 days for prothrombin to fall to an effective antithrombotic level (roughly 20% of normal), Coumadin should not be used alone in the acute setting.

2. **Monitoring.** An INR of 2.5 should be targeted for most patients.

3. **Duration of treatment.** Six weeks of Coumadin is sufficient for calf vein thrombosis. Three to six months are recommended for patients with proximal DVT and for patients with PE. Patients with idiopathic venous thrombosis are likely to exhibit recurrence even after 6 months of Coumadin (2-year incidence up to 27%), and 6 to 12 months of anticoagulation is reasonable in this setting. Lifelong anticoagulation is considered for recurrent episodes or a first event with a nonreversible risk factor such as cancer, homozygous factor V Leiden carriers, or antiphospholipid antibody syndrome.

F. Thrombolytic therapy

1. **Indications.** Thrombolytic therapy is approved for proximal DVT and massive PE (emboli causing hemodynamic instability). Some authors recommend lytic therapy for patients with echocardiographic evidence of RV dysfunction during acute embolization along with biomarker evidence of RV injury (troponin) or strain (BNP). However, randomized trials are needed to determine if such a strategy improves short- or long-term outcomes with an acceptable risk to benefit profile. Because mortality appears to be similar and complications are less with heparin, we favor the use of thrombolytic therapy only for acute massive PE with hemodynamic compromise. We favor Alteplase at the FDA recommended dose of 100 mg IV over 2 hours.

2. **The objective** of thrombolysis for DVT is complete and rapid removal of thrombus and preservation of venous valvular function, leading to a reduction in postphlebitic complications. Severe postphlebitic complications (e.g., edema, pain, and ulceration) are probably reduced with streptokinase compared to heparin, but the effect is small. The objective of thrombolytic agents for PE is to accelerate clot lysis, reduce pulmonary artery pressure, improve RV function, and improve survival. Although no reduction in mortality has been shown in comparison with heparin in large prospective series, a recent smaller study of tissue plasminogen activator (tPA) hinted at a survival advantage with

lysis, though the heparin dosing schedule was suboptimal. Thrombolytic therapy may allow improved pulmonary function after recovery, and a recent long-term follow-up study suggested improved exercise tolerance 7 years after thrombolysis.

3. **Contraindications.** Absolute contraindications include intracranial bleeding or a strong possibility thereof, or other major bleeding. Relative contraindications are recent (10 days) surgery or trauma.

4. **Complications.** Bleeding complications correlate poorly with coagulation parameters but are increased by performing invasive procedures. Patients in whom thrombolytic therapy is considered should have procedures performed in distal vessels, if possible. As many as one-third of patients treated with streptokinase develop mild fever, and a smaller number have allergic reactions, usually manifested by urticaria, itching, or flushing. Hypotension may occur in approximately 10% and limits the use of this agent in unstable patients.

G. **Inferior vena caval filters.** If anticoagulation is strongly contraindicated or if emboli recur despite adequate anticoagulation, an inferior vena cava interruption procedure should be performed to prevent further embolization from leg or pelvic veins. Removable inferior vena caval filters are now available. These offer an attractive alternative because there is increased risk of new or recurrent DVT post–vena caval filter placement. Depending on the type, filters can be removed 2 weeks to 3 months after placement. More data are needed on their efficacy and long-term outcomes.

H. **Pulmonary embolectomy.** The utility of emergency pulmonary embolectomy for massive PE is uncertain. Eighty percent of those who die from emboli do so in the first hour. Only rarely can an embolectomy be accomplished in this time frame. Published mortality during thromboembolectomy is as high as 57% in emergency procedures and 25% in semiurgent procedures. Randomized comparison with thrombolytic therapy has not been performed. Transvenous catheter embolectomy or catheter fragmentation can be considered as an alternative to operative embolectomy in nonsurgical candidates. The use of newer techniques of pulmonary embolectomy in patients with large clot burden and RV dysfunction has been evaluated in a small number of patients, with only 11% mortality, but the use of these techniques in the critically ill patient needs further investigation.

Selected References

Aklog L, Williams CS, Byrne JG, et al. Acute pulmonary embolectomy: a contemporary approach. *Circulation* 2002;105:1416–1419.

Anderson FA, Spender FA. Risk factors for venous thromboembolism. *Circulation* 2003;107: 9–16.

Brender E. Use of emboli-blocking filters increases, but rigorous data are lacking. *JAMA* 2006;295:989.

Dauphine C, Omari B. Pulmonary embolectomy for acute massive pulmonary embolism. *Ann Thorac Surg* 2005;79:1240.

Decousus H, Leizorovicz A, Parent F, et al. A clinical trial of vena caval filters in the prevention of pulmonary embolism in patients with proximal deep-vein thrombosis. *N Engl J Med* 1998;338:409–415.

de Gregorio MA, Gamboa P, Gimeno MJ, et al. The Gunther Tulip retrievable filter: prolonged temporary filtration by repositioning within the inferior vena cava. *J Vasc Interv Radiol* 2003;14:1259–1265.

Ghignone M, Girling L, Prewitt RM. Volume expansion versus norepinephrine in treatment of a low cardiac output complicating an acute increase in right ventricular afterload in dogs. *Anesthesiology* 1984;60:132.

Gulba DC, Schmid C, Borst HG, et al. Medical compared with surgical treatment for massive pulmonary embolism. *Lancet* 1994;343:576–577.

Horlander KT, Leeper KV. Troponin levels as a guide to treatment of pulmonary embolism. *Curr Opin Pulm Med* 2003;9:374.

Jardin F, Genevray B, Brun-Ney D, Margairaz A. Dobutamine: a hemodynamic evaluation in pulmonary embolism shock. *Crit Care Med* 1985;13:1009.

Kanne JP, Lalani TA, et al. Role of computed tomography and magnetic resonance imaging for deep venous thrombosis and pulmonary embolism. *Circulation* 2004;109:I15–I21.

Kucher N, Goldhaber SZ. Management of massive pulmonary embolism. *Circulation* 2005; 112:e28.

Koning R, Cribier A, Gerber L, et al. A new treatment for severe pulmonary embolism: percutaneous rheolytic thrombectomy. *Circulation* 1997;96:2498–2500.

Kostantinides S, Geibel A, Heusel G, et al. Heparin plus alteplase compared with heparin alone in patients with submassive pulmonary embolism. *N Engl J Med* 2002;347:1143–1150.

Meyer G, Tamisier D, Sors H, et al. Pulmonary embolectomy: a 20-year experience at one center. *Ann Thorac Surg* 1991;51:232–236.

Mismetti P, Rivron-Guillot K, Quenet S, et al. A prospective long-term study of 220 patients with a retrievable vena cava filter for secondary prevention of venous thromboembolism. *Chest* 2007;131:223.

Rocha AT, Tapson VF. Venous thromboembolism in intensive care. *Clin Chest Med* 2003;24: 103–122.

Sohne M, Ten Wolde M, Boomsma F, et al. Brain natriuretic peptide in hemodynamically stable acute pulmonary embolism. *J Thromb Haemost* 2006;4:552.

Stein PD, Fowler SE, Goodman LR, et al. Multidetector computed tomography for acute pulmonary embolism. *N Engl J Med* 2006;354:2317.

Tapson VF. Acute pulmonary embolism. *N Engl J Med* 2008;358:1037.

Tapson VF, Carroll BA, Davidson BL, et al. The diagnostic approach to acute venous thromboembolism: a clinical practice guideline. *Am J Respir Crit Care Med* 1999;160:1043–1066.

Velmahos GC, Vassiliu P, Wilcox A, et al. Spiral computed tomography for the diagnosis of pulmonary embolism in critically ill surgical patients: a comparison with pulmonary angiography. *Arch Surg* 2001;136:505–511.

Wells PS, Anderson DR, Rodger M, et al. Evaluation of D-dimer in the diagnosis of suspected deep-vein thrombosis. *N Engl J Med* 2003;349:1227–1235.

Wood KE. Major pulmonary embolism: review of a pathophysiologic approach to the golden hour of hemodynamically significant pulmonary embolism. *Chest* 2002;121:877–905.

23

Discontinuation of Mechanical Ventilation

Bishr Haydar and Jean Kwo

I. Prolonged intubation and mechanical ventilation are associated with significant complications and an increase in mortality—they should be discontinued as soon as the conditions that caused the patient to require it stabilize and begin to resolve.

    A. Reintubation of the trachea is associated with an eightfold increase in pneumonia and a six- to twelvefold increase in mortality.

    B. A reintubation rate of 5% to 15% likely reflects an optimal balance between the risks of prolonged intubation and reintubation.

II. **Definitions**

    A. Weaning is the gradual withdrawal of ventilator support.

    B. Discontinuation or **liberation** refers to the removal of ventilator support. Many patients can be successfully liberated from mechanical ventilation without weaning.

    C. Extubation is the removal of the endotracheal tube.

    D. Decannulation is the removal of a tracheostomy tube.

    E. Ventilator dependence is the need for mechanical ventilation beyond 24 hours or a failure to respond to attempts at discontinuation of mechanical ventilation.

III. **Ventilator dependence** is often multifactorial, and identifying all potential contributing causes is of the highest importance.

    A. Respiratory issues leading to continued ventilator dependence can be due to respiratory pump insufficiency, an elevated respiratory muscle load, or a mismatch between these two factors. Patients with an imbalance between respiratory pump capacity and load often exhibit rapid shallow breathing during a spontaneous breathing trial (SBT).

        1. Respiratory load (see Chapter 4) depends on both respiratory system (resistance and compliance) and ventilatory drive (estimated by the minute ventilation) mechanics.

            a. Airways resistance (R_{aw}) is due to bronchoconstriction, airway inflammation, or secretions in the airway. Increased R_{aw} is treated with bronchodilators, airway clearance, and steroids.

                (1) In patients with airways obstruction, the load imposed by **dynamic hyperinflation** ("auto-PEEP" or "intrinsic PEEP," **Chapter 4**) can be an important contributor to ventilator dependence.

            b. Respiratory system compliance (C_{RS}) determines the pressure needed to inflate the lungs and chest wall by a given volume once static conditions have been reached.

                (1) Decreased lung compliance may be due to pulmonary edema, lung consolidation, infection, or fibrosis.

                (2) Decreased chest wall compliance can be due to either chest wall abnormalities or intra-abdominal processes.

    c. Minute ventilation (V_E) is normally <10 L/min. An increase in carbon dioxide production (Vco_2) (e.g., sepsis or acute burn injuries) or an increase in dead space (V_D) requires an increased V_E to maintain a normal $Paco_2$.

2. **Respiratory pump insufficiency**
   a. **Metabolic factors** such as nutrition, electrolyte imbalances, and hormones may affect ventilatory muscle function.
      (1) Adequate **nutritional support** is necessary to prevent respiratory muscle protein catabolism and loss of muscle performance.
         i. **Overfeeding,** particularly with carbohydrates, can lead to excess CO_2 production and an increased V_E requirement.
      (2) **Electrolyte imbalances** can impair respiratory muscle function.
         i. Phosphate depletion has been associated with muscle weakness and failure of the patient to liberate from the ventilator.
         ii. Magnesium deficiency has also been associated with muscle weakness.
      (3) **Hormonal factors** such as severe hypothyroidism can lead to diaphragm weakness and a decreased respiratory drive (i.e., decreased response to hypercapnia and hypoxia).
         i. Insulin, glucagon, and adrenal corticosteroids are necessary for optimal ventilatory muscle function—their role in ventilator dependence is unclear.
3. **Sedative and narcotic drugs** are often used to treat anxiety, agitation, pain, and patient–ventilator dyssynchrony. Sedatives are usually infused continuously to provide a constant level of sedation and improve patient comfort.
   a. Prior to starting an SBT, sedatives should be adjusted to allow sleep at night and maximum alertness and cooperation during the day.
   b. Protocols for the management of analgesia and sedation are associated with a reduction in the duration of mechanical ventilation.
   c. Coordination of SBTs with daily awakenings has been shown to expedite ventilator liberation.
4. **Neurologic diseases** such as brainstem stroke, central apnea, or occult seizures can decrease central respiratory drive from the ventilatory pump controller in the brainstem.
5. **Critical illness polyneuropathy** (CIP) and **critical illness myopathy** (CIM) **(Chapter 35)** often become apparent when patients have difficulty liberating from the ventilator.
   a. CIP occurs in patients with a history of sepsis, multiorgan failure, respiratory failure, prolonged immobility, steroids, or systemic inflammatory response syndrome (SIRS), and causes sensory motor nerve dysfunction.
   b. CIM is associated with the above, along with neuromuscular blockade, and is associated with muscle atrophy and decreased excitability.
6. **Cardiovascular issues** may hinder weaning in patients with limited cardiac reserve.
   a. With the transition from positive pressure ventilation to spontaneous ventilation, the lower intrathoracic pressure increases venous return and may overload a previously dysfunctional myocardium, precipitating acute congestive heart failure in susceptible patients.
   b. Increases in heart rate, blood pressure, and arrhythmias may occur during weaning. This may induce ischemia or myocardial dysfunction in patients with coronary artery disease.

7. **Psychologic factors** such as fear of the loss of a life support system may be an important factor in ventilator dependence. Frequent communication and reassurance for the patient and family can minimize stress.

8. As clinical data are imperfect predictors of patient readiness for ventilator discontinuation, clinicians may inadvertently prolonged mechanical ventilation. **Protocols** for ventilator weaning may reduce this effect (**Fig. 23-1**).

   a. Nurse-implemented protocols that allow for the adjustment of the level of sedatives based on either a scale or the ability to awaken a patient are associated with a shorter duration of mechanical ventilation and decreased ICU stay.

   b. Respiratory therapist- and nurse-directed protocols consisting of a **daily screening procedure followed by an SBT** can allow for the early identification of patients ready for the discontinuation of mechanical ventilation.

      (1) Multiple randomized controlled trials have shown that use of these protocols are associated with fewer days on the ventilator, fewer complications related to the ventilator, and lower ICU costs.

IV. Assessment for ventilator discontinuation potential

A. A few simple criteria should be evaluated before the patient undergoes an assessment of discontinuation potential.

1. There should be some evidence of **resolution of underlying disease** that led to respiratory failure and the need for mechanical ventilation.

2. There should be **adequate gas exchange,** both adequate oxygenation (Pao_2 >60 mm Hg on PEEP <8 cmH_2O and Fio_2 <50%) and adequate ventilation (pH ≥7.25).

3. The patient should be **hemodynamically stable** with no evidence of active myocardial ischemia or significant vasopressor support.

4. The patient should be able to initiate an **inspiratory effort.**

   a. **Sedation** should be adjusted such that the patient is awake and able to be cooperative with the weaning process.

B. **Weaning parameters** are objective measures used to assess a patient's readiness to successfully maintain spontaneous ventilation. Most of these parameters reflect only a single component of the respiratory system and are at best poor predictors of weaning outcome.

1. A V_E >15 L/min is a reasonable but weak predictor of continued ventilator dependence.

2. The **Rapid Shallow Breathing Index (RSBI)** is obtained by dividing the respiratory rate by the tidal volume (f/V_T) during the first minute of spontaneous breathing.

   a. A high RSBI >105 (i.e., rapid shallow breathing) has been used to predict the need for continued ventilator dependence, but it has not been shown to decrease the time to extubation.

3. **Maximal inspiratory pressure** (P_imax or MIP), also called the negative inspiratory force (NIF), is a **measure of respiratory muscle strength**. Because it measures the pressure generated against a prolonged airway occlusion, this maneuver requires no patient coordination and cooperation. A P_imax <−30 cmH_2O has been used to predict successful ventilator liberation, but it is often of limited usefulness.

4. The $P_{0.1}$ is the **airway occlusion pressure** measured 0.1 s after initiation of inspiration against an occluded airway and is an **index of respiratory drive**.

   a. A high respiratory drive ($P_{0.1}$ of −4 to −10 cmH_2O) has been used to predict patients with continued ventilator dependence.

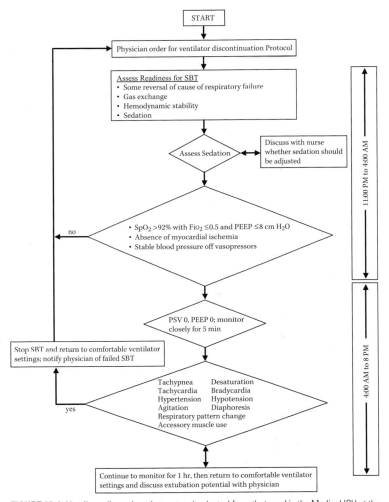

FIGURE 23-1 Ventilator discontinuation protocol, adapted from that used in the Medical ICU at the Massachusetts General Hospital. Note several characteristics of this protocol: (1) It emphasizes collaboration between the respiratory therapist, nurse, and physician. (2) After receiving a physician order, it is implemented by nonphysicians. (3) It stresses bedside assessment and spontaneous breathing trials. (4) It is completed before morning rounds, so a decision regarding extubation can be made at rounds.

      b. Measurement of the $P_{0.1}$ usually requires specialized equipment, but can be measured directly by some ventilators.
   5. Work of breathing indices (Chapter 4) have generally been limited to research applications and still need further study before they can be applied to predict weaning outcome. Because respiratory failure is

often multifactorial, individual parameters are poor predictors of weaning. A comprehensive evaluation of the patients as outlined in the preceding sections is a necessary component of successful weaning outcome. **SBTs**, where ventilator support is greatly reduced or withheld for a set period of time to assess the patient's own respiratory efforts, are the best predictor of successful ventilator discontinuation.

V. **Strategies for ventilatory management: Ventilator modes and weaning (see also Chapter 7)**

   A. There is no evidence that the gradual weaning of ventilator support, which will gradually load the respiratory system, hastens ventilator discontinuation.

   B. Newer ventilator modes such as **proportional assist ventilation** or **adaptive support ventilation (Chapter 7)** provide automated, computer-controlled weaning of ventilator support as patient effort increases, but no data yet show that they are superior to SBT.

   C. With **pressure support ventilation** (PSV), the level of inspiratory pressure assistance can be gradually decreased until the patient is able to breathe without assistance (usually a pressure support of <10 cmH_2O).

   D. With **synchronized intermittent mandatory ventilation** (SIMV), the mandatory rate is decreased gradually until the patient is able to breathe without assistance (usually when the patient receives <4 mandatory breaths/min). Several studies suggest that SIMV weaning is inferior to PSV and may prolong the duration of mechanical ventilation.

   E. An **SBT** is the best way to assess a patient's performance without ventilator support. An SBT is more predictive of a patient's readiness to breathe without ventilator support than any weaning parameter reported to date. Most patients who tolerate an SBT of 30 to 120 minutes can be discontinued from mechanical ventilation. The initial few minutes of an SBT should be closely monitored since the detrimental effects of ventilatory muscle overload usually occur early.

   F. No new mode on the ventilator has been shown to produce better outcomes for discontinuation of mechanical ventilation than an SBT.

VI. Several technical approaches for the SBT can be used.

   A. An SBT performed with a **T-piece** or **tracheostomy collar** is the technique most commonly reported in the literature. With older ventilators, there was a concern of increased resistance of the ventilator system while breathing spontaneously, but this is not an issue with modern ventilators.

   B. Several **on-ventilator approaches** to the SBT can be used. With these approaches, the monitoring capabilities of the ventilator (tidal volume, respiratory rate, minute ventilation, apnea alarms) remain active.

      1. The **PSV 0/PEEP 0** setting on the ventilator simulates a T-piece trial.

      2. A **low level of PSV** (5–7 cmH_2O) is acceptable and has been shown to have little effect on the outcome of the SBT. This approach may be useful if there is concern about the resistance through the endotracheal tube.

      3. A **low-level CPAP** (5 cmH_2O) is acceptable in many patients.

         a. An SBT with CPAP may facilitate breath triggering in patients with auto-PEEP. However, this may disguise the patient's inability to breathe adequately after extubation.

         b. An SBT with CPAP may not decrease the preload in a patient with left ventricular dysfunction. In this case, the patient may develop

TABLE 23-1	Criteria to Determine Tolerance of a Spontaneous Breathing Trial
Objective Criteria	
Gas exchange	pH >7.32; ↑Pco_2 ≤10 mm Hg; PO_2 ≥50–60 mm Hg; SpO_2 ≥85%–90%
Hemodynamics	HR <120–140/min or not changed >20%; SBP <180–200 mm Hg and >90 mm Hg; SBP not changed >20%
Ventilatory pattern	RR ≤30–35 breaths/min or not changed >50%
Subjective Criteria	
Mental status	No new or excessive somnolence, anxiety, agitation
Discomfort	No new or worsened
Diaphoresis	
Increased work of breathing	No accessory respiratory muscle use, thoracoabdominal paradox

acute cardiogenic pulmonary edema immediately following extubation.

4. **Tube compensation** is available on newer-generation ventilators (Chapter 7). With this mode, the ventilator adds pressure to overcome resistance through the endotracheal tube or tracheostomy tube.

C. **SBT duration**

1. The duration of SBT most commonly reported in the literature is 120 minutes.

2. There is no benefit of a prolonged SBT (>120 minutes) and this may contribute to a greater likelihood of failure.

3. It is possible that an SBT of 30 minutes is as predictive of readiness for ventilator discontinuation as an SBT of 120 minutes. Because most patients who fail an SBT do so early after its initiation, an SBT of 30 to 60 minutes is usually sufficient.

D. How to recognize a **failed SBT**

1. The patient must be monitored closely during the SBT and ventilator support should be promptly restored if there is clinical evidence of failure.

2. There is no single parameter to indicate whether an SBT is successful but rather a constellation of physiologic and clinical parameters is used to judge tolerance of the SBT (**Table 23-1**).

3. Common objective measurements include maintenance of acceptable gas exchange, hemodynamic stability, and a stable ventilatory pattern throughout the trial.

4. Subjective parameters include mental status, degree of discomfort, diaphoresis, and signs of increased work of breathing.

E. **Ventilator settings after a failed SBT**

1. The ventilator should be set to a nonfatiguing, comfortable mode while a search for the cause of the failed SBT is underway.

2. The clinician should take into account patient effort, ease of triggering the ventilator, flow demand, and the presence of auto-PEEP when selecting the appropriate ventilator settings.

F. Our approach to ventilator discontinuation using the SBT is shown in **Fig. 23-2**. In this protocol, the patients are closely monitored throughout the

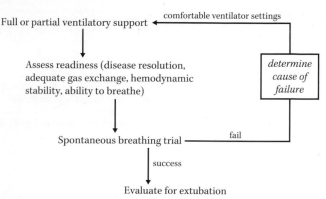

FIGURE 23-2 A simple approach to ventilator discontinuation that is independent of weaning parameters or ventilator mode.

SBT, but especially for the first 2 minutes objective and subjective criteria of respiratory insufficiency or patient distress are continually reassessed. If the SBT is judged as a failure, patients have their ventilator support temporarily increased, as they may have fatigue or subjective respiratory distress due to the SBT.

VII. **The cause of a failed SBT** is the same factors that led to the initiation of mechanical ventilation in the first place.
   A. Most often, **further resolution of underlying disease** is needed.
   B. **Other contributory causes** such as dynamic hyperinflation, cardiac disease and myocardial ischemia, and critical illness neuropathy/myopathy should be thoroughly investigated.
   C. **Malposition** of the tracheostomy tube should be suspected when patients fail to wean off a low level of support or develop respiratory distress quickly after removal of positive pressure ventilation. Bronchoscopic examination often reveals occlusion of the airway device by the posterior membrane of the trachea. One study found a 10% incidence of tracheostomy tube malposition and this was associated with a 10-day prolongation of mechanical ventilation.
   D. Once the cause for the failed SBT is corrected, the SBT should be repeated.
   E. An SBT once per day is usually sufficient unless the cause of the failed SBT is rapidly resolved.

VIII. **Extubation.** Once a patient successfully completes an SBT, the clinician needs to assess whether there is a continued need for an artificial airway.
   A. Prior to extubation, patients should be evaluated for their ability to **protect the airway.**
      1. Patients with a poor cough, a large amount of secretions, poor mental status, or significant neurologic deficits may fail extubation because the endotracheal tube allows easy suctioning of the airway.
      2. Assessment of a patient's ability of clear airway secretions includes noting the quality of cough during suctioning, the absence of excessive secretions, and the frequency of suctioning (e.g., less than every 2 hours).

3. The **white card test** assesses the ability of a patient to expel secretions unto a white card held 1 to 2 cm from the endotracheal tube. Patients who are unable to do so are more likely to fail extubation.
4. Low **cough peak flows** (<60 L/min) have been associated with a five-fold increase in extubation failure and increased mortality.
5. If the ability to protect the airway is not expected to recover, these patients may require tracheostomy prior to ventilator liberation.

B. **Upper airway edema** can lead to extubation failure.
   1. This most commonly occurs with prolonged mechanical ventilation, smaller airways (female gender, children), trauma, and repeated or traumatic intubation.
   2. A **leak test** performed with the cuff of the endotracheal tube deflated can identify patients at risk for upper airway obstruction.
      a. The presence of leak with cuff deflation suggests absence of significant upper airway swelling.
      b. Absence of a leak is affected by factors in addition to upper airway swelling which limits its ability to predict postextubation stridor.
   3. Intravenous steroids given 12 hours before planned extubation may reduce extubation failure and reintubation.
   4. Patients who develop postextubation stridor can be treated with nebulized epinephrine and/or steroids.
      a. Heliox may also be used temporarily to improve airflow through the upper airway.
      b. Mask CPAP may stent the airway open.
      c. Heliox and CPAP treat only the symptom of stridor and do not reduce upper airway swelling.
   5. **Patient cooperation** is a key component to a successful extubation.
      a. Ideally, the patient is alert, comfortable, and able to follow instructions to cough.
      b. Judicious use of anxiolytics and pain medicines can help achieve that goal.

C. For borderline cases, the difficulty of initial intubation should also be considered.

IX. The role of **noninvasive positive pressure ventilation** (NPPV) periextubation
A. **Extubation to NPPV**
   1. Selected patients, particularly those with COPD who fail an SBT, may be considered for extubation to NPPV.
   2. Postextubation support with NPPV in carefully selected patients is associated with decreased duration of mechanical ventilation, decreased incidence of nosocomial pneumonia, decreased ICU stay, and increased survival.

B. The available evidence **does not support the use of NPPV as a rescue** to patients who develop respiratory failure following a planned extubation and may potentially be harmful.

X. Approach to the **long-term ventilated patient**
   A. As many as 20% of medical ICU patients require prolonged mechanical ventilation (defined as >6 hours per day for >21 days).
   B. Patients at risk for prolonged mechanical ventilation include those with underlying lung disease, chest wall trauma, neuromuscular disease, and prolonged hospitalization for multiorgan system failure or postoperative complications.
   C. **Setting the ventilator** in the long-term ventilated patient.

1. The **etiology** of prolonged mechanical ventilation is almost universally multifactorial, and it differs from patient to patient.
2. The approach to the patient with prolonged mechanical ventilation must be **tailored** to the individual patient's needs.
3. These patients are unlikely to have problems that will resolve over 24 hours, and daily SBTs to identify discontinuation potential are of limited utility.
4. These patients benefit from protocols that gradually reduce ventilator support.
   a. Daily SBTs of increasing duration may be resumed once the patient's support has been reduced past a preset threshold, determined by the physician or the protocol itself.

D. These patients have **problems that require special attention** since they are often debilitated after a long critical illness.
1. Patients benefit from a **multidisciplinary approach** involving physicians, nurses, respiratory therapists, physical therapists, and speech therapists.
2. Close attention to **nutritional status** with the adequate administration of calories and protein without overfeeding is needed.
3. **Physical therapy** is needed for muscle strengthening and to prevent contractures and improves patients' functional status.
4. **Speech therapy** is needed since these patients often have swallowing dysfunction after a prolonged intubation.
5. For some patients, **palliative care** services may be greatly beneficial, as some patients and their families may change their treatment goals.

E. **Long-term weaning units** that specialize in the care and weaning of patients on long-term mechanical ventilation have been shown to be safe and effective for weaning ICU patients from mechanical ventilation.
1. These units provide a **structured program** for the medically complex patient with frequent physician monitoring and nursing skilled in the care of the ventilated patient.
2. These units become appropriate when the patient has become hemodynamically stable and the comorbidities requiring an acute level of care have been reduced.
3. Because they generally have less intensive staffing, these units are less costly. They can be freestanding long-term acute care hospitals and thus serve many hospitals in a geographic area, or they may be units within a host hospital.

F. Some patients may require **life-long mechanical ventilation.**
1. A home-ventilator support program should be established.
2. Available data from long-term weaning hospitals suggest that unless the patient has evidence for clearly irreversible disease (e.g., high spinal cord injury, amyotrophic lateral sclerosis), several months may be needed for a patient with respiratory failure to be discontinued from mechanical ventilation.

XI. **Decannulation** is the removal of a tracheostomy tube
A. A tracheostomy improves patient comfort, facilitates talking, improves mouth care, and may decrease airways resistance. This may promote weaning from mechanical ventilation.
B. The optimal time of tracheostomy tube placement has not yet been established. A meta-analysis showed tracheostomy placement within 7 days of intubation decreased patient days on the ventilator and ICU length of stay. However, there was no difference in patient mortality.

C. Timing of decannulation

1. The tracheostomy stoma may narrow or close within 48 to 72 hours of removal of the tracheostomy tube, leading to difficulty in replacement of the tube should respiratory difficulties arise after decannulation.

2. A systematic assessment of a patient's readiness for decannulation is needed.

   a. The patient should have a **stable respiratory status** after discontinuation of mechanical ventilation.

   b. The patient should be able to **protect the airway.**

      (1) This can be assessed by deflation of the tracheostomy cuff and observation for signs of aspiration.

      (2) A small amount of blue dye can be introduced into the oral cavity and suctioning of the tracheostomy tube undertaken at regular intervals. The presence of any blue color at the tracheostomy site or within the suction catheter indicates that the patient is at risk for aspiration.

   c. **Anatomic abnormalities of the airway** such as granulation tissue, strictures, and vocal cord injuries are a complication of long-term intubation.

   d. Adequacy of the native airway can be assessed by deflating the tracheostomy cuff and capping the tube.

      (1) Adults who can breathe around a capped size 7.0 or 8.0 tracheostomy tube have adequate respiratory muscle function and a sufficiently preserved native airway to tolerate decannulation.

      (2) Patients who fail breathing trials with capped tracheostomy tubes should be evaluated by **flexible fiberoptic bronchoscopy** above and below the tracheostomy tube for evidence of airway lesions.

   e. Patients with limited ventilatory reserve due to neuromuscular disease or COPD may benefit from stepwise **downsizing and capping** of the tracheostomy tube.

      (1) Patients who can breathe and clear secretions around a small, capped tube may be decannulated.

      (2) Occasionally, the patient with moderate secretions may have difficulty because the presence of the tracheostomy impairs secretion clearance through the native airway. These patients may benefit from placement of a **stomal obturator.**

XII. Successful liberation from mechanical ventilation improves patient survival—in one review, successful weaning in a specialized unit reduced mortality by sevenfold. Severity of acute illness (i.e., APACHE III score), multiple comorbidities, and poor prehospital functional status were all predictors of poor outcome.

Selected References

Bigatello LM, Stelfox HT, Berra L, et al. Outcomes of patients undergoing prolonged mechanical ventilation after critical illness. *Crit Care Med* 2007;35:2491–2497.

Brochard L, Rauss A, Benito S, et al. Comparison of three methods of gradual withdrawal from ventilatory support during weaning from mechanical ventilation. *Am J Respir Crit Care Med* 1994;150:896–903.

Ely EW, Meade MO, Haponik EF, et al. Mechanical ventilator weaning protocols driven by nonphysician health-care professionals: evidence-based clinical practice guidelines. *Chest* 2001;120:454S–463S.

Epstein SK. Decision to extubate. *Intensive Care Med* 2002;28:535–546.

Esteban A, Alia I, Gordo F, et al. Extubation outcome after spontaneous breathing trials with T-tube or pressure support ventilation. *Am J Respir Crit Care Med* 1997;156:459–465.

Esteban A, Frutos F, Tobin MJ, et al. A comparison of four methods of weaning patients from mechanical ventilation. *N Engl J Med* 1995;332:345–350.

Esteban A, Frutos-Vivar F, Ferguson ND, et al. Noninvasive positive-pressure ventilation for respiratory failure after extubation. *N Engl J Med* 2004;350:2452–2460.

Ferrer M, Esquinas A, Arancibia F, et al. Noninvasive ventilation during persistent weaning failure: a randomized controlled trial. *Am J Respir Crit Care Med* 2003;168:70–76.

Francois B, Bellissant E, Gissot V, et al. 12-h pretreatment with methylprednisolone versus placebo for prevention of postextubation laryngeal oedema: a randomized double-blind trial. *Lancet* 2007;369:1083–1089.

Griffiths J, Barber VS, Morgan L, et al. Systematic review and meta-analysis of studies of the timing of tracheostomy in adult patients undergoing artificial ventilation. *BMJ* 2005;330:1243–1248.

Hurford WE, Favorito F. Association of myocardial ischemia with failure to wean from mechanical ventilation. *Crit Care Med* 1995;23:1475–1480.

Keenan SP, Powers C, McCormack DG, et al. Noninvasive positive-pressure ventilation for postextubation respiratory distress: a randomized controlled trial. *JAMA* 2002;287:3238–3244.

MacIntyre NR, Cook DJ, Ely EW Jr, et al. Evidence-based guidelines for weaning and discontinuing ventilatory support. *Chest* 2001;120:375S–395S.

MacIntyre NR, Epstein SK, Carson S, Scheinhorn D, Christopher K, Muldoon S. A NAMDRC Consensus Conference. *Chest* 2005;128:3937–3954.

Meade M, Guyatt G, Cook D, et al. Predicting success in weaning from mechanical ventilation. *Chest* 2001;120:400S–424S.

Petter AH, Chiolero RL, Cassina T, et al. Automatic "Respirator/Weaning" with adaptive support ventilation: the effect on duration of endotracheal intubation and patient management. *Anesth Analg* 2003;97:1743–1750.

Schmidt U, Hess D, Kwo J, et al. Tracheostomy tube malposition in patients admitted to a respiratory acute care unit following prolonged ventilation. *Chest* 2008;134:288–294.

Schweickert WD, Gehlbach BK, Pohlman AS, et al. Daily interruption of sedative infusions and complications of critical illness in mechanically ventilated patients. *Crit Care Med* 2004; 32:1272–1276.

Smina M, Salam A, Khamiees M, et al. Cough peak flows and extubation outcomes. *Chest* 2003;124:262–268.

24

Acute Kidney Injury

Beverly Newhouse

I. Terminology and classification

   A. The term **acute kidney injury (AKI)** has replaced the term acute renal failure and is used to define the spectrum from minor decreases in glomerular filtration rate (GFR) to severe renal dysfunction requiring renal replacement therapy (RRT).

   B. Recently, the **RIFLE criteria** were developed to standardize the definition and classification of AKI. The acronym RIFLE denotes three increasing classes of severity—risk (R), injury (I), and failure (F), and two outcome classes—loss (L) and end-stage renal disease (E). **Table 24-1** shows the RIFLE classification system.

II. Epidemiology

   A. Depending on the definition used, it is estimated that up to 20% of all hospitalized patients and up to **65% of all critically ill patients develop some level of AKI**. Approximately, **35% of critically ill patients reach the level of failure (F) by RIFLE** criteria.

   B. AKI is an independent predictor of mortality in critically ill patients, with an **associated mortality of 15% to 60%**. In patients who have had a myocardial infarction, AKI is a major risk factor for further cardiovascular complications.

   C. Increasing RIFLE class is associated with increasing length of hospital stay and increasing mortality.

   D. Of those patients with AKI who survive, most regain kidney function to dialysis independence within 30 days.

III. Risk factors

   A. **Risk factors** for development of AKI in the **ICU** include age >65, infection, cardiac failure, respiratory failure, liver disease, and a history of lymphoma/leukemia. The most common factor contributing to AKI is **sepsis,** followed by **hypotension** and **IV contrast**.

   B. **Risk factors** for the **perioperative** development of AKI include prolonged aortic clamping, emergency rather than elective surgery, baseline creatinine clearance less than 47 mL/min, diabetes, and the use of higher volumes (>100 mL) of intravenous (IV) contrast media.

IV. Etiology and pathophysiology

   A. AKI has traditionally been divided into **prerenal, intrinsic renal,** and **postrenal** etiologies (**Table 24-2**). These categories are useful in understanding the pathophysiology of AKI, but rarely is the etiology of purely one category, nor is any category more benign than the others. Most hospitalized patients who develop AKI exhibit a combination of two or more etiologies.

   1. **Prerenal injury** is caused by **reduced renal perfusion** secondary to systemic hypotension, hypovolemia, heart failure, renal artery disease, or maldistribution of blood flow.

	Creatinine or GFR Criteria	Urine Output Criteria
R = Risk	Cr >1.5× baseline or GFR <25% baseline	UOP <0.5 mL/kg/h × 6 h
I = Injury	Cr >2× baseline or GFR <50% baseline	UOP <0.5 mL/kg/h × 12 h
F = Failure	Cr >3× baseline or GFR <75% baseline OR Cr ≥ 4 mg/dL or acute rise ≥ 0.5 mg/dL	UOP <0.3 mL/kg/h × 24 h OR anuria × 12 h
L = Loss	Persistence of failure criteria >4 weeks but <3 mo	
E = ESRD	Persistence of failure criteria >3 mo	

GFR, glomerular filtration rate; Cr, creatinine; UOP, urine output; ESRD, end-stage renal disease.
Adapted with permission from Bellomo R, Ronco C, et al; The Second International Consensus Conference of the Acute Dialysis Quality Initiative (ADQI) Group. Acute renal failure: definition, outcome measures, animal models, fluid therapy and information technology needs. *Crit Care* 2004;8:R204–R212.

    a. Renal hypoperfusion activates numerous neurohumoral responses that help to maintain renal perfusion pressure and GFR.

    b. **Efferent arteriolar vasoconstriction** is produced by the activation of the sympathetic and renin–angiotensin system.

    c. **Afferent arteriolar vasodilation** is produced by activation of prostaglandins, the kallikrein system, nitric oxide, and direct myogenic influences.

    d. Oliguria develops when the reduction in renal perfusion pressure exceeds the compensatory ability of these autoregulatory mechanisms to maintain adequate GFR.

  2. With sustained hypoperfusion, prerenal azotemia can lead to intrinsic renal injury. **Intrinsic renal injury** is caused by **renal parenchymal injury** resulting from **acute tubular necrosis (ATN)**, interstitial nephritis, embolic disease, glomerulonephritis, vasculitis, or small vessel disease. In critically ill patients, intrinsic renal injury most commonly results from **ischemic** or **nephrotoxic** injury.

    a. **ATN** is the most common cause of intrinsic acute renal injury, resulting from ischemia (50%), toxins (35%), or multifactorial causes.

      (1) **Ischemic ATN** results from prolonged renal hypoperfusion, including prolonged prerenal azotemia.

      (2) **Nephrotoxic ATN** can result from endogenous (e.g., myoglobin, hemoglobin) or exogenous (e.g., aminoglycoside, contrast) toxins.

    b. The **pathophysiology** of ATN involves

      (1) **Intrarenal vasoconstriction** leading to decreased blood flow to the renal cortex and outer medulla.

      (2) **Tubular cell injury** involving loss of the apical brush border, loss of polarity, and disruption of intercellular tight junctions.

      (3) **Leukocyte infiltration.**

      (4) **Reperfusion injury.**

T A B L E	
24-2	Etiologies of Acute Kidney Injury in the Intensive Care Unit

Prerenal	Intrinsic Renal	Postrenal (Obstructive)

Intravascular volume depletion
 • GI fluid loss (e.g., vomiting, diarrhea, EC fistula)
 • Renal fluid loss (e.g., diuretics)
 • Burns
 • Blood loss
 • Redistribution of fluid (e.g., "third-spacing," pancreatitis, cirrhosis)
	Acute tubular necrosis
	 • Ischemic
	 • Toxin-induced
	   − Drugs
	   − IV contrast
	   − Rhabdomyolysis
	   − Massive hemolysis
	   − Tumor lysis syndrome
		Upper urinary tract obstruction
		 • Nephrolithiasis
		 • Hematoma
		 • Aortic aneurysm
		 • Neoplasm

Decreased renal perfusion pressure • Shock (e.g., sepsis) • Vasodilatory drugs • Preglomerular (afferent) arteriolar vasoconstriction • Postglomerular (efferent) arteriolar vasodilation	Acute interstitial nephritis • Drug-induced • Infection-related • Systemic diseases (e.g., SLE) • Malignancy	Lower urinary tract obstruction • Urethral stricture • Hematoma • Benign prostatic hypertrophy • Neurogenic bladder • Malpositioned urethral catheter • Neoplasm
Decreased cardiac output • Congestive heart failure • Myocardial ischemia	Acute glomerulonephritis • Postinfectious • Systemic vasculitis • TTP/HUS • Rapidly progressive GN Vascular • Atheroembolic disease • Renal artery or vein thrombosis • Renal artery dissection • Malignant hypertension Hepatorenal syndrome Increased intra-abdominal pressure	

GI, gastrointestinal; EC, enterocutaneous; IV, intravenous; SLE, systemic lupus erythematosus; TTP, thrombotic thrombocytopenic purpura; HUS, hemolytic uremic syndrome; GN, glomerulonephritis.
Adapted with permission from Barozzi L, Valentino M et al. Renal ultrasonography in critically ill patients. *Crit Care Med* 2007;35(5 suppl):S198–S205 and Acute renal failure. In: Glassock RJ, ed. *Nephrology self-assessment program (NephSAP)*, Vol. 2, No. 2. Philadelphia: Lippincott Williams & Wilkins, 2003:42–43.

    c. Phases of ATN:

      (1) Initiation phase, the period immediately following the renal insult, during which tubular injury has not occurred and the process is still potentially preventable.

      (2) Maintenance phase, which begins with the onset of tubular injury and defines the onset of a decrease in GFR. This phase can last from days to weeks and can manifest with variable urine output.

      (3) Recovery phase, in which cellular regeneration restores tubular integrity and function, with improvement in GFR and return of renal function to baseline or near baseline.

3. Postrenal injury is caused by **obstruction** to the urinary tract at the level of the ureters, bladder, or urethra with resultant renal congestion and hydronephrosis. Complete obstruction results in anuria, whereas incomplete obstruction results in variable urine output.

    a. GFR can be maintained by continued salt and water absorption, **dilation of the collecting system** (with a resulting decrease in intratubular pressure), and changes in renal hemodynamics.

    b. Following relief of the obstruction, a **postobstructive diuresis** can ensue from the elimination of retained salt and water and from tubular defects incurred during the obstructive process.

    c. Upper urinary tract obstruction may require a ureteral stent or percutaneous nephrostomy to relieve the obstruction, while lower urinary tract obstruction is treated with bladder catheterization, either transurethral or percutaneous.

    d. Recovery of renal function is dependent on the duration of obstruction. Complete recovery can usually be expected with an obstructive duration of less than 1 week, whereas minimal recovery is expected with obstructive duration exceeding 12 weeks.

V. Prevention of AKI

  A. Objectives are to **limit dehydration, maintain adequate circulating blood volume and renal perfusion,** and **minimize exposure to nephrotoxins.**

  B. Studies have found the following interventions to be beneficial in the **prevention** of AKI:

    1. Hydration with **0.9% sodium chloride** in patients who will receive IV contrast to prevent contrast nephropathy. The use of a **sodium bicarbonate** solution given as a bolus of 3 mL/kg/h for 1 hour before contrast administration, followed by an infusion of 1 mL/kg/h for 6 hours after the procedure showed benefit in one randomized controlled trial. However, these results were not repeated in a more recent, similar trial of patients undergoing coronary angiography, which found no benefit to sodium bicarbonate versus normal saline.

    2. Administration of oral *N*-acetylcysteine (NAC), either 600 or 1,200 mg PO twice per day for 2 days, plus hydration (versus hydration alone) in patients at high risk for contrast nephropathy. NAC plus sodium bicarbonate infusion was more effective than NAC plus sodium chloride in one study.

    3. Use of **low osmolality** (e.g., iopromide, 607 mOsm/kg) or **iso-osmolar** (e.g., iodixanol, 290 mOsm/kg) contrast media compared to high osmolality media. This benefit has been greatest in patients with underlying renal impairment.

    4. Use of **nonionic** versus ionic contrast.

    5. Single daily dosing of aminoglycosides rather than multiple doses.

    6. Use of **lipid formulations** of amphotericin B compared to standard formulations.

C. There are either conflicting or insufficient data for the following interventions and their role in **prevention** of AKI:

1. **Fenoldopam** is a selective dopamine-1 receptor agonist that causes vasodilation. While it has been shown to increase renal blood flow and creatinine clearance, no clear benefit in outcome has been shown, and potential harm may occur secondary to hypotension and decreased renal perfusion pressure.

2. **Mannitol** with hydration has not been found to decrease the incidence of AKI.

3. Prophylactic **renal replacement therapy (RRT)** with **continuous hemofiltration (CVVH)** pre- and post-contrast was shown in one controlled trial to reduce the incidence of contrast-induced AKI and mortality in patients with renal insufficiency who underwent coronary interventions. Prior to widespread endorsement of this technique, more data are necessary because of the high associated cost of RRT.

4. **Natriuretic peptides** given to patients receiving IV contrast. Atrial natriuretic peptide (ANP) increases GFR and causes natriuresis and diuresis, but there have been conflicting results in prevention of AKI and dialysis-free survival. ANP also decreases angiotensin II, potentially leading to decreased systemic vascular resistance and systemic hypotension.

D. Multiple studies have found the following interventions to be ineffective or harmful when used for the **prevention** of AKI:

1. Low-dose **dopamine** infusion.

2. **Loop diuretics**.

3. **Calcium channel blockers** in patients undergoing renal **transplant** who will receive calcineurin inhibitor immunosuppressants.

VI. Evaluation and diagnosis

A. A focused **history** seeks to identify baseline renal function, risk factors, and precipitating events.

B. The **physical examination** aims to assess **intravascular volume**, evaluating for hypervolemia (e.g., jugular venous distention) or hypovolemia (e.g., tachycardia, hypotension). Because physical signs of intravascular volume may be unreliable, invasive measurements such as central venous pressure or pulmonary capillary wedge pressure and stroke volume may be helpful (see **Chapter 1**).

C. **Evaluation of renal function.** There are two physiologic functions of the kidney that can be evaluated objectively: (1) production of urine and (2) excretion of metabolic waste products.

1. **Urine output** is commonly measured in the ICU, and is highly sensitive to changes in renal hemodynamics. However it is very nonspecific, except when significantly reduced or absent, in which case it can signify oliguric or anuric AKI. Conversely, severe AKI can exist despite normal urine output.

2. **Excretion of metabolic waste products** is the result of the **glomerular filtration rate (GFR)**. GFR is the traditional parameter used to quantify renal function. It is important to note that GFR can vary significantly with normal renal physiology. It can be difficult to accurately measure GFR, especially in critically ill patients.

   a. **Laboratory indices of GFR**

      (1) **Blood urea nitrogen (BUN)** is a poor correlate for GFR because it is a highly nonspecific indicator of renal function. The BUN will be elevated with protein loading, steroid therapy, tetracyclines, gastrointestinal bleeding, or a hypermetabolic state. Conversely, the BUN can be lowered with severe liver disease or malnutrition.

(2) **Serum creatinine concentration (Cr)** is far more specific in the assessment of renal function, but still only weakly corresponds to GFR. While it is a reasonable estimate of GFR in most patients with normal renal function, it is not accurate during the progression of AKI. The change in serum Cr from a patient's baseline may be more useful in the diagnosis of AKI than the absolute value. Cr production depends on muscle mass and may be relatively decreased in cachectic patients. Certain drugs including cimetidine, trimethoprim, and methyldopa can falsely elevate Cr.

(3) The current gold standard for quantification of GFR is measurement of **24-hour creatinine clearance.** Even this method will not accurately reveal the GFR because it tends to overestimate as creatinine excretion exceeds the filtered load. Determination of accurate GFR requires measuring inulin clearance which is not clinically feasible.

3. New **biomarkers** of renal function/injury include plasma neutrophil gelatinase-associated lipocalin, plasma cystatin C, urine neutrophil gelatinase-associated lipocalin, urine interleukin 18, and urine kidney injury molecule-1. While further study of these biomarkers is necessary, it is hoped that their measurement may lead to earlier diagnosis, prevention, and treatment of AKI.

D. **Evaluation of the urine**
1. **Urinalysis** and **determination of urine indices** are simple tests that may provide useful diagnostic information. A summary is given in **Table 24-3.**
2. **Urine indices**
   a. **Prerenal kidney injury** is associated with urine that reflects intact renal mechanisms of salt and water balance. The body's effort to augment intravascular volume results in elevation of the ratio of serum BUN to Cr concentration, high urine osmolality, and low fractional excretion of sodium (**FENa <1%**). FENa reflects the ratio of urine to serum concentration of sodium (Na) and Cr:

$$FENa = (urine\ Na/urine\ Cr)/(serum\ Na/serum\ Cr)\%$$

TABLE 24-3 Diagnostic Studies and Indices of Urine

	Prerenal	**Renal**	**Postrenal**
Dipstick	0 or trace protein	Mild-moderate protein, hemoglobin, leukocytes	0 or trace protein, red and white cells
Sediment	Few hyaline casts	Granular and cellular casts[a]	Crystals and cellular casts possible
Serum BUN/Cr	20	10	10
Urine osmolality	>500	<350	<350
Urine sodium	<20	>30	
Urine/serum Cr	>40	<20	<20
Urine/serum urea	>8	<3	<3
FENa	<1%	>1%	>1%
FEUr	<35%	>50%	

FENa, fractional excretion of sodium = (urine Na/urine Cr)/(serum Na/serum Cr)%; Cr, creatinine; FEUr, fractional excretion of urea
[a]Composition of casts depends on cause of renal failure.
Adapted with permission from Thadhani R, Pasqual M, Bonventre JV. Acute renal failure. *N Engl J Med* 1996;334:1448–1460.

      b. Disruption of tubular function with **intrinsic renal injury** usually produces a defect in urinary concentrating ability and the production of isotonic urine. The associated FENa is typically $\geq 1\%$.

  3. Specific limitations of urinary indices

      a. Pre-existing renal disease may affect salt and water homeostasis, making interpretation of urine electrolytes difficult. Patients with chronic kidney disease, adrenal insufficiency, and cerebral salt wasting may have a FENa $>1\%$ even when they are volume depleted.

      b. Diuretic administration blocks tubular reabsorption of solute, and can complicate data interpretation for up to 24 hours. When diuretics elevate the FENa, a fractional excretion of urea $<35\%$ can be an indicator of prerenal azotemia.

      c. Urinary tract obstruction, acute **glomerulonephritis,** or renal **emboli** may present with decreased GFR with normal tubular function. Highly concentrated urine is expected in these settings.

  4. Urine dipstick

      a. Proteinuria is usually associated with glomerular lesions, but may also be seen with tubular injury. Glomerular injury permits large proteins to pass into the urine as indicated by a reading of 3 to 4+ on dipstick testing. Tubular injury may prevent the normal reabsorption of small, filtered proteins as indicated by mild proteinuria of 1 to 2+.

      b. Heme-positive dipstick tests, without red blood cells in the urinary sediment, suggest hemoglobinuria or myoglobinuria.

      c. Microscopic examination of the urine sediment provides insight into the pathogenesis of AKI. Tubular casts are an indirect indication of ongoing processes in the kidney.

          (1) Hyaline casts are acellular and are consistent with prerenal azotemia. They can often be seen in healthy patients.

          (2) Granular casts contain degenerating renal tubular epithelial cells and are seen in ATN due to ischemic or nephrotoxic injuries.

          (3) Pigmented casts can be seen in hemoglobin- and myoglobin-induced AKI.

          (4) White blood cell casts indicate an inflammatory process and may be seen in pyelonephritis or acute interstitial nephritis.

          (5) Red blood cell casts indicate glomerular pathology such as glomerulonephritis.

E. Imaging techniques

  1. Imaging techniques generally are used to exclude reversible causes of urinary tract obstruction, traumatic injury, or vascular perturbations. Newer modalities also have the potential to aid in the diagnosis and evaluation of other forms of AKI.

      a. Ultrasonography is the most valuable tool for initial evaluation of postrenal obstruction (by visualization of **hydronephrosis**) and can be performed at the bedside in unstable patients. False-negative results can arise in approximately 10% of cases, early in the disease process (insufficient time for hydronephrosis to develop), with hypovolemia, or when obstruction is caused by retroperitoneal disease.

          (1) The use of ultrasound has expanded recently and is being used to evaluate **renal parenchyma** for evidence of tubular necrosis, cystic masses, and other pathology. Color **Doppler** flow can be used to assess **renal perfusion** and rule out thrombosis/occlusion.

      b. Abdominal computed tomography (CT) scan is more sensitive and can be used when ultrasonography is indeterminate. CT can provide useful detailed anatomic information on the kidneys, bladder, and urinary collecting system.

c. **Antegrade** and **retrograde pyelography** may be used for exact localization of urinary tract obstruction and to accomplish drainage.

d. **Nuclear medicine scans** may be used to assess renal function with the use of radioisotopes. Renal scintigraphy is usually applied for the assessment of renal function expressed as GFR, effective renal plasma flow, or overall kidney perfusion.

e. **Magnetic resonance imaging (MRI)** of the kidneys has potential because of the combined value of anatomical and functional information provided. MRI is able to show infiltrative kidney disorders, assess alterations in renal function, and reveal obstruction or inflammation. Ongoing studies will evaluate the value of various MRI sequences in the diagnosis of AKI. Critical care practitioners must be aware of the newly recognized syndrome of **nephrogenic systemic fibrosis (NSF),** which is associated with use of **gadolinium** contrast in patients with chronic kidney disease. This disease causes progressive fibrosis of the skin and connective tissues, leading to joint contractures, impaired mobility, and deformity. Other manifestations may include fibrosis of the heart, lungs, liver, and central nervous system. Currently, the disease has no treatment, is progressive, and can be lethal. For this reason, the U.S. FDA cautions against the use of gadolinium contrast in patients with estimated GFR 15 to 60 mL/min or those who are on dialysis and recommends consideration of prompt dialysis for those who have received gadolinium in this setting.

f. **Angiography** can be used to assess the integrity of the renal arteries and veins.

g. **Renal biopsy** is not indicated in most cases because history, physical examination, and noninvasive testing will indicate the cause of the renal injury. Biopsy may be indicated in cases of intrinsic AKI not caused by ischemia or toxins or for determining the cause of graft dysfunction after renal transplantation. The morbidity of renal biopsy is relatively low.

VII. Specific etiologies
A. Drug-related AKI
1. **Angiotensin-converting enzyme (ACE) inhibitors** and **angiotensin receptor blockers (ARBs)**

a. **Angiotensin-II** is a potent constrictor of the efferent arteriole that maintains glomerular perfusion pressure and GFR during renal hypoperfusion.

b. Inhibition of the production of angiotensin-II by ACE inhibitors or blockade of the receptor by ARBs decreases intraglomerular pressure, which is beneficial in slowing the progression of proteinuric or diabetic renal disease. Inhibition/blockade of angiotensin-II also decreases systemic vascular resistance, and these agents are commonly used in the management of hypertension and heart failure.

c. However, the decrease in intraglomerular pressure increases the risk of AKI during periods of renal hypoperfusion. Patients with **bilateral renal artery stenosis,** shock, or decreased intravascular volume are particularly susceptible.

d. Other risk factors for ACE inhibitor or ARB-induced AKI include older age, depressed ventricular function, concurrent diuretic

therapy, cirrhosis, chronic kidney disease, or the use of cyclooxygenase inhibitors, cyclosporine, or tacrolimus.

2. **Nonsteroidal anti-inflammatory drugs (NSAIDs)**
   a. **NSAIDs** can be divided into nonselective (cyclooxygenase [COX]-1
      and -2) or selective (COX-2) inhibitors of the enzyme cyclooxyge-
      nase, which is involved in the synthesis of prostaglandin precur-
      sors. COX-1 and -2 are constitutively produced in the kidneys,
      where **vasodilatory prostaglandins** are important to the maintenance
      of normal intrarenal hemodynamics.
   b. In most circumstances, there is minimal risk of injury from the use of
      NSAIDs in patients with normal renal function. However, in situa-
      tions of renal hypoperfusion, which are relatively common in criti-
      cally ill patients, the inhibition of prostaglandin-induced vasodila-
      tion with NSAIDs can further reduce renal blood flow and exacerbate
      injury.
   c. Common nonselective COX inhibitors include ibuprofen, aspirin,
      ketorolac, and indomethacin. Indomethacin is the most likely
      NSAID to cause renal impairment, and aspirin is the least likely.
   d. While *selective* COX-2 inhibitors were initially thought to be "renal
      sparing," recent data suggest that their nephrotoxic effects are sim-
      ilar to their nonselective counterparts. Furthermore, some of these
      agents have been taken off the market for their potential cardiovas-
      cular toxicity.
   e. **Risk factors** for NSAID-induced AKI include the following:
      (1) Old age.
      (2) Congestive heart failure (CHF).
      (3) Concurrent use of other potential nephrotoxins, such as amino-
          glycosides, ACE inhibitors, or ARBs.
      (4) Advanced liver disease.
      (5) Atherosclerotic vascular disease.
      (6) Chronic kidney disease.

3. **Calcineurin inhibitors (CNIs)**
   a. **CNIs** include the immunosuppressants **cyclosporine** and **tacrolimus,**
      which are used in the management of patients who have undergone
      renal transplant. These agents have led to marked improvement in
      allograft and overall patient survival since their introduction in the
      1980s. However, the use of CNIs is often limited by their potential
      for nephrotoxicity.
   b. AKI induced by CNIs leads to decreased GFR, hyperkalemia, hyper-
      tension, renal tubular acidosis (RTA), increased reabsorption of
      sodium, and decreased urine output. Often, this syndrome can be
      managed by dose reduction, but occasionally an irreversible
      chronic nephropathy develops.

4. **Aminoglycosides (AGs)**
   a. These antimicrobial agents are often used in the intensive care unit
      for the management of **severe gram-negative infections,** despite well-
      known nephrotoxicity and ototoxicity.
   b. AGs are not metabolized and are excreted unchanged by glomeru-
      lar filtration. Renal pathophysiology is related to proximal tubular
      cell toxicity with the development of **ATN.** AG-induced AKI is usu-
      ally nonoliguric with decreased urine concentrating ability, FENa
      >1%, and urinary magnesium wasting. Prognosis is usually good
      with return of renal function to baseline or near-baseline levels in
      most patients after discontinuation of the drug. Occasionally,

supportive RRT may be necessary, especially if AG-induced injury is exacerbated by other renal insults.

c. **Risk factors** include the type of AG, cumulative dose, duration and frequency of administration, and patient-related factors such as pre-existing kidney dysfunction or decreased renal perfusion.

d. AG-induced AKI occurs in approximately 10% to 20% of patients treated with these agents. Neomycin has been associated with the most toxicity; streptomycin with the least toxicity; and gentamicin, tobramycin, and amikacin with intermediate toxicity.

e. The only strategy that has been clearly shown to reduce the risk of AG-induced AKI is **once-daily dosing.** Other proposed strategies which require further study include calcium supplementation, calcium channel blockers, and antioxidants.

f. The appropriate monitoring strategy of AG serum levels in critically ill patients with unstable renal function has been the subject of debate. Traditionally, it has been recommended to monitor trough levels. However, the correlation between trough levels and toxicity can vary, and renal toxicity can occur despite careful monitoring and maintenance of levels within accepted guidelines.

5. **Amphotericin B** (see **Chapter 12**)

a. **Amphotericin B** is used in the treatment of **fungal infections** and is associated with a high incidence of nephrotoxicity. Approximately 80% of patients treated with amphotericin B experience some renal injury.

b. Pathophysiology involves injury to multiple tubular segments including the proximal tubule, ascending limb, and collecting system from direct toxicity and preglomerular vasoconstriction. The resulting abnormalities can include a type I (distal) **renal tubular acidosis (RTA)** and sodium, potassium, and magnesium wasting.

c. **Risk factors** include large dosages, duration of therapy, pre-existing renal disease, hypokalemia, hypovolemia, and concurrent use of other nephrotoxins.

d. The availability of newer alternative antifungal agents has led to a marked reduction in the use of amphotericin B. If it must be used, **preventive strategies** include IV saline loading, slower infusion rates, and use of less nephrotoxic preparations such as liposomal amphotericin B or amphotericin B colloid dispersion (see **Chapter 12**).

6. **Vancomycin**

a. **Vancomycin** is the standard agent used for the treatment of methicillin-resistant *Staphylococcus aureus* (MRSA) infections.

b. Vancomycin-induced renal injury has been reported to occur in approximately 6% to 30% of patients treated with the drug. However, most reported cases were confounded by additional risk factors for AKI, and the clinical evidence of independent renal toxicity from vancomycin is lacking. The mechanism of vancomycin-induced injury is unknown.

7. **Drugs associated with acute interstitial nephritis (AIN)**

a. **Drug-induced AIN** is an inflammatory process in the renal tubules and interstitium caused by a hypersensitivity reaction to certain medications, most commonly **β-lactam antibiotics** and **sulfonamides.**

b. Although an extensive list of agents has been implicated, the most common offenders include penicillins, cephalosporins, sulfonamides (including loop and thiazide diuretics), fluoroquinolones, phenytoin, rifampin, allopurinol, cimetidine, omeprazole, and NSAIDs (AIN with proteinuria).

    c. AIN usually occurs 1 to 2 weeks after exposure to the drug and may be characterized by systemic symptoms including fever, rash, arthralgias, eosinophilia, eosinophiluria, hematuria, and pyuria. Although the importance of **eosinophilia** in making the diagnosis of AIN is frequently emphasized, data suggest that it has a low sensitivity, albeit with a high specificity. The pathognomonic finding of AIN remains the identification of an inflammatory infiltrate by renal biopsy.

    d. Therapy involves the discontinuation of any possible offending medications and supportive care. In most cases, AIN is reversible and patients will have a gradual return to their baseline renal function. Although steroid therapy is often used and may hasten the recovery, the data for the utility of steroids in treating AIN remain controversial.

    e. It should be noted that AIN can also develop as a complication following bacterial or viral infection or as a consequence of systemic diseases such as lupus or sarcoidosis.

8. Other drugs

    a. Intravenous immune globulin (IVIG) is used for the management of immune-mediated disorders in the intensive care unit and has been associated with nephrotoxicity, most often in elderly patients with pre-existing renal dysfunction.

    b. Hydroxyethyl starches are often used as plasma volume expanders in critically ill patients, and have been associated with renal injury in the form of osmotic nephrosis.

    c. Antiretroviral agents used in the management of patients with human immunodeficiency virus have dramatically improved survival rates. Case reports have described nephropathies associated with the use of these agents, most frequently the protease inhibitor indinavir and the reverse transcriptase tenofovir.

B. Abdominal compartment syndrome (ACS, see **Chapter 9)**

    1. ACS is a multifactorial syndrome resulting from intra-abdominal hypertension. **Causes of ACS** include trauma, pancreatitis, intra-abdominal/retroperitoneal bleeding, and bowel ischemia. Primary ACS usually occurs in the setting of traumatic injury from hemorrhage and visceral edema. Secondary ACS occurs after vigorous volume resuscitation leading to the formation of ascites and visceral edema.

    2. Intra-abdominal pressure can be estimated by measuring intragastric or bladder pressure. While a normal intra-abdominal pressure is <5 to 7 mm Hg, the generally accepted upper limit is 12 mm Hg.

    3. The **hemodynamic effects** result from decreased preload (decreased venous return), increased afterload, and extrinsic compression leading to decreased oxygen delivery to organs. Signs associated with ACS include hypovolemic shock, AKI, respiratory failure with increased intrathoracic pressures, increased intracranial pressure, and acute hepatic failure.

    4. Renal injury results from a combination of hypoperfusion, aberrant intrarenal hemodynamics from the neurohumoral response to increased intra-abdominal pressure, and increased renal venous pressure. Oliguria typically occurs at bladder pressures above 15 mm Hg, while anuria occurs at pressures exceeding 25 to 30 mm Hg. Ureteral obstruction typically is not seen with ACS.

    5. Treatment of ACS is **abdominal decompression.** If the duration of insult is limited, renal function generally recovers shortly after decompression.

C. Septic AKI

    1. Sepsis is the most common cause of AKI in critically ill patients and may account for more than 50% of cases.

2. Septic AKI is defined by the presence of both **RIFLE** criteria and consensus criteria for sepsis and by the absence of other non–sepsis-related causes of AKI. The **mortality** of septic AKI is high, varying from 20% to 57% depending on the severity of AKI.

3. **Pathophysiology** of septic AKI traditionally has been related to decreased renal blood flow, vasoconstriction, ischemia, and ATN. More recent data describe renal vasodilation, hyperemia, reperfusion, and tubular cell apoptosis.

4. Routine evaluation of the urine (see **Section VI.D.1** and **Table 24-3**) has been shown to lack diagnostic accuracy, prognostic value, or clinical utility when used in the assessment of septic AKI. Emerging biomarkers of AKI may become more clinically valuable, but at this time still need further validation.

D. **Contrast-induced AKI**

1. The increasing use of highly advanced imaging and interventional procedures for diagnosis and management of illness and injury means that more patients will be exposed to **IV iodinated contrast media.**

2. **Contrast-induced AKI is defined** as a rise in serum Cr of ≥0.3 mg/dL with oliguria after exposure to iodinated IV contrast media. This typically occurs within 24 to 48 hours following exposure with a peak in Cr at 4 to 5 days, and return of near-baseline renal function within 7 to 10 days.

3. Established patient **risk factors** for contrast-induced AKI are chronic kidney disease, diabetes mellitus, volume depletion, heart failure, hemodynamic instability, and concomitant use of other nephrotoxins. The osmolality, ionicity, and volume of contrast media are important risk factors. The risk of AKI may be higher after intra-arterial administration than after IV administration.

4. The **pathogenesis** of contrast-induced AKI involves a combination of direct cytotoxicity to renal tubular cells, intrarenal vasoconstriction, and free radical–mediated injury.

5. Strategies aimed at prevention of contrast-induced AKI are illustrated in **Section V.**

E. **Ischemic AKI**

1. Ischemic insult to the kidneys typically results from states of systemic **hypoperfusion,** such as heart failure or hypovolemic shock, but can also occur with relative normotension and euvolemia.

2. Mechanisms for normotensive (or hypertensive) ischemic renal injury include thromboembolic phenomena, atherosclerotic narrowing of renal vessels, malignant hypertensive crisis, and hypercalcemia-induced vasoconstriction. These processes are characterized by impaired vasodilatory capacity of the renal vessels.

3. Ischemic injury is often exacerbated by other causes of AKI, such as septic or drug-induced nephrotoxicity.

F. **Atheroembolic disease**

1. **Embolization** of cholesterol crystals from atheromatous plaques and their subsequent lodging in renal arteries and arterioles leads to AKI from inflammation and ischemia.

2. AKI secondary to atheroembolic disease is often seen in conjunction with contrast-induced injury in patients undergoing angiographic or surgical manipulation of the aorta.

3. The **clinical signs and symptoms** of atheroembolic disease depend on the distribution of emboli. The classic syndrome includes livedo reticularis and manifestations of digital ischemia of the lower extremities,

the "blue toe syndrome." Other manifestations can include neurologic deficits, coronary ischemia, intestinal ischemia, and rhabdomyolysis. The pathognomonic finding is the identification of biconcave cholesterol crystals within blood vessels or skin lesions (most common) on biopsy. Although eosinophilia, eosinophiluria, and proteinuria have been described with this process, their sensitivity and specificity are poor.

4. Disease onset is typically subacute, and can manifest with a staggered deterioration in renal function for up to 6 to 8 weeks after an inciting event. Unlike contrast-induced AKI, **renal function rarely returns to baseline**, although it may improve after a period of deterioration.

5. Therapy is primarily supportive. Steroids have been associated with increased mortality. Mortality associated with atheroembolization has been estimated as high as 80% but is heavily weighted toward the most severe cases.

G. Small vessel vasculitis

1. **Other vascular etiologies** of AKI include antiphospholipid antibody syndrome, scleroderma, polyarteritis nodosa (PAN), hemolytic uremic syndrome (HUS), and thrombotic thrombocytopenic purpura (TTP).

H. Glomerulonephritis

1. **Glomerular disease** can be postinfectious (poststreptococcal, etc), primary immune mediated, or vasculitic (lupus, Wegener's granulomatosis, etc). **Rapidly progressive glomerulonephritis** is increasingly being identified as a cause of intrinsic AKI in the elderly.

I. Hepatorenal syndrome (HRS)

1. **HRS** describes the syndrome of AKI in the setting of severe hepatic dysfunction.

2. The **pathophysiology** involves marked arterial vasodilation (particularly of the splanchnic vasculature) and profound renal vasoconstriction with histologically normal kidneys. The intense renal vasoconstriction is a consequence of the depressed effective circulating volume and activation of neuroendocrine mediators (angiotensin, vasopressin, nitric oxide, etc) that follows the intense mesenteric vasodilation associated with advanced liver disease.

3. HRS is classified into two types:

   a. **Type I** is associated with rapid and profound deterioration in renal function (increase in serum Cr to >2.5 mg/dL or reduction in Cr clearance by 50% or to <20 mL/min over <2 weeks). It is typically seen with end-stage liver disease and often has an identifiable precipitating event, such as large-volume paracentesis, spontaneous bacterial peritonitis, or gastrointestinal bleeding. The prognosis is extremely poor with a median survival of approximately 2 weeks and >90% mortality at 3 months.

   b. **Type II** has a more insidious onset and modest deterioration in renal function without obligatory progression. Prognosis is better than that of type I HRS with a median survival of approximately 6 months.

   c. The diagnosis of HRS is typically one of exclusion. Indices of function may suggest prerenal azotemia, but response to volume loading is typically poor. The urine sediment is usually bland.

   d. Therapy is primarily supportive. Renal vasodilator therapy has not been shown to be of benefit. However, some studies suggest that mesenteric vasoconstrictors (midodrine, octreotide, the vasopressin analogues terlipressin and ornipressin), and the antioxidant NAC may be of benefit in select patients. **Transjugular intrahepatic portosystemic shunt (TIPS, Chapter 25)** has also shown benefit in treating patients with HRS who are not candidates for liver transplantation. The role of dialysis remains controversial.

    e. Liver transplantation is the definitive treatment. Renal function usually recovers following transplantation.

J. Rhabdomyolysis

1. **Rhabdomyolysis** is a syndrome of skeletal muscle breakdown which releases myoglobin, creatine phosphokinase (CPK), and electrolytes into the intravascular space.

2. **Rhabdomyolysis** causes include trauma, burns, crush injuries, ischemia, severe muscle overuse or prolonged muscle immobilization, medications, toxins, myopathies, or metabolic disorders that result in muscle breakdown.

3. **Diagnosis** is made by elevated CPK, usually more than five times the normal value. The pathognomonic finding is **cola-colored urine** with a heme-positive dipstick result but without red blood cells on microscopic examination of the urine sediment (indicating myoglobinuria). Hyperkalemia, hyperphosphatemia, hyperuricemia, hypocalcemia, and an anion-gap metabolic acidosis are frequently present.

4. **Complications** include AKI (when CPK levels exceed 5,000 U/L), compartment syndromes, electrolyte abnormalities, cardiac dysrhythmias, hepatic dysfunction, and disseminated intravascular coagulopathy.

5. The **pathophysiology** of myoglobin-induced nephrotoxicity is related to hypovolemia (fluids shift into injured muscle), intrarenal vasoconstriction, direct tubular toxicity, and intratubular cast formation.

6. The most important method to prevent AKI following rhabdomyolysis is **vigorous saline hydration** to induce a brisk urine output. Mannitol and bicarbonate are often used to induce diuresis and alkalization of the urine, respectively. While experimental studies suggest these measures may be protective, clinical evidence does not support a benefit from these agents over and above aggressive fluid resuscitation.

7. **Treatment** is primarily supportive. Calcium should only be administered to treat symptomatic hypocalcemia or hyperkalemia because during the recovery phase, hypercalcemia often occurs as calcium is released from recovering tissues. If AKI occurs, it may be necessary to initiate RRT.

VIII. Management of AKI. The **goals** of AKI management include the following:

- Avoidance of further renal injury.
- Treatment and reduction of complications such as volume overload and electrolyte disturbances.
- Facilitation of renal recovery and reduction of the need for chronic dialysis.

A. Pharmacologic treatment

1. There is no evidence supporting the use of any particular agent in the **treatment** of AKI.

2. When infused at low doses (0.03–0.1 μg/kg/min), **fenoldopam** has been shown to increase renal plasma flow and reduce the aberrant renal hemodynamics seen with aortic cross-clamping without significantly affecting systemic hemodynamics. However, there are no controlled data confirming these anecdotal observations.

3. Although it is known that nonoliguric renal failure is associated with a better prognosis than oliguric renal failure, there is no evidence to show that using diuretics to convert oliguric renal failure to a nonoliguric form has any benefit in any outcome. In fact, some studies suggest that **high-dose loop diuretics may worsen outcome with AKI.**

4. **Atrial natriuretic peptide (ANP)** increases GFR, decreases renin, angiotensin II, and aldosterone, and induces natriuresis and diuresis. One small randomized trial found that infusion of ANP improved dialysis-free survival, but larger studies have shown no benefit or worse survival. Therefore, current evidence does not support the use of ANP in the treatment of AKI.

5. **Insulin-like growth factor 1 (IGF-1)** has been shown to accelerate renal recovery in experimental models of ischemic AKI. However, the clinical evidence in humans shows no benefit in terms of renal recovery, need for renal replacement, or mortality.

6. Pharmacologic agents that continue to be studied for their potential use in the management of AKI include antiapoptosis/antinecrosis agents, anti-inflammatory agents, antisepsis agents, growth factors, and renal vasodilators.

B. **RRT** is often indicated in the management of patients with AKI in the ICU.

1. **Conventional indications for RRT include**

   a. Volume overload unresponsive to diuretics.

   b. Hyperkalemia refractory to medical therapy.

   c. Metabolic acidosis refractory to medical therapy.

   d. Intoxication with a dialyzable drug/toxin.

   e. Progressive azotemia, especially if uremic symptoms are present (e.g., encephalopathy, pericarditis, bleeding).

2. **Intermittent hemodialysis (IHD)** uses a concentration gradient between blood and a dialysate to enable solute clearance by across a semipermeable membrane (see **Fig. 24-1**). This remains a viable and efficient option for hemodynamically stable patients, although the optimal frequency for patients with AKI has not been determined.

   a. IHD requires the establishment of vascular access in the femoral, internal jugular, or subclavian vein.

   b. Anticoagulation can be avoided in the acute setting by periodically flushing the filter.

   c. **Complications** of IHD include hypotension, arrhythmias, bleeding, and infection at the access site. Rapid solute removal can cause disequilibrium syndrome, which leads to confusion and other mental status changes.

   d. The use of **synthetic biocompatible membranes** leads to improved recovery rates and mortality rates over bioincompatible membranes.

3. **Continuous venovenous hemofiltration (CVVH)** is the most common modality utilized in the unstable patient as it is associated with a more even control of fluid shifts, better blood pressure tolerance, and better 24-hour solute clearance. It may be preferred over IHD in patients who have or are at risk for intracranial hypertension and edema. The relative risks versus benefits of CVVH must be weighed in context.

   a. **Access** is the same as for IHD.

   b. **Anticoagulation** can be with heparin or citrate serving as a regional anticoagulant. Argatroban may be used in the critically ill patient with heparin-induced thrombocytopenia.

   c. Solute clearance is achieved via **convection**, with a transmembrane pressure gradient across a semipermeable membrane (see **Fig. 24-1**). The primary determinant of clearance is the rate of **ultrafiltration**, such that CVVH efficacy is dependent on the hourly ultrafiltrate volume. Replacement fluid can then be added back in a volume to achieve the desired hourly body balance.

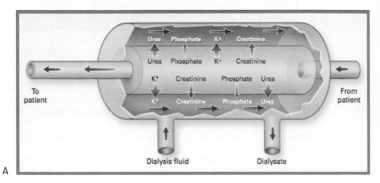

A

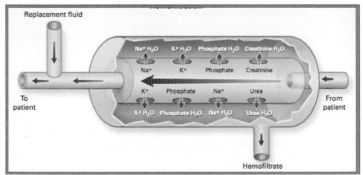

B

FIGURE 24-1 A. Hemodialysis achieves solute clearance by *diffusion* across a semipermeable membrane from a higher concentration (in patient's blood) to a lower concentration (in the dialysis fluid). **B.** Hemofiltration (which is the mechanism used in CVVH) achieves solute clearance by *convection* across a semipermeable membrane from a higher hydrostatic pressure (in patient's blood) to a lower hydrostatic pressure (in the hemofiltrate). (From: Forni LG, Hilton PJ. Continuous hemofiltration in the treatment of acute renal failure. *N Engl J Med* 1997;336:1303–1309, with permission).

    d. Severely catabolic patients may require high ultrafiltration rates to effectively control azotemia. The convective clearance of ultrafiltration can be supplemented with a diffusion component by adding a dialysate flow through the membrane. This form of CVVH is termed **continuous venovenous hemodiafiltration (CVVHDF)**.

    e. Several single-center RCTs have suggested that dialysis at higher doses can improve survival. Although these results have been confuted by a larger multicenter trial, it is possible that a higher dose of CVVH may be more effective.

    f. Complications of CVVH

        (1) Citrate toxicity can occur when citrate is used, particularly in patients with liver disease. Features of citrate toxicity include normal serum total calcium, low ionized calcium, a high anion gap, and worsening metabolic acidosis.

        (2) Bleeding may be seen, requiring halting or reversal of anticoagulants if they are used.

(3) Conversely, **clotting** of the filter or circuit may occur, resulting in interruption of hemofiltration and potential loss of extracorporeal blood as the circuit is replaced.

(4) Under- or overdosing of medications may occur, especially with antimicrobials, since clearance of many agents in patients receiving CVVH is not yet defined.

(5) **Other complications** include infection, bleeding, metabolic alkalosis (due to hepatic conversion of citrate to bicarbonate), and hypophosphatemia, especially with prolonged therapy.

4. **Sustained low-efficiency dialysis (SLED)** is an adjustment to IHD that involves slower blood and dialysate flow rates in order to improve hemodynamic stability. Reduced flow rates decrease the effectiveness of solute clearance, but this is offset by longer dialysis times. SLED is usually applied for 8 to 12 hours daily, thereby achieving adequate solute clearance and volume control while avoiding hypotensive episodes. SLED is technically easier than CVVH and avoids the need for replacement fluid.

5. **Peritoneal dialysis (PD)** uses the peritoneum as a natural semipermeable membrane for removal of solutes via diffusion. The use of PD is very limited in surgical critically ill patients because of low peritoneal surface for exchange in many patients, potential for abdominal distention, and complications from catheter leakage and infection.

IX. **Management of the complications of AKI**
   A. **Volume overload** (see also **Chapter 8**)
   1. In patients with AKI, the **inability to balance fluid intake by urinary elimination** may lead to volume overload.
   2. Treatment options for minimizing the risk of or for treating fluid overload include the following:
      a. **Induced diuresis.** Fluid management often can be facilitated when oliguria responds to diuretic therapy. Forced diuresis may have specific benefits in a limited number of conditions such as rhabdomyolysis and tumor lysis syndrome, but should never be attempted prior to adequate volume resuscitation. It should also be emphasized that while diuretics may treat fluid overload, there is no evidence to suggest that diuretics are of value in the treatment of AKI.
      b. **Minimize exogenous fluid administration**
         (1) Use low-flow, constant-flush systems on pressure-monitoring catheters and infusion pumps.
         (2) Concentrate drugs to their solubility or safety limits.
         (3) Avoid any unnecessary fluid administration (e.g., convert medications to enteral formulations whenever practical).
      c. **RRT** will inevitably be required in the anuric patient or when conservative therapy fails.
   B. **Metabolic acidosis** (see also **Chapter 8**)
   1. Metabolic acidosis is typically associated with an increased anion gap from the retention of organic acids.
   2. Organic acids are normally produced at a rate of 1 mEq/kg/d, but production may be greatly increased in the catabolic critically ill patient. Serum bicarbonate may decrease at a daily rate of 2 mEq/L or more.
   3. Treatment is usually not necessary, and overaggressive correction of acidosis may precipitate metabolic alkalosis and acute hypocalcemia.
   4. When acidosis is severe (pH <7.2), sodium bicarbonate may be used temporarily to maintain pH within the normal range. If impaired

alveolar ventilation impedes the patient's ability to eliminate carbon dioxide produced by sodium bicarbonate, other nonbicarbonate buffers are available (e.g., trometamol or THAM). However, these compounds may have other undesirable side effects in the patient with AKI, including respiratory depression, hypoglycemia, and hypotension.

5. Dialysis may be necessary when the acid load is very high or when volume overload or hypernatremia limits the amount of sodium bicarbonate that can be safely administered.

C. Electrolyte abnormalities (see also **Chapter 8**)

1. **Hyperkalemia**

   a. Treatment depends on the degree of hyperkalemia and the severity of ECG changes. The presence of a widened QRS complex is an indication for immediate treatment with IV calcium, bicarbonate, glucose, and insulin. Less pronounced changes such as T-wave peaking may be managed with the more slowly acting cation exchange resins.

   b. **Specific treatment guidelines**

      (1) **Calcium gluconate** (15–30 mg/kg intravenously [IV]) or **calcium chloride** (5–10 mg/kg IV), administered over 2 to 5 minutes, directly antagonizes the effect of potassium on the myocardium.

      (2) **Sodium bicarbonate**, 50 to 100 mEq IV, will partly reverse the acidosis and cause a redistribution of potassium into cells. In mechanically ventilated patients, hyperventilation can be used to create a respiratory alkalosis, which will have the same effect.

      (3) **Glucose and insulin.** One to two ampules of 50% glucose (dextrose) in water and 10 U of regular insulin IV should be given over a 5-minute period. Redistribution of potassium into the cell occurs within minutes.

      (4) Sodium polystyrene sulfonate **(Kayexalate)** is a sodium–potassium ion exchange resin given via the gastrointestinal tract that directly removes potassium from the body. Kayexalate (25–50 g in 100 mL of a 20% sorbitol solution) may be given orally or as a retention enema. Because of its slow rate of potassium removal, it should not be used as sole therapy for life-threatening hyperkalemia.

      (5) **RRT** is indicated for the urgent treatment of life-threatening hyperkalemia. HD is far more effective than CVVH for acute management of hyperkalemia.

2. **Hyponatremia** most often results from excessive antidiuretic hormone (ADH) secretion, but may also develop as a result of defective concentrating mechanisms. The first line of treatment in either of these cases is fluid restriction (< 800 mL/d). Treatment with normal saline and a loop diuretic may be necessary.

3. **Hypermagnesemia** is rarely seen in renal failure, except when supplemental magnesium is administered.

4. **Hyperphosphatemia** is common in AKI. Although phosphorus has no toxic effects, in excess it decreases serum calcium concentration. Severe elevations of phosphate, as seen in tumor lysis syndrome, can be associated with metastatic calcifications. Phosphorus-binding antacids usually are given to decrease plasma phosphorus levels and maintain calcium levels within a normal range. Calcium-based phosphate binders such as calcium acetate and non–calcium-based binders such as sevelamer can also be used. Overuse of antacids may produce hypophosphatemia.

D. Anemia in patients with AKI has many causes. Erythropoietin (EPO) is produced by the kidney and stimulates erythrocyte production within the bone marrow. Absence of EPO likely contributes to anemia in AKI. EPO therapy is used routinely for patients with chronic renal failure.

E. Uremic encephalopathy
1. Manifestations range from tremor, myoclonus, asterixis, and frank seizures to lethargy, disorientation, and coma.
2. Uremic encephalopathy usually improves with dialysis.
3. Many other metabolic derangements and drug effects during AKI can contribute to encephalopathy in critically ill patients.

F. Decreased drug elimination. A large number of drugs are eliminated by the kidneys, including several antibiotics, neuromuscular blocking agents and potentially toxic drugs such as aminoglycosides and digoxin. The doses of renally excreted drugs must be adjusted when renal function is impaired. It is important to recognize that early in AKI, the serum creatinine concentration does not fully reflect the reduction in GFR.

G. Uremic pericarditis occurs for unknown reasons and can be complicated by cardiac tamponade and infective pericarditis. Patients should be examined daily for the presence of a **pericardial friction rub**. Cardiac tamponade should be considered if unexplained cardiovascular decompensation occurs. Pericarditis may be an indication for urgent dialysis.

H. Bleeding abnormalities secondary to uremic platelet dysfunction are common in patients with renal failure and are generally attributed to abnormal platelet function. Management of uremic bleeding problems is discussed in **Chapter 26**.

I. Infectious complications are responsible for the majority of deaths in patients with AKI. Uremia impairs the ability to fight infection and may blunt the usual manifestations of infection that allow early diagnosis.

J. Nutritional support (see **Chapter 11**) is an important ancillary measure in critically ill patients with AKI.
1. Management of nutritional support in AKI is complicated by the need for volume restriction and the concern that supplemental protein may result in production of additional nitrogenous wastes.
2. Carbohydrates have a protein-sparing effect. Nutritional supplements, when administered with essential amino acid preparations, can be provided without significantly increasing the serum urea nitrogen concentration.
3. Enteral nutrition is preferred to parenteral nutrition when possible.
4. Continuous renal replacement therapies permit an increased volume of feedings with less concern about volume overload. Renal replacement therapies also eliminate nutrients, as they do wastes. Glucose is usually infused with the replacement fluid, and amino acid solutions may be increased to compensate for the loss.

Selected References

Aspelin P, Aubry P, Fransson SG, et al; Nephrotoxicity in High-Risk Patients Study of Iso-Osmolar and Low-Osmolar Non-Ionic Contrast Media Study Investigators. Nephrotoxic effects in high-risk patients undergoing angiography. *N Engl J Med* 2003;348(6):491–499.

Bagshaw SM, Langenberg C, Bellomo R. Urinary biochemistry and microscopy in septic acute renal failure: a systematic review. *Am J Kidney Dis* 2006;48(5):695–705.

Bell M, Granath F, et al; Swedish Intensive Care Nephrology Group (SWING). Continuous renal replacement therapy is associated with less chronic renal failure than intermittent haemodialysis after acute renal failure. *Intensive Care Med* 2007;33(5):773–780.

Bellomo R, Ronco C, Kellum JA, et al; The Second International Consensus Conference of the Acute Dialysis Quality Initiative (ADQI) Group. Acute renal failure: definition, outcome measures, animal models, fluid therapy and information technology needs. *Crit Care* 2004;8:R204–R212.

Fabrizi F, Martin P, Messa P. Recent advances in the management of hepato-renal syndrome (HRS). *Acta Clin Belg Suppl* 2007;(2):393–396.

Forni LB, Hilton PJ. Continuous hemofiltration in the treatment of acute renal failure. *N Engl J Med* 1997;336:1303–1309.

Huerta-Alardín AL, Varon J, Marik PE. Bench-to-bedside review: rhabdomyolysis—an overview for clinicians. *Crit Care* 2005;9(2):158–169.

Marenzi G, Marana I, Lauri G, et al. The prevention of radiocontrast-agent-induced nephropathy by hemofiltration. *N Engl J Med* 2003;349(14):1333–1340.

Merten GJ, Burgess WP, Gray LV, et al. Prevention of contrast-induced nephropathy with sodium bicarbonate: a randomized controlled trial. *JAMA* 2004;291(19):2328–2334.

Ostermann M, Chang RW. Acute kidney injury in the intensive care unit according to RIFLE. *Crit Care Med* 2007;35(8):1837–1843.

Palevsky PM, Zhang JH, O'Connor TZ, et al; VA/NIH Acute Renal Failure Trial Network. Intensity of renal support in critically ill patients with acute kidney injury. *N Engl J Med* 2008;359(1):7–20.

Pannu N, Nadim MK. An overview of drug-induced acute kidney injury. *Crit Care Med* 2008;36(4 suppl):S216–S223.

Parikh CR, Devarajan P. New biomarkers of acute kidney injury. *Crit Care Med* 2008;36 (4 suppl):S159–S165.

Prins JM, Weverling GJ, de Blok K, et al. Validation and nephrotoxicity of a simplified once-daily aminoglycoside dosing schedule and guidelines for monitoring therapy. *Antimicrob Agents Chemother* 1996;40(11):2494–9249.

Ronco C, Bellomo R, Homel P, et al. Effects of different doses in continuous veno-venous haemofiltration on outcomes of acute renal failure: a prospective randomised trial. *Lancet* 2000;356(9223):26–30.

Schortgen F, Lacherade JC, Bruneel F, et al. Effects of hydroxyethyl starch and gelatin on renal function in severe sepsis: a multicentre randomised study. *Lancet* 2001;357(9260):911–356.

Uchino S, Bellomo R, Kellum JA, et al; Beginning and Ending Supportive Therapy for the Kidney (BEST Kidney) Investigators Writing Committee. Patient and kidney survival by dialysis modality in critically ill patients with acute kidney injury. *Int J Artif Organs* 2007;30:281–292.

Uchino S, Kellum JA, Bellomo R, et al. Acute renal failure in critically ill patients: a multinational, multicenter study. *JAMA* 2005;294:813–818.

Vinsonneau C, Camus C, Combes A, et al; Hemodiafe Study Group. Continuous venovenous haemodiafiltration versus intermittent haemodialysis for acute renal failure in patients with multiple-organ dysfunction syndrome: a multicentre randomised trial. *Lancet* 2006;368(9533):379–385.

25

Liver Dysfunction

Daniel Johnson and William Benedetto

I. **Liver dysfunction in the ICU** is commonly seen. The spectrum of severity ranges from mild elevations in transaminases to fulminant hepatic failure. The non-specific **symptoms** of liver dysfunction (right upper quadrant pain, nausea, indigestion, pruritus, fatigue, and confusion) may not be readily evident in critically ill and postoperative patients who are sedated and have comorbidities with similar findings. Patients with known hepatic disease exhibiting cirrhosis, splenomegaly, and ascites may be admitted to an ICU postoperatively or for exacerbations related to their disease.

II. **Acute liver failure**

A. **Acute liver failure** (ALF, also called **fulminant hepatic failure**) affects approximately 2,000 patients per year in the United States and is characterized by **encephalopathy** and **coagulopathy** in the setting of an acute hepatic disease. Based on the time interval between first signs of liver disease (e.g., jaundice) and the onset of hepatic encephalopathy, ALF may be subdivided into **hyperacute** (0–7 days), **acute** (8–28 days), and **subacute** (29 days–12 weeks). Transplant-free short-term survival is lower in the subacute patient population than in the hyperacute or acute population.

B. **Causes of ALF.** The most common etiologies are acetaminophen overdose, idiosyncratic drug reactions, viral hepatitis, and indeterminate causes. Overall patient survival is poor.

1. **Drugs/chemicals/toxins**
   a. **Acetaminophen** is the most common cause in the United States and United Kingdom, often related to a suicide attempt. Acetaminophen overdose associated with ethanol intoxication increases hepatotoxicity.
   b. A partial list of other **drugs/chemicals/toxins** that can lead to ALF includes carbon tetrachloride, mushroom toxins (e.g., *Amanita phalloides*), isoniazid, valproic acid, halothane, phenytoin, amiodarone, ethanol, and MDMA ("ecstasy").

2. **Viral infections**
   a. **Hepatitis B** (with or without hepatitis D) and **hepatitis A** are relatively common causes of ALF. Hepatitis E, an uncommon cause in the United States, is a significant risk during pregnancy in Asia, Africa, the Middle East, and Central America. Hepatitis C is not thought to be a significant cause of ALF.
   b. Unusual causes of ALF include Epstein-Barr virus, cytomegalovirus, herpes simplex virus, and varicella zoster virus.

3. **Ischemia** secondary to passive congestion due to heart failure, Budd-Chiari syndrome, trauma, or tumors that may occlude the hepatic arterial supply or portal veins, in addition to generalized prolonged **hypoxia**, are causes of ALF.

4. **Other** etiologies include Reye's syndrome, acute fatty liver of pregnancy (± HELLP), Wilson's disease, oral contraceptive drugs, and heat stroke.

TABLE 25-1	Clinical Stages of Hepatic Encephalopathy
Stage 1.	Altered behavior, impairment of sleep, change of handwriting, slurred speech
Stage 2.	Drowsiness, disorientation, restlessness, brisk tendon reflexes, increased muscle tone, clonus
Stage 3.	Somnolent but arousable, marked confusion, disturbance of speech, hyperreflexia, miosis
Stage 4.	Coma, mydriasis, hypo- or areflexia, unresponsiveness to painful stimuli

C. **Complications of ALF**

1. **Cerebral edema** is the leading cause of death in ALF. Cerebral edema with or without elevations in intracranial pressure is present in 75% to 80% of cases of hepatic failure that progress to stage IV encephalopathy (**Table 25-1**). Focal neurologic signs are infrequently seen and may indicate intracranial bleeding or early herniation. Theories for the development of cerebral edema include impaired cerebral autoregulation, compromise of the blood–brain barrier, and intracellular accumulation of osmotically active molecules.

2. **Cardiovascular** changes in ALF include vasodilation, decreased systemic vascular resistance, hypotension, tachycardia, **increased cardiac output,** and arteriovenous shunting. Sepsis must be considered in the differential diagnosis.

3. **Respiratory** compromise with or without hypoxia may occur secondary to hypoventilation, hyperventilation, atelectasis, pleural effusion, aspiration, pulmonary shunting, and pulmonary edema.

4. **Coagulopathies** can be secondary to decreased production of clotting factors and/or pathologic thrombolysis. Thrombocytopenia and impaired platelet function are common.

5. **Renal failure** complicates about half of cases of ALF and commonly is due to **hepatorenal syndrome (HRS)**. Renal failure and hepatic disease are discussed in detail in **Section V.**

6. **Electrolyte and acid–base disorders** are varied and include
   a. Respiratory alkalosis: From central hyperventilation.
   b. Metabolic acidosis as a sign of acetaminophen intoxication or a late sign of lactic acidosis when the liver is no longer able to metabolize lactic acid adequately.
   c. Hypokalemia as a renal response to respiratory alkalosis.
   d. Hyponatremia due to reduced free water clearance.
   e. Hypernatremia secondary to dehydration after mannitol therapy.
   f. Hypoglycemia due to impaired glycogen mobilization, gluconeogenesis, and insulin metabolism.

D. **Management**

1. Respiratory failure or inability to protect the airway (due to encephalopathy) necessitate **tracheal intubation and mechanical ventilation.**

2. Intracranial pressure monitoring, attention to **maintenance of adequate cerebral perfusion pressure,** and **management of cerebral edema** are discussed in Chapter 10.

3. Cardiovascular stability depends on maintenance of **euvolemia,** and frequently requires **vasopressor therapy.** Invasive hemodynamic monitoring is typically necessary.

4. **Transfusion** of coagulation factors or platelets in the absence of active bleeding is controversial, but may be indicated prior to invasive procedures or when ICP monitors are in place.

5. **Renal replacement therapy** is frequently necessary. Continuous hemofiltration is generally better tolerated than intermittent hemodialysis. Worsening metabolic acidosis when citrate is used in the hemofiltration regimen indicates end-stage hepatic disease that is usually terminal.

6. Prophylaxis against ulcers with an H2-blocking agent or a proton pump inhibitor should be initiated.

7. **Consultation of a liver transplantation team** should be considered early in the course of severe ALF.

E. **Liver transplantation in ALF**

1. **Indications.** Orthotopic liver transplantation may be an option for patients with ALF. The intensivist and transplantation team have the challenge of making an accurate prediction of whether a patient will be able to recover with medical treatment alone or will need early transplantation, which may improve outcome. The **King's College criteria for liver transplantation** (**Table 25-2**) is the most often used tool for repeated, fast, and inexpensive assessment of liver function to predict who will require transplantation. Some hepatologists advocate that all patients with ALF should be listed for transplantation upon diagnosis with reevaluation when a donor graft becomes available.

2. **Contraindications** to transplantation include sepsis, acute respiratory distress syndrome, and cerebral edema that is unresponsive to treatment. **Relative contraindications** include rapidly developing hemodynamic instability requiring increasing vasopressor support, history of certain psychiatric disturbances (e.g., noncompliance, suicide attempts), known malignancy outside of the liver, and advanced age.

3. **Ex vivo liver support systems** analogous to renal replacement therapy have been proposed as a bridge to transplantation. Experience with these devices remains limited. An early meta-analysis of studies demonstrated a benefit for acute-on-chronic liver failure but did not find a demonstrable effect on ALF.

| TABLE 25-2 | King's College Criteria for Liver Transplantation in Acute Liver Failure |

Acetaminophen intoxication
    Arterial pH <7.3 irrespective of grade of encephalopathy
    Or a combination of:
        Encephalopathy grade III or IV
        Prothrombin time >35 s
        Serum creatinine >3.4 mg/dL

Nonacetaminophen patients
    INR >7.7 irrespective of grade of encephalopathy
    Or any three of the following variables:
        Age <10 or >40 years
        Etiology is hepatitis C, halothane hepatitis, or idiosyncratic drug reaction
        Duration of jaundice before onset of encephalopathy >7 days
        Prothrombin time >25 s
        Serum bilirubin >18 mg/dL

III. Postoperative complications of liver surgery

A. Hemorrhage

1. **Insufficient surgical hemostasis.** Bleeding must be anticipated. Surgical techniques respecting the segmental structure of the liver (i.e., anatomic resection) and the use of argon beam coagulators have decreased intra- and postoperative blood loss. Wedge resections tend to bleed more postoperatively than lobectomies because more of the raw surface remains.

2. **Coagulopathy** (see **Chapter 26**) may occur secondary to dilution associated with massive transfusion, inadequate replacement of components, hypothermia, hyperfibrinolysis, or decreased production of clotting factors by the remaining hepatic tissue. Correction of coagulopathy is carried out with transfusion of fresh frozen plasma, platelets, and cryoprecipitate, as guided by clinical situation and laboratory data.

3. **Management**

   a. Restoration of **normovolemia** with crystalloids, colloids, and blood products as needed.

   b. Restoration of **normothermia** with warming modalities.

   c. If the hematocrit does not stabilize or hemodynamics do not stabilize despite the aforementioned measures, ongoing bleeding must be suspected that requires **surgical reintervention**. Hepatic **angiography and embolization** are also options.

B. Fever may reflect resorption of hematoma or necrotic tissue or may be a sign of infection, peritonitis, or abscess formation.

C. Leaking bile ducts may form bile collections. Existing drains should be left in place or new drains should be inserted. Typically, biliary fistulae close on their own within 3 weeks.

D. Hepatic pseudoaneurysm refers to the development of a pseudoaneurysm after an injury of the hepatic vasculature; a potential late complication after hepatic trauma; and is indicated by anemia, leukocytosis, and abdominal pain. Therapeutic embolization is considered the treatment of choice.

E. Intra- or perihepatic abscess. The risk of abscess formation is increased with concomitant colonic or pancreatic injury, large collections of hematoma or bile, and open drains. Prolonged postoperative pyrexia in combination with leukocytosis and increasing right upper quadrant pain should raise the suspicion of an intra- or perihepatic abscess. Treatment includes intravenous antibiotics and drainage via interventional radiology or surgery.

F. Postoperative liver failure. In otherwise normal livers (e.g., liver surgery for removal of a metastatic lesion or adenoma), resections of up to 80% of the liver mass can generally be tolerated. Complications may arise in the following circumstances:

1. The remaining liver is too small to maintain full hepatic function.
2. Alterations in hepatic blood flow lead to ischemia.

IV. Postoperative liver dysfunction after nonhepatic surgery

A. Etiologies include

1. Infection (e.g., viral hepatitis, exacerbation of chronic hepatitis, sepsis).
2. Ischemia secondary to hypotension, congestive heart failure, or hepatic artery ligation or injury.
3. Hypoxia.
4. Drugs and toxins (see **Section VI**).
5. Bile duct obstruction or injury.

6. Pancreatitis.
7. Bilirubin overload secondary to hematoma, blood transfusions, or hemolysis.
B. **Pre-existing liver disease** makes the liver more vulnerable to perioperative stresses.
C. **Management:** See **Section II.D.**

V. **Chronic liver disease. Cirrhosis** can be seen as an irreversible common pathway of different chronic liver diseases. Hepatocyte necrosis and destruction of the connective tissue network lead to irregular nodular regeneration of hepatic parenchyma, extensive fibrosis, and distortion of the hepatic vasculature.
A. **Most common etiologies** include **alcoholic** liver disease (by far the most common in the Western world) and **chronic hepatitis** following viral hepatitis B or C infection (20% of chronic hepatitis C infections progress to cirrhosis). Additional etiologies of liver cirrhosis are listed in **Table 25-3.**
B. **Portal hypertension** and **bleeding from gastroesophageal varices.** Although other causes exist (e.g., Budd-Chiari syndrome, portal vein thrombosis), cirrhosis is the most common underlying disease leading to portal hypertension. Cirrhosis leads to portosystemic collaterals that may form varices with a risk of bleeding.
   1. **Patients with esophageal bleeding** (see also **Chapter 27**) present with hematemesis, melena, and hematochezia. The diagnosis must be confirmed by esophagogastroscopy because bleeding frequently occurs from duodenal or gastric ulcers or the Mallory-Weiss syndrome.
   2. **Endoscopic sclerotherapy and variceal ligation** are commonly used to manage esophageal varices and esophageal bleeding. The procedures are highly successful and can immediately follow diagnostic esophagogastroscopy.
   3. **Nonselective β-adrenergic antagonists** such as **propranolol** administered prophylactically reduce the risk of bleeding, although mortality is unaffected. Propranolol reduces portal flow by constriction of the splanchnic vasculature (via β_2 blockade) and by cardiac output reduction (via β_1 blockade).
   4. **Vasopressin** reduces blood flow and pressure in the portal system including its collaterals. It improves acute variceal bleeding, but has not been shown to decrease mortality. The infusion dose is typically 0.1 to 0.4 U/min (**note** that, this dose is 10 times higher than the dose of

TABLE 25-3	Other Etiologies of Liver Cirrhosis
Primary biliary cirrhosis	From T-cell mediated attack on bile ducts
Biliary cirrhosis	From prolonged obstruction of the biliary tract
Primary sclerosing cholangitis	Strongly associated with inflammatory bowel disease
Metabolic diseases	Hemochromatosis, Wilson's disease, glycogen storage diseases, α-1-antitrypsin deficiency
Drug-related toxicity	e.g., methotrexate, isoniazid, methyldopa
Parasitic infections	e.g., *Echinococcus* infection, schistosomiasis
Nonalcoholic fatty liver disease	
Longstanding congestive heart failure	
Autoimmune hepatitis	

vasopressin suggested as therapy in septic shock). Side effects include myocardial ischemia, gastrointestinal ischemia, acute renal failure, and hyponatremia. Vasopressin should be administered through a central line because infiltration may cause tissue necrosis. Concomitant infusion of **nitroglycerin** may reduce the potential harmful effects of vasopressin.

5. **Somatostatin,** a naturally produced peptide hormone, acts as a vaso-constrictor in supraphysiologic doses and is effective in reducing acute bleeding. Fewer side effects are reported with somatostatin than with vasopressin. **Octreotide** is a synthetic analogue of somatostatin with a much longer half-life. The typical dose is 25 to 50 µg/h.

6. **Balloon tamponade** is only recommended if medical or sclerotherapy/variceal ligation is unsuccessful (see **Chapter 27**).

7. **Emergency surgical shunt operations** and **surgical ligations** are only used as a last resort. **Transjugular intrahepatic portosystemic shunt (TIPS)** procedures use a percutaneously placed expandable metal stent to form a direct portocaval channel within the liver. These procedures are associated with high complication rates, and are usually reserved for patients who have recurrent bleeding despite repeated sclerotherapies.

C. **Hepatic encephalopathy** is caused by multiple factors. In liver failure, hepatic clearance of cerebrotoxic substances such as ammonia, mercaptans, and short-chain fatty acids is reduced. Experimental evidence suggests that the damaged liver is no longer able to produce certain substances that are crucial for normal brain function. The isolation of benzodiazepine-like compounds from brains of patients with hepatic encephalopathy and partial antagonism of hepatic encephalopathy by flumazenil suggest that the γ-aminobutyrate (GABA)-ergic system may be altered.

1. **Diagnosis of hepatic encephalopathy** is made clinically. Ammonia levels do not correlate with the severity of the encephalopathy. In contrast to ALF, increased intracranial pressure is only rarely associated with chronic hepatic encephalopathy.

2. **Management**
   a. **Elimination of precipitating factors** (such as gastrointestinal bleeding or infection) if possible. A **nasogastric tube** should be inserted to document and evacuate any upper gastrointestinal bleeding (if present) and to permit administration of medications.
   b. **Lactulose** is a disaccharide that is degraded into acids by colonic bacteria. The acidic environment ionizes ammonia to ammonium ion, which cannot cross the colonic membrane and thus is excreted in stool. This decreases plasma levels of ammonia, which usually improves the patient's mental status. The typical initial dose is 20 mL q hour orally or by nasogastric tube until catharsis occurs. The dose is then adjusted to produce three to four soft stools per day. Lactulose also can be administered as a 1-L enema (300 mL of lactulose plus 700 mL of water three times daily; enema should be retained for 30–60 minutes). Side effects include hypokalemia, dehydration, and hypernatremia.
   c. **Neomycin,** 1 g PO or PNGT q 6 hours, may be helpful. After clinical response is noted, the dose can be reduced to 1 to 2 g daily. The mechanism of improvement may be decrease in flora (and ammonia) and/or decrease in intestinal absorption.

D. **Ascites** is produced by the combination of portal hypertension, hypoalbuminemia, and fluid retention. More than 500 mL of ascites can usually be detected clinically by a distended abdomen, bulging flanks, everted umbilicus, shifting abdominal dullness, and an abdominal fluid wave. The diagnosis can be confirmed by ultrasonography. Other causes of ascites should be excluded by a diagnostic paracentesis. Ascites can be classified as transudative or exudative.

1. **Transudative ascites** is caused by movement of fluid across the hepatic sinusoids and the intestinal capillaries and is due to increased hydrostatic pressure from portal hypertension. In transudative ascites due to portal hypertension, the total protein concentration tends to be less than 2.5 g/dL and the serum to ascites albumin gradient (SAAG) is frequently greater than 1 g/dL. **Noncirrhotic causes** of transudative ascites include congestive heart failure, inferior vena cava occlusion, Budd-Chiari syndrome, and Meigs syndrome.

2. **Exudative ascites** develops secondary to exudation of fluid from the peritoneum, and is not the norm in patients with portal hypertension. In exudative ascites (with normal portal pressure), the total protein concentration usually exceeds 2.5 g/dL and the SAAG is less than 1 g/dL. **Causes** of exudative ascites include neoplasms (e.g., peritoneal carcinomatosis), peritoneal infections (e.g., tuberculosis, pyogenic peritonitis), chylous ascites, pancreatitis, and nephrogenic ascites.

3. Ascites fluid obtained by paracentesis should be sent for cell count with differential, albumin, total protein, glucose, Gram stain, bacterial culture (in blood culture bottles), amylase, lactate dehydrogenase, carcinoembryonic antigen, and triglycerides. Serum albumin should be sent for calculation of SAAG.

4. **Mainstays of therapy for ascites** in cirrhosis are a salt-restricted diet, containing as little as 11 mmol of sodium per day to induce a negative sodium balance and limit ascitic fluid accumulation. Diuretics are added if necessary. Because one cause for fluid retention in cirrhosis is secondary hyperaldosteronism, **spironolactone** is the diuretic of first choice. Other diuretics may be added cautiously if needed. Overly aggressive diuresis may result in azotemia and hypotension secondary to hypovolemia. The effectiveness of the treatment is monitored by daily weighing. Daily weight loss should not exceed 0.5 to 1 kg. Patients refractory to medical therapy may require repeated paracenteses. Plasma and urinary electrolytes should be monitored regularly, especially during diuretic treatment.

E. **Splenomegaly** may produce thrombocytopenia or pancytopenia, but rarely requires treatment.

F. **Spontaneous bacterial peritonitis (SBP)** is an infection of ascitic fluid without a primary intra-abdominal focus (see also **Chapter 29**).

1. **Signs and symptoms** may range from subtle to severe abdominal pain with rebound tenderness, fever, chills, nausea, and vomiting. Because symptoms may be absent, **diagnostic paracentesis** is recommended in the assessment of patients with ascites. Gastrointestinal hemorrhage, which is often associated with bacteremia, puts the cirrhotic patient at risk of developing SBP. The most important sources of contamination of the ascites are the gastrointestinal tract, urinary tract, pneumonias, and endoscopic procedures. More than 90% of cases of SBP are caused by a single organism. Enteric gram-negative bacteria are most frequently isolated (70%), followed by gram-positive cocci (*Streptococcus pneumoniae, Enterococcus, Staphylococcus*) in approximately 20% of the cases and anaerobes in approximately 5%. **Polymicrobial infections in SBP are rare** and should trigger a search for bowel perforation.

   2. **Treatment.** Because the mortality of untreated SBP is high, antibiotic therapy should be initiated immediately after samples of the ascites are taken. Potential regimens include the following:
      a. A third-generation nonpseudomonal cephalosporin such as **cefotaxime** 2 g intravenously (IV) q 8 to 12 hours or **ceftriaxone**. This is currently considered to be the treatment of choice.
      b. A β-lactam such as **ampicillin** plus an **aminoglycoside**.
      c. **Vancomycin** should be added to the regimen if methicillin-resistant *Staphylococcus aureus* (**MRSA**) is suspected.
   3. **Prophylaxis.** Patients with cirrhosis who are admitted with gastrointestinal bleeding may be prophylactically treated with cefotaxime. To prevent recurrence of SBP, prophylactic treatment with fluoroquinolone or trimethoprim–sulfamethoxazole may be considered, especially for liver transplant candidates.

G. **Hepatopulmonary syndrome.** Pathologic **dilation of intrapulmonary vessels** in cirrhosis increases right-to-left shunting of blood flow through the lungs. Dyspnea and arterial hypoxemia may be worsened by standing and improved by lying down. The diagnosis can be made with contrast-enhanced echocardiography or radiolabeled macroaggregated albumin. The degree of hypoxemia is variable, and is inconsistently improved by administration of supplemental oxygen. Partial or complete improvement of hypoxemia after liver transplantation has been reported.

H. **Hepatorenal syndrome (HRS)** is characterized by worsening renal function, sodium retention, and oliguria without an identifiable cause in a patient with cirrhosis and ascites. Renal failure is thought to be caused by inappropriate renal **vasoconstriction**, which reduces renal blood flow and glomerular filtration rate. Significant morphologic abnormalities are absent. Clinical signs usually include oliguria, azotemia, hyperkalemia, and hyponatremia (due to impairment of water excretion). Other causes of renal failure, such as prerenal azotemia, acute tubular necrosis, and glomerulonephritis, must be excluded (**Chapter 24**). In HRS, the urinary sediment is unremarkable, and significant sodium retention is present. The urinary sodium is often less than 5 mmol/L, which is less than that observed in prerenal azotemia, and is not improved by fluid administration. Treatment of HRS syndrome is often unsuccessful and the mortality rate is high. Treatments with TIPS and arteriolar vasoconstrictors have been attempted, but have met with limited success. Liver transplantation remains the only definitive therapy.

I. **Grading of liver disease.** Originally designed to assess the surgical risk in patients undergoing surgery, the Child-Turcotte-Pugh classification (**Table 25-4**) is also used to assess severity of disease in patients with cirrhosis.

VI. **Drug-induced liver disease**
A. The liver is the central organ for the metabolism of most drugs. Drug excretion through the kidneys and the bile is made possible by transformation to more hydrophilic compounds (biotransformation). In most cases, hepatotoxicity is not caused by the originally administered drug, but by its metabolites.

B. **Hepatotoxicity** has been classified into direct hepatotoxic reactions and idiosyncratic reactions.
   1. **Direct hepatotoxins** damage the liver in a dose-dependent fashion and characteristically produce hepatocyte necrosis in a particular region of the liver lobule. Such hepatotoxins include acetaminophen, ethanol, chemotherapeutic agents, carbon tetrachloride, and certain metals.

TABLE 25-4	Child–Turcotte–Pugh Classification		
	Classification Points		
	1	**2**	**3**
Encephalopathy	None	Grades 1 and 2	Grades 3 and 4
Ascites	Absent	Slight–moderate	Tense
Bilirubin (mg/dL)	<2.0	2–3	>3.0
Bilirubin (mg/dL) if primary biliary cirrhosis	<4	4–10	>10
Albumin (g/dL)	>3.5	2.8–3.5	<2.8
PT (seconds above control)	1–4	4–6	>6

Points from each of the five categories are summed to yield a total score: class A, 5–6 points; class B, 7–9 points; class C, 10–15 points. The mortality of cirrhotic patients rises dramatically with increasing scores. The 1-year mortality rate is 0%–10% for class A, 20%–30% for class B, and 50%–60% for class C. PT, prothrombin time.

2. **Idiosyncratic reactions** account for the majority of cases, are unpredictable, and occur even when the drugs are administered in the normal therapeutic range. Diffuse liver injury consists of necrosis and/or cholestasis, and usually is associated with a significant inflammatory reaction. Rash, fever, eosinophilia, or a serum sickness syndrome may be present. In some instances, autoantibodies to cytochrome P-450 and other microsomal enzyme groups can be demonstrated. Drugs implicated in idiosyncratic hepatotoxicity include isoniazid, chlorpromazine, dantrolene, ketoconazole, phenytoin, amoxicillin–clavulanate, and nitrofurantoin.

3. Considerable interindividual variation exists in susceptibility to direct hepatotoxins. Some idiosyncratic reactions seem to occur when a combination of host factors and/or environmental factors is present. Variables such as enzyme polymorphism, interactions among drugs, age, history of ethanol use, and obesity influence the extent of both direct and idiosyncratic hepatotoxic reactions.

C. **Diagnosis** is based on a history of exposure to a certain drug (reactions usually occur within 90 days after first administration), but is especially difficult in the ICU setting, where patients are exposed to multiple drugs. Clinical and laboratory data are used to support the diagnosis. Other causes of liver dysfunction must be excluded.

D. Some drugs are associated with characteristic histologic lesions, whereas others may vary or show considerable overlap in their histologic presentation. Results of liver biopsies often are inconclusive. **Table 25-5** lists some examples of drugs associated with liver disease. Virtually any drug, however, may injure the liver.

VII. **Total parenteral nutrition (TPN) and liver disease**

A. **Steatosis ("fatty liver").** Parenteral feeding may be associated with complications that affect the liver. Increasing serum hepatic aminotransferases and bilirubin concentrations may be observed with increasing duration of TPN. The histopathologic correlate in adults usually is a fatty liver (i.e., macro- and microvesicular steatosis). It is usually asymptomatic and benign in character.

B. **Cholestasis.** Cholecystokinin (CCK), a hormone derived from the intestine, is released after stimulation by food. TPN creates a fasting-like state for the gut and decreases CCK release. This diminishes gallbladder emptying and promotes biliary sludge formation. Acalculous and calculous forms of cholecystitis may be distinguished by ultrasonography.

TABLE 25–5 Classification of Drug-Induced Hepatic Disease

Type of Lesion	Examples	Comments
Acute viral hepatitis–like reaction	Diclofenac, halothane, isoflurane, isoniazid, methyldopa, phenytoin	Mortality rate much higher than that of viral hepatitis; histologic pattern of bridging necrosis in severe cases
Zonal necrosis	Acetaminophen, carbon tetrachloride	Dose dependent; negligible inflammatory response; lesions predominantly restricted to one lobular zone
Steatohepatitis, alcoholic hepatitis–like reaction	Amiodarone, perhexiline, nifedipine, valproic acid	
Steatohepatitis, microvesicular	Aspirin, tetracycline, zidovudine	
Cholestasis	Angiotensin-converting enzyme inhibitors, carbamazepine, chlorpromazine, cimetidine, cotrimoxazole, dextropropoxyphene, erythromycin, estrogens, flucloxacillin, haloperidol, sulfonamides, tricyclic antidepressants	Histologically, inflammatory, noninflammatory, and forms with bile duct destruction can be recognized
Granulomatous hepatitis	Allopurinol, diltiazem, quinidine, phenytoin, procainamide, sulfonamides	Histiocytes and eosinophiles in the granulomas reflect a hypersensitivity reaction
Veno-occlusive disease	Chemotherapeutic drugs	Lesions are dose dependent
Chronic hepatitis	Amiodarone, aspirin, diclofenac, isoniazid, methyldopa, phenytoin, nitrofurantoin, trazodone	Occurs with continued exposure to a drug; in most cases, hepatitis resolves after discontinuation of the drug
Adenomas, hepatocellular carcinomas	Estrogens, anabolic hormones	

Selected References

Caraceni P, Van Thiel DH. Acute liver failure. *Lancet* 1995;345:163–169.

Christenson E, Schlichting P, Fauerholdt L, et al. Prognostic value of Child-Turcotte criteria in medically treated cirrhosis. *Hepatology* 1984;4:430–435.

Kjaergard L, Lise L, Liu J, et al. Artificial and bioartificial support systems for acute and acute-on-chronic liver failure: a systematic review. *JAMA* 2003;289:217–222.

Lee WM. Acute liver failure. *N Engl J Med* 1993;329(25):1862–1872.

Lee WM. Drug-induced hepatotoxicity. *N Engl J Med* 2003;349:474–485.

McCormick PA. Improving prognosis in hepatorenal syndrome. *Gut* 2000;47:166–167.

Menon KVN, Kamath PS. Managing the complications of cirrhosis. *Mayo Clin Proc* 2000;75: 501–509.

O'Grady JG, Alexander GJ, Hayllar KM, et al. Early indicators of prognosis in fulminant hepatic failure. *Gastroenterology* 1989;97:439–445.

O'Grady JG, Schalm SW, Williams R. Acute liver failure: redefining the syndromes. *Lancet* 1993;342:273–275.

Ostapowicz G, Fontana RJ, Schiodt FV, et al. Results of a prospective study of acute liver failure at 17 tertiary care centers in the United States. *Ann Intern Med* 2002;137(12):947–954.

Patzer JF. Advances in bioartificial liver assist devices. *Ann N Y Acad Sci* 2001;944:320–333.

Polson J, Lee WM. AASLD position paper: the management of acute liver failure. *Hepatology* 2005;41:1179–1197.

Schiff E, Sorrell MF, Maddrey W, eds. *Schiff's diseases of the liver*. 9th ed. Philadelphia: Lippincott, Williams & Wilkins, 2003.

Shellman R, Fulkerson W, DeLong E, et al. Prognosis of patients with cirrhosis and chronic liver disease admitted to the medical intensive care unit. *Crit Care Med* 1988;16:671–678.

Sherlock S, Dooley J. *Diseases of the liver and biliary system*. 10th ed. Oxford: Blackwell Science, 1997.

26

Coagulopathy and Hypercoagulability

Lorenzo Berra and Rae Allain

I. **Laboratory assessment of patient's coagulation.** The most important clue to a clinically significant bleeding disorder in an otherwise healthy patient remains the *history*. Prior surgical bleeding, gingival bleeding, easy bruising, epistaxis, or menorrhagia should raise concern. There are many tests available to assess the coagulation, but no single test measures the integrity of the entire coagulation system.

A. **Partial thromboplastin time (PTT or aPTT)** is performed by adding particulate matter to a blood sample to activate the intrinsic coagulation system. Normal values of PTT vary by laboratory, depending upon the reagent used, and require normal levels of clotting factors in the intrinsic coagulation system. The test is sensitive to decreased amounts of coagulation factors and is elevated in patients on *heparin therapy*. The PTT will also be abnormal if there is a circulating anticoagulant present (e.g., lupus anticoagulant, antibodies to factor VIII). The clinician should remember that an abnormal PTT does not necessarily correlate with clinical bleeding. Aggressive correction of an abnormal PTT in surgical patients is not always indicated unless the patient is actively bleeding. Recently, study of the "*PTT waveform*" (**Fig. 26-1**), the biphasic waveform which represents the change in light transmittance through the plasma sample as the PTT reaction takes place, has been shown to be abnormal in early disseminated intravascular coagulation (DIC) associated with sepsis and to be predictive of mortality. The PTT waveform is generated only by laboratory coagulation analyzers which use an optical (not mechanical) method of clot detection.

B. **Prothrombin time (PT)** is a measure of the extrinsic coagulation system and is measured by adding a thromboplastin reagent to a blood sample. While both PT and PTT are affected by levels of factors V and X, prothrombin, and fibrinogen, PT is specifically sensitive to deficiencies of factor VII. PT is normal in deficiencies of factors VIII, IX, XI, and XII, prekallikrein, and high-molecular-weight kininogen. The **international normalized ratio (INR)** standardizes PT values to permit comparisons of PT value among laboratories or within one laboratory but at different times for patients anticoagulated with warfarin. The INR is the ratio of patient PT to control PT that would be obtained if international reference reagents had been used to perform the test. Warfarin therapy may be guided by a target INR value that is independent of laboratory variability. Although the INR is frequently used to assess coagulation impairment in patients with liver disease (e.g., the MELD score), it may not be valid since liver disease affects both vitamin K-dependent and independent factors.

C. **Activated clotting time (ACT)** is a modified whole-blood clotting time in which diatomaceous earth or kaolin is added to a blood sample to activate the intrinsic clotting system. The ACT is the time until clot formation. Normal ACT depends upon the equipment used for performing the test

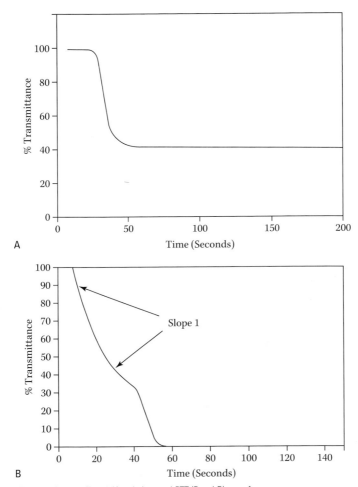

FIGURE 26-1 Normal (Panel A) and abnormal PTT (Panel B) waveforms.

and should be standardized by institution. ACT is usually a point-of-care test performed to monitor heparin therapy in the acute setting (e.g., during cardiopulmonary bypass).

D. The **bleeding time** is thought to be a crude assay of platelet function. Results are poorly reproducible and do not predict either bleeding or hemostasis during surgical procedures. For this reason, it has been abandoned for routine preoperative testing.

E. **Fibrinogen** may be depleted by excessive consumption as in massive hemorrhage (see **Chapter 35**) or DIC. A normal fibrinogen level is 150 to 400 mg/dL. It is an acute-phase reactant, and is often elevated in postoperative patients or following trauma or inflammation. For extensive surgical procedures associated with bleeding or in cases of massive transfusion, it is prudent to maintain the fibrinogen level above 100 mg/dL via transfusion of fresh frozen plasma (FFP) or cryoprecipitate.

F. **Fibrin(ogen) degradation products (FDPs)** are peptides produced from the action of plasmin on fibrinogen or fibrin monomer. They are measurable by serum assays and may aid in the diagnosis of primary fibrinolysis or DIC. FDPs modulate further clotting/lysis by interfering with fibrin monomer polymerization and by impairing platelet function. FDPs are often elevated in severe hepatic disease due to failed clearance from the circulation.

G. **D-Dimer** is a specific fragment produced when plasmin digests cross-linked fibrin (clot). It is measurable by serum assay and is elevated in many conditions, including venous thromboembolism, malignancy, pregnancy, DIC, and in postsurgical patients.

H. **Factor assays** are specialized tests that quantify the activity of individual coagulation factors. Most of these are performed in the setting of an unexplained coagulopathy that has not improved after attempted repletion of coagulation factors, and are usually obtained in concert with a clinical pathology or hematology consultation. Classically, factor assays are used to confirm the diagnosis of hemophilia A or B.

I. **Antifactor Xa assay.** Low-molecular-weight heparins (LMWH) and fondaparinux, when present at therapeutic levels, do not or minimally prolong PTT. Therefore, when laboratory tests are used to monitor therapeutic anticoagulant levels of these drugs, antifactor Xa assays are necessary. In addition, in some instances, the PTT cannot be used to monitor unfractionated heparin. For example, lupus anticoagulants or certain factor deficiencies (e.g., factor XII deficiencies) may prolong the baseline PTT and/or accentuate the PTT prolongation when heparin is added. In these cases, unfractionated heparin may be monitored with antifactor Xa assays.

J. **Thromboelastography (TEG)** is a point-of-care test most commonly used in the operating room, because it gives real-time, dynamic information on all aspects of coagulation. It is performed by placing a small amount of blood into a heated oscillating cup. Inside the cup is a pin attached to a wire. As clot forms, torque on the wire is detected and translated into an electrical signal, which a computer converts into a tracing (**Fig. 26-2**). Specific patterns of the trace are characteristic of coagulation abnormalities (e.g., factor deficiencies, fibrinolysis), assisting the clinician with the diagnosis and proper treatment.

II. Common coagulopathies in critical ill patients

A. **Disseminated intravascular coagulation (DIC)** refers to the abnormal, diffuse systemic activation of the clotting system. Its presentation can range from mild and asymptomatic to severe and marked by massive hemorrhage, thrombosis, and multiorgan failure. There are many potential causes of DIC (**Table 26-1**), with the common pathogenesis thought to involve coagulation activation by tissue factor, which may be expressed by multiple cell types when exposed to inflammatory cytokines. Thus, endothelial cell damage with exposure of collagen may be the cause of DIC seen in *shock* and *severe infections*; similarly, DIC is common in extensive *head injury* because of the high content of thromboplastin in brain tissue.

1. **Pathophysiology** of DIC involves excessive formation of thrombin resulting in fibrin formation throughout the vasculature, platelet activation, fibrinolysis, and consumption of coagulation factors.

2. **Clinical features** of DIC include petechiae, ecchymoses, bleeding from venipuncture sites, and hemorrhage from operative incisions. The bleeding manifestations of DIC are clinically obvious, but more common are the diffuse microvascular and macrovascular thromboses,

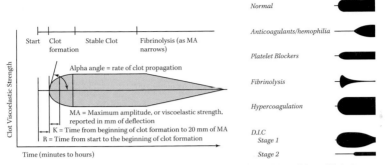

FIGURE 26-2 Thromboelastography and characteristic waveforms. Adapted from *Clinical anesthesia procedures of the Massachusetts General Hospital.* 7th ed, and reprinted from Mallett SV, Cox DJ. Thromboelastography. *Br J Anaesth* 1992;69:307–313, with permission.

which are difficult to treat and are frequently life threatening because of ischemia to vital organs.

3. **Laboratory features** of DIC include an elevated D-dimer, indicating fibrin degradation by plasmin, in all cases. The PT and PTT are prolonged in the majority of cases. FDPs are elevated, but this is not specific to DIC because FDPs may be present from the formation of fibrin by fibrinogen or from the degradation of fibrinogen by plasmin. For laboratories that use an optical coagulation analyzer, the PTT waveform (see **Section I.A, Fig. 26-1**) may be an early indicator of DIC, with abnormality manifesting before prolongation of the PTT. PTT waveform offers improved specificity of the diagnosis over

TABLE 26-1	Causes of Disseminated Intravascular Coagulation (DIC)
Acute	**Chronic**
Sepsis	Malignancy (hematologic or solid organ)
Shock	Liver disease
Trauma	Vascular abnormalities
Head injury	Aortic aneurysm
Crush injury	Aortic dissection
Burns (extensive)	Peritoneovenous shunt
Extracorporeal circulation (e.g., ECMO)	Intra-aortic balloon pump
Pregnancy catastrophes	
Placental abruption	
Amniotic fluid embolus	
Septic abortion	
Embolism of fat or cholesterol	
Hepatic failure (severe)	
Toxic/immune reactions (severe)	
Snake bites	
Hemolytic transfusion reactions	

D-dimer, which is often elevated in the critically ill, and over fibrinogen, which may be initially elevated in critically ill patients because it is an acute phase reactant. For laboratories with mechanical coagulation analyzers (unable to perform PTT waveform), serial measurements demonstrating a falling fibrinogen level and platelet count are characteristic of DIC. Examination of the peripheral blood smear in the patient with DIC reveals schistocytes in approximately 50% of cases; these are formed from the shearing of RBCs by intravascular fibrin strands.

4. **Treatment**
   a. The primary treatment of DIC involves treating the precipitating cause.
   b. Transfusion of appropriate blood components is indicated to correct bleeding. **Fibrinogen levels** should be maintained at more than 50 to 100 mg/dL. **Platelets** should be transfused in bleeding patients if the count is $<$50,000/mm^3; in nonbleeding patients, a cutoff of $<$10,000–20,000 mm^3 may be used.
   c. **Pharmacologic treatment** of DIC is controversial, but anticoagulant treatment may be beneficial based on the pathophysiology. Low-dose heparin treatment has been effective for chronic DIC with thrombosis. Trials of tissue factor inhibitor and antithrombin III treatment of septic patients have as yet not shown a reduced mortality.
   d. Inhibitors of fibrinolysis (e.g., aminocaproic acid) administered during DIC have some theoretical value but are risky given the possibility of diffuse intravascular thrombosis. Hematologic consultation is generally recommended for cases of DIC-related bleeding, which are unresponsive to transfusion and for which the intensivist is considering using antifibrinolytics.

B. **Chronic liver disease.** With the exception of factor VIII and von Willebrand's factor, which are manufactured by the endothelium, coagulation factors are synthesized by the liver. Patients with hepatic dysfunction may have decreased production of coagulation factors and decreased clearance of activated factors. Many, however, will respond to vitamin K (see **Section II.C**) and thus should receive a trial of vitamin K therapy. Failed response to vitamin K and the immediate need to correct coagulopathy require FFP transfusions until the PT has responded sufficiently (INR $<$1.5) or the bleeding has stopped. Thrombocytopenia also occurs frequently in liver disease due to splenic sequestration of platelets. This may be treated with platelet transfusion.

C. **Vitamin K deficiency** can be treated with vitamin K, 2.5 to 25 mg subcutaneously (SQ) once, or 10 mg SQ once daily for 3 days. Intravenous administration of vitamin K can correct the PT slightly faster, but is accompanied by a rare risk of anaphylaxis. If used, intravenous vitamin K should be administered very slowly. If faster correction of PT.

D. **Uremia.** Despite hemodialysis, abnormal platelet function in uremia remains a clinical issue because it may contribute to serious bleeding in patients with renal failure, particularly following surgical procedures or trauma. Treatment of uremic bleeding should include
   1. **Hemodialysis,** which is the primary therapy and which should be performed prior to emergent surgery or invasive procedures. It is also important to seek and correct other coexisting coagulopathies, such as vitamin K deficiency.

2. **IV desmopressin** (1-desamino-8-D-arginine vasopressin, DDAVP), which increases the release of factor VIII: von Willebrand's factor multimers from endothelium. The dose is 0.3 μg/kg infused slowly over 15 to 30 minutes to avoid hypotension.

3. **Treatment of anemia.** Acutely, this should be accomplished with transfusion of packed red blood cells (**pRBCs**) to a target hemoglobin approximately >10 mg/dL. The mechanism is believed to be a change in blood rheologic properties with a higher hematocrit tending to push platelets to the outer regions of the column of blood flow, closer to the blood vessel wall, and therefore enabling platelet interaction and adherence at the site of vessel injury. For the long-term treatment or prevention of uremic bleeding, erythropoietin should be considered.

4. **Cryoprecipitate,** 10 U every 12 hours until bleeding stops (see Chapter 35).

5. **Conjugated estrogens.** Onset of action is slower than DDAVP, but estrogens provide a more prolonged effect (4–7 days). The mechanism remains unclear; dose is 0.6 mg/kg/d IV or 50 mg/d orally for a total course 4 to 7 days.

E. **Massive transfusion** is discussed in **Chapter 35.**

III. **Common abnormalities of hemostasis in critical ill patients**
   A. **Bleeding disorders**
      1. **Hemophilias A and B** are rare congenital abnormalities of factors VIII and IX respectively.
         a. Clinical features. The diagnosis should be suspected in a patient with the appropriate history and an **elevated PTT** and normal PT.
         b. Because these patients have normal platelet function, they are able to form an initial clot. Because they are unable to stabilize the blood clot, however, bleeding will recur.
         c. Treatment consists of lyophilized factor VII, rFVIIa, factor IX concentrates, FFP, cryoprecipitate, or desmopressin. In critically ill bleeding patients, hematologic input is recommended.
      2. **von Willebrand's disease** is associated with abnormalities of von Willebrand's factor, a glycoprotein manufactured by megakaryocytes and endothelial cells that has multiple functions. It serves as an anchor for platelet adhesion to collagen, it interlinks platelets in clot formation, and it protects and stabilizes factor VIII. von Willebrand's disease is most commonly inherited in an autosomal dominant pattern with variable penetrance. Treatment includes DDAVP and/or cryoprecipitate. If cryoprecipitate is unavailable, FFP may be used. In patients with acquired von Willebrand's disease, high-dose IV γ-globulin (1 g/kg for 2 days) has been used successfully.
      3. **Other rare factor deficiencies** that predispose patients to bleeding have been described, including deficiencies of fibrinogen, factors II (prothrombin), V, VII, X, XI, and XIII. Treatment usually consists of factor concentrate or blood component replacement, and is best guided by hematology consultation.
   B. **Clotting disorders**
      1. **Congenital hypercoagulability abnormalities,** which predispose to clotting, may cause thrombosis and concurrent critical illness. Many specialized tests are available for diagnosing these abnormalities and guide therapy, which usually consists of lifelong anticoagulation. Test results may affect not only the patient, but also family members, because many of

these disorders are genetically transmitted. For patients presenting with venous thromboembolism, consideration should be given to testing for factor V Leiden (activated protein C resistance), AT III defects, proteins C and S deficiency, antiphospholipid antibodies, and hyperhomocysteinemia. The exact tests to be performed may be best determined by patient and family history. Many of these tests are unreliable during an acute illness because of the presence of acute-phase reactants. For these reasons, a hematology consultation is advisable when a congenital hypercoagulable state is suspected.

2. **Acquired disorders,** such as surgery, pregnancy, and trauma, all predispose to thrombosis. The cause is multifactorial. In surgical patients, venous stasis during perioperative immobility contributes. In addition, surgery and trauma produce a systemic response marked by an increase in acute-phase reactants, including increases in fibrinogen, factor VIII, and α-1-antitrypsin. Fibrinolytic proteins and coagulation inhibitors are decreased. Platelet activation and aggregation are enhanced. All of the preceding events promote a hypercoagulable state in surgical and trauma patients and mandate aggressive prophylaxis for thromboembolism (see Chapter 13). Prophylaxis may include pneumatic compression boots, early ambulation, and treatment with heparin, LMWH, fondaparinux, warfarin, or direct thrombin inhibitors.

3. **Heparin-induced thrombocytopenia (HIT)** occurs in two forms:

   a. HIT type I, a common, non–immune-mediated phenomenon, is a benign drop in platelet count within 5 days of institution of heparin therapy. Platelet counts rarely fall to less than $100,000/mm^3$ and recover to normal after approximately 5 days. HIT type I does not require discontinuation of heparin and does not carry a risk of thrombosis.

   b. HIT type II, hereafter referred to as HIT, is an immune-mediated thrombocytopenia triggered by IgG antibodies, which may form against heparin–platelet factor 4 (PF 4) complexes. The heparin–PF 4 complexes are seen as antigens and are bound to the Fc receptor on the platelet, activating the platelet and causing platelet aggregation and further PF 4 release. The result is thrombocytopenia, platelet aggregation, and the potential for arterial and venous thromboses (**Fig. 26-3**). In addition, HIT antibodies may bind to PF 4 complexes attached to endothelial cell surfaces, leading to injury, tissue factor expression, and a prothrombotic state.

      (1) The spectrum of HIT is best described by the "iceberg model" (**Fig. 26-4**), which suggests that a significant number of patients who are exposed to heparin develop the heparin–PF 4 complex antibody; a subset of these develop platelet aggregation and thrombocytopenia, and a small fraction of this subset develop vascular thrombosis. Data suggest that up to 50% of cardiac surgery patients and 15% of orthopedic surgery patients who are exposed to unfractionated heparin develop the HIT antibody as assessed by the enzyme-linked immunosorbent assay (ELISA). Of these, approximately 1% and 3%, respectively, go on to develop clinical HIT with thrombosis. The risk for HIT is greater with use of bovine versus porcine unfractionated heparin and may be dramatically reduced by use of low-molecular-weight heparins. Use of fondaparinux or the direct thrombin inhibitors for parenteral anticoagulation is not associated with development of HIT.

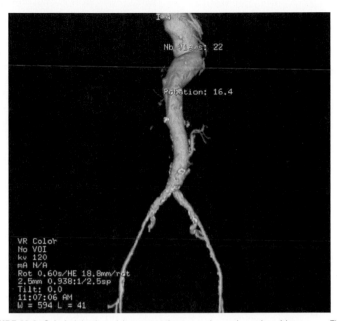

FIGURE 26-3 Spiral abdominopelvic computed tomography angiography with contrast. Three-dimensional aortic reconstruction shows complete failure of opacification of the celiac, superior mesenteric, and right renal aortic grafts. (Reprinted from Crimi C, Berra L, et al. *J Cardiothorac Vasc Anesth.* 2008;22:732–734, with permission.)

(2) The diagnosis of HIT should be suspected in a patient noted to have a more than 50% drop in platelet count from baseline, with the onset of the drop usually occurring 5 to 14 days after heparin exposure, but potentially sooner if the patient has a circulating antibody and is reexposed to heparin. The heparin exposure may occur in any form, including SQ prophylactic dosing, heparin flushes for indwelling catheters, or heparin coatings on indwelling central lines (e.g., pulmonary artery catheters). **Unexplained tachyphylaxis** or resistance to heparin anticoagulation may be suggestive of HIT, as may recovery of the platelet count after discontinuing heparin. The diagnosis is usually easy to make with ELISA testing in the proper clinical setting. Confirmation with a functional test of platelet aggregation such as the platelet serotonin release assay may be desirable because of the imperfect specificity of ELISA, but is in general impractical because of the limited availability of this test.

(3) The clinical course of HIT is notable for a median nadir of the platelet count of 50,000/mm^3. Despite the thrombocytopenia, the hallmark of the syndrome is platelet activation, aggregation, and a cascade of procoagulant effects resulting in thrombosis.

(4) **Treatment** of suspected or diagnosed HIT consists of (a) discontinuing all heparin exposure, including stopping heparin flushes and removing heparin-coated vascular catheters and (b) initiating

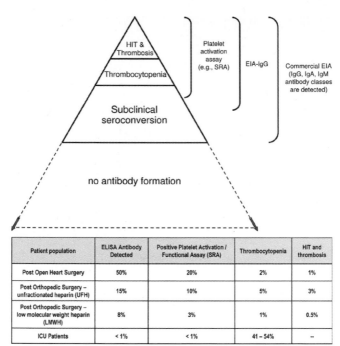

Patient population	ELISA Antibody Detected	Positive Platelet Activation / Functional Assay (SRA)	Thrombocytopenia	HIT and thrombosis
Post Open Heart Surgery	50%	20%	2%	1%
Post Orthopedic Surgery – unfractionated heparin (UFH)	15%	10%	5%	3%
Post Orthopedic Surgery – low molecular weight heparin (LMWH)	8%	3%	1%	0.5%
ICU Patients	< 1%	< 1%	41 – 54%	--

FIGURE 26-4 Iceberg model of HIT. Note the considerable differences in diagnostic specificity among the laboratory assays to detect HIT antibodies, thus, there is the potential to overdiagnose HIT (false positive). (Reprinted from Napolitano LM, Warkentin TE, et al. *Crit Care Med* 2006;34: 2898–2911, with permission.)

alternate anticoagulation, usually with a direct thrombin inhibitor (e.g., argatroban, lepirudin). **Table 26-2** describes dosing guidelines. Prophylactic platelet transfusions are contraindicated and usually unnecessary because thrombosis is a far greater clinical problem than bleeding. The importance of alternate anticoagulation in these patients must be emphasized because approximately 50% to 75% of patients with HIT will develop thrombotic complications with an attributable mortality estimated at 10% to 20%.

(5) Thromboses due to HIT are more commonly venous (DVT or PE) than arterial, but data suggest that the ratio of venous to arterial clots may be reversed in cardiovascular patients where arterial events are more than eight times as likely. Sites of severe atherosclerosis or recent arterial trauma (e.g., vascular access catheters) are particularly at risk. Arterial thromboses may present as mesenteric or limb ischemia, stroke, or myocardial infarction.

(6) No consensus exists as to the required duration of anticoagulant therapy for HIT, but most consultants recommend at least 6 weeks of treatment with an endpoint possibly marked by disappearance of the HIT antibody on ELISA. Oral anticoagulation should not be used to treat acute HIT and should not be initiated

TABLE 26-2	Dosing Guidelines for Treatment of Heparin-induced Thrombocytopenia (HIT)		
Drug	**Initial Dose**	**Adjustment**	**Comment**
Argatroban	[a]0.1 μg/kg/min	Titrate to target PTT 1.5–3.0 times baseline	Careful use in patients with hepatic dysfunction
Lepirudin	Bolus 0.2 mg/kg Infusion 0.1 mg/kg/h	Titrate to target PTT 1.5–2.0 times baseline	Initial IV bolus to be given only in case of perceived life- or limb-threatening thrombosis. Consider argatroban if renal dysfunction

PTT, partial thromboplastin time.
[a]This low dose range is suggested for critically ill patients with multiorgan failure.

until the platelet count is greater than $100,000/mm^3$. When initiating oral anticoagulation, it is critical to overlap therapy with a direct thrombin inhibitor because warfarin treatment is associated with an initial brief period of hypercoagulability due to decreased levels of protein C preceding adequate suppression of prothrombin levels. Thus, initiation of warfarin without overlapping anticoagulation can trigger venous limb gangrene. Reference to an algorithm for the transition to oral anticoagulation in HIT or consultation with a hematologist is recommended.

c. **Sickle cell disease** has a prevalence of approximately 1% in the African American population of the United States. Sickle cell disease is caused by the substitution of valine for glutamic acid at the sixth position on the β-chain of hemoglobin. Homozygotes for this substitution (as well as double heterozygotes for SC or β-thalassemia) have the clinical syndrome.

   (1) Clinical features. The abnormal hemoglobin polymerizes and causes a sickling deformity of the red cell under certain conditions (e.g., hypoxia, hypothermia, acidosis, and dehydration). Sickle cells cause microvascular occlusion with tissue ischemia and infarction. A sickle cell crisis typically presents with excruciating chest or abdominal pain, fever, tachycardia, leukocytosis, and hematuria. The red cells have a shortened survival time of 12 days (normal being 120 days), leading to anemia and extramedullary hematopoiesis. Neonates are usually protected from sickle crisis for the first few months of life due to persistent fetal hemoglobin (hemoglobin F). Patients with sickle cell trait are usually asymptomatic.

   (2) **Perioperative management.** It has been common practice to transfuse these patients perioperatively, to reduce the relative proportion of Hgb S. Past guidelines suggested transfusing to an endpoint of 70% of the patient's hemoglobin being Hgb A, measured by hemoglobin electrophoresis, prior to major surgery. Recently, this practice has been questioned, and routine preoperative transfusion of asymptomatic patients is not recommended. Perioperative care should be directed at reducing the risks of sickling, including hypoxia, acidosis, dehydration, and hypothermia.

Recent understanding of the pathobiology cascade caused by intravascular hemolysis provides new targets for potential therapeutic intervention, including inhaled nitric oxide, arginine, sodium nitrite, phosphodiesterase-5 inhibitors, inhaled carbon monoxide, niacin, and endothelin receptor blockade.

IV. **Anticoagulation treatment.** Indications for anticoagulation include the prevention or treatment of DVT, PE, intracardiac thrombus in atrial fibrillation or severe ventricular dysfunction, and vascular graft thrombosis (see Chapters 18, 19, 22, and 39 among others). Anticoagulation also may be required for renal replacement therapy (dialysis or hemofiltration), extracorporeal circulation, or cardiac support (intra-aortic balloon pump).

A. **Heparin** (see also **Appendix**) is a naturally occurring anticoagulant produced from bovine lung or porcine intestine that acts by accelerating the effect of AT III. Structurally, heparin is a heterogeneous mixture of glycosaminoglycans with molecular weights ranging from 3,000 to 30,000 Da. A repetitive pentasaccharide glucosamine sequence that is present in only one-third of the heparin molecules is necessary for AT III binding. The heparin–AT III complex inactivates several factors in the coagulation cascade, but most importantly thrombin (factor II) and factor X. Longer heparin chains are required for thrombin inhibition than for X inhibition. For full anticoagulation, as in the treatment of DVT or PE, heparin may be administered by a continuous intravenous infusion. The 2008 Antithrombotic and Thrombolytic Therapy Guidelines of the American College of Chest Physicians recommend that after an initial IV bolus (80 U/kg or 5,000 U), heparin should be administered by continuous infusion (initially at a dose of 18 U/kg/h or 1,300 U/h), with dose adjustment to achieve and maintain a PTT prolongation ranging from 1.5 to 2 times baseline. The PTT should be determined every 6 hours until the level of anticoagulation is stable and therapeutic PTT should be reached within the first 24 hours of treatment. Heparin has a short life (approximately 90 minutes). Stopping a heparin infusion for 2 to 4 hours will usually reverse the effect. If faster reversal is required, protamine, a natural antagonist, may be used. Dosage is 1 mg for every 100 U of heparin estimated to be remaining in the patient, and it should be given slowly because adverse reactions (e.g., hypotension, pulmonary hypertension, hypersensitivity reactions) are common. Institution-wide heparin protocols promote safe and effective anticoagulation practices.

1. Heparin resistance occurs frequently in critically ill patients because circulating acute-phase reactants nonspecifically bind heparin and limit its anticoagulant effect. The resulting tachyphylaxis to heparin can usually be overcome with increasing doses of the drug. Occasionally, AT III levels may be depleted in critically ill patients, also contributing to heparin failure. If AT III levels are low, AT III concentrate or, alternatively, FFP may be administered to replete AT III and restore heparin efficacy. Of note, HIT should always be considered in the differential diagnosis of heparin tachyphylaxis.

2. Heparin may be administered SQ in low dose for DVT prophylaxis. The usual dose is 5,000 U SQ every 8 to 12 hours. This dose usually does not prolong the PTT.

B. **Anti-factor Xa inhibitors**

1. **Low-molecular-weight heparins (LMWH)** are commercially prepared by fractionating heparin into molecules of 2,000 to 10,000 Da. Most of these lower-molecular-weight molecules are incapable of cross-linking to both antithrombin and thrombin and thus exert their

anticoagulant effect primarily by inhibiting factor X. Treatment with LMWH generally does not prolong the PTT and usually does not require laboratory monitoring of anticoagulation. The anticoagulant effect may be assessed by measuring anti-Xa levels, if desired.

- **a.** Advantages. LMWH is superior to unfractionated heparin in DVT prophylaxis of certain high-risk patients, including patients undergoing elective hip or knee replacement or hip replacement due to fracture. Studies also support a therapeutic advantage in trauma and spinal cord–injured patients. LMWH has a more predictable dose–response relationship for anticoagulation than unfractionated heparin, because LMWH has much less nonspecific binding to acute-phase reactants than unfractionated heparin. The more predictable effect of LMWH decreases or eliminates the need for laboratory monitoring of drug effect. LMWH anticoagulation may be associated with fewer bleeding complications than standard heparin. Finally, the incidence of HIT is less with LMWH than with unfractionated heparin.
- **b.** Disadvantages of LMWH include a half-life of 4 hours, incomplete reversal with protamine, renal clearance, and cost.
- **c.** Several commercially available preparations of LMWH are available with slightly different mean molecular weights and anti-Xa activity. LMWH may be administered IV, but excellent bioavailability and long half-life permit convenient SQ dosing. Dosing for DVT prophylaxis is 30 mg SQ every 12 hours for **enoxaparin** and 2,500 to 5,000 anti-Xa U SQ once daily for **dalteparin.** Dosing for DVT treatment is 1 mg/kg SQ every 12 hours for enoxaparin and 100 U/kg SQ every 12 hours for dalteparin.
- **d.** **Fondaparinux** is a pentasaccharide molecule that selectively inhibits factor Xa by binding to antithrombin and inducing a conformational change that increases antithrombin's binding affinity for Xa. The drug is administered SQ, has a long half-life (14–16 hours), and has a predictable anticoagulant effect. Prophylactic doses (2.5 mg daily) normally do not prolong the PT or PTT, and laboratory monitoring of anticoagulant effect is usually unnecessary. In critically ill patients, the drug may be used for either prophylaxis or treatment of DVT. Fondaparinux does not interact with platelets or platelet factor 4, and thus, unlike heparin, is not expected to induce HIT. Therefore, routine platelet count monitoring for patients receiving fondaparinux is not recommended. Disadvantages to use of fondaparinux in the critically ill include its irreversibility and diminished clearance in the elderly and patients with renal dysfunction.
- **e.** **Idraparinux** is a longer-acting analogue of fondaparinux, administered SQ once per week, and currently under investigation in clinical trials. While idraparinux was not inferior to vitamin K antagonists in terms of the primary efficacy outcome of stroke prevention, it did show a significantly increased risk of clinically relevant bleeding.
- **f.** The oral agents **rivaroxaban, apixaban,** and **razaxaban** are newly available factor Xa inhibitors under investigation, and are not yet FDA approved. Preliminary studies have shown that this class of anticoagulants are relatively safe and effective for prevention and treatment of thromboembolism.

C. Vitamin K antagonists. Warfarin (Coumadin) *inhibits vitamin K epoxide reductase.* This produces a deficiency of vitamin K, preventing the hepatic carboxylation of factors II, VII, IX, and X and proteins C and S to the active form. The half-life of warfarin is approximately 35 hours, requiring days for reversal. If quick reversal of warfarin is required, active factors can be given in the form of FFP (5–15 mL/kg). Vitamin K (2.5–25 mg IV or SQ) can also be given for warfarin reversal, but its effect requires 6 or more hours. Warfarin may be administered enterally or parenterally once daily. Anticoagulation does not occur for approximately 3 to 4 days and may require a week or more to achieve a stable level. Therapy is guided by measurement of INR (see **Section I.B**). Cautious dosing should be undertaken in patients who are vitamin K depleted to avoid over-anticoagulation and possible bleeding complications.

D. Direct thrombin inhibitors (DTIs) act independently of cofactors (e.g., AT III) to inhibit not only circulating thrombin, but also clot-bound thrombin, thereby inhibiting clot enlargement. These drugs are useful for the treatment of HIT or for prevention of HIT with thrombosis in patients at risk. Dosage of DTIs is guided by prolongation of the ACT or PTT to therapeutic range (see **Table 26-2**). The drugs have no reversal agents.

1. **Lepirudin** was originally isolated from the salivary gland of leeches and was approved for the treatment of HIT. The short half-life (80 minutes) of this agent allows relatively rapid reversal of anticoagulation by stopping the drug. Lepirudin undergoes renal excretion, and thus its use should be avoided or the dose carefully adjusted in patients with renal failure due to the risk for bleeding (see **Table 26-2**).

2. **Bivalirudin** is hirudin analogue with a short (25 minute) half-life that is administered via intravenous infusion for percutaneous coronary interventions. Anecdotal reports suggest its efficacy in the treatment of patients with HIT, and it has been successfully used for cardiopulmonary bypass with patients with HIT, although it is not approved for this use.

3. **Argatroban** is a small, synthetic molecule derived from L-arginine. Argatroban's half-life is 40 minutes, allowing relatively rapid reversal of anticoagulation by solely stopping the drug. Argatroban is approved by the Food and Drug Administration (FDA) for treatment of HIT complicated by thrombosis and for prophylaxis against thrombosis in patients with HIT. Argatroban undergoes hepatobiliary excretion and requires dose adjustment in patients with hepatic dysfunction. The drug prolongs the INR, complicating assessment of warfarin anticoagulant effect when patients are transitioned from parenteral to enteral anticoagulation. Argatroban has a greater pharmacodynamic predictability than lepirudin and may have a greater safety profile in critically ill patients due to its reliable excretion even in moderate renal failure. In addition, argatroban crosses the blood–brain barrier and may serve a role in the treatment of ischemic or thrombotic stroke.

4. **Oral direct thrombin inhibitors** are now under development and investigation. Dabigatran etexilate was as effective as enoxaparin in reducing risk of DVT after total hip replacement in a randomized trial.

E. Platelet inhibitors may be useful for reducing thromboembolic events in patients with arterial vascular disorders (e.g., carotid stenosis), prosthetic heart valves, or recent invasive arterial procedures (e.g., percutaneous coronary angioplasty or stenting). **Aspirin** and **nonsteroidal anti-inflammatory drugs (NSAIDs)** inhibit platelet aggregation by interfering with the cyclooxygenase pathway. Aspirin permanently inhibits the pathway for the lifespan of the platelet. Because the half-life of platelets in circulation is approximately 4 days, at least 10 days are required before platelet function returns to normal after aspirin. The other NSAIDs reversibly inhibit the cyclooxygenase pathway; their effects dissipate within 3 days of discontinuing the drug. **Ticlopidine** and **clopidogrel** are oral antiplatelet agents that inhibit ADP-mediated platelet aggregation and are frequently used following percutaneous coronary interventions. The intravenous glycoprotein IIb/IIIa receptor inhibitors **abciximab** and **eptifibatide** are drugs that bind to the key platelet receptor that mediates aggregation. Fibrinogen, von Willebrand's factor, and other adhesive molecules are thereby blocked from binding to the platelet, inhibiting platelet aggregation and resulting in anticoagulation. Both drugs may be used for treatment of acute coronary syndromes or during percutaneous coronary interventions. Abciximab remains in the circulation bound to platelets 15 days following dosing, although platelet function is usually recovered within 48 hours after a dose. Eptifibatide has a reversible antiplatelet effect that normalizes approximately 4 hours after discontinuation of the infusion. The use of glycoprotein IIb/IIIa receptor inhibitors is contraindicated within 6 weeks of major surgery or trauma due to bleeding risk. Immediate reversal of platelet inhibitors may require platelet transfusion, although even this treatment may result in only partial reversal of the effect (see **Chapter 25**).

F. **Thrombolytic agents** act by dissolving thrombi via conversion of plasminogen to plasmin, which lyses fibrin clots. They are intended to reverse thrombosis and recanalize blood vessels. These agents are used to treat acute occlusion of coronary, cerebral, pulmonary, and peripheral arteries, typically in combination with heparin to prevent reocclusion. Three thrombolytic agents, **tissue plasminogen activator (tPA), streptokinase, and urokinase,** are used commonly in clinical practice, each with slightly different pharmacodynamic and side effect profiles. Each of these drugs results in a hypofibrinogenemic state and carries a substantial risk of bleeding. They are generally contraindicated perioperatively. If emergent surgery is required following thrombolytic therapy, the effect may be reversed by administration of aminocaproic or tranexamic acid (see **Section V.A**). Additionally, the fibrinogen level may be restored by transfusion of cryoprecipitate or FFP (see **Chapter 35**).

V. Hemostatic agents

A. **Lysine analogues—aminocaproic acid and tranexamic acid.** The lysine analogues **aminocaproic acid (Amicar)** and tranexamic acid inhibit fibrinolysis, the endogenous process by which fibrin clot is broken down. They act by displacing plasminogen from fibrin, diminishing plasminogen conversion to plasmin, and preventing plasmin from binding to fibrinogen or fibrin monomers. *Aminocaproic acid* is used to provide prophylaxis for dental surgery in hemophiliacs, prevent bleeding in prostatic surgery, and reduce hemorrhage in cases of excessive fibrinolysis (e.g., during orthotopic liver transplantation). Because cardiopulmonary bypass can initiate fibrinolysis, aminocaproic acid has been used during cardiac surgery to diminish postoperative bleeding, but its effects on transfusion requirements have been variable. The dose is **10 g IV load over 1 hour followed by 1 to 2 g/h.** Thrombotic risks of aminocaproic acid have been suggested via case reports, but have not been substantiated by clinical trial. Nevertheless, because normal function of the coagulation cascade involves a balance between pro- and anticoagulant effects, using aminocaproic acid in circumstances where uninhibited clotting may be disastrous (e.g., DIC) is ill advised and should be undertaken only with expert guidance.

B. **DDAVP** increases endothelial cell release of von Willebrand's factor, factor VIII, and plasminogen activator, and thus has utility in certain bleeding disorders, including hemophilia A (factor VIII deficiency), classic von Willebrand's disease, and uremic bleeding (see **Section II**).

C. Aprotinin is a serine protease inhibitor which had been used to decrease blood loss from complicated cardiac procedures and major surgeries associated with massive hemorrhage, including orthotopic liver transplantation. The drug was withdrawn from the market in 2007 based on studies in cardiac patients showing an increased risk of death.

Selected References

Bousser MG, Bouthier J, et al. Comparison of idraparinux with vitamin K antagonists for prevention of thromboembolism in patients with atrial fibrillation: a randomised, open-label, non-inferiority trial. *Lancet* 2008;371:315–321.

Buller HR, Cohen AT, et al. Extended prophylaxis of venous thromboembolism with idraparinux. *N Engl J Med* 2007;357:1105–1112.

Eriksson BI, Dahl OE, et al. Dabigatran etexilate versus enoxaparin for prevention of venous thromboembolism after total hip replacement: a randomised, double-blind, non-inferiority trial. *Lancet* 2007;370:949–956.

Ganter MT, Hofer CK. Coagulation monitoring: current techniques and clinical use of viscoelastic point-of-care coagulation devices. *Anesth Analg* 2008;106:1366–1375.

Hirsh J, Guyatt G, et al; American College of Chest Physicians. Antithrombotic and thrombolytic therapy: American College of Chest Physicians Evidence-Based Clinical Practice Guidelines (8th Edition). *Chest* 2008;133:110S–112S.

Kato JG; Gladwin TM. Evolution of novel small-molecule therapeutics targeting sickle cell vasculopathy. *JAMA* 2008;300:2638–2646.

Lassen MR, Ageno W, et al. Rivaroxaban versus enoxaparin for thromboprophylaxis after total knee arthroplasty. *N Engl J Med* 2008;358:2776–2786.

Napolitano L, Warkentin T, et al. Heparin-induced thrombocytopenia in the critical care setting: diagnosis and management. *Crit Care Med* 2006;34:2898–2911.

O'Connell NM, Perry DJ, et al. Recombinant FVIIa in the management of uncontrolled hemorrhage. *Transfusion* 2003;43:1711–1716.

Schneewiss S, Seeger JD, et al. Aprotinin during coronary-artery bypass grafting and risk of death. *N Engl J Med* 2008;358:771–783.

Warkentin TE, Greinacher A, et al. Treatment and prevention of heparin-induced thrombocytopenia: American College of Chest Physicians Evidence-Based Clinical Practice Guidelines (8th Edition). *Chest* 2008;133:340S–380S.

27

Acute Gastrointestinal Diseases

Eugene Fukudome and Jean Kwo

I. Patients may be admitted to the ICU for management of gastrointestinal (GI) diseases, such as acute pancreatitis, perforation, and bleeding, or following a major surgical procedure involving the GI tract. Alternatively, critically ill patients may develop GI pathology while undergoing treatment for an unrelated condition, often as part of multisystem organ dysfunction. This chapter will first address the evaluation of suspected GI diseases in an ICU setting, and will then focus on management of commonly encountered GI pathology.

II. **Evaluation of suspected GI pathology:** Critically ill patients may develop new GI pathology during their hospitalization. The diagnosis of a new GI disorder in the ICU is challenging as these patients may not be able to articulate their symptoms, and often do not present with classic clinical findings. A nonspecific finding such as change in mental status, fever, leukocytosis, hypotension, or decreased urine output may be the only sign of intra-abdominal pathology. Physical examination may be unreliable, and the patient may be too unstable to leave the ICU to undergo diagnostic studies. Thus, clinicians must maintain a high index of suspicion for an undiagnosed GI problem when ICU patients have a change in their clinical course.

A. **Signs and symptoms** that suggest GI pathology are numerous and can include abdominal pain, chest pain, bleeding (hematemesis, melena, rectal bleeding), emesis, change in bowel habits, and tube feed intolerance.

B. **Initial evaluation** includes assessing for abdominal tenderness and distension, fever, tachycardia, hypotension, and/or change in vasopressor requirement. Correct positioning and function of existing nasogastric tubes and abdominal drains must be confirmed. Laboratory tests such as a complete blood count (CBC), serum chemistries, liver function tests (LFTs), and amylase may be helpful.

C. Increased vigilance is required when caring for solid **organ transplant** recipients or patients with chronic inflammatory or autoimmune disorders treated with immunosuppressive medications. These chronically **immunosuppressed** patients may have no signs or symptoms of ongoing GI pathology.

D. **Further diagnostic studies and procedures** are often necessary to establish a diagnosis and are guided by the initial assessment. Portable plain radiographs can reveal the presence of pneumoperitoneum, intestinal obstruction, or confirm the correct placement of an enteral tube (**Fig. 27-1**). However, more sophisticated studies are often required to establish a diagnosis. The risks associated with a diagnostic study must be weighed against the expected benefits. Commonly performed tests such as an abdominal CT scan pose a higher risk to the critically ill patient who is at increased risk for contrast-induced nephropathy (**Chapter 24**), ventilator-associated pneumonia, as well as airway and hemodynamic complications while traveling to the radiology department. Commonly available

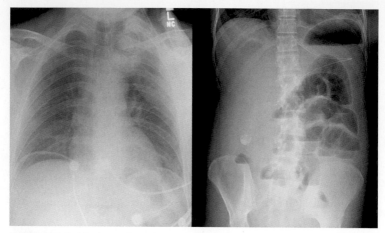

FIGURE 27-1 A plain chest radiograph demonstrating pneumoperitoneum (left) and an abdominal film demonstrating small bowel obstruction and nasogastric tube placement (right). Courtesy of Hasan Alam, MD.

diagnostic modalities and their advantages and disadvantages in an ICU setting are summarized in **Table 27-1**.

III. **GI bleeding** is commonly seen in an ICU setting (**Table 27-2**). GI bleeding may originate from the upper (proximal to the ligament of Treitz) or lower GI tract. Risk factors include liver disease, alcoholism, uremia, diverticulosis, peptic ulcer disease, and the intake of a variety of medications, including nonsteroidal anti-inflammatory drugs (NSAIDs), antiplatelet agents, and anticoagulants.

A. **Signs and symptoms** include shock, hematemesis, coffee ground emesis, melena, hematochezia, or hematocrit drop with occult blood present in the stool.

B. **Initial evaluation** may need to proceed simultaneously with stabilization depending on the rate of blood loss and hemodynamic stability of the patient.

1. A **history** focusing on risk factors for GI bleeding, prior abdominal operations, and significant medical comorbidities should be obtained.

2. **Physical examination** should focus on assessing end organ perfusion. Certain physical findings such as stigmata of liver disease may suggest an underlying etiology.

3. **Laboratory studies** including CBC, coagulation studies, and chemistries should be obtained. Initial hemoglobin values will not reflect the degree of acute blood loss.

C. **Stabilization** is accomplished by ensuring an adequate airway, hemodynamic stability, and adequate monitoring. A patient with an altered level of consciousness and copious hematemesis will likely require endotracheal intubation. Adequate peripheral intravenous access should be secured. Central venous access, an arterial catheter, and a urinary catheter placement may be appropriate for patients in shock. Initial resuscitation with isotonic crystalloid solution is appropriate while preparations for blood transfusions are made. Severe coagulopathy should be corrected (**Chapter 26**).

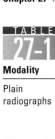

TABLE 27-1	Diagnostic Modalities for Acute Gastrointestinal Diseases in the ICU	
Modality	**Advantages and Usefulness**	**Disadvantages**
Plain radiographs	• Portable and fast • Assess for free air • Confirm tube placement (nasogastric, postpyloric)	• Findings are usually nonspecific • Overlying tubes, monitors, cables and other ICU equipment often obscure images
Ultrasound	• Portable • Assess gall bladder/biliary tree • Can guide procedures (paracentesis, biliary drains)	• Image quality is operator dependent • Air-filled intestines can obscure images
CT	• Characterizes many forms of intra-abdominal pathology • CT angiography can assess mesenteric vessels	• Patient transport out of the ICU • Optimum study requires IV contrast which can cause nephropathy and allergic reactions
MRI	• Noninvasive method to assess for choledocholithiasis	• Patient transport out of the ICU • Time consuming • Requires patient cooperation
Angiography	• Diagnostic and therapeutic in mesenteric ischemia, GI bleeding and intra-abdominal/pelvic bleeding following trauma	• Patient transport out of the ICU • Requires IV contrast • Risk of vascular injury (arterial injury at the access site, pseudoaneurysms, hematoma, bleeding, arterial dissection, and embolization of vessel plaque)
Radionuclide imaging	• HIDA scan may help characterized suspected biliary pathology such as cholecystitis • Technetium scan can confirm ongoing GI bleeding	• Never an initial diagnostic test • Patient transport out of the ICU • Limited utility in an ICU setting
Endoscopy	• Diagnostic and therapeutic • EGD and colonoscopy can be performed portably • ERCP can be life-saving in cholangitis	• Requires sedation • Colonoscopy requires colonic purge for optimum study • Small risk of intestinal perforation • ERCP can cause pancreatitis
Bedside laparoscopy	• Direct visualization facilitates diagnosis of acalculous cholecystitis and mesenteric ischemia, according to several reports (small case series) • Can potentially avoid nontherapeutic laparotomy	• Invasive • Inability to evaluate some areas (retroperitoneum) • Patient must be mechanically ventilated and sedated • Utility as a diagnostic modality in the ICU has not been rigorously studied

Causes of Gastrointestinal (GI) Bleeding	
Upper GI Source	**Lower GI Source**
Variceal bleeding	Diverticulum
• Esophageal, gastric, duodenal	• Small bowel, colonic
Mallory–Weiss tears	Inflammatory bowel disease
Peptic ulcers	Mesenteric ischemia including ischemic colitis
• Gastric, duodenal	Infectious colitis
Gastritis and erosions	Malignancy
Malignancy	Angiodysplasia
Dieulafoy's lesions	• Colonic, small bowel
Arterial-enteric fistula	Hemorrhoids
• Rupture of aneurysm or ulcer	
• Postaortic surgery	
Diverticulum (duodenal)	
Angiodysplasia (duodenal)	
Hemobilia	
Pancreatic bleeding	

D. **Localization of bleeding**
1. **Nasogastric tube lavage** of the stomach is easy to perform and may help localize the hemorrhage. **Clear lavage fluid with bile** staining makes gastric, duodenal, and biliopancreatic sources of bleeding unlikely.
2. **Endoscopy**
    a. **Esophagogastroduodenoscopy (EGD)** is the diagnostic test of choice for suspected upper GI bleeding, and is diagnostic in 90% to 95% of cases. Often, the precise source of bleeding is identified, allowing for immediate endoscopic therapy; however, this can be challenging if a copious amount of blood and clot is present.
    b. **Colonoscopy** for lower GI bleeding is diagnostic in 53% to 97% of cases, depending on the patient population of each study. Colonoscopy is usually undertaken after a colonic purge to increase diagnostic accuracy and visualization. Complications, including perforation, are rare, but the index of suspicion for their occurrence must be high in critically ill, elderly, and immunosuppressed patients.
3. **Angiography** may be required if endoscopy cannot localize bleeding.
    a. Requires ongoing bleeding for successful angiographic detection (0.5–1 mL/min, approximately 3 U of blood per day).
    b. Angiography may direct endoscopic or surgical treatment, or may be therapeutic via embolization or selective intra-arterial vasopressin infusion.
    c. Complications associated with angiography include contrast-induced nephropathy, distal embolization of vessel wall plaque, and access site complications.
4. **Radionuclide imaging** involves the use of one of two available tracers: technetium-99 m–labeled sulfur colloid (^{99m}Tc-SC), and technetium-99 m–labeled red blood cells (^{99m}Tc-RBC). ^{99m}Tc-SC can be used immediately, but is taken up by the liver and spleen, which can obscure interpretation of the images when bleeding is located adjacent to these structures. ^{99m}Tc-RBC is not taken up by the liver and spleen, but requires preparation prior to use.

     a. ^{99m}Tc-labeled scans are sensitive and can confirm ongoing bleeding. Their specificity in determining a precise anatomic site of bleeding is debatable.

     b. Their utility in an ICU setting is limited, but may be helpful in hemodynamically stable patients with slow lower GI bleeding not localized by colonoscopy.

   5. A **capsule study** can occasionally help identify a bleeding source in the small bowel of hemodynamically stable patients.

E. Specific therapy for common causes of GI bleeding

  1. Upper GI bleeding

    a. Variceal bleeding may originate in the esophagus, stomach, or duodenum, and is usually the result of cirrhosis and portal hypertension. Splenic vein thrombosis can also result in the development of gastric varices.

     (1) Prognosis is related mainly to the severity of the patient's underlying liver disease. Mortality following an episode of variceal bleeding ranges from 10% to 70%. The risk of rebleeding is 70% within 6 months.

     (2) Early endoscopy is crucial for diagnosis and management. Thirty to fifty percent of patients with known varices bleed from other upper GI sources. Endoscopic variceal band ligation and sclerotherapy can control bleeding in 80% to 90% of cases.

     (3) Balloon tamponade is indicated when endoscopic interventions cannot control esophageal or gastric variceal bleeding. Because of the risk of pressure necrosis, balloon deflation must occur within 24 to 48 hours, and should be followed by another attempt at endoscopy with band ligation or sclerotherapy.

     (4) Medical management should occur concurrently with endoscopy or balloon tamponade. **Somatostatin** and its synthetic analog **octreotide,** as well as **vasopressin**, have been used.

     (5) After the bleeding has stopped and the patient is stabilized, treatment with **nonselective β-blockers** (propranolol or nadolol) should be initiated. These agents decrease the risk of rebleeding and have a proven survival benefit.

     (6) Transjugular intrahepatic portosystemic shunting (TIPS) controls refractory variceal bleeding in up to 90% of cases by reducing the portal pressure gradient to <15 mm Hg. Using a transjugular approach, a stent is placed in the liver to connect a branch of the portal vein with a hepatic vein. Complications include occlusion, accelerated liver failure, and hepatic encephalopathy.

     (7) Surgical therapy for refractory bleeding includes splenorenal shunt and portacaval shunt, and should generally be undertaken after the patient is determined to not be a liver transplant candidate.

     (8) Splenectomy is indicated in patients who are bleeding from gastric varices due to splenic vein thrombosis.

    b. Mallory-Weiss tears are mucosal lacerations within 2 cm of the gastroesophageal (GE) junction that are likely due to increases in pressure occurring during vomiting. Most of these lesions stop bleeding spontaneously and have less than a 10% chance of rebleeding. However, actively bleeding Mallory-Weiss tears are best addressed endoscopically.

    c. Peptic ulcer disease can manifest as duodenal or gastric ulcers.

(1) **EGD** is the initial diagnostic and therapeutic choice. The **endoscopic appearance** of an ulcer has prognostic significance. Ulcers with a spurting artery or a visible vessel have a high rebleeding risk (50%–100%). Ulcers with adherent clot or a red or black spot are at moderate risk, while ulcers with a clean base are at low risk (<5%) for rebleeding. Repeat EGD may be necessary to control bleeding in some circumstances. In refractory cases, angiographic embolization has been reported to stop bleeding in 80% to 88% of cases. Uncontrolled bleeding in a hemodynamically unstable patient may necessitate surgical intervention.

(2) **Acid suppression** with proton pump inhibitors (PPIs) has evolved as a crucial component in the management of ulcer disease. In the acute setting, PPIs are administered intravenously as a continuous infusion or twice-daily boluses. Patients are then transitioned to an oral regimen. PPIs produce more consistent acid suppression than histamine receptor (H2) blockers.

(3) *H. pylori* **infection** (see **Section IV.B.2**), if present, should be eradicated to decreases the rate of future rebleeding.

(4) Mucosal ulcerations may be due to **neoplasm** rather than peptic ulcer disease. The endoscopic appearance in conjunction with a biopsy will help establish the correct diagnosis.

d. **Stress ulceration,** also called stress-related erosive syndrome, erosive gastritis, or hemorrhagic gastritis, leads to upper GI bleeding in 1% to 7% of ICU patients. Mucosal hypoperfusion and increased gastric acidity occurring in critically ill patients are postulated to play a role in pathogenesis.

(1) **Endoscopic** findings include mucosal erosions.

(2) **Management** is with PPIs as discussed above. *Helicobacter pylori* infection should be excluded. Rarely, angiography with selective embolization (often of the left gastric artery) is necessary. Operative management is reserved for severe refractory hemorrhage.

e. **Aortoenteric fistulae** are communications between the GI tract, most commonly the distal duodenum, and either the native aorta (primary) or an aortic vascular graft (secondary). Secondary fistulas are more common, occurring in 0.6% to 1.5% of patients after aortic reconstructive surgery. An initial "herald" bleed followed by massive hemorrhage has been described. Patients may also present with graft infection. Accurate and timely diagnosis is facilitated by a high index of suspicion.

(1) **Endoscopy** demonstrating an eroding aortic graft is uncommon. CT scan is the diagnostic study of choice and may demonstrate hematoma or air at the aortic graft. Once the diagnosis is established, emergency operative exploration is indicated. Endovascular techniques utilizing stent grafts may be an option for patients without evidence of infection.

f. **Dieulafoy's lesion** is an abnormally large artery protruding through the mucosa, most often into the gastric lumen (fundus or body). There is no mucosal ulceration. Bleeding can be massive and can recur in 5% to 15% despite endoscopic therapy. When rebleeding occurs despite endoscopic intervention, surgical ligation or excision of the vessel is indicated.

g. **Duodenal diverticulum** is a rare cause of upper GI bleeding. The diagnosis can be made endoscopically. Bleeding duodenal diverticula are treated with surgical excision.

h. **Angiodysplasia** can be located throughout the entire GI tract and can cause brisk bleeding. Endoscopy can detect and treat these lesions. Surgical excision is indicated when lesions continue to bleed despite medical management.

i. **Pancreatic bleeding** can occur from erosion of a pancreatic pseudocyst into an adjacent vessel, resulting in upper GI bleeding.

j. **Hemobilia** can result from trauma, procedures such as liver biopsy, biliary stent placement, malignancy, gallstones or erosion of blood vessels into the biliary tree.

2. **Lower GI bleeding** accounts for approximately 25% of GI bleeding, and has a mortality rate of 2% to 4%.

a. **Intestinal ischemia** can involve either the small bowel or the colon, and can present with lower GI bleeding. Intestinal ischemia is discussed later in greater detail (Section IV.F.1).

b. **Small bowel bleeding** is suspected after two negative EGDs and a negative colonoscopy.

   (1) **Angiodysplasia** is the most common cause of GI hemorrhage between the ligament of Treitz and the ileocecal valve. Other causes include tumors, inflammatory bowel disease, Meckel's diverticulum, NSAID-induced ulcers, and Dieulafoy's lesions.

   (2) **Diagnosis** is difficult but may be made in approximately 50% to 70% of cases by push enteroscopy (which examines the jejunum) or capsule study. If the bleeding is brisk, radionuclide scans or angiography may be useful.

   (3) **Treatment** of small intestinal sources of bleeding is directed at the underlying disease.

c. **Diverticular bleeding** accounts for 20% of colonic bleeding. Hemorrhage occurs when the *vasa recta* ruptures into an adjacent diverticular lumen. Bleeding is usually self-limited but can recur in 14% to 53% of patients. Colonoscopy can locate the site of bleeding, but therapeutic maneuvers are difficult. Angiography can also localize the bleeding, and is potentially therapeutic. Urgent operative resection is indicated when bleeding and hemodynamic instability persists. Elective colectomy is considered after multiple episodes of diverticular bleeding.

d. **Colonic angiodysplasias** are more frequent in patients over the age of 60. Most lesions are found in the ascending colon, and most patients have multiple lesions. Colonoscopy and angiography are very successful for diagnosis and treatment, and colon resection is reserved for failures of these modalities.

e. **Colorectal neoplasm** (adenocarcinoma as well as polyps) can present with acute lower GI bleeding, although chronic or occult blood loss and microcytic anemia is a more common presentation. Treatment is multidisciplinary including surgical resection. Postpolypectomy bleeding can be treated with colonoscopy and coagulation.

f. **Hemorrhoids and other benign anorectal diseases** make up nearly 10% of acute hematochezia. In patients with portal hypertension, hemorrhoidal bleeding can be life threatening, and treatment must be aggressive and may involve a portosystemic shunting procedure.

g. **Colitis** may be ischemic, infectious, or a result of inflammatory bowel disease (**Crohn's disease** or **ulcerative colitis**), and can present with bloody diarrhea, hematochezia, or melena. Colonoscopy usually reveals diffuse mucosal inflammation. Management of inflammatory bowel disease is best directed by a gastroenterologist and consists of hydration, bowel rest, and steroids. Ischemic and infectious colitis are discussed in **Sections IV.F.1** and **IV.F.4.**

IV. Specific GI problems by organ

A. Esophagus

1. **Esophageal perforation** is most often iatrogenic and may follow upper endoscopy procedures, NG tube placement, balloon tamponade of bleeding varices, endotracheal tube placement, or transesophageal echocardiography. Abnormal anatomy such as a Zenker's diverticulum may predispose the patient to this complication. Perforation can occur in the cervical, thoracic, or abdominal esophagus, leading to cervical abscess, mediastinitis, empyema, or peritonitis.

   a. **Diagnosis.** Patients may have pain, fever, subcutaneous crepitus, leukocytosis, pneumomediastinum, or a pleural effusion. A contrast swallow study, CT scan, or esophagoscopy can confirm and localize esophageal perforations.

   b. **Treatment** is urgent and includes broad-spectrum antibiotics, drainage, and gastric acid suppression. Some patients may be candidates for primary repair at the time of drainage. Most patients will be fasted for a prolonged period, and will require nutritional support via a feeding tube.

2. **Boerhaave's syndrome** refers to spontaneous esophageal perforation, which may have no obvious precipitant or may be related to retching/vomiting, blunt trauma, weightlifting, or childbirth. Predisposing factors include reflux esophagitis, esophageal infections, peptic ulcer disease, and alcoholism.

3. **Ingestion** of foreign bodies and caustic substances can cause significant esophageal injury.

   a. Ingested **foreign bodies,** most commonly food boluses, can present with dysphagia, odynophagia, chest pain, or airway obstruction. Blunt objects less than 2 cm in size traverse the GI tract uneventfully, while objects larger than 6 cm will obstruct within the duodenum if not in the esophagus. Most objects that do not pass spontaneously may be removed endoscopically—this should be done early to minimize the risk of perforation from pressure-induced necrosis of the esophageal wall.

   b. **Acids** (pH <2) and **alkalis** (pH >12) cause severe burns when ingested. Vomiting after the ingestion exposes the esophagus to the caustic substance a second time.

      (1) **Initial management** includes a careful assessment of the airway. Intraoral burns, edema of the uvula, and inability to swallow saliva may suggest impending airway compromise. Assessment of the airway should be ongoing as the injury evolves. Patients may also require significant **resuscitation** due to inflammation of the mediastinal tissues. Radiographs of the chest and abdomen are helpful to evaluate for perforation. There is no role for gastric lavage, induced emesis, or activated charcoal.

      (2) **Endoscopy** early in the patient's course is controversial but can be helpful to assess the degree of injury. Endoscopy is helpful in evaluating and managing esophageal strictures that develop later on as a complication of caustic ingestions.

B. Stomach

1. **Stress ulceration** is discussed in **Section III.E.1.**

2. **Peptic ulcer disease** (PUD) refers to gastric and duodenal ulcers. Risk factors include *H. pylori* infection, NSAIDs, and aspirin use. Patient can present with pain, upper GI bleeding, obstruction, or peritonitis from perforation.

   a. The **diagnosis** of active *H. pylori* infection can be made during endoscopy utilizing the biopsy specimen, and include histology, culture, urease testing, and polymerase chain reaction.

   b. **Treatment** of *H. pylori* is indicated in most patients based on its association with peptic ulcers, gastric carcinoma, and gastric lymphoma. First-line regimens consist of a PPI plus two antibiotics such as amoxicillin + clarithromycin (first-line therapy), amoxicillin + metronidazole (for macrolide allergy), or metronidazole + clarithromycin (for penicillin allergy).

   c. **Complications** of PUD include upper GI bleeding (**Section III.E.1**), perforation, and obstruction. Perforation requires an operation with either a laparoscopic or an open approach.

C. Pancreas

1. **Acute pancreatitis**

   a. Most common **etiologies** are alcohol and gallstones (70%–80% of cases). Other causes include biliary reflux, contrast reflux, hypercalcemia, hyperlipidemia, trauma, and so on.

   b. The **pathogenesis** of acute pancreatitis is related to the release of activated pancreatic enzymes that autodigest the pancreatic parenchyma and cause inflammation, microvascular injury, and necrosis. Activated enzymes may also circulate to distant organs, causing activation of the complement and coagulation cascades, vasodilatation, and endothelial injury. Systemic consequences may include shock, acute lung injury and acute respiratory distress syndrome (ALI/ARDS), and acute renal failure.

   c. **Symptoms** of acute pancreatitis include severe epigastric pain radiating to the back, nausea and vomiting, and fever.

   d. The **diagnosis** is established with a consistent history and physical examination, increased serum amylase or lipase levels, and an abdominal CT scan demonstrating pancreatic inflammation, edema, or necrosis (**Fig. 27-2**).

   e. The **prognosis** for the majority of patients is good and they experience mild, self-limiting disease. Severe acute pancreatitis, defined as acute pancreatitis with organ dysfunction, develops in 10% to 20% of patients, necessitating admission to the ICU. Various tools have been developed to assess the severity of acute pancreatitis—the most commonly used is Ranson's criteria (**Table 27-3**).

   f. **Clinical course**

      (1) **The early phase** is characterized by local inflammation, significant retroperitoneal fluid sequestration, and a systemic inflammatory response that can be robust and may lead to **multiple organ system failure.**

         i. **Initial treatment** is largely supportive. Aggressive fluid resuscitation and electrolyte repletion should be undertaken. Nasogastric tube decompression can be helpful to alleviate nausea but does not shorten the clinical course. Pain relief, supplemental oxygen, invasive monitoring, mechanical ventilation, and inotropic support may be necessary.

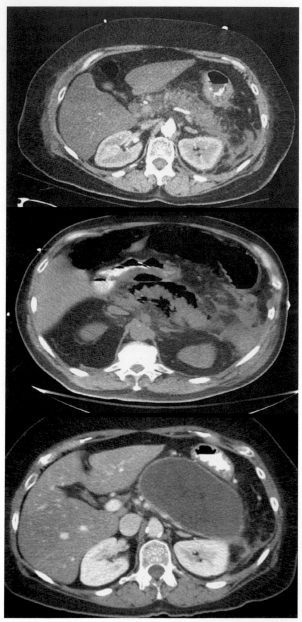

FIGURE 27-2 Acute pancreatitis. Axial CT images demonstrating: acute pancreatitis with prominent pancreatic inflammation (top); pancreatic necrosis with air around the pancreas (middle), and a giant pancreatic pseudocyst that developed several weeks after the acute episode (bottom). Courtesy of Hasan Alam, MD.

| TABLE 27-3 | Ranson's Criteria for Prognosis of Acute Pancreatitis |

At admission
- Age >55 years
- WBC count >16,000/μL
- Blood glucose >200 mg/dL
- Serum lactate dehydrogenase (LDH) >350 IU/L
- Serum glutamic oxaloacetic transaminase (SGOT, AST) >250 IU/L

During initial 48 hours
- Hematocrit decrease of >10%
- Blood urea nitrogen (BUN) increase of >5 mg/dL
- Serum calcium <8 mg/dL
- Arterial PaO$_2$ <60 mmHg
- Base deficit >4 mEq/L
- Estimated fluid sequestration >6 L

Number of Criteria Met	Expected Mortality
Less than 3	Less than 1%
3 or 4	15%
5 or 6	40%
7 or 8	90%

    ii. **Prophylactic antibiotics** are not indicated for mild pancreatitis and are controversial in severe pancreatitis. In patients with a large amount of necrosis (30% or more), antibiotics are often used but recent clinical trials do not support this practice.

    iii. **Nutrition** should be provided. Several trials support the use of early enteral feeding via a nasojejunal tube once the initial resuscitation phase is completed. Total parenteral nutrition (TPN) may be required for patients who cannot tolerate adequate enteral nutrition.

    iv. Patients with mild gallstone pancreatitis should undergo **cholecystectomy** to prevent recurrence. The type of intervention and timing for patients with severe gallstone pancreatitis must be individualized. Patients who are too sick to undergo cholecystectomy may be treated with ERCP and sphincterotomy.

  (2) The later phase of severe acute pancreatitis is characterized by local complications, and can carry on for weeks or months.

    i. **Pancreatic necrosis (Fig. 27-2)** should be suspected in patients who fail to improve or suffer clinical deterioration. Necrosis is not present in the first 2 to 3 days of symptoms. The extent of pancreatic necrosis correlates well with the amount of devascularized pancreas as demonstrated by a contrast-enhanced CT scan. By the second week, infected necrosis is common (30%–50%). New organ failure, new fever, or an increasing leukocytosis should prompt CT-guided aspiration of necrotic tissue. Gram stain and culture aid in establishing the diagnosis of infected pancreatic necrosis. Patients with infected pancreatic necrosis should be treated with antibiotics and surgical debridement. Early debridement may result in incomplete debridement and the need for a second operation. The ideal timing for surgical debridement appears to be between 21 and 27 days. The management of a patient with sterile pancreatic necrosis is controversial.

ii. **Pancreatic pseudocysts** (**Fig. 27-2**) are encapsulated fluid collections, rich in pancreatic enzymes, which form 4 to 6 weeks after an episode of acute pancreatitis. Typically, they communicate with the pancreatic duct. Collections that are observed earlier are referred to as acute fluid collections and may spontaneously regress. Small, asymptomatic pseudocysts can be observed safely.

(a) Large (>6 cm) or symptomatic pseudocysts can be drained either endoscopically or surgically.

(b) **Complications** associated with pseudocysts include rupture into the peritoneal cavity resulting in pancreatic ascites, or into the pleural space resulting in pancreaticopleural fistula, erosion into an adjacent vessel resulting in upper GI bleeding, compression of intra-abdominal structures, and infection resulting in abscess formation.

iii. **Pseudoaneurysms** occur most commonly in the **splenic artery** due to the proximity of this structure to the inflamed pancreas. Splenic artery pseudoaneurysms have a 75% bleeding rate and may rupture into a pseudocyst or intraperitoneally. Hemorrhage requires immediate intervention, either angiographically or surgically.

iv. **Splenic vein thrombosis** may occur and lead to the later development of portal hypertension. Patients may require splenectomy if variceal bleeding develops. Thrombosis of the mesenteric vessels leading to gut ischemia is rare.

D. Biliary tree

1. **Acute acalculous cholecystitis** (**AAC**) is an inflammatory disease of the gallbladder occurring in the absence of gallstones. Predisposing factors include critical illness, trauma, sepsis, burns, hypotension, TPN, atherosclerosis, and diabetes.

a. The **pathogenesis** of AAC is multifactorial and appears to be related to chemical and ischemic injury of the gallbladder. Pathology specimens reveal an occluded or impaired gallbladder microcirculation, possibly due to inflammation or inappropriate activation of the coagulation cascade.

b. **Diagnosis** requires a high index of suspicion, as fever may be the only symptom. Other signs and symptoms can include right upper quadrant or epigastric pain, nausea/vomiting, and new intolerance of enteral feeding. Laboratory findings may be limited to leukocytosis and LFT abnormalities, which may already be present in the critically ill ICU patient. Ultrasound and CT scans are used to confirm the diagnosis.

(1) **Ultrasound** can be performed at the bedside. Diagnostic findings include gallbladder wall thickness >3.5 mm, gallbladder distension >5 cm, sludge or gas in the gallbladder, pericholecystic fluid, mucosal sloughing, and intramural gas or edema. However, the sensitivity of ultrasound in diagnosing AAC may be as low as 30%.

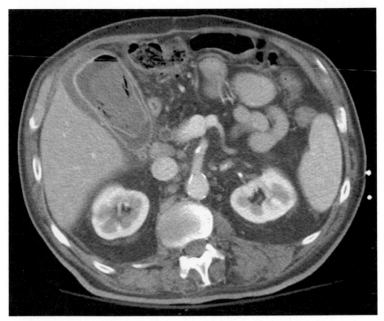

FIGURE 27-3 Acute acalculous cholecystitis (AAC). Axial CT image demonstrating several common findings of AAC, including an enhancing gallbladder wall, distended gallbladder, pericholecystic fluid, and air within the gallbladder. Courtesy of Hasan Alam, MD.

> (2) **CT** scan (**Fig. 27-3**) may be helpful when the diagnosis is uncertain and other intra-abdominal pathology needs to be excluded.
>
> (3) **HIDA** scan is another option to establish the diagnosis. A nonfilling gallbladder confirms the diagnosis.
>
> c. **Treatment** involves antibiotics and cholecystectomy if the patient can tolerate an operation, or placement of a percutaneous **cholecystostomy** tube for drainage.
>
> 2. **Cholangitis** is an infection of the biliary tract, often associated with septic shock, and is described in **Chapter 29**.

E. **Spleen:** Patients may be admitted to the ICU for management of a splenic laceration or rupture following blunt abdominal trauma. Other splenic pathology encountered in the ICU includes splenomegaly, infarction, or abscess. Splenic infarct usually occurs in patients with pre-existing splenomegaly due to portal hypertension or hematologic disorders such as leukemia, sickle cell disease, polycythemia, or hypercoagulable states. **Splenic abscess** usually requires splenectomy, and can be due to direct extension of infection or hematogenous seeding. Thus, the possibility of endocarditis should be entertained. Patients who undergo splenectomy should receive vaccination against *Streptococcus pneumoniae*, *Haemophilus influenzae*, and *Neisseria meningitides*, and should be counseled about their immunocompromised state and the need for revaccination.

F. Intestines
1. **Intestinal ischemia** may be acute or chronic and may affect the small or large intestine.
   a. **Acute mesenteric ischemia (AMI)** occurs as a result of arterial obstruction (embolic, thrombotic, or due to aortic dissection) or venous obstruction. AMI can also be nonocclusive and result from hypoperfusion, vasoconstriction, or vasospasm.
      (1) AMI typically presents with severe abdominal pain out of proportion to physical examination findings. Other signs include sudden intolerance of enteral feeding, nausea, vomiting, fever, intestinal bleeding, abdominal distension, and altered mental status.
      (2) **Leukocytosis** and **metabolic acidosis** are common early laboratory abnormalities, while elevated serum lactate and amylase are late findings.
      (3) **Abdominal radiograph** may show an ileus. **CT scan** may show thickened bowel. Portal venous gas and *pneumatosis intestinalis* are late findings of intestinal ischemia and suggest infarction. **CT angiography** may reveal the site of arterial occlusion. **Conventional angiography** can also be used to establish the diagnosis and may be therapeutic. **Duplex ultrasound** can be used to assess proximal celiac and superior mesenteric artery (SMA) flow. However, overlying edematous bowel can make ultrasonography nondiagnostic.
      (4) **Treatment** of acute mesenteric ischemia should be prompt and is aimed at restoring intestinal blood flow to avoid intestinal infarction. Patients should be given volume resuscitation, correction of hypotension, broad-spectrum antibiotics, and nasogastric drainage. Systemic anticoagulation is appropriate after aortic dissection is ruled out as a cause of mesenteric ischemia. Depending on the cause of ischemia, patients may require surgical or endovascular revascularization or observation. A second-look laparotomy may be necessary in 12 to 24 hours to reassess bowel viability.
         i. **SMA emboli** cause 50% of AMI. Emboli typically originate from the left atrium, left ventricle and cardiac valves. The SMA is susceptible due to its anatomy (large caliber, nonacute angle off aorta). Vasoconstriction of surrounding nonobstructed arteries further exacerbates intestinal hypoperfusion. Treatment involves aggressive resuscitation and anticoagulation. Intra-arterial administration of **papaverine** may improve bowel viability. Laparotomy and embolectomy is performed prior to evaluating bowel viability.
         ii. **SMA thrombosis** generally occurs acutely in patients with chronic mesenteric ischemia from atherosclerosis. Blunt trauma to the abdomen is also a risk factor, presumably from endothelial disruption. As with SMA embolism, intra-arterial **papaverine** can improve bowel viability. Surgical revascularization usually requires thrombectomy or a bypass graft.
         iii. **Nonocclusive mesenteric ischemia** results from mesenteric arterial vasospasm and accounts for 20% to 30% of AMI. Vasopressors, diuretics, cocaine, arrhythmia, and shock predispose patients to this condition. Therapy involves anticoagulation, administration of vasodilator agents, and discontinuation of the offending agent.

  iv. Mesenteric venous thrombosis is a less common cause of intestinal ischemia. Risk factors include inherited or acquired hypercoagulable states, abdominal trauma, portal hypertension, pancreatitis, and splenectomy. Diagnosis is by CT scan. Treatment is with systemic **anticoagulation** (heparin followed by warfarin). Laparotomy is indicated only in cases of suspected bowel infarction.

 b. Ischemic colitis is a common form of mesenteric ischemia typically affecting the "watershed" areas (splenic flexure and rectosigmoid junction) of the colon. It is usually caused by underlying atherosclerotic disease in the setting of hypotension, although embolism, vasculitis, hypercoagulable states, vasospasm, and inferior mesenteric artery (IMA) ligation during aortic surgery are other causes.

  (1) The **diagnosis** of ischemic colitis is suspected in patients with left-sided crampy abdominal pain, often associated with mild lower GI bleeding, diarrhea, abdominal distension, nausea, and vomiting. Other signs and symptoms include fever, leukocytosis, and abdominal tenderness to palpation. The diagnosis is confirmed by CT scan or by endoscopy.

  (2) Most cases resolve within days to weeks with **supportive care** including bowel rest, fluid resuscitation, and broad-spectrum antibiotics. Fifteen percent of patient will develop transmural necrosis. Indications for colon resection include peritonitis, colonic perforation, and clinical deterioration despite adequate medical therapy. Long-term complications include chronic colitis and colonic strictures.

2. Adynamic or paralytic ileus refers to an alteration in GI motility that leads to failure of intestinal contents to pass. Ileus can affect the entire GI tract or a localized segment.

 a. Ileus may be related to a number of predisposing factors. After an uncomplicated abdominal operation, small bowel motility generally returns within 24 hours. Gastric motility follows within 48 hours and colonic motility returns in 3 to 5 days.

 b. Diagnosis is clinical and radiologic. Patients may present with nausea/vomiting, abdominal distension, intolerance of enteral feeding, and diffuse abdominal discomfort. Abdominal radiographs show distension of the affected part of the GI tract with intraluminal air throughout. Contrast studies are sometimes needed to exclude mechanical obstruction.

 c. Complications of ileus depend on the portion of the GI tract involved. A severe ileus can lead to increased intra-abdominal pressure, and even abdominal compartment syndrome. Ileus can also lead to bacterial overgrowth, and reflux of bowel contents into the stomach can predispose to aspiration. **Fluid sequestration** due to intestinal wall edema can compromise the gut's microcirculation. **Colonic dilation** can lead to ischemia, necrosis, and perforation. Patients with a cecal diameter more than 12 cm are at higher risk for perforation, although perforations have been reported with smaller cecal diameters. Patients with chronic colonic dilation may tolerate much larger diameters.

 d. Treatment begins with **supportive care,** which consists of fluid and electrolyte repletion and nasogastric tube drainage. Potential causes of ileus should be reviewed and corrected (**Table 27-4**). If tolerated, fiber-containing enteral diets or minimal enteral nutrition

TABLE 27-4	Causes of Ileus

Postoperative
Intraperitoneal or retroperitoneal pathology:
• Inflammation, infection
• Hemorrhage
• Intestinal ischemia
• Bowel wall edema (may be due to massive fluid resuscitation)
• Ascites
Systemic sepsis
Trauma
Uremia
Sympathetic hyperactivity
Electrolyte derangements
Drugs:
• Catecholamines
• Calcium channel blockers
• Narcotics
• Anticholinergics
• Phenothiazines
• β-blockers

can promote GI motility. Patients should be encouraged to ambulate. Medications such as metoclopramide, erythromycin, and neostigmine have been used with mixed results.

(1) **Neostigmine** (2–2.5 mg IV given over 3 minutes) can successfully treat Ogilvie syndrome in approximately 80% of cases. Close monitoring for bradycardia is required.

(2) If conservative measures fail or if perforation appears imminent, **colonoscopic** or **operative decompression** is indicated.

3. **Bowel obstruction** presents with signs and symptoms similar to ileus. As with ileus, plain x-rays (**Fig. 27-1**) and CT scan (**Fig. 27-4**) can confirm the diagnosis.

a. **Small bowel obstruction** (**SBO**) is most often due to adhesions. Other causes include abdominal wall and internal hernias, tumors, foreign bodies, and gallstones. Patients with partial SBO often respond to nonoperative management, which consists of fluid and electrolyte repletion and nasogastric tube drainage. Fevers, leukocytosis, persistent pain, and tenderness on examination are indications to proceed with exploratory laparotomy. Complete SBO should be managed surgically due to high risk for bowel ischemia, necrosis, and perforation.

b. **Large bowel obstruction** (LBO) is commonly due to malignancy, and develops insidiously over time. Other causes include sigmoid or cecal volvulus (**Fig. 27-5**), diverticular strictures, and fecal impaction. **Treatment** of large bowel obstruction is usually operative. Sigmoid volvulus may respond to decompression via contrast enema or colonoscopy.

4. **Diarrhea** occurs when fluid intake into the gut lumen does not match fluid absorption from the GI tract.

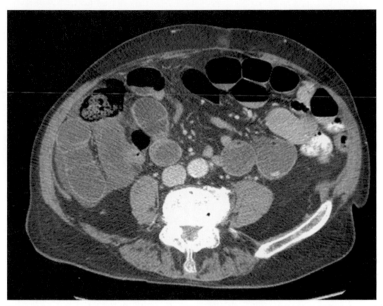

FIGURE 27-4 Small bowel obstruction. Axial CT image demonstrating several dilated loops of small bowel, consistent with small bowel obstruction.

a. Under normal conditions, 9 to 10 L of fluid enters the bowel lumen each day from oral intake and intestinal secretions. The majority is absorbed in the small bowel, leaving the remaining 1 to 1.5 L to be absorbed in the proximal half of the colon, with approximately 100 mL lost daily in stool.

b. Water is absorbed secondary to osmotic flow as well as active and passive transport of sodium. Changes in GI motility and epithelial mucosal integrity can drastically affect fluid absorption.

c. Common **etiologies** of diarrhea in the critically ill patient include infections, enteral nutrition, medications, ischemic colitis, fecal impaction, intestinal fistula, pancreatic insufficiency, and hypoalbuminemia.

   (1) **Infectious diarrhea** in the ICU setting is usually due to *Clostridium difficile* infection in patients treated with antibiotics.

      i. **Clinical presentation** varies from asymptomatic leukocytosis to severe colitis and toxic megacolon.

      ii. Because the sensitivity of the toxin assay for *C. difficile* is no greater than 90%, testing three separate stool samples is the standard for diagnosis if the clinical suspicion is there. Treatment is with metronidazole or oral vancomycin, as described in **Chapter 27.**

   (2) **Enteral nutrition** causing diarrhea is a diagnosis of exclusion. Osmotic diarrhea is secondary to malabsorption of nutrients and usually stops with fasting. Malnutrition and hypoalbuminemia can also cause malabsorption.

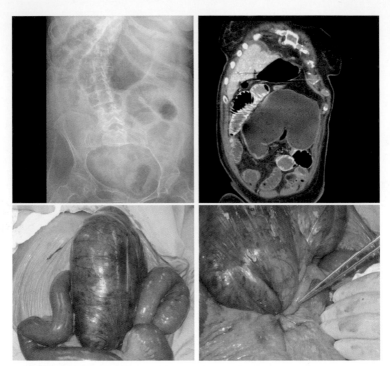

FIGURE 27-5 Cecal volvulus. A plain abdominal radiograph (left upper) and a coronal CT image (right upper) demonstrating cecal volvulus. Intra-operative photographs reveal a dilated and ischemic cecum (left lower), as well as the site of torsion (right lower). Courtesy of Hasan Alam, MD.

      i. An **osmolar gap** in the stool of >70 mOsm suggests an osmotic diarrhea. The osmolar gap is the difference between the measured stool osmolarity and the predicted osmolarity, which is $2 \times ([Na^+] + [K^+])$, based on serum electrolyte measurements.

     ii. **Treatment** of enteral nutrition–related diarrhea involves slowing the rate of feeding, diluting the tube feeds, changing the formula, or temporarily stopping enteral nutrition. Enteral nutrition should be lactose-free. In some patients, peptide-based, fiber-rich, or elemental diets with reduced fat and residue may be helpful.

   (3) Fecal impaction can paradoxically lead to diarrhea as a result of decreased fecal tone, mucus secretion, and impaired anorectal sensation.

   (4) An **altered enterohepatic circulation,** leading to increased bile acid in the colon, can induce net fluid secretion. This is seen in diseases of the ileum, fatty acid malabsorption, and altered bowel flora.

  d. Management of diarrhea consists of replacement of lost fluids and electrolytes, and treatment of the underlying cause. After excluding infectious etiologies, diarrhea can be treated symptomatically with agents such as **diphenoxylate with atropine** (Lomotil 5 mg/dose,

4 doses/d, reduce dose once controlled), **loperamide** (Imodium 4–16 mg/d), **bismuth subsalicylate** (Pepto-Bismol 262 mg/dose up to 8 doses/d), and **deodorized or camphorated opium tincture** (0.3–1 mL/dose every 2–6 hours up to 6 mL/d).

5. **Constipation** may affect up to 83% of ICU patients, and has been associated with prolonged ICU length of stay, infectious complications, pulmonary complications, and increased mortality in some studies.

    a. The **etiology** of constipation in the ICU is incompletely understood. Proinflammatory mediators, poor perfusion, dehydration, immobilization, and medications (vasopressors and opiates) likely contribute to the problem.

    b. A **bowel regimen** should be initiated and titrated to avoid constipation, and can include **stool softeners** (Colace), **bulking agents** (methylcellulose, psyllium), **stimulants** (castor oil, senna), **lubricants** (mineral oil), or **osmotic agents** (lactulose, magnesium).

Selected References

Batke M, Cappell MS. Adynamic ileus and acute colonic pseudo-obstruction. *Med Clin North Am* 2008;92:649–670.

Cheatham ML, Malbrain ML, Kirkpatrick A, et al. Results from the International Conference of Experts on intra-abdominal hypertension and abdominal compartment syndrome. II. Recommendations. *Intensive Care Med* 2007;33:951–962.

Chey WD, Wong BC; Practice Parameters Committee of the American College of Gastroenterology. American College of Gastroenterology guideline on the management of *Helicobacter pylori* infection. *Am J Gastroenterol* 2007;102:1808–1825.

Crandall M, West MA. Evaluation of the abdomen in the critically ill patient: opening the black box. *Curr Opin Crit Care* 2006;12:333–339.

Dellinger EP, Tellado JM, Soto NE, et al. Early antibiotic treatment for severe acute necrotizing pancreatitis. A randomized, double blind, placebo-controlled study. *Ann Surg* 2007;245: 674–683.

Haney JC, Pappas TN. Necrotizing pancreatitis: diagnosis and management. *Surg Clin North Am* 2007;87:1431–1446.

Heinrich S, Schafer M, Rousson V, Clavien P. Evidence-based treatment of acute pancreatitis. *Ann Surg* 2006;243:154–168.

Jaramillo EJ, Treviño JM, Berghoff KR, et al. Bedside diagnostic laparoscopy in the intensive care unit: a 13-year experience. *JSLS* 2006;10:155–159.

Maerz L, Kaplan LJ. Abdominal compartment syndrome. *Crit Care Med* 2008;36:S212–S215.

Proctor DD. Critical issues in digestive diseases. *Clin Chest Med* 2003;24:623–632.

Raju GS, Gerson L, Das A, et al; American Gastroenterological Association. American Gastroenterological Association (AGA) Institute technical review on obscure gastrointestinal bleeding. *Gastroenterology* 2007;133:1697–1717.

Ramasamy K, Gumaste VV. Corrosive ingestion in adults. *J Clin Gastroenterol* 2003;37:119–124.

Stewart D, Waxman K. Management of postoperative ileus. *Am J Ther* 2007;14:561–566.

Villatoro E, Bassi C, Larvin M. Antibiotic therapy for prophylaxis against infection of pancreatic necrosis in acute pancreatitis. *Cochrane Database Syst Rev* 2006Oct 18;(4):CD002941.

Endocrine Disorders and Glucose Management

Steven Russell and B. Taylor Thompson

I. **Glucose homeostasis, insulin resistance, and insulin deficiency**
   A. **Normal blood glucose dynamics.** In the normal fasting state, blood glucose (BG) is regulated between **70 and 110 mg/dL** and does not increase to more than 200 mg/dL despite significant fluxes of glucose into the bloodstream after meals. Absorption of a typical meal may require 150 g of glucose (a 30-fold excess of the steady-state amount in the blood) to move through the circulation and into storage within a few hours. A rise in BG of twofold (more than 200 mg/dL) during this movement is abnormal and is sufficient to diagnose **diabetes mellitus (DM)** in the outpatient setting.
   B. **Endocrine control of blood glucose.** Pancreatic β-cells secrete **insulin** directly into the portal circulation in response to the BG level. Glucose is converted to glycogen for storage in the liver and muscle and to triglycerides for storage in the adipose tissue. During fasting, pancreatic α-cells secrete **glucagon** to promote breakdown of glycogen stores and release of glucose into the blood. Glucagon is also the first line of defense against hypoglycemia.
   C. **Insulin resistance and deficiency.** Insulin binds a cell surface receptor to stimulate glucose uptake and promote cell growth and survival. In states of insulin resistance, such as type 2 DM and critical illness, much higher levels of insulin can be required for the same degree of glucose uptake. Postreceptor signaling events can be inhibited by the **counter-regulatory hormones** glucagon, epinephrine, norepinephrine, cortisol, and growth hormone, as well as inflammatory cytokines and intracellular free fatty acids. These same counter-regulatory hormones can stimulate glycogen breakdown, glucose production from amino acids, and release of fatty acids from lipids. If pancreatic β-cells cannot sufficiently increase insulin production in response to insulin resistance, relative insulin deficiency leads to hyperglycemia. Toxicity of cytokines and hyperglycemia itself can lead to β-cell failure and absolute insulin deficiency superimposed on insulin resistance.

II. **Hyperglycemia of critical illness**
   A. **Pathophysiology.** Critically ill patients without pre-existing DM frequently become insulin resistant and hyperglycemic due to elevated levels of cytokines and stress hormones such as cortisol, glucagon, and adrenergic hormones. Treatment with glucocorticoids and sympathomimetic drugs, increased nutrition to compensate for a catabolic state, and administration of intravenous (IV) dextrose all contribute to hyperglycemia. Patients with pre-existing DM almost always need higher levels of insulin for a given calorie intake to maintain normal glucose levels when they are ill.
   B. **Hyperglycemia and outcomes.** Hyperglycemia appears to be a **marker for severity of illness** and is **associated with poor outcomes** including increased infarct volume after stroke, decreased cardiac function after myocardial infarction, increased wound complications after heart surgery, and

increased mortality. Unfortunately, it remains unclear whether intervention to control hyperglycemia can improve outcomes, and if so, what populations of critically ill patients may benefit.

C. **Intensive insulin therapy (IIT).** A series of clinical trials that started in 2001 has tested the efficacy of using **IV insulin to tightly regulate BG to normal or near normal,** a much narrower range than it had been customary in the ICU. This approach reduced in-hospital mortality of surgical ICU patients by as much as 34%, as well as reducing the incidence of acute renal failure, bloodstream infections, critical illness polyneuropathy, and the duration of mechanical ventilation and of ICU stay. Based on these remarkable findings, IIT became the de facto standard of care in most ICUs, and is recommended by practice guidelines by professional societies. However, not all studies have confirmed such beneficial effect of IIT, and have shown an alarmingly high incidence of severe **hypoglycemia.** Recently, two multicenter trials designed to test the benefits of IIT were interrupted before reaching full enrollment because of either futility or possible harm (from hypoglycemia). **Another trial found a small increase in mortality associated with a target of normal BG (80–110 mg/dL) versus a higher blood glucose target (140–180 mg/dL) for patients treated with IIT.** The reason for such wide discrepancy among large, controlled clinical trials is not entirely clear. Confounding factors may include the different ranges of BG goals tested, the proportions of medical versus surgical patients, and the different provision of total calories as well as their source (enteral vs. parenteral).

D. **Risks of IIT.** The primary risk of IIT is **hypoglycemia.** Throughout the various IIT trials severe hypoglycemia (BG <40 mg/dL) occurred in 5% to 19% of study patients, and was in some cases identified as an independent risk factor for death in patients treated with IIT. Severe hypoglycemia may cause neurologic damage because the brain depends on glucose. The risk of hypoglycemia to other organs systems is not as well defined, but hypoglycemia due to excess insulin is also associated with low blood levels of free fatty acids, the preferred fuel for the heart. This may be particularly problematic because of increased cardiac demand during critical illness. The consequences of hypoglycemia may counteract some or all of the benefits of IIT. In the ICU, the most common cause of hypoglycemia is **interruption of nutrition** without stopping the insulin infusion. This can occur due to occlusion of feeding tubes, depletion of TPN or IV glucose bags, or accidental removal of tubes or lines. The BG level can fall very rapidly when feeding is interrupted, requiring a **high degree of vigilance** from staff. If enteral feeding or TPN is interrupted, a D10 infusion should be started immediately and the rate of insulin infusion decreased to prevent a precipitous fall in blood glucose (see **Chapter 11**).

E. **Implementation of IIT.** To reduce the risk of hypoglycemia and achieve adequate BG control, most ICU protocols specify point-of-care testing of BG every 1 to 2 hours, although this approach requires up to 2 hours of nursing time each day. Given the lack of uniformity of the results of the IIT trials, a wider target range for blood glucose control may confer most of the potential benefit with less risk of hypoglycemia. The recent international guidelines from the **Surviving Sepsis Campaign** (see also **Chapter 30**) sponsored by a number of critical care societies suggest a few main points in implementing IIT:

   1. Following initial stabilization, hyperglycemia should be treated with IV insulin.
   2. A validated protocol should be used to treat hyperglycemia, with a suggested target of maintaining BG levels between 110 and 150 mg/dL.

3. All patients receiving IV insulin must also receive a glucose calorie source, and must have BG monitored as frequently as every 1 to 2 hours until BG values are stable, then every 4 hours.

4. Low BG levels obtained from capillary blood by point-of-care testing should be confirmed with a full blood or plasma sample, as the former may overestimate BG level.

F. **Dosing algorithms for insulin.** No consensus has emerged on the best algorithms to use for control of BG with IV insulin, and many forms of paper-based algorithms have been used. At least two computerized decision support tools have been approved by the FDA (http://www.glucotec.com/glucommander/safe_insulin_administration.asp and http://www.hospira.com/Products/endotool.aspx), and another one used in one of the IIT trials is available on the Web (https://studies.thegeorgeinstitute.org/nice/docs/algorithm.pdf). There has been interest in developing automated "closed-loop" systems for glucose regulation in the ICU to improve quality of BG control and safety. When such a system becomes available, it will be much easier to conduct the studies required to resolve the many remaining uncertainties about IIT. Very high doses of insulin may be required to control BG in critically ill patients. Insulin infusion rates of greater than 10 U/h are not uncommon and some patients require rates in excess of 50 U/h.

G. **Appropriate use of IIT algorithms.** IIT protocols are not appropriate for all hyperglycemic patients. IIT protocols have as their only goal control of BG and typically suspend delivery of insulin when blood glucose nears the bottom of the target range. They are not appropriate for treatment of patients with type 1 DM who need a basal rate of insulin administration to prevent lipolysis and ketone body formation. IIT protocols are also not appropriate for treatment of diabetic ketoacidosis (DKA) and hyperosmolar hyperglycemic states (HHS) where the primarily goals are closure of the anion gap and normalization of the serum osmolarity, respectively (see below).

H. **Transition from IV to subcutaneous (SC) insulin.** The transition from IIT therapy to SC insulin injections requires careful attention. The first dose of a long-acting analog of insulin (usually **NPH insulin, twice daily**) should be given at least **2 hours prior to discontinuation of the infusion**. The total daily dose of long-acting insulin (divided into two daily doses if using NPH insulin) should be at least half of the total insulin dose administered IV over the last 24 hours. The remainder of the insulin requirement may be provided with a sliding scale of **regular** or **rapid-acting** formulation (insulin aspart, lispro, or glulisine). A sliding scale order alone, without any standing insulin, is not sufficient and will result in recurrent hyperglycemia. The dose of long-acting insulin should be re-evaluated every day. A useful rule of thumb is to add at least half of the sliding scale given on the previous day to the basal insulin dosing for the upcoming day, and repeat the process until all or most of the blood glucose values are in the desired range. Conversely, hypoglycemia should usually prompt reduction in the basal insulin dose unless it occurred after a large sliding scale bolus to treat hyperglycemia. **All type 1 diabetic patients require basal insulin,** whether or not they are eating, to prevent development of DKA. A modest reduction from the home basal insulin dose may be appropriate upon hospital admission depending on the form of basal insulin and tightness of control.

III. Diabetic ketoacidosis (DKA)

A. **Pathophysiology.** In DKA, a relative or absolute lack of insulin, usually in the setting of an excess of counter-regulatory hormones or inflammatory cytokines, leads to elevated BG, lipolysis, and production of **ketoacids** from fatty acids, **metabolic acidosis, hyperosmolarity, volume depletion,** and **electrolyte imbalances.** Hyperkalemia is common despite whole-body potassium depletion because insulin in an important mediator of potassium uptake into cells. Glucosuria results in an osmotic diuresis with prominent potassium and phosphate wasting. There is loss of water in excess of sodium resulting in both dehydration and volume depletion. Decreased peripheral vascular resistance, nausea, vomiting, and abdominal pain are likely due to elevated levels of prostaglandins.

B. **The syndrome of DKA.** Symptoms may include polyuria, polydipsia, polyphagia, weight loss, vomiting, abdominal pain, dehydration, weakness, confusion, or coma. The examination may find poor skin turgor, ileus, Kussmaul respirations (very deep breaths without tachypnea), tachycardia, and hypotension, the fruity aroma of ketones on the breath, coffee ground emesis (hemorrhagic gastritis), altered mental status, shock, and coma. The patient may have a warm and well-perfused periphery despite severe volume depletion. Full-blown DKA can evolve in less than 24 hours.

C. **Causes of DKA.** DKA occurs when **insulin is mistakenly withheld or reduced,** when insulin is inactive, or when an **acute illness** increases insulin requirements. Patients with type I DM are most at risk but patients with type 2 DM can also develop DKA in the setting of a catastrophic illness or as the initial presentation of the disease. The possibility of DKA should be considered in any patient with diabetes and critical illness. Drugs can uncommonly precipitate DKA. A partial list of causes for DKA is shown in **Table 28-1.**

TABLE 28-1	Causes of Diabetic Ketoacidosis

- Omission of insulin, inappropriate reduction in dose, inadvertent use of denatured insulin (insulin exposed to heat)
- Infection/sepsis
- Infarction
  - MI, bowel ischemia, stroke
- Endocrine abnormalities:
  - Pheochromocytoma
  - Acromegaly
  - Thyrotoxicosis
  - Glucagonoma
  - Pancreatectomy
- Medications/drugs:
  - Ethanol abuse (DKA can be confused with alcoholic ketosis)
  - Atypical antipsychotics—olanzapine, clozapine, risperidone
  - Anti-calcineurin drugs—FK506
  - HIV protease inhibitors
  - α-Interferon/ribavirin therapy
  - Corticosteroids
  - Sympathomimetics (cocaine, terbutaline, dobutamine)
  - Pentamidine
  - Thiazides
- Other conditions that may predispose to DKA:
  - Pancreatitis (reduced insulin secretion and insulin resistance)
  - Surgery
  - Trauma
  - Pregnancy
  - Eating disorder

D. **Diagnosis of DKA.** Diagnosis requires the presence of serum ketones and is supported by anion gap >12 mEq/L (AG = Na − [Cl + HCO]), plasma glucose >250 mg/dL, pH <7.3, serum bicarbonate <18 mEq/L, and moderate to large ketones in the urine. Patients who have been able to keep up with volume and water losses by drinking may have been able to excrete enough ketones as sodium salts with retention of chloride so that they present with a hyperchloremic nonanion gap metabolic acidosis. Treatment of DKA with extra insulin by the patient or another provider can decrease BG to <200 mg/dL without clearing ketones to produce "normoglycemic DKA." Concurrent insulin and glucose infusions are usually necessary to clear the ketones. See **Table 28-2** for the differential diagnosis of anion gap acidosis. See **Fig. 28-1** for summary of diagnosis and management of hyperglycemic emergencies.

E. **Measurement of serum ketones.** Measurement of serum ketones with traditional methods such as the nitroprusside test may initially underestimate ketone levels. Treatment may increase the apparent levels of ketones in the blood by converting a poorly detected form (β-hydroxybutyrate) to a more easily detected form (acetoacetate). Therefore, ketone levels should be used to make the diagnosis, but not to follow the progress of therapy.

F. **Goals of therapy and search for the cause of DKA.** Normalization of glucose is not sufficient treatment of DKA. The **primary goals of therapy are to treat hypovolemia, to normalize blood potassium concentration and replete potassium stores, to close the anion gap, and to identify and treat the underlying cause of DKA.** Even if insulin omission is suspected, a full workup for other causes is mandatory. Certain laboratory anomalies are common in DKA, which may obscure the underlying cause. Amylase and lipase elevations of less than threefold are not sufficient to diagnose pancreatitis in DKA. Leukocytosis with elevated PMNs may be due to stress and proportional to ketonemia, or secondary to underlying infection. Creatinine is often elevated due to hypovolemia (with elevated BUN/Cr ratio), but ketone bodies may also interference with the creatinine assay. Liver enzymes may be elevated. All of these abnormalities should resolve with treatment of DKA if there is not another underlying cause.

G. **Volume repletion.** Typical volume deficits in DKA are 10% of body mass. Fluid repletion should **begin with approximately 2 L of NS** administered at a rate of 500 cm^3/h. After the initial hydration, fluids should change to 1/2NS, assuming the corrected serum sodium (taking serum glucose into account) is normal or high. The rate should be reduced with a goal of correcting half of the volume deficit in the first 12 hours and the remainder in

TABLE 28-2	Differential Diagnosis of Anion Gap Acidosis

- Starvation ketosis—bicarbonate rarely <18, no hyperglycemia
- Alcoholic ketoacidosis—glucose usually <250, may be hypoglycemic
- Lactic acidosis—serum lactate
- Renal failure—BUN, Cr (note that the measured Cr can be artifactually elevated by acetoacetate depending on the assay used)
- Salicylate intoxication—salicylate level
- Methanol—methanol level
- Ethylene glycol—calcium oxalate and hippurate crystals in urine
- Paraldehyde ingestion—usually hyperchloremic, strong odor on breath

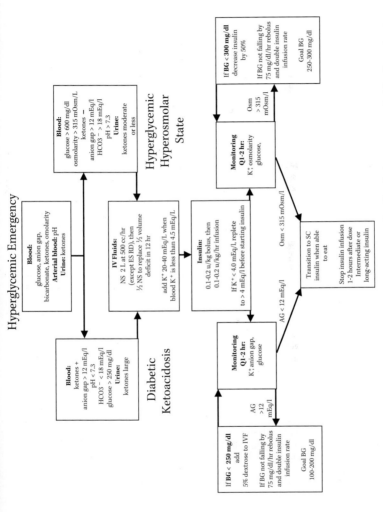

FIGURE 28-1 Diagnosis and management of hyperglycemic emergencies. Not all elements are required for diagnosis – key elements for DKA are blood ketones and anion gap >12, for HHS BG >600 and Osm >315 mOsm/L.

the next 12 hours. More rapid administration of fluid may delay resolution of acidemia by diluting bicarbonate. In children, too rapid repletion of volume has been associated with cerebral edema, which can be fatal. In adults, excess administration of NS can delay resolution of the **hyperchloremic metabolic acidosis,** which may underlie or follow treatment of the anion gap acidosis. End-stage renal failure patients who are anuric are a special case and are likely to need little or no IV fluid, as they are not capable of osmotic diuresis in response to hyperglycemia.

H. **Potassium repletion.** Potassium (K^+) depletion is almost universal in DKA (with the exception of oliguric or anuric patients) with a typical deficit of 3 to 5 mEq K^+ per kilogram body weight that requires aggressive repletion. The initial serum K is often elevated despite severe total body depletion due to shifts from within cells to the extracellular fluid. Insulin administration will lower the potassium concentration in the blood. Potassium should be added at 20 to 40 mEq/L to the IVF when the serum K^+ is 4.5 or less. The serum K^+ should be followed closely and repleted aggressively with cardiac monitoring. If the patient is hypokalemic on presentation, potassium should be repleted to the lower limit of normal before insulin is given to avoid severe hypokalemia and life-threatening arrhythmias.

I. **Insulin therapy.** Insulin is given IV with an initial bolus of 0.1 to 0.2 U/kg (or **10 U**) followed by a **continuous IV infusion of approximately 0.1 U/kg/h (or 10 U/h).** Insulin is typically mixed at 1 U/mL. Lower concentrations may lead to proportionally large losses by adherence to the infusion bag or IV tubing. In-line filters may bind and deplete insulin. The combined effect of insulin effect and fluid repletion will usually lead to a decrease in the blood glucose of 75 to 100 mg/dL/h. If the decrease in BG is less than 75 mg/dL/h, the insulin dose may be doubled. If the decline is still too slow, a new bottle of insulin should be used.

J. **Closure of the anion gap. The endpoint of therapy should be closure of the anion gap** (<12 mEq/L) **and resolution of the acidosis** (pH >7.3, bicarbonate >18 mEq/L). If glucose falls to less than 250 mg/dL but the anion gap is not closed, 5% dextrose should be added to the IV fluids (e.g., D51/2NS at 100 cm^3/h) and the insulin dose should be decreased to 0.05 to 0.1 U/kg/h (or 5 U/h). The insulin dose should then be adjusted as needed to hold the glucose at 100 to 200 mg/dL until the anion gap is closed. Measurement of ketones should not be used to determine the endpoint of therapy. It is not necessary to eliminate ketonemia and ketonuria as long as the anion gap is closed. A hyperchloremic, non-anion gap acidosis is a very common consequence of aggressive hydration with saline. It does not need to be treated and will correct itself over several days by renal excretion of ammonium chloride if renal function is adequate.

K. **Phosphorus and bicarbonate.** Phosphate is often normal to high in DKA, but falls with treatment. Phosphorus repletion is only indicated in patients with phosphorous less than 1.0 mEq/L and with a clinical syndrome consistent with hypophosphatemia, which may include hemolytic anemia, platelet dysfunction with petechial hemorrhage, rhabdomyolysis, encephalopathy, seizure, heart failure, and weakness of respiratory or skeletal muscles. There is **no benefit of bicarbonate treatment in patients with pH greater than 6.9.** Administration of insulin will result in utilization of ketones in the TCA cycle and regeneration of bicarbonate. Extra bicarbonate can increase potassium requirements, may increase hepatic production of ketones, and may delay resolution of cerebral acidosis.

L. **Complications of DKA.** The most feared complication of DKA is **cerebral edema,** which occurs in up to 1% of children with DKA, but rarely, if ever, in adults. Cerebral edema as a complication of DKA is a diagnosis of exclusion in adults and other causes of depressed mental status should be carefully investigated.

M. Transition from IV to SC insulin (see **Section II.H**) should begin when the patient is able to eat. A dose of the long-acting insulin (NPH, glargine, or detemir) should be given, or continuous SC infusion should be started 1 to 2 hours before the insulin infusion is stopped. In cases of uncomplicated DKA (i.e., due to insulin omission), the patient's home regimen can be restarted if home control (as judged by the HgbA1c) was good. Making the transition to SC insulin in the morning or evening is strongly preferred so that there is a smooth transition to the patient's usual insulin schedule.

IV. Hyperosmolar hyperglycemic state (HHS)

A. Pathophysiology. Insulin is able to suppress lipolysis and ketogenesis at much lower concentrations than is required to stimulate glucose uptake. In contrast to patients with type 1 DM, patients with type 2 DM usually have sufficient insulin production to prevent the excessive production of ketones. When **severe hyperglycemia occurs in the absence of ketosis,** the syndrome is called **HHS** or hyperosmolar nonketotic coma **(HONKC)**. BG may rise to levels that are unusual in DKA, often greater than 1,000 mg/dL. The blood pH and bicarbonate levels are typically normal and tests for ketones are negative. Both HHS and DKA are associated with hyperosmolarity, polyuria, polydipsia, volume depletion, and whole-body potassium depletion, although the serum potassium is usually normal or elevated before treatment. The two syndromes are part of a spectrum and some patients have some aspects of both syndromes. **Altered mental status**, including obtundation and coma, are more common in HHS because the degree of hyperglycemia and hyperosmolarity are higher. Patients with HHS may also develop seizures or focal neurologic signs, and up to 50% of patients present with coma. As in DKA, patients with oliguric renal failure have a different presentation. Although glucose levels are high, the serum sodium is reduced to compensate so that there is minimal hyperosmolarity and few neurologic symptoms.

B. Diagnosis. The diagnosis of HHS requires **severe hyperglycemia** (>600 mg/dL, often >1,000 mg/dL) and **hyperosmolarity without an anion gap acidosis**. HHS exists on a spectrum with DKA and some patients with HHS may have modest ketonemia, while some patients with DKA may have more severe hyperosmolarity than is typical of DKA. See **Fig. 28-1** for summary of diagnosis and management of hyperglycemic emergencies.

C. Treatment. IV fluid replacement and insulin therapy are the mainstays of treatment for HHS, just as they are for DKA, but the goals of insulin therapy differ. Fluid replacement in HHS is similar to that in DKA, although the fluid requirement may be greater due to the more extreme hyperosmolarity. **Insulin therapy starts** similarly **with an initial bolus of 0.1 to 0.2 U/kg and an infusion rate of approximately 0.1 to 0.2 U/kg/h,** but instead of closing the anion gap **the goal is to bring the glucose into a reasonable range and then to normalize the osmolarity**. While most patients with DKA are insulin sensitive, **many patients with HHS are very insulin resistant**. Much higher doses of insulin may be required. Once the BG falls to less than 300 mg/dL, the insulin infusion rate should be reduced by 50%. The serum glucose should be maintained between 250 and 300 mg/dL by adjusting the insulin infusion rate until the plasma osmolarity is less than 315 mOsm/L. **Potassium repletion** is similar to that in DKA with ½ NS being used for fluid repletion if potassium is added at 20 to 40 mEq/L.

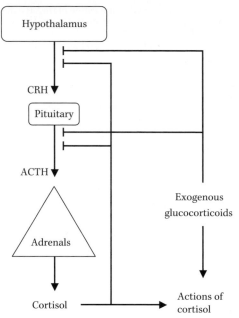

FIGURE 28-2 Regulation of adrenal hormone secretion. Arrows indicate positive action, production, or conversion. Lines ending in cross-bars indicate inhibition.

V. Normal adrenal physiology and pathophysiology of adrenal insufficiency

    A. Adrenal functional anatomy. Each adrenal gland is made up of a **cortex**, which produces sex steroids, aldosterone, and glucocorticoids—primarily cortisol—and a **medulla**, which produces adrenergic hormones—primarily epinephrine. The term "adrenal insufficiency" is commonly used to describe deficiency of both **cortisol** (which may be isolated) and of **aldosterone** (which is almost always associated with cortisol deficiency).

    B. Regulation of adrenal hormone production (**Fig. 28-2**). Cortisol production by the adrenal glands is dependent on **adrenocorticotrophic hormone (ACTH),** which is produced by the pituitary gland under control of corticotropin-releasing hormone (CRH), produced in the hypothalamus. Cortisol feeds back to inhibit CRH and ACTH release, closing the control loop. Cortisol deficiency may be caused by injury either to the adrenal cortex (primary adrenal insufficiency with elevated ACTH) or to the pituitary or hypothalamus (secondary or central adrenal insufficiency with low or "inappropriately normal" ACTH). Primary adrenal insufficiency is often associated with aldosterone deficiency, but central forms of adrenal insufficiency are limited to a deficit in cortisol production because aldosterone production is not dependent on ACTH.

    C. Consequences of adrenal insufficiency. Cortisol deficiency is acutely dangerous, and causes **circulatory collapse** with **refractory hypotension** that may be fatal within hours to days without glucocorticoid replacement. Symptoms and signs of glucocorticoid deficiency including nausea, vomiting, anorexia, weight loss and wasting, weakness, hyponatremia, and eosinophilia. Suspicion of glucocorticoid deficiency is sufficient cause to begin

TABLE 28-3	Differential Diagnosis of Adrenal Insufficiency

Primary Adrenal Insufficiency	Central Adrenal Insufficiency

• Hemorrhagic infarction
  • Sepsis
  • Adrenal vein thrombosis
  • Anticoagulation
  • Coagulopathy
  • Thrombocytopenia
  • Hypercoagulable state
  • Trauma
  • Postoperative
  • Severe stress
• Cancer metastasis/lymphoma
• Autoimmune
  • Addison's disease
  • Polyglandular autoimmune
    syndromes I and II
• Infections process
  • Disseminated fungal infections
    (histoplasmosis)
  • Tuberculosis
  • HIV (CMV, MAI, Cryptococcus)
• Infiltrative process
• Iatrogenic
  • Ketoconazole
  • Etomidate
  • Metyrapone
  • Suramin
	• Iatrogenic
	  • Glucocorticoids
	  • Megestrol acetate (glucocorticoid activity)
	• Tumor or other mass lesion
	  • Pituitary adenoma
	  • Metastasis
	  • Lymphoma
	  • Primary tumor of brain or meninges
	  • Rathke's cleft cyst
	  • Empty sella
	• Pituitary apoplexy
	  • Sheehan's syndrome (post-partum hemorrhage)
	• Infiltrative process
	  • Hemachromatosis
	  • Histiocytosis
	  • Tuberculosis

treatment immediately; treatment can be discontinued if adequate adrenal function is demonstrated.

    D. "Functional" adrenal insufficiency. A "functional" or "relative" deficiency in cortisol secretion **may occur in critical illness,** but this is controversial and there are no universally accepted criteria for diagnosis of this condition. Adrenal insufficiency may be caused by drugs that inhibit cortisol production, notably ketoconazole and etomidate. Drugs that accelerate the metabolism of cortisol, such as phenytoin, barbiturates, and rifampin, can contribute to the development of adrenal insufficiency in patients with limited reserve. The **most common cause of adrenal insufficiency is exogenous glucocorticoids** (or drugs with glucocorticoid activity such as megestrol acetate) that cause feedback inhibition of ACTH production, which in turn causes atrophy of the cortisol producing cells in the adrenal gland. **Complete recovery** from iatrogenic adrenal insufficiency **may take months or even years.** Causes of adrenal insufficiency are listed in **Table 28-3.**

    E. Aldosterone deficiency. Aldosterone production is regulated by the **renin–angiotensin system.** The most important action of aldosterone is to promote sodium retention by the kidney. Deficiency of aldosterone causes sodium wasting, hypovolemia, and hypotension. Aldosterone deficiency can be managed in the short term with sufficient sodium and fluid intake, but long-term deficiency is managed with medications having aldosterone receptor agonist activity, such as fludrocortisone. The most common cause of aldosterone deficiency is injury to the adrenal gland itself, which is typically also associated with glucocorticoid deficiency. Isolated aldosterone deficiency is unusual except as a consequence of medications that affect the renin–aldosterone axis.

VI. Adrenal insufficiency

A. **Diagnosis of adrenal insufficiency in critical illness.** The diagnosis of cortisol deficiency in the setting of critical illness is much more challenging than in the outpatient setting. Cortisol secretion is normally increased during times of physiologic stress, and critical illness may unmask pre-existing, subclinical adrenal insufficiency. Critical illness may also cause a functional deficiency in cortisol production or responsiveness. Improvement of critical illness in response to glucocorticoids does not necessarily imply that the patient had diminished adrenal function. It is important to make a conceptual distinction between treatment of adrenal insufficiency and pharmacological treatment with glucocorticoids, which may improve clinical outcomes independent of adrenal functional status. These two concepts are sometimes confused in literature on this topic.

B. **Total versus free cortisol.** Widely available assays for cortisol measure total cortisol, but free cortisol is responsible for the physiological effects of the hormone. Critical illness is often associated with reductions in the level of cortisol-binding proteins, so total cortisol may be reduced without reduction of free cortisol, **leading to overdiagnosis of adrenal insufficiency.** Therefore, it is not clear how useful a diagnosis of "relative" adrenal insufficiency using total cortisol measurements actually is in selecting candidates for glucocorticoid treatment. Unfortunately, free cortisol assays are not widely available.

C. **Selection of patients to test for adrenal insufficiency.** The index of suspicion for adrenal insufficiency should be high in the ICU given the severe consequences of untreated insufficiency. Severe cortisol deficiency decreases response to vasopressors, so patients who remain hypotensive despite aggressive fluid and vasopressor therapy should be evaluated for adrenal insufficiency. Iatrogenic adrenal insufficiency can be very prolonged after treatment with glucocorticoids, so the diagnosis should be considered in all patients with a significant history of glucocorticoid use (e.g., more than 5 mg prednisone daily for more than 3 weeks within the previous year). Adrenal insufficiency should be ruled out in any critically ill patient with known lesions of the adrenal glands, pituitary, or hypothalamus. Adrenal insufficiency can cause hyponatremia, so adrenal insufficiency must be ruled out before a diagnosis of SIADH (syndrome of inappropriate antidiuretic hormone) can be made.

D. **ACTH stimulation test.** The main test for cortisol deficiency is the ACTH stimulation test. A blood sample for cortisol and ACTH determination is obtained and synthetic ACTH (cosyntropin) is administered IV or IM. A blood sample for a second cortisol measurement is obtained 60 to 90 minutes later. This test does not determine whether sufficient cortisol is being produced by the hypothalamic–pituitary–adrenal axis; it measures only the ability of the adrenal cortex to respond to exogenous ACTH. In the case of recent-onset central adrenal insufficiency, the adrenal cortex may not yet have atrophied and the stimulated cortisol response may be normal, although the baseline cortisol should be low in this case.

1. The amount of cosyntropin used in the stimulation test is a matter of debate. The typical test uses an IV dose of 250 µg cosyntropin. Some studies suggest use of a lower dose (e.g., 1 µg) identifies more patients

who benefit from glucocorticoid treatment, but it is not clear whether all of the identified patients are actually cortisol deficient and in need of replacement.

2. **Diagnostic criteria for adrenal insufficiency.** Glucocorticoid levels are normally elevated in response to stress, so a very low baseline plasma cortisol (**<3 μg/dL**) in the setting of critical illness is diagnostic of adrenal insufficiency. Moderate levels of baseline cortisol (**<10 μg/dL**) suggest adrenal insufficiency but may be misleading in the setting of a low CBG where free cortisol may be appropriately elevated. A **baseline (nonstimulated) cortisol of >18 μg/dL** effectively rules out adrenal insufficiency in most patients and a baseline cortisol value of <3 μg/dL is sufficient to diagnose adrenal insufficiency. In between, **a rise from baseline of less than 9 μg/dL has been proposed to identify patients who would benefit from glucocorticoid therapy.** Cortisol-binding globulin can be elevated in response to oral estrogen and liver inflammation so cortisol more than 18 μg/dL cannot rule out adrenal insufficiency in these settings.

E. **Therapy.** Ideally, cortisol and ACTH levels should be drawn before any empiric therapy is begun. If cosyntropin is available, it should be given immediately. If not, a second baseline sample (cortisol only) should be drawn just before injection of cosyntropin. In either case, empiric therapy with dexamethasone (1–2 mg IV every 8–12 hours) does not interfere with the ACTH stimulation test. Once the postcosyntropin cortisol sample has been drawn, **hydrocortisone,** which provides complete glucocorticoid and mineralocorticoid replacement, should be used at a total daily dose of **300 mg daily, divided every 6 or 8 hours,** unless there is no suspicion for primary adrenal insufficiency. It should be noted that what is the appropriate "stress" dose of glucocorticoids is a matter of controversy, and this generally used dose may provide glucocorticoid activity in excess of that produced by the normal adrenal gland during critical illness. As the clinical situation improves, the glucocorticoid dose should be tapered. There is no reliable test to determine the appropriateness of the replacement dose, so the dosing must be adjusted empirically. Doses of hydrocortisone should not be reduced below a replacement dose for a hospitalized patient with known adrenal insufficiency (50–60 mg orally divided in two doses, roughly twice the replacement dose in health) until follow-up testing demonstrates adequate adrenal function. An equivalent minimal dose of prednisone is 10 to 15 mg every morning or dexamethasone 1.5 to 2.5 mg daily. Doses of hydrocortisone less than 50 mg daily do not provide sufficient mineralocorticoid activity for patients with primary adrenal insufficiency, and prednisone and dexamethasone have essentially no mineralocorticoid activity. Patients requiring mineralocorticoid replacement should be treated with fludrocortisone at doses of 0.1 to 0.2 mg orally daily.

F. **Identifying the cause of adrenal insufficiency.** Once the diagnosis of adrenal insufficiency is made, an adrenocorticotropin (ACTH) sample drawn before initiation of empiric glucocorticoid therapy can help to localize the cause of adrenal insufficiency. An elevated ACTH suggests primary adrenal insufficiency and a low or (inappropriately, in this case) "normal" ACTH is consistent with central adrenal insufficiency. If the test suggests primary cortisol insufficiency (elevated ACTH levels), the evaluation should include imaging of the adrenal glands (usually with CT) to evaluate for metastatic, inflammatory, or infiltrative processes. In the setting of central cortisol deficiency, imaging of the pituitary and hypothalamus is indicated. Pituitary protocol MRI is the most appropriate test, but CT can rule out large tumors or gross hemorrhage. See **Table 28-3** for differential diagnosis of adrenal insufficiency.

G. **Pituitary apoplexy.** Pituitary apoplexy is a clinical syndrome caused by hemorrhage or infarct within a pre-existing pituitary mass lesion. It is rare cause of adrenal insufficiency but it deserves special mention in the ICU because it is one of the true **endocrine emergencies.** Pituitary apoplexy can lead to abrupt and severe adrenal insufficiency in the setting of severe physiologic stress, a combination that may prove fatal if not treated promptly. In addition, mass effect on surrounding structures, including the optic nerve and cranial nerves III and VI, can lead to permanent visual deficits or blindness. Case reports and series suggest that conditions and interventions common to the ICU, including anticoagulation or anti-platelet therapy, coagulopathy, thrombocytopenia, renal failure, throm-bolysis, hypertension, hypotension, and head trauma may precipitate apoplexy in patients with undiagnosed pituitary tumors. Therefore, pitu-itary apoplexy should always be considered in the differential diagnosis of adrenal insufficiency. Unfortunately, the signs and symptoms of apoplexy (headache, visual disturbance) may be masked in critically ill patients, so imaging must be the mainstay of diagnosis. A noncontrast head CT does not reliably allow detection of hemorrhage or infarction in pituitary tumor, but is sensitive for pituitary masses larger than 1 cm, the substrate for most cases of apoplexy. MRI can be used to identify hemorrhage or infarction if a mass is found. High-dose glucocorticoids and rapid surgical decompression are the therapies of choice for pituitary apoplexy and pro-vide favorable neurological outcomes.

VII. Cushing's syndrome

A. **Diagnosis.** Cushing's syndrome is defined by excessive production of corti-sol and loss of the normal diurnal rhythm of cortisol production. The nor-mal response to critical illness is to dramatically increase cortisol produc-tion, with loss of the normal diurnal rhythm. Therefore, the usual screening tests for Cushing's syndrome, which rely on measuring total uri-nary excretion or cortisol or abnormal excretion of cortisol in the late evening, cannot be used in the ICU. Suspicion of Cushing's syndrome may arise in the setting of a typical body habitus, but the most specific signs are the presence of enlarged supraclavicular and dorsal cervical fat pads, wide (>1 cm) violaceous (not pink) striae, and proximal weakness. Cushing's syndrome may be a cause for hypertension, but is rarely the cause of a hypertensive emergency. Suspicion for Cushing's syndrome should prompt endocrine consultation, but it would be unusual for treatment for Cushing's syndrome to begin in the ICU setting unless the cause of the ill-ness was thought to be hypercortisolism itself.

B. **Treatment.** Definitive treatment of Cushing's syndrome is usually surgical, involving removal of an ACTH secreting pituitary tumor, an adrenal tumor, or in rare cases an ectopic ACTH-secreting tumor. Temporizing treatment would most commonly be with **ketoconazole** or other drugs that inhibit synthesis of cortisol. This would uncommonly be started in the ICU due to the risk of provoking an adrenal crisis, but would be delayed until resolution of the acute illness.

VIII. Pheochromocytoma and paraganglioma

A. **Diagnosis.** These are tumors of neural crest origin that secrete cate-cholamines (norepinephrine, epinephrine, and/or dopamine) in an unpre-dictable manner. They are found arising from the medulla of the adrenal gland or from the sympathetic ganglia along the aorta up to the carotic bifurcation. The classical history is one of "spells" of palpitations, headache, and pallor, classically associated with **hypertension**, but tonic hypertension without spells is an equally likely presentation. The normal physiological response to critical illness is to increase production of the same catecholamines (and their metabolites) that are produced by pheochromocytomas. No "normal" ranges for these hormones exist for hospital inpatients, much less ICU patients. Therefore, the appropriate strategy in most cases of suspected pheochromocytoma is to wait until the patient has recovered from their acute illness to perform diagnostic testing. Occasionally, empirical treatment may be indicated, such as in the setting of hypertension or labile blood pressure and a newly discovered mass in an adrenal gland or along the aorta or neck vessels. Approximately 5% of all incidentally discovered adrenal masses are pheochromocytomas. Characteristics of the mass on MRI imaging and specialized tests such as meta-iodobenzylguanidine (MIBG) scintiscanning can be used to support the diagnosis in patients for whom biochemical testing is not appropriate.

B. **Treatment.** All patients with catecholamine-secreting tumors require **preparation for surgery.** Even external palpation of these masses may provoke a crisis, so no manipulations should not be done (even as a diagnostic measure) without careful thought, and unless appropriate monitoring (arterial pressure monitoring) and countermeasures (such as nitroprusside for IV administration) are in place. Definitive treatment of pheochromocytoma involves surgical resection, but the same methods used for surgery preparation can be used as temporizing measures until a definitive diagnosis can be made or until other medical issues are resolved. The usual regimen includes loading with **phenoxybenzamine,** which inhibits vasoconstriction in response to catecholamines secreted by the tumor. Pheochromocytoma is often accompanied by tonic vasoconstriction and volume contraction, and phenoxybenzamine-mediated vasodilation may cause hypotension. Therefore, administration of phenoxybenzamine must be accompanied by volume repletion. In the ICU setting, phenoxybenzamine can be rapidly titrated up to 40 mg twice a day with the appropriate monitoring of arterial blood pressure. An alternative is a **continuous IV infusion of a calcium channel blocker** starting before surgery and continuing until the tumor is resected.

C. **Postoperative management of pheochromocytoma.** After successful surgical resection, phenoxybenzamine can be discontinued. Autodiuresis should occur as the vasodilatory effects of the phenoxybenzamine dissipate. Patients treated with calcium channel blockers prior to surgery may need volume repletion to prevent hypotension as the chronically constricted vasculature relaxes. Hypoglycemia can complicate the immediate postoperative period, so glucose monitoring should occur at regular intervals in the first postoperative day.

IX. **Thyroid function and disease**
   A. **Physiology** (**Fig. 28-3**). There are two forms of thyroid hormone, **T4 (levothyroxine),** which contains four iodine atoms, and **T3 (triiodothyronine),** which contains three iodine atoms. Both T4 and T3 are produced in the thyroid gland and are stored in the form of thyroglobulin. The production and release of thyroid hormone is controlled by **thyroid-stimulating hormone (TSH)** secreted by the pituitary gland. TSH stimulates the breakdown of thyroglobulin to release T3 and T4 and promotes the conversion of some

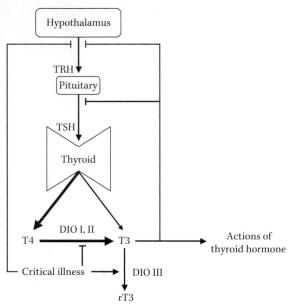

FIGURE 28-3 Regulation of thyroid hormone secretion and activity. Arrows indicate positive action, production, or conversion. Lines ending in cross-bars indicate inhibition. TRH, thyrotropin releasing hormone; TSH, thyroid-stimulating hormone; T4, levothyroxine (prohormone, minimal activity); T3, triiodothyronine (active thyroid hormone); rT3, reverse T3 (inactive); DIO I, II, III, deiodinase types I, II, and III.

T4 to T3 prior to release into the bloodstream. TSH secretion is regulated by thyrotropin-regulating hormone (TRH), which is secreted by the hypothalamus. TRH and TSH secretion are under negative regulation by thyroid hormone, thereby completing a feedback regulatory loop. Thyroid hormone acts through receptors for T3, which are widely distributed. T4 has little activity of its own and is essentially a prohormone. Some T3 is directly released by the thyroid, but the large majority of T3 is produced in other tissues by conversion of T4 to T3 by deiodinase enzymes (types I and II). T4 can also be converted to reverse T3 (rT3), which contains three iodine atoms in a different configuration and has no thyroid hormone activity, by a third deiodinase (type III). Production of T3 outside of the thyroid gland by deiodinase activity is suppressed by conditions common to the ICU, including poor nutrition, diabetes (insulin resistance or relative insulin deficiency), high levels of free fatty acids, inflammatory cytokines, illness in general, and drugs including β-blockers and amiodarone. The production of active T3 is increased by high calorie intake and glucose plus insulin. The conversion of T4 to inactive rT3 is increased by illness.

B. **Functions of thyroid hormone and symptoms and signs of thyroid dysfunction.** Thyroid hormone is an important modulator of metabolic rate and the rate of protein synthesis and turnover. Thyroid hormone increases both cardiac contractility and heart rate and promotes relaxation of arteries, reducing systemic vascular resistance. **Hyperthyroidism** is associated with tachycardia, systolic hypertension, widened pulse pressure, high-output heart failure, increased risk of atrial fibrillation, and myocardial ischemia. **Hypothyroidism** is associated with bradycardia and hypertension and can precipitate congestive heart failure in those with underlying cardiac disease. Myopathy associated with hypothyroidism and hyperthyroidism can cause respiratory muscles to become weak in both conditions, which can cause inadequate ventilation. Poor ventilation can be especially problematic in hyperthyroidism, in which oxygen consumption and CO_2 production are increased. Thyroid hormone promotes gut motility; hypothyroidism is associated with constipation and hyperthyroidism with frequent stools or diarrhea which may be associated with malabsorption. Thyroid hormone is important for free water clearance and hypothyroidism is associated with hyponatremia. Consequently, hypothyroidism must be ruled out before a diagnosis of SIADH can be made. The metabolism of many drugs and endogenous hormones is regulated by thyroid hormone. Drug dosages may need to be reduced in hypothyroidism due to slow clearance or increased with hyperthyroidism due to increased clearance. Cortisol clearance is promoted by thyroid hormone so that treatment of hypothyroidism with thyroid hormone can precipitate adrenal crisis in individuals with adrenal insufficiency. Hypothyroidism is associated with accumulation of matrix glycosaminoglycans in many tissues, which can lead to coarse skin and hair, enlargement of the tongue, hoarseness, and nonpitting edema **(myxedema)**. Graves disease, the most common cause of hyperthyroidism, can also cause autoimmune infiltration of the fatty tissue of the orbit and autoimmune attack on the eyes, which can cause ocular inflammation and protrusion of the eyes from the orbits.

X. Thyroid function in critical illness
   A. Nonthyroidal illness syndrome. In contrast to the outpatient setting, TSH levels in hospitalized patients can be misleading, and particularly so in patients with critical illness. Several drugs and hormones affect TSH secretion. Dopamine suppresses TSH and dopamine antagonists such as metoclopramide stimulate TSH secretion. Elevated glucocorticoid levels, both endogenous in response to stress and from glucocorticoid therapy, suppress both TRH and TSH secretion. A more fundamental problem is that low TSH levels as well as low T4 and T3 levels are very common in critical illness so that normal thyroid studies are the exception rather than the rule in the ICU. This syndrome used to be called "euthyroid-sick syndrome," but it is now thought that **critically ill patients may indeed be hypothyroid** as a result of TRH and TSH suppression. The preferred name for the syndrome of abnormal thyroid function during illness is the **"nonthyroidal illness syndrome" (NTIS)**. Even though this state is no longer thought to be "euthyroid," the weight of evidence suggests that **treatment of critically ill patients with NTIS is not beneficial** and may be harmful, perhaps because relative hypothyroidism reduces catabolism and is therefore protective.
   B. When to send thyroid studies in the ICU. Because NTIS is so common in critical illness, **thyroid studies should not be sent on hospitalized patients unless there is a strong suspicion of thyroid dysfunction**. In patients receiving therapy with T4 before hospitalization, the dose of T4 should generally not be changed. It may be useful to confirm that the dose was appropriate before the onset of critical illness by reviewing historical (premorbid) TSH values. If gut absorption is compromised, orally administered levothyroxine should be replaced with IV levothyroxine, reducing the dose by 20% to account for increased bioavailability by the IV route. In patients on therapy

for hyperthyroidism prior to their critical illness the dose of medications to treat their disorder should not be changed unless there is evidence of new toxicity. Confirmation that the hyperthyroidism was well controlled prior to hospitalization is recommended, and endocrine consultation is appropriate in all critically ill patients with hyperthyroidism.

C. **Laboratory diagnosis of thyroid dysfunction in patients with critical illness.** For patients without a prior diagnosis of thyroid dysfunction but a strong suspicion of new or undiagnosed thyroid dysfunction, the diagnosis of the thyroid state can be very challenging. In this setting, the **TSH alone is of little use.** TSH is typically normal or suppressed in NTIS, although TSH levels can be elevated during the recovery from NTIS as the system seeks a new equilibrium. A full panel of thyroid function studies including TSH, total T4, free T4 (or free thyroxine index), and T3 should be ordered. **The TSH must be interpreted not only in light of the T4 and T3 values, but also in the clinical context.** It is important to decide *a priori* what kind of thyroid dysfunction (hyperthyroidism or hypothyroidism) is suspected on clinical grounds before thyroid laboratories are ordered.

D. **Interpretation of a low TSH.** A normal or low TSH is an expected component of the NTIS. A low TSH alone should not be interpreted to mean the patient is hyperthyroid or that the dose of thyroid hormone should be reduced. If the TSH is low and hyperthyroidism is suspected on clinical grounds, the **serum T3** may be helpful. Patients with NTIS should have low or low normal T3 values, while those with hyperthyroidism should have high or high normal T3 values. A patient with an **undetectable TSH** using a modern high sensitivity assay is likely to have hyperthyroidism, and this diagnosis can be supported by an elevated or high normal T3. If central hypothyroidism (deficiency of TSH due to a hypothalamic or pituitary lesion) is suspected and the TSH is normal or low, measurement of **serum rT3** may be helpful. Levels of rT3 are usually elevated in NTIS, but are likely to be low in severe central hypothyroidism.

E. **Interpretation of an elevated TSH.** An elevated TSH can be seen in patients recovering from NTIS, although the TSH rarely rises to more than 20 mU/L. In a patient who is still critically ill, an elevated TSH is suggestive of **primary hypothyroidism** due a defect in thyroid hormone synthesis or release by the thyroid gland. A diagnosis of hypothyroidism can be supported by a low or low-normal T3.

F. **Interpretation of T4 levels.** T4 is highly bound by serum proteins, primarily by thyroid-binding globulin, but also transthyretin, albumin, and lipoproteins; only a tiny fraction of T4 is unbound. Reductions in levels or modifications of binding proteins, which reduce T4 binding and total T4 levels, are common in critical illness. Therefore, **total T4 levels are low in up to half of ICU patients.** Depending on the degree of binding protein reduction, a free thyroxine index may be normal or low. "Direct" free T4 assays are variably affected by drugs and circulating substances such as free fatty acids. A total T4, free thyroxine index, or direct free **T4 measurement that is elevated** in a critically ill patient **can support a diagnosis of hyperthyroidism.** If a direct free T4 is obtained in a critically ill patient, a total T4 measurement should also be obtained to increase the likelihood that an artifactual elevated free T4 measurement can be recognized as such. **Low or normal values for total T4, free thyroxine index, or direct free T4 are generally not helpful.** An exception to the general rule of illness reducing thyroid hormone–binding proteins is the association of hepatitis and hepatoma with abnormally high blood levels of thyroid-binding proteins and total T4 levels.

XI. **Treatment of thyroid dysfunction In ICU patients**
   A. **Treatment of hypothyroidism.** Although NTIS is probably a state of relative hypothyroidism, **treatment with thyroid hormone does not improve outcomes in patients with critical illness** or in postsurgical patients. This may be because a mild degree of hypothyroidism is protective in the face of a catabolic state. Patients with pre-existing hypothyroidism should not have their usual dose of thyroid hormone adjusted. Treatment of newly diagnosed hypothyroidism should be with T4, and initial dosing should be weight based. A **replacement dose of T4 by the enteral route** is approximately **1.6 μg/kg daily,** although individual patients may require substantially more or less. A somewhat lower initial dose is appropriate for patients who are elderly and frail or if there is concern for precipitating cardiac ischemia or atrial fibrillation. **T4 should be given separately from all other medications and enteral feeds should be paused** until there is minimal gastric residual before the thyroid hormone is given, and should not be started for 30 minutes afterward. **In cases where this is not practical** (such as in patients receiving insulin therapy) or when enteral feeds are not tolerated, **IV administration is preferred.** In this case, the **dose should be reduced by 20%** to account for improved bioavailability. It takes at least 6 weeks after a change in dose before the T4 and TSH to reach a new equilibrium, so dosage changes based on measurements made earlier than this should be made with caution. Treatment of hypothyroidism with T3 is generally not indicated except in cases of myxedema coma.
   B. **Treatment of hyperthyroidism.** Patients under active treatment for hyperthyroidism before developing critical illness should be monitored by an endocrine consultant because antithyroid medications can have significant toxicities, and because large iodine loads from medications (such as amiodarone) or from imaging contrast can change the thyroid state and may necessitate changes in therapy. If a new diagnosis of hyperthyroidism is suspected, endocrine consultation should be obtained to confirm the diagnosis and to monitor treatment. Thyroid hormone action **increases the number of β-adrenergic receptors** in many tissues, explaining many of the symptoms of hyperthyroidism. Therapy for hyperthyroidism typically includes treatment with a β-blocker to counteract the increased β-adrenergic action. **Propranolol and metoprolol** both can be given IV, and have the additional advantage of inhibiting T4 to T3 conversion by deiodinase. Other therapies should be initiated in consultation with an endocrinologist. A typical course of therapy includes treatment with thionamide antithyroid drugs such as **methimazole** (more potent) and **propylthiouracil** (**PTU,** less potent). These drugs **block new production of thyroid hormone but do not prevent release of thyroid hormone** that has already been synthesized, so thionamide drugs have little immediate effect on their own. However, once the thionamide has blocked new thyroid hormone synthesis, large doses of **iodine may be given to block release of T3 and T4** from the thyroid. If new synthesis of thyroid hormone is not first blocked by a thionamide, the iodine will be converted into new thyroid hormone, so the order of administration is critical.

XII. **Myxedema coma**
   A. **The clinical syndrome.** The manifestations of extreme hypothyroidism can include altered mental status (usually lethargy but occasionally psychosis; actual coma is rare), hypothermia, bradycardia, hypotension, hypoventilation, hyponatremia, and hypoglycemia. All of these manifestations are reversible by thyroid hormone. **Myxedema coma can occur acutely** in

persons with pre-existing untreated or inadequately treated hypothyroidism who are exposed to the stress of an illness, cold ambient temperatures, or sedative drugs. Age and cardiovascular disease are risk factors for mortality, which can be as high as 40%. Myxedema coma will not occur quickly after **discontinuation of thyroid hormone** even in a patient with severe hypothyroidism because the **half-life of thyroid hormone is long** (approximately 1 week).

B. Diagnosis and treatment. The severity of hypothyroidism required to produce this clinical syndrome is extreme, so high levels of TSH are to be expected. An exception is hypothyroidism of central origin in which the TSH may be normal or low. The mortality of true myxedema coma is high and treatment with thyroid hormone reduces mortality. Therefore, if the suspicion for myxedema coma is high, treatment should begin immediately, without waiting for the laboratory test. Confirmatory tests must be drawn before treatment is started, however. Myxedema coma can be associated with adrenal insufficiency, either due to an endocrine autoimmune syndrome or pituitary dysfunction. **Administration of thyroid hormone** to a patient with adrenal insufficiency can acutely **precipitate an adrenal crisis.** Therefore, a cosyntropin test should be performed at the time thyroid tests are obtained and **stress-dose glucocorticoid therapy** must be started before initiation of thyroid hormone therapy. Glucocorticoids can be discontinued if the cosyntropin stimulation test demonstrates sufficient adrenal reserves. The appropriate treatment for myxedema coma is controversial, with different authorities preferring T3 alone, T4 alone, or both hormones together. Treatment of myxedema coma should be initiated in consultation with an endocrinologist and doses should be adjusted both for weight and the presence of cardiac illness. Supportive care may include passive warming, volume resuscitation, vasopressors, ventilatory support, and IV glucose. Treatment of the precipitating illness is essential.

XIII. Thyroid storm

A. The clinical syndrome and diagnostic criteria. Thyroid storm is a syndrome of severe hyperthyroidism with exaggerated symptoms and signs, usually occurring as an acute exacerbating of pre-existing hyperthyroidism. Because the diagnosis is a matter of degree (once biochemical hyperthyroidism is established), diagnostic criteria include calculation of a score, with more points for increasing degrees of **hyperpyrexia, tachycardia,** severity of **congestive heart failure,** presence of **atrial fibrillation,** altered mental status (with higher scores for seizure or coma), and GI symptoms (including diarrhea, vomiting, abdominal pain, and jaundice). Points are also given for history of an event that may have precipitated the thyroid storm, such as an iodine load (from medications or IV contrast), thyroid surgery, trauma, infection, or any other severe stress including nonthyroidal surgery.

B. Treatment consists of supportive therapy and medications targeted specifically at the excessive action, production, and release of thyroid hormone. Initial therapy should include an IV β-blocker titrated to control tachycardia. Stress-dose **glucocorticoids** (100 mg hydrocortisone IV every 8 hours) are administered to reduce T4 to T3 conversion by deiodinase and to ensure thyroid storm is not complicated by adrenal insufficiency due to rapid glucocorticoid metabolism. The use of thionamide medications such as methimazole and propylthiouracil to reduce the production of thyroid hormone, followed by iodine to inhibit thyroid hormone release, is similar to the treatment of less severe hypothyroidism, except that the doses are larger. Supportive care includes aggressive treatment of hyperpyrexia, fluid resuscitation, ventricular rate control in atrial fibrillation, and diagnosis and treatment of any precipitating conditions.

XIV. Carcinoid syndrome

A. **Carcinoid tumor physiology.** Carcinoid tumors are most frequently found in the **bronchi** and in the **gastrointestinal (GI) tract.** The liver inactivates most of the products of carcinoid tumors, so GI tumors typically do not cause symptoms without metastasis to the liver. Lung tumors can cause symptoms without metastasis because the carcinoid products are secreted directly into the systemic circulation, but lung tumors are less common than primary GI tumors. Carcinoid tumors can secrete a wide variety of products including serotonin, histamine, tachykinins, kallikrein, and prostaglandins. Less common products having relevance in the ICU setting include norepinephrine, dopamine, gastrin, glucagon, ACTH, and growth hormone. Almost all carcinoid tumors take up and metabolize tryptophan. In most cases, they convert it to **serotonin,** which is then metabolized to 5-hydroxyindoleacetic (5-HIAA) acid, but in some cases no serotonin is produced and the primary metabolites are 5-HIAA and **histamine.** The characteristic production of 5-HIAA by carcinoid tumors allows their detection by measurement of 5-HIAA in the blood and urine.

B. **Features of carcinoid syndrome.** Secretory diarrhea and flushing and itching of the skin are the most common manifestations, caused by excess of serotonin, histamine, and kinins. The diarrhea can be explosive and result in substantial fluid loss and malabsorption. Peripheral vasodilation may lead to hypotension and tachycardia. Episodes are usually spontaneous and last less than 30 minutes. However, flushing episodes can be precipitated by drugs, especially anesthesia, or palpation of the tumor, and this "carcinoid crisis" can last for hours and be associated with severe hypotension, bronchoconstriction, arrhythmias, and death. Flushing may be associated with bronchospasm, particularly when associated with arise from bronchial carcinoids. β-Agonists (but not albuterol) can provoke persistent vasodilation and hypotension. High levels of serotonin may lead to cardiac valvular abnormalities, typically involving fibrous thickening of the right heart valves and leading most commonly to tricuspid regurgitation and/or pulmonic stenosis or regurgitation. Depletion of tryptophan (by conversion to serotonin and 5-HIAA) may lead to muscle wasting due to poor protein synthesis and nicotinic acid deficiency, which may result in overt pellagra (rough skin, glossitis, angular stomatitis, and altered mental status).

C. **Diagnosis.** In patients with the carcinoid syndrome, typical levels of 5-HIAA in urine are more than 10-fold above the upper limit of normal. Many drugs and foods can give falsely elevated levels of 5-HIAA including acetaminophen, phenobarbital, and ephedrine. False-negative tests can also be caused by cosyntropin, levodopa, MAO inhibitors, phenothiazines, ASA, and heparin. Bronchial and gastric carcinoids may have normal urinary 5-HIAA levels even in the absence of interfering substances. In such cases, blood measurements of chromogranin A and serotonin may be helpful. In the ICU, the provocation of paradoxical flushing and hypotension by epinephrine should prompt consideration of carcinoid syndrome.

D. **Treatment.** Definitive treatment of carcinoid syndrome involves surgical removal of the tumor. However, most patients who develop the classic syndrome have gut carcinoids with metastasis to the liver, so definitive surgical management is not possible. **Flushing and diarrhea are treated primarily with octreotide,** which is highly effective. Octreotide is also used to prevent progression of carcinoid cardiac valvular disease. Octreotide can be used prophylactically to prevent carcinoid crisis due to anesthesia and surgery. Levels of urinary 5-HIAA can be followed to monitor the effectiveness of treatment. Wheezing can be treated with albuterol. The treatment of hypotension in carcinoid crisis is unusual because **catecholamines can worsen the crises** and further lower blood pressure. Hypotension should be treated with intravenous octreotide (IV bolus of 300 μg followed by an infusion of up to 150 μg/h) and fluid resuscitation. A paradoxical fall in blood pressure upon treatment with sympathomimetic agents should prompt consideration of the carcinoid syndrome.

XV. **Regulation of calcium homeostasis**
   A. **Calcium uptake from the gut and secretion by the kidney.** Under ordinary circumstances, the intake and excretion of calcium are balanced. From a typical daily intake of 1,000 mg, there may be 200 mg net absorption from the gut and a similar amount excreted in the urine. All calcium is filtered by the glomerulus and must be actively reabsorbed so that only a few percent of the filtered load is actually excreted. The absorption of calcium (along with phosphate) from the gut and liberation of calcium and phosphorus from bone both are promoted by the **parathyroid hormone (PTH).** In addition to direct effects on the gut, PTH promotes the activation of vitamin D to **1,25-dihydroxyvitamin D,** which also promotes calcium and phosphorus absorption from the gut. In the kidney, PTH promotes calcium reabsorption but phosphate excretion. The net effect of increasing PTH is to raise the serum calcium and reduce serum phosphorus. Most of the **calcium reabsorption** by the kidney occurs in the proximal tubule and **is associated with sodium absorption.** Calcium absorption is promoted in sodium avid states (dehydration) and calcium excretion is promoted by saline infusion. A smaller amount of calcium absorption occurs in the thick ascending limb of the loop of Henle, and loop diuretics inhibit this. Finally, a small proportion of calcium is reabsorbed in the distal tubule, and this is regulated by PTH. Reduced renal function plays an important role in many hypercalcemia syndromes.
   B. **Calcium equilibrium between the blood and bone.** A small fraction (approximately 1%) of the total body calcium is found within cells and in the extracellular fluid. The remainder, approximately 1 kg, is found along with phosphorus in hydroxyapatite crystals within the bone. If bone reabsorption is increased out of proportion of bone mineralization, quite large amounts of calcium can be released into the blood. Equilibrium between the blood and the bone is primarily regulated by PTH, but mechanical stress also promotes bone formation. In the setting of **immobilization,** the equilibrium can shift dramatically to bone reabsorption, causing hypercalcemia in bed-bound patients.

XVI. **Causes of hypercalcemia**
   A. **Primary hyperparathyroidism.** This syndrome is typically caused by **benign parathyroid tumors.** It is the most common cause of hypercalcemia in the outpatient setting. The sensitivity of parathyroid tumors to the ambient calcium levels is reduced so that higher levels of calcium are required to fully suppress PTH production. A new equilibrium is reached in which serum calcium levels are elevated, yet PTH levels are not fully suppressed. **PTH levels are not usually elevated, but are not appropriately suppressed to undetectable levels** in the setting of elevated calcium levels.
   B. **Secondary hyperparathyroidism (renal osteodystrophy).** Renal insufficiency reduces the ability to excrete phosphorus. **Elevated phosphorus,** like low

calcium, is a **stimulus to PTH secretion**. PTH promotes phosphorus excretion and the absorption of calcium from the gut and liberation of calcium from bone. The elevation of calcium may be exacerbated by administration of calcium containing phosphate binders. PTH is usually not elevated, but is inappropriately high ("normal") in the setting of hypercalcemia.

C. **Tertiary hyperparathyroidism.** Long-standing secondary hyperparathyroidism may lead to a degree of **parathyroid autonomy** from calcium feedback regulation. Once this occurs, PTH production is not appropriately suppressed even if phosphate levels are controlled by dialysis or phosphate binders. The consequence is inappropriately high ("inappropriately normal") PTH levels in the setting of hypercalcemia.

D. **Hypercalcemia of malignancy.** This syndrome may develop in the setting of large lytic lesions of bone, but more commonly is associated with secretion of **PTH-related protein (PTHrP)** from tumors, which circulates systemically and acts similarly to PTH. PTHrP is classically associated with multiple myeloma and breast, lung, and squamous cell cancer, but may be found with tumors of many types. PTH production from the parathyroid glands is suppressed by the elevated calcium and PTH is typically undetectable.

E. **Milk-alkali syndrome.** The renal **excretion of calcium is inhibited by alkaline urine.** When intake of calcium and alkali are increased together, typically in the setting of at least mild renal insufficiency, hypercalcemia may occur. Hypercalcemia can lead to further decrease in GFR, so the syndrome can be self-perpetuating. The name is derived from patients who develop the syndrome while taking large quantities of milk and/or calcium carbonate antacids to treat gastritis or peptic ulcer disease. PTH is suppressed and typically undetectable.

F. **Hypervitaminosis D.** Vitamin D conversion to 25-hydroxyvitamin D in the liver is largely unregulated. Conversion to the active form of vitamin D, 1,25-dihydroxyvitamin D, occurs in the kidney and is regulated by PTH. In granulomatous diseases, including sarcoidosis, tuberculosis, and fungal infections, macrophages may produce **excess 1,25-dihydroxyvitamin D**, leading to excess calcium absorption from the gut. Some hematologic malignancies can also produce 1,25-dihydroxyvitamin D.

G. **Immobilization.** When the bones are unweighted, as in bed rest, bone formation may no longer balance bone resorption in states of **high bone turnover** (see **Section XV.B.**) The amount of calcium liberated into the circulation may dramatically increase, resulting in hypercalcemia. If PTH is regulated appropriately and renal function is normal, immobilization alone should not cause hypercalcemia. Unless hyperparathyroidism is the cause of increased bone turnover, PTH should be completely suppressed. Elevated levels of cytokines, as found in sepsis, may promote bone turnover.

H. **Paget's disease of bone.** Localized patches of increased bone resorption and disorganized re-formation are the hallmark of Paget's disease. By itself, Paget's disease usually does not cause hypercalcemia because bone resorption is balanced by bone formation. However, **immobilization** can lead to the abrupt development of hypercalcemia. Paget's disease is present in up to 3% of individuals older than 50 years.

I. **Drugs and ingestions.** Excess ingestion of vitamin D or vitamin D metabolites such as 1,25-hydroxyvitamin D can cause hypercalcemia. Other drugs that may cause hypercalcemia include vitamin A (increased bone turnover), lithium (increasing PTH secretion), theophylline (increased bone turnover), and thiazide diuretics (reduced calcium excretion).

J. **Endocrinopathies.** Nonparathyroid endocrinopathies that may cause hypercalcemia include hyperthyroidism (increased bone turnover), adrenal insufficiency (decreased calcium excretion), and pheochromocytoma (PTHrP secretion).

K. **Parathyroid carcinoma.** Cancerous parathyroid tissue may be extremely resistant to suppression by calcium. Both PTH levels and calcium levels may become extremely elevated. By the time the diagnosis is made, parathyroid carcinoma has often metastasized, making calcium control extremely difficult.

L. **Familial hypocalciuric hypercalcemia (FHH).** In this relatively common syndrome, the **set point for calcium suppression of PTH production is higher than normal** due to a mutation in the calcium sensing receptor. Serum calcium is typically mildly elevated, but **urine excretion of calcium is low or normal,** rather than elevated as in hyperparathyroidism. PTH levels are normal or slightly elevated. Differentiating this syndrome from mild primary hyperparathyroidism can be difficult. The inheritance of the syndrome is **autosomal dominant,** so family history or measurement of serum calcium in family members can be helpful. The syndrome is not progressive and serum **calcium levels are consistent throughout life.** Historical calcium measurements, if available, may be very helpful. **No treatment** is indicated for this disorder.

M. **Overlap syndromes.** It is common for patients with critical illness to develop hypercalcemia that results from a combination of causes, and severe hypercalcemia can result from a "perfect storm" of increased calcium release from the bone and decreased excretion. For instance, mild primary hyperparathyroidism may not result in hypercalcemia until the patient is immobilized, at which point the net release of calcium from the bone may increase markedly. Even this might not lead to hypercalcemia in the setting of normal kidney function, but if renal function is compromised for some reason severe hypercalcemia may develop. Likewise, elevated cytokine levels may promote bone turnover, which in combination with immobilization and renal insufficiency may result in hypercalcemia.

XVII. Diagnosis of hypercalcemia

A. **Signs and symptoms associated with severe hypercalcemia** include polyuria, abdominal pain, nausea, vomiting, constipation, headache, altered mental status, lethargy, weakness, and depression. Hyporreflexia, hypertension, and bradycardia may occur. In the critical care setting, hypercalcemia is primarily diagnosed by laboratory studies.

B. **Measurement of serum calcium.** Approximately 50% of serum calcium in found as free, ionized calcium, while approximately 40% is bound to albumin and 10% is complexed with anions. Total serum calcium levels can be corrected for the serum albumin level [corrected Ca^{2+} = total Ca^{2+} + $0.8 \times$ (normal albumin $-$ patient albumin)], but this correction is not entirely reliable. It is preferable to **directly measure the ionized calcium** and make diagnostic and therapeutic decisions on this basis.

C. **Differential diagnosis of hypercalcemia.** It is critical to **draw appropriate laboratory studies before any treatment is begun.** Hypercalcemia is never so much of an emergency that several tubes of blood cannot be obtained before treatment is initiated. **Once calcium is normalized** by any means it is very difficult to make a definitive diagnosis. Hypercalcemia acts as a "stress test" for the calcium control system and once the stress is removed, most diagnostic tests become useless. For instance, an elevated PTH is only "abnormal" if the calcium is also abnormal. In the setting of normal or low calcium, an elevated PTH might be the appropriate homeostatic response to increased calcium excretion and/or poor calcium intake or absorption. Initial workup should include ionized calcium (preferred) or total serum calcium and albumin, phosphorus, BUN and creatinine, and intact PTH.

D. **PTH-dependent hypercalcemia.** Serum PTH is not usually elevated even when PTH is the cause of the hypercalcemia. Rather, PTH is **"inappropriately normal"** in the setting of hypercalcemia. A frankly elevated PTH may also be found, but extreme elevations of PTH are rare and suggest the diagnosis of parathyroid carcinoma. In the setting of hypercalcemia, **any detectable PTH** suggests hyperparathyroidism as the cause. Primary hyperparathyroidism can be distinguished from secondary and tertiary hyperparathyroidism by renal function studies and history. If primary hyperparathyroidism is diagnosed, identification of the parathyroid adenoma can usually be delayed until the critical illness has resolved.

E. **PTH-independent hypercalcemia.** If PTH is undetectable, past medical history and medication history will provide important clues. Additional laboratory workup should include PTHrP (for hypercalcemia of malignancy), 25-hydroxyvitamin D (if ingestion is suspected), 1,25-dihydroxyvitamin D (for granulomatous disease), and thyroid studies (TSH, free T4, T3). A corticotropin stimulation test and/or morning cortisol values may be considered to rule out adrenal insufficiency. Alkaline phosphatase is usually strikingly elevated in Paget's disease and less so in other causes of increased bone turnover such as hyperthyroidism. A plain film skeletal survey can be used to look for bone metastasis or Paget's disease of bone. Milk-alkali syndrome is associated with alkalosis and renal insufficiency, and will be associated with a characteristic medication history.

XVIII. Treatment of hypercalcemia

A. **Promotion of renal calcium excretion.** Calcium is freely filtered into the urine and most of it is actively reabsorbed along with sodium. Delivery of sodium in the form of **saline hydration** can be very effective in lowering serum calcium in volume-depleted patients. The goal in most cases should be to adequately hydrate the patient, although saline therapy may be limited by development of volume overload and edema. In such cases, a loop diuretic such as furosemide may be required and may further promote calcium excretion. Loop diuretics should not be used without saline treatment, as dehydration may worsen hypercalcemia. The combination of saline and furosemide for **forced diuresis has fallen out of favor** as the first-line therapy for hypercalcemia. In the setting of renal failure, renal replacement therapy with dialysis or continuous hemofiltration with a low calcium dialysate is usually necessary to treat hypercalcemia. **Dialysis** may also be used for emergency treatment of severe hypercalcemia in patients with normal or only modestly impaired renal function.

B. **Inhibiting calcium release from bone. Calcitonin** inhibits bone resorption as well as renal calcium resorption. Treatment with calcitonin, at 4 to 8 U/kg subcutaneously every 6 hours, can be very effective in **rapidly lower serum calcium,** often within hours. The combination of calcitonin and saline hydration is probably the most appropriate **first-line therapy** for hypercalcemia. **Tachyphylaxis** to the effects of calcitonin usually occurs after a few days of treatment, so it is usually used in the acute phase of treatment only. Rebound hypercalcemia can occur upon development of tachyphylaxis when calcitonin is the sole therapy. Either the underlying cause should be treated or **bisphosphonates** should be given concurrently with calcitonin and saline hydration. Bisphosphonates are deposited in the mineral matrix of bone and inhibit the release of calcium from bone. Pamidronate and zoledronic acid can be administered IV. **Pamidronate is given at 60 to 90 mg IV over 4 hours, zoledronic acid at 4 mg IV over 15 minutes.** The peak effect of both drugs occurs after 48 to 72 hours. These drugs are clearly indicated for treatment of **hypercalcemia of malignancy,** but should be used cautiously in other settings because their effects may last for years. They inhibit bone loss in high turnover states, but also retard bone formation when conditions would otherwise favor it. Bisphosphonates may cause **hypocalcemia** in certain clinical situations, such as patients with **vitamin D deficiency.** These drugs should be used when the ultimate cause of the hypercalcemia cannot be reversed in the short-to-medium term (malignancy) or when they directly address the pathophysiology of the hypercalcemia (Paget's disease of bone). In cases where the primary cause is reversible, such as milk-alkali syndrome, or can be treated more directly, such as hyperthyroidism or granulomatous disease, bisphosphonates are not appropriate. Bisphosphonates are relatively contraindicated in the setting of renal failure. Glucocorticoid may also provide benefit, in combination with bisphosphonates, for hypercalcemia of malignancy due to osteolytic lesions.

C. **Inhibition of PTH and active vitamin D production. Cinacalcet** is a drug that increases the sensitivity of the **calcium sensing receptor,** found on parathyroid cells, to extracellular calcium. It is useful in PTH-dependent hypercalcemia by decreasing PTH secretion and serum calcium levels. Cinacalcet is approved for the treatment of secondary hyperparathyroidism and parathyroid carcinoma. It is also clinically used for treatment of primary hyperparathyroidism. It has no role in the treatment of PTH-independent hypercalcemia. **Glucocorticoids** are the treatment of choice for treatment for hypercalcemia due to granulomatous disease, but may obscure a pathological diagnosis if used prior to a biopsy.

Suggested References

Arafah BM. Hypothalamic pituitary adrenal function during critical illness: limitations of current assessment methods. *J Clin Endocrinol Metab* 2006;91:3725–3745.

Baird TA, Parsons MW, Phanh T, et al. Persistent poststroke hyperglycemia is independently associated with infarct expansion and worse clinical outcome. *Stroke* 2003;34:2208–2214.

Beall DP, Henslee HB, Webb HR, Scofield RH. Milk-alkali syndrome: a historical review and description of the modern version of the syndrome. *Am J Med Sci* 2006;331:233–242.

Bendelow J, Apps E, Jones LE, Poston GJ. Carcinoid syndrome. *Eur J Surg Oncol* 2008;34:289–296.

Brunkhorst FM, Engel C, Bloos F, et al. Intensive insulin therapy and pentastarch resuscitation in severe sepsis. *N Engl J Med* 2008;358:125–139.

Devos P, Preiser J, Melot C. Impact of tight glucose control by intensive insulin therapy on ICU mortality and the rate of hypoglycaemia: final results of the Glucontrol study. *Intensive Care Med* 2007;33:S189.

Dickstein G. On the term "relative adrenal insufficiency"—or what do we really measure with adrenal stimulation tests? *J Clin Endocrinol Metab* 2005;90:4973–4974.

Fietsam R Jr, Bassett J, Glover JL. Complications of coronary artery surgery in diabetic patients. *Am Surg* 1991;57:551–557.

Grinspoon SK, Biller BM. Clinical review 62: laboratory assessment of adrenal insufficiency. *J Clin Endocrinol Metab* 1994;79:923–931.

Hamrahian AH, Oseni TS, Arafah BM. Measurements of serum free cortisol in critically ill patients. *N Engl J Med* 2004;350:1629–1638.

Ilias I, Pacak K. Current approaches and recommended algorithm for the diagnostic localization of pheochromocytoma. *J Clin Endocrinol Metab* 2004;89:479–491.

Jacobs TP, Bilezikian JP. Clinical review: rare causes of hypercalcemia. *J Clin Endocrinol Metab* 2005;90:6316–6322.

Kitabchi AE, Umpierrez GE, Murphy MB, et al. Hyperglycemic crises in diabetes. *Diabetes Care* 2004;27(suppl 1):S94–S102.

Krinsley JS, Grover A. Severe hypoglycemia in critically ill patients: risk factors and outcomes. *Crit Care Med* 2007;35:2262–2267.

Kwaku MP, Burman KD. Myxedema coma. *J Intensive Care Med* 2007;22:224–231.

LeGrand SB, Leskuski D, Zama I. Narrative review: furosemide for hypercalcemia: an unproven yet common practice. *Ann Intern Med* 2008;149:259–263.

Lumachi F, Brunello A, Roma A, Basso U. Medical treatment of malignancy-associated hypercalcemia. *Curr Med Chem* 2008;15:415–421.

Mebis L, Debaveye Y, Visser TJ, Van den Berghe G. Changes within the thyroid axis during the course of critical illness. *Endocrinol Metab Clin North Am* 2006;35:807–821.

Meijering S, Corstjens AM, Tulleken JE, et al. Towards a feasible algorithm for tight glycaemic control in critically ill patients: a systematic review of the literature. *Crit Care* 2006;10:R19.

Mesotten D, Vanhorebeek I, Van den Berghe G. The altered adrenal axis and treatment with glucocorticoids during critical illness. *Nat Clin Pract Endocrinol Metab* 2008;4:496–505.

Mundy GR, Edwards JR. PTH-related peptide (PTHrP) in hypercalcemia. *J Am Soc Nephrol* 2008;19:672–675.

Nayak B, Burman K. Thyrotoxicosis and thyroid storm. *Endocrinol Metab Clin North Am* 2006;35:663–686.

Nayak B, Hodak SP. Hyperthyroidism. *Endocrinol Metab Clin North Am* 2007;36:617–656.

NICE-SUGAR Study Investigators. Intensive versus conventional glucose control in critically ill patients. *N Engl J Med* 2009;360:1283–1297.

Pacak K. Preoperative management of the pheochromocytoma patient. *J Clin Endocrinol Metab* 2007;92:4069–4079.

Shepard MM, Smith JW III. Hypercalcemia. *Am J Med Sci* 2007;334:381–385.

Van den Berghe G, Wilmer A, Hermans G, et al. Intensive insulin therapy in the medical ICU. *N Engl J Med* 2006;354:449–461.

Van den Berghe G, Wouters P, Weekers F, et al. Intensive insulin therapy in critically ill patients. *N Engl J Med* 2001;345:1359–1367.

Wiener RS, Wiener DC, Larson RJ. Benefits and risks of tight glucose control in critically ill adults: a meta-analysis. *JAMA* 2008;300:933–944.

Wilson M, Weinreb J, Hoo GW. Intensive insulin therapy in critical care: a review of 12 protocols. *Diabetes Care* 2007;30:1005–1011.

Wisneski LA. Salmon calcitonin in the acute management of hypercalcemia. *Calcif Tissue Int* 1990;46(suppl):S26–S30.

Young WF Jr. Adrenal causes of hypertension: pheochromocytoma and primary aldosteronism. *Rev Endocr Metab Disord* 2007;8:309–320.

Infectious Diseases—Specific Considerations

Aranya Bagchi and Judith Hellman

This chapter provides an overview of specific infections encountered in critically ill patients and emphasizes their clinical presentation, microbiology, and diagnostic and therapeutic approaches. The reader is referred to **Chapter 12** for a review of antimicrobial agents and infectious disease issues in immunocompromised patients, and to Chapter 30 for a review of sepsis. Unless otherwise indicated, the potential antibiotic regimens presented are for the initial empiric treatment of infection. Subsequent therapy should be appropriately tailored to culture data as they become available. Because of the complexity of infectious complications in critically ill patients, management sometimes requires the consultation of infectious disease specialists. Also, please **refer to Chapter 12 for abbreviations** of the names of microorganisms used herein.

I. Thoracic infections

A. Community-acquired pneumonia (CAP)
is an infection of the lower respiratory tract that is acquired outside of the hospital. Although the overall mortality of CAP is low, the mortality in ICU patients with CAP is quite high. Risk factors for poor outcome include advanced age, coexisting chronic diseases (such as heart disease, pulmonary disease, diabetes), immunosuppression, and neoplastic disease. Clinical findings on admission also predict outcome. Increased respiratory rate, hypotension, fever, altered mental status, high or low white blood cell (WBC) count, hypoxemia, and multilobar or extrapulmonary involvement are associated with higher mortality.

1. **Microbiology.** The most frequent pathogen is *Streptococcus pneumoniae*. CAP is also caused by *Haemophilus influenzae* and other gram-negative bacteria such as *Klebsiella pneumoniae* and *Pseudomonas aeruginosa* (particularly in patients with underlying lung disease), gram-positive bacteria such as *Staphylococcus aureus*, atypical pathogens such as *Legionella pneumophila*, *Mycoplasma pneumoniae*, and *Chlamydia pneumoniae*, and viruses. *Moraxella catarrhalis* may cause CAP in patients with chronic obstructive pulmonary disease and chronic bronchitis. Immunocompromised patients can develop pneumonia due to the standard pathogens as well as opportunistic organisms.

2. **Diagnosis.** Findings on chest radiography may be variable depending on the pathogen and the underlying condition of the host. Infiltrates may be unilobar or multilobar, and may not be apparent on initial chest radiographs of severely hypovolemic patients. Whenever possible, the causative microorganism should be identified. Analysis of the sputum by Gram stain should reveal more than 25 neutrophils and fewer than 10 epithelial cells per low-power field. The causative organism may be suggested by the abundance and morphology of the bacteria on a well-collected sample. In some cases, it may be necessary to perform a bronchoscopy to obtain adequate sputum samples. Sputum cultures may be helpful in identifying the organism and defining the antimicrobial sensitivity. Blood cultures may also be helpful in defining the organism. If pneumonia is accompanied by a significant pleural

effusion, the pleural fluid should be analyzed for Gram stain and culture, pH, lactate dehydrogenase, glucose, and protein concentration. Serologic tests may be useful for identifying infection due to atypical pathogens. *Legionella pneumophila* antigen may be detected in the sputum or urine.

3. **Treatment.** Initial management of CAP is generally empiric, guided by patient condition and the results of Gram stained sputum specimens, if available. Outcome is improved with early administration of antibiotics. Clinical presentation does not reliably predict the pathogens involved, and frequently the causative microorganism is not identified. The potential for antibiotic resistance should influence the choice of antibiotics (e.g., *S. pneumoniae* may be penicillin resistant). Antibiotics for early broad empiric therapy should cover typical as well as atypical microorganisms. Therapy should be adjusted based on results of cultures and serologic tests. Potential empiric regimens for severely ill patients in the ICU include the following:

   a. A third- or fourth-generation cephalosporin such as cefotaxime, ceftriaxone, or cefepime plus an intravenous (IV) macrolide such as azithromycin.

   b. A third- or fourth-generation cephalosporin plus a fluoroquinolone such as levofloxacin.

   c. A β-lactam/β-lactamase inhibitor such as ampicillin/sulbactam plus IV macrolide or fluoroquinolone.

   d. If *Pseudomonas* is a possibility, a β-lactam/β-lactamase inhibitor such as piperacillin/tazobactam or a carbapenem such as imipenem or meropenem plus IV macrolide or fluoroquinolone.

B. **Hospital-acquired pneumonia** (HAP) is common in surgical and trauma patients and is associated with the highest mortality of all nosocomial infections. **Ventilator-associated pneumonia (VAP)** is a subset of HAP that occurs more than 48 hours after intubation. VAP affects between 9% and 27% of intubated patients and doubles the risk of dying compared to similar patients without VAP. The mortality attributable to VAP varies among different studies and is estimated to be in the range of 33% to 50%. Bacteria enter the lungs through various routes, including aspiration of oropharyngeal secretions or esophageal/gastric contents, inhalation of airborne droplets, hematogenous spread from other sites, and direct inoculation from colonized hospital personnel or contaminated equipment or devices.

1. **Microbiology.** The microorganisms causing nosocomial pneumonia differ substantially from those causing CAP. Infections are often polymicrobial. Common pathogens include aerobic gram-negative bacilli, such as *P. aeruginosa*, *Escherichia coli*, *K. pneumoniae*, and *Acinetobacter* species. Infections due to MRSA are becoming increasingly common in the United States, particularly in patients with diabetes mellitus and head injuries. Other pathogens include enteric gram-negative rods, such as *Proteus* spp and *Enterobacter* spp, and gram-positive cocci, such as *Enterococcus* spp. Antibiotic-resistant bacteria are very common. Risk factors for multidrug-resistant (MDR) infections include being hospitalized for ≥5 days, use of antibiotics during the preceding 90 days, a high frequency of antibiotic resistance in the specific hospital/unit, and immunosuppressive disease or immunosuppressive therapy.

2. **Diagnosis** of VAP can be difficult because many conditions (e.g., sepsis, ARDS, CHF, atelectasis, thromboembolic disease, pulmonary hemorrhage, etc) that are common in critically ill patients also produce similar clinical signs. The most accurate clinical criteria for VAP diagnosis

include the presence of new or progressive radiographic infiltrates in addition to at least two of three clinical features: fever >38°C, leucocytosis or leucopenia, and purulent tracheal secretions. Progressive hypoxemia is a necessary, but insufficient and nonspecific criterion to diagnose VAP. Patients meeting these criteria should be considered for empiric antibiotic therapy. Blood cultures and cultures of lower respiratory tract secretions should be obtained prior to giving the first dose of antibiotics. Controversies persist over whether or not to use invasive methods for collection of sputum samples, and quantitative cultures to assist with the diagnosis of VAP. With all sampling techniques, the sensitivity of sputum cultures decreases with even short courses of antibiotics prior to sample collection. Current evidence indicates that quantitative cultures of bronchoalveolar lavage (BAL) fluid do not improve survival compared with nonquantitative cultures of endotracheal aspirate. Availability of clinical and microbiologic expertise for bronchoscopy and quantitative culture should determine which method is chosen.

a. **Nonquantitative cultures** are often performed on sputum samples (obtained by noninvasive and invasive means). Most agree that cultures of expectorated sputum and samples from blind endotracheal suctioning are unreliable for definitive diagnosis of pneumonia or for defining with certainty the etiologic microorganism. It is likely, however, that the pathogen will be among the bacteria cultured, and sensitivity data may help to define the antimicrobial resistance patterns.

b. **Invasive collection** using protected-brush bronchoscopy and/or BAL provides lower respiratory tract samples for **quantitative cultures.** Quantitative cultures may be more reliable for diagnosis of infection and identification of the specific pathogen(s). Pneumonia is diagnosed for protected-brush bronchoscopy concentrations of more than 10^3 colony-forming units/mL and BAL concentrations of more than 10^4 or 10^5 colony-forming units/mL. These samples may also be more useful in defining the specific pathogen. Negative cultures of lower respiratory secretions in the absence of a new antibiotic in the preceding 72 hours virtually rules out a bacterial pneumonia (although *Legionella* is still possible). Unfortunately, these techniques can be limited by the invasiveness of the procedures, the lack of standardization for obtaining such samples, and the potential failure to diagnose pneumonia in the early stages when bacterial counts may be lower.

3. **Prophylaxis** of **VAP** is of paramount importance in decreasing morbidity and mortality in the ICU, and is discussed in **Chapter 12**.

4. **Treatment** (**Fig. 29-1**). Principles for managing VAP include use of early, appropriate empiric antibiotics in adequate doses, de-escalation of initial antibiotic therapy based on culture data and patient response, and shortening duration of therapy to minimum effective dose. Use of a unit-specific broad-spectrum antibiotic regimen can reduce the incidence of inappropriate initial therapy to <10%.

a. **Uncomplicated mild to moderate disease** (i.e., without respiratory failure, hemodynamic instability, or signs of injury to other organs) occurring early during hospitalization (<5 days) is often treated with a single antibiotic such as a third- or fourth-generation cephalosporin, a carbapenem, or a fluoroquinolone in patients who are allergic to penicillins. Numerous studies suggest that **monotherapy** is safe and effective when used properly and may decrease the

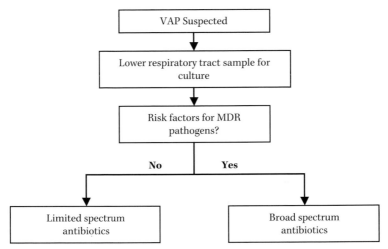

FIGURE 29-1 Clinical approach to the management of VAP. VAP, ventilator-associated pneumonia.

likelihood of infection due to antibiotic-resistant microorganisms. If anaerobes are a possibility, a β-lactam/β-lactamase inhibitor combination such as ampicillin/sulbactam or ticarcillin/clavulanate can be used as monotherapy. Alternatively, clindamycin or metronidazole may be used in combination with a β-lactam or fluoroquinolone for adequate anaerobic coverage.

   b. **Severe HAP** (i.e., respiratory failure, hemodynamic instability, extrapulmonary organ damage) is treated with **combination therapy.** Combination therapy should also be considered when **mild to moderate pneumonia** occurs later in the hospitalization, occurs in patients with significant comorbidities, or occurs in patients with recent antibiotic exposure. These situations increase the likelihood that pneumonia is caused by *P. aeruginosa,* other **multiresistant enteric gram-negative bacilli** such as *Enterobacter* spp, *Klebsiella* spp, and/or methicillin-resistant *S. aureus* **(MRSA).** Generally, combination therapy includes any empiric monotherapy agent mentioned previously plus a fluoroquinolone or an aminoglycoside. Linezolid or vancomycin should be added if there is a possibility of MRSA pneumonia. Some data suggest that linezolid leads to better outcomes than vancomycin, especially in patients with diminished renal function. *Acinetobacter* spp infections can be treated with carbapenems, sulbactam (ampicillin–sulbactam combinations), or inhaled colistin (polymyxin). Combination therapy is recommended for the treatment of *P. aeruginosa* pneumonia. Inhaled aminoglycoside or polymyxin treatment may be considered in MDR gram-negative pneumonias in patients who are not improving with systemic therapy.

C. **Lung abscess** results from destruction of the pulmonary parenchyma leading to large, fluid-filled cavities. The most frequent predisposing factor for lung abscess is **aspiration pneumonia,** followed by periodontal disease and gingivitis. Bronchiectasis, pulmonary infarction, septic embolization, and bacteremia also predispose to lung abscess.

1. **Microbiology.** Bacteria causing aspiration pneumonia and subsequent abscess formation differ depending on whether aspiration occurs as an outpatient or as an inpatient. Hospital-acquired aspiration pneumonia is caused by anaerobes, gram-positive bacteria such as *S. aureus,* and gram-negative bacteria such as *P. aeruginosa* and *K. pneumoniae.* Abscesses resulting from hematogenous spread of infection are usually peripheral and multifocal and are most commonly caused by *S. aureus.* Anaerobes and gram-negative bacteria also cause abscesses in this setting. *Mycobacterium tuberculosis, Nocardia,* amebas, and fungi are less frequent causes of lung abscess.

2. **Diagnosis** of lung abscess may be made based on chest radiograph or chest computed tomography (CT). Cultures of expectorated sputum are unreliable. Samples should be collected using protected-brush bronchoscopy or BAL.

3. **Treatment.** With some exceptions, witnessed aspiration rarely requires antibiotics. Exceptions include patients whose stomachs are colonized with enteric flora (such as patients with small bowel obstruction), and patients who may have bacterial colonization of the stomach and are severely immunocompromised. Lung abscesses require prolonged (2–4 months) antibiotic therapy. Antibiotic choices will depend on culture isolates. Postural drainage is an important aspect of the management, and bronchoscopy can be helpful in facilitating drainage or removing foreign bodies. Occasionally, a lung abscess is treated with surgical resection; however, this is not a first-line therapy. Complications of lung abscess include empyema, bronchopleural fistula formation, and bronchiectasis.

D. **Empyema** usually originates from intrapulmonary infection such as lung abscess or pneumonia, but also can be introduced from extrapulmonary sites as in trauma or thoracic surgery.

1. **Microbiology.** The most common bacterial cause of empyema is *S. aureus.* Enteric and nonenteric gram-negative bacteria, gram-positive bacteria, anaerobic bacteria, fungi, and *M. tuberculosis* also can cause empyema.

2. **Diagnosis** requires direct analysis of pleural fluid for pH, total protein, red blood cells (RBC), and leukocyte (WBC) count and differential, Gram-stained and bacterial cultures (anaerobic and aerobic) and possibly fungal smear and culture. Smears and cultures for acid-fast bacilli should be performed if *M. tuberculosis* is suspected.

3. **Treatment.** Empyema is treated with a combination of antibiotics and drainage via a thoracoscopy tube. Occasionally, open drainage or decortication of the empyema sac may be required.

E. **Mediastinitis** can result from spontaneous perforation of the esophagus, leakage from an esophageal anastomosis, trauma, cardiothoracic surgery, head and neck infections, and dental procedures.

1. **Microbiology.** Mediastinitis following cardiothoracic surgery that does not involve the esophagus is generally monomicrobial and is most often due to gram-positive bacteria, although gram-negative bacteria and fungi also cause mediastinitis. Mediastinitis arising from infections in the head and neck or disruption of the esophagus is usually polymicrobial and is caused by mixed anaerobic bacteria (*Peptococcus* spp, *Peptostreptococcus* spp, *Fusobacterium* spp, and *Bacteroides* spp), gram-positive bacteria, enteric and nonenteric gram-negative bacteria, and fungi (*Candida albicans, Candida glabrata*).

2. **Diagnosis.** Chest pain may be a presenting symptom. Other manifestations include fever and other systemic signs, crepitus and edema of the head and neck, and sepsis. Widening of the mediastinum, pleural

effusion, and subcutaneous or mediastinal emphysema may be evident on chest radiograph and chest CT.

3. **Treatment** must be initiated rapidly, in most cases with a combination of antibiotics and surgical intervention, including drainage, debridement, and removal or repair of the source of infection. In some situations, contained rupture or small perforations of the esophagus can be treated medically. Broad empiric antibiotic coverage should be employed initially. Antibiotics should then be adjusted based on results of intraoperative cultures. Coverage for head and neck sources (including esophageal disruption) should include anaerobes, gram-positive aerobes, gram-negative aerobes, and facultative anaerobes. Combination therapy with penicillin G or clindamycin plus agents against gram-negatives (such as a third-generation cephalosporin or a fluoroquinolone) is effective. Metronidazole will also provide adequate anaerobic coverage. Broadly active β-lactams such as ticarcillin/clavulanate or carbapenems such as imipenem/cilastatin or meropenem also offer reasonable early coverage. Empiric coverage for postsurgical mediastinitis should include an antistaphylococcal agent such as nafcillin or vancomycin (for MRSA or for patients who are allergic to penicillin).

II. **Intra-abdominal infections** usually arise from sources within the gastrointestinal (GI) tract. Infection can also result from contiguous spread from the urogenital/reproductive tract or hematogenous or lymphatic spread, and can be introduced from the outside (as occurs with trauma or surgery). Infections are often polymicrobial and include enteric gram-negative rods (*E. coli, Klebsiella, Enterobacter,* and *Proteus* spp), *P. aeruginosa,* aerobic gram-positive cocci (*Enterococcus* and *Streptococcus* spp), and gram-positive and gram-negative anaerobes (*Clostridium, Bacteroides, Fusobacterium,* and *Peptostreptococcus* spp). Management of intraabdominal infection depends on the cause and the site(s).

A. **Microflora of abdomen and pelvis**

1. **GI tract.** Normally, concentrations of bacteria increase progressively from the stomach through the small bowel and colon. Bacteria in the stomach and proximal small bowel include *Streptococcus* spp and *Lactobacillus* spp as well as anaerobes such as *Peptostreptococcus* spp but generally not *Bacteroides* spp. The concentrations of enteric gram-negative rods such as *E. coli* and anaerobic gram-negatives such as *Bacteroides* spp increase progressively in the distal small bowel and colon. Colonic bacteria include enteric gram-negative rods, gram-positive bacteria such as *Enterococcus* and *Lactobacillus,* and anaerobes such as *Bacteroides* spp, *Clostridium* spp, and *Peptostreptococcus* spp. Many factors alter either the quantity or the quality of the GI microflora, resulting in increases in the concentration as well as a shift in the spectrum of bacteria to include antibiotic-resistant bacteria, including nonenteric strains such as *P. aeruginosa.* Such factors include the following:

   a. pH (antacids, histamine-2 blockers).
   b. Antibiotics.
   c. GI dysmotility.
   d. Small-bowel obstruction, ileus, regional enteritis.
   e. Bowel resection or intestinal bypass procedures.
   f. Hospitalization or residence in a chronic nursing facility prior to developing infection.

2. **Genital tract microflora** include gram-positive aerobic bacteria such as *Streptococcus* spp, *Lactobacillus* spp, and *Staphylococcus* spp as well as anaerobic bacteria such as *Peptostreptococcus* spp, *Clostridium* spp, and *Bacteroides* spp.

B. **Peritonitis.** Peritoneal infections can occur spontaneously, can result from perforation of an abdominal viscus, or can be introduced from the outside (as with trauma or the presence of foreign bodies such as peritoneal dialysis catheters).

1. **Spontaneous bacterial peritonitis (SBP)** occurs in susceptible individuals, including those with ascites from chronic liver disease or congestive heart failure, and is believed to result from hematogenous or lymphatic spread or translocation of bacteria across the bowel wall. Symptoms/signs of SBP include fever, abdominal pain, GI dysmotility, worsening liver function/hepatic encephalopathy, and renal failure. However, patients with SBP may be asymptomatic or have only minor symptoms.

   a. **Microorganisms.** Generally SBP is caused by a single organism. Enteric gram-negatives followed by nonenterococcal streptococci are most common. SBP is sometimes caused by enterococci. Anaerobes rarely cause SBP. The presence of anaerobic bacteria or mixed flora suggests the possibility of secondary peritonitis.

   b. **Diagnosis.** A diagnostic paracentesis should be performed prior to the administration of antibiotics if SBP is suspected. Ascites fluid should, at minimum, be sent for cell counts and Gram stain and culture. A polymorphonuclear leukocyte (PMN) count of more than 250 is highly suggestive of SBP. If the ascites fluid is hemorrhagic, the PMN per mm^3 count should be adjusted based on the RBC count by subtracting 1 WBC for every 250 RBCs. Cultures of ascites fluid are often negative despite a cell count that is consistent with SBP. Use of blood culture bottles (anaerobic and aerobic) to culture ascites fluid may increase the likelihood of detecting the bacteria. Blood cultures should also be obtained.

   c. **Treatment.** Empiric antibiotic therapy should be initiated prior to obtaining the results of cultures if the ascites fluid PMN counts are greater than 250 cells/mm^3. Antibiotics should be modified appropriately when culture and sensitivity data become available. Potential empiric regimens include the following:

      (1) Cefotaxime is the primary regimen for SBP. High doses (2 g IV every 4 hours) are used for life-threatening SBP.

      (2) A β-lactam/β-lactamase inhibitor combination, such as ampicillin/sulbactam, piperacillin/tazobactam, or ticarcillin/clavulanate.

      (3) Ceftriaxone.

      (4) Ertapenem.

      (5) If resistant enteric gram-negatives are a possibility, imipenem or meropenem, or a fluoroquinolone should be considered

2. **Secondary peritonitis** usually results from perforation or necrosis of a solid viscus or suppurative infections of the biliary and female reproductive tracts.

   a. **Diagnosis** is often made with assistance of plain abdominal radiograph films and scans (e.g., CT, magnetic resonance [MR] imaging, ultrasonography). Exploratory laparotomy may be necessary to diagnose and treat the source of peritonitis.

   b. **Treatment** requires identification and control of the source of infection. Treatment usually involves a combination of surgery or placement of drainage catheters and broad-spectrum antibiotics that are active against gram-negative and gram-positive bacteria and anaerobes. Knowledge of local resistance patterns should influence the ultimate choice of empiric antibiotics.

(1) Peritonitis that occurs very early in the hospitalization and without recent antibiotic therapy in patients who are not in chronic care facilities is unlikely to result from antibiotic-resistant bacteria. Potential regimens include the following:

i. A β-lactam/β-lactamase inhibitor such as ampicillin/sulbactam.

ii. A third-generation cephalosporin (ceftriaxone, cefotaxime) plus an antianaerobe (clindamycin or metronidazole).

iii. A carbapenem.

iv. Fluoroquinolone plus an antianaerobe (clindamycin, metronidazole).

v. The traditional "triple-antibiotic" regimen of ampicillin, gentamicin, and metronidazole.

vi. Ampicillin, levofloxacin, metronidazole.

(2) Peritonitis that develops during hospitalization or residence in a chronic nursing facility or in the context of recent therapy with antibacterial agents may be caused by antibiotic-resistant microorganisms.

i. Monotherapy with a carbapenem (imipenem/cilastatin or meropenem).

ii. A third- or fourth-generation cephalosporin (ceftazidime or cefepime if *Pseudomonas* spp are suspected) plus an antianaerobe. Consider adding a fluoroquinolone if infection with *Pseudomonas* spp or *Enterobacter* spp is suspected. If ceftazidime is used, an additional agent with gram-positive coverage should be added.

iii. An antianaerobe with coverage of aerobic gram-positives (clindamycin) and a fluoroquinolone may be useful in patients who are allergic to β-lactams or if infection with *Pseudomonas* spp is suspected.

iv. Vancomycin or linezolid should be added to each of the aforementioned regimens if infection with MRSA is a possibility.

C. Intra-abdominal abscess may result from persistence of bacteria after secondary peritonitis or hematogenous spread of extra-abdominal infection. Abscesses can cause fever, peritonitis, sepsis, and multiple-organ dysfunction syndrome.

1. Microorganisms commonly cultured from abscesses include *Bacteroides* spp (especially *Bacteroides fragilis*), gram-negative and gram-positive bacteria such as *Enterococcus* spp and *S. aureus*.

2. Diagnosis. CT is useful for diagnosing and localizing abscesses. Ultrasonography can be done at the bedside, and can be particularly useful in diagnosis of right upper quadrant, renal, and pelvic abscesses. Indium-labeled WBC and gallium scans are occasionally useful in localizing abscesses but have low specificity and must be followed up with more definitive tests. Rarely, exploratory laparotomy must be performed for diagnosis.

3. Treatment of intra-abdominal abscess includes drainage and antibiotics. The method of drainage (percutaneous under CT or ultrasound guidance versus operative) depends on a variety of factors including the abscess location, whether the abscess is associated with perforation or gangrene, and the presence of loculations that make drainage with a single catheter unlikely. Often culture data are available to guide antibiotic selection. For initial empiric coverage, it is reasonable use one of the combinations suggested previously for treating secondary peritonitis in hospitalized patients. Ceftazidime or cefepime may be favored over ceftriaxone because they have better activity against *P. aeruginosa.*

D. Infections of the hepatobiliary system

1. **Acute cholecystitis** results from biliary tract obstruction or instrumentation of the biliary tract and involves the gall bladder (GB) and cystic duct.

   a. **Complications** include GB perforation with subsequent peritonitis, empyema of the GB from cystic duct obstruction, emphysematous cholecystitis, and empyema of the GB, which can cause gram-negative sepsis.

   b. **Microbiology.** Bacteria include enteric gram-negative bacteria such as *E. coli, Klebsiella, Proteus,* and *Enterobacter* spp, gram-positive bacteria such as *Enterococcus* spp, and anaerobes such as *Clostridium* and *Bacteroides* spp. Emphysematous cholecystitis is caused by *Clostridium* spp and gram-negative bacteria.

   c. **Diagnosis.** Abdominal ultrasonography may reveal gallstones, thickening of the GB wall, a dilated gallbladder, or a pericholecystic fluid collection.

   d. **Treatment** includes antibiotics and surgery. The timing of surgery depends on a number of factors. Surgery is often performed on an urgent basis when the more severe complications of acute cholecystitis as just described occur. Surgery may be delayed for stabilization of the patient or for preparation of the patient with serious medical conditions. Cholecystitis can be treated with the antibiotic regimens previously described for secondary peritonitis.

2. **Cholangitis** is usually caused by partial or complete common bile duct (CBD) obstruction.

   a. **Diagnosis.** The classic presentation is jaundice, fevers, chills, and biliary colic. Blood cultures are often positive.

   b. **Treatment** differs depending on whether there is partial or complete CBD obstruction. **Nonsuppurative cholangitis,** which results from partial CBD obstruction, will often respond to antibiotic therapy. **Suppurative cholangitis,** which is due to complete CBD obstruction causing pus under pressure, bacteremia, and septic shock, must be treated as early as possible with a combination of antibiotics and surgical or endoscopic decompression. Cholangitis can be treated with the antibiotic regimens described previously for secondary peritonitis.

3. **Liver abscess.** Abscesses can be solitary or multiple. Manifestations range from fever with leukocytosis and right upper quadrant pain to sepsis. Liver abscesses can result from local or hematogenous spread of infection. The most common local source is the biliary system.

   a. **Microbiology.** The organisms depend on the source.

      (1) **Biliary tract:** Gram-negative bacteria and *Enterococcus* spp.

      (2) **Peritoneal infections:** Gram-positive and gram-negative bacteria and anaerobes.

      (3) **Hematogenous spread:** Generally a single organism such as *S. aureus* or *Streptococcus* spp. Candidal abscesses also occur.

   b. **Diagnosis** is generally made by CT scan or ultrasonography.

   c. **Treatment** includes drainage and antibiotics. The initial antibiotic choice depends on the origin of the infection. Abscess arising from the biliary tract or peritoneum should be treated with antibiotics directed against the organisms involved in the initial infection. Abscess resulting from hematogenous spread should be treated with agents active against gram-positive bacteria.

E. **Splenic abscess** is rare, but has high mortality if left untreated. It usually results from hematogenous spread, but can result from splenic trauma or contiguous spread. The diagnosis of splenic abscess should prompt a search for **bacterial endocarditis** as the source.
   1. **Microbiology.** The most common organisms isolated on culture are *Streptococcus* spp followed by *S. aureus*. *Salmonella* spp and, rarely, anaerobic bacteria also cause splenic abscess.
   2. The **diagnosis** is suggested by left upper quadrant pain, fever, leukocytosis, and a left-sided pleural effusion.
   3. **Treatment.** Splenic abscess is usually treated with splenectomy and antibiotics.

F. ***Clostridium difficile*–associated diarrhea (CDAD)** occurs as a complication of antibiotic therapy and is caused by overgrowth of *C. difficile,* an anaerobic, gram-positive, spore-forming bacillus that produces toxins that damage the bowel wall. The carrier rate is 1% to 3% in the general population and 20% in patients treated with antibiotics. Although clindamycin, cephalosporins, and ampicillin are the most frequent offenders, almost all antibiotics have been implicated, including vancomycin and metronidazole. Since 2000, a hypervirulent strain (NAP1/027) has been implicated in epidemics of severe CDAD in the United States and Canada, and in Europe and Japan. Some of these epidemics have been associated with an increased use of fluoroquinolones. Antibiotics alter the normal flora, providing an environment for the conversion of *C. difficile* spores to vegetative forms leading to rapid replication and toxin production. **Risk factors** include exposure to antibiotics in the last 8 weeks, advanced age, and hospitalization. Nosocomial diarrhea arising more than 72 hours after hospitalization in patients who are receiving antibiotics should be assumed to be due to CDAD until proven otherwise. **Manifestations** include watery and/or bloody diarrhea, abdominal cramps, toxic megacolon, perforation of the bowel, and peritonitis. Leukocytosis can be marked, sometimes in excess of 50,000 cells/μl.
   1. **Diagnosis.** The *C. difficile* **toxin cytotoxicity assay** is the best available test, with a sensitivity and specificity of 98% and 99% in one trial. However, it is technically demanding and has a turnover time of 24 to 72 hours, and therefore is not used routinely. Commercially available **ELISAs for toxin A and toxin B** are the most commonly used diagnostic tests. These tests were relatively less sensitive (75%–85%) and are typically repeated up to three times. Newer versions of the test are reported to be >90% sensitive and 100% specific compared to the cytotoxicity assay, and many hospitals do not repeat this test. **Stool cultures** for *C. difficile* are not helpful. **CT imaging** in fulminant CDAD may show colonic thickening and pericolic stranding with "accordion sign" with enteral contrast or a "double halo/target sign" with IV contrast. **Sigmoidoscopy and/or colonoscopy** with visualization of "pseudomembranes" can be helpful in making the diagnosis if serologic tests are inconclusive.
   2. **Treatment.** Discontinue the causative antibiotics, if possible. Begin empiric treatment after a stool sample has been sent if the clinical suspicion is high. Medical treatment options are outlined in **Table 29-1**. Treatment is usually continued for 10 to 14 days. **Surgical consultation** is indicated in patients who have signs of shock or organ failure, or who have not responded to 24 to 72 hours of maximal medical therapy. The surgical treatment of choice is a total abdominal colectomy with an end ileostomy. Experimental therapies include the anion exchange resin Tolevamer, antimicrobials (Nitazoxanide, Ramoplanin, Difimicin, and Rifamixin), IV immunoglobulin, and monoclonal antibodies

TABLE 29-1	Medical Management of *C. difficile*–Associated Diarrhea (CDAD)
Severity	**Treatment**
Initial/mild CDAD	Metronidazole PO 250 mg Q6 H or 500 mg Q8 H
Severe CDAD[a]	Vancomycin PO 125 to 500 mg Q6 H
Complicated CDAD (ileus/toxic megacolon)	Vancomycin PO/NGT or enema[b] + IV Metronidazole

[a]Criteria for severe CDAD include WBC count >15,000/mL, >50% rise in serum creatinine, hypoalbuminemia, severe diarrhea, and temperature >38.3°C.
[b]Vancomycin enema—Instill 500 mg Vancomycin in 100 cm³ saline into rectum via a Foley catheter (18G, 30 cm³ balloon). Keep catheter clamped for 1 hour, then remove Foley. Repeat Q6 H. **IV Vancomycin is not effective.**

against toxins A and B. Treatment for recurrent CDAD is primarily with vancomycin. In addition, measures for repopulation of GI flora with probiotics such as *Lactobacillus* spp, *Saccharomyces boulardii*, or administration of stool from healthy subjects may be considered. Probiotics should be used with caution in immunocompromised patients as *S. boulardii* fungemia has been reported in this population.

III. **Wound infections.** Multiple factors influence the development and severity of wound infections. The incidence of postoperative wound infection due to antibiotic-resistant bacteria increases with the length of hospitalization prior to surgery. Prophylactic measures are effective in preventing wound infections.
   A. **Classification of surgical wounds**
      1. **Clean.** No entry into internal organs that harbor bacteria.
      2. **Clean-contaminated.** Organs are entered in elective surgery without spillage of contents.
      3. **Contaminated.** Spillage of organ contents occurs without formation of pus.
      4. **Dirty.** Spillage of contents occurs with pus formation.
   B. **Microbiology.** Microorganisms reflect the site of origin and are altered by recent treatment with antibiotics, prolonged preoperative hospitalization, and coexisting diseases. **Clean surgical wound infections** are most often caused by *S. aureus*, coagulase-negative *Staphylococcus*, and *Streptococcus* spp. Severe wound infections that occur in the first 48 hours after surgery may be caused by *Clostridium* or group A streptococcus (*Streptococcus pyogenes*). Infections of **contaminated wounds** will reflect the origin of contamination (respiratory, GI, or genitourinary [GU] tract).
   C. **Clinical presentation and diagnosis.** Wound infections vary in severity from superficial infections of the skin and subcutaneous tissues to deep and severe infections involving the underlying fascia and/or muscles. Superficial wound infections are most frequently manifested by erythema, warmth, and swelling. Fever is variably present.
   D. **Prevention.** Detection and treatment of infection at other sites, limiting the duration of hospitalization before surgery, proper surgical technique, and proper preoperative scrubbing of the patient and the surgical team are important measures. While recommendations vary for clean procedures that do not involve placement of foreign material, **prophylactic antibiotics** are routinely administered for clean procedures involving placement of foreign material and for all procedures that enter, or are complicated by spillage from, internal organs. Prophylactic antibiotics should be given within the 30 minutes prior to incision, and for clean or clean-contaminated operations

should be discontinued within 24 hours of surgery to minimize the risk of colonization with antibiotic-resistant organisms. Longer courses of antibiotics are generally given for contaminated or dirty wounds. Choices of prophylactic antibiotics are guided by site and type of surgery, duration of hospitalization prior to surgery, and recent use of antibiotics. Many institutions have established specific guidelines for prophylactic antibiotics.

E. **Treatment**

1. **Mild superficial wound infections** may be treated with removal of sutures or staples and opening of the wound to drain fluid collections.

2. **Severe wound infections** are usually treated with a combination of parenteral antibiotics and surgical debridement. Cultures of fluid or tissue collected in a sterile fashion should be used to guide antimicrobial therapy. Initial empiric antibiotic coverage will be dictated by the setting. First-generation cephalosporins offer reasonable coverage for uncomplicated postoperative wound infections. Clindamycin is an alternative in patients allergic to β-lactams. Vancomycin, linezolid, or daptomycin should be reserved for cases where there is a reasonable possibility that the infection is caused by MRSA. Gram-negative coverage should be considered for infections originating in the GI, GU, and respiratory tracts.

F. **Necrotizing soft tissue infections. Necrotizing fasciitis** and **myonecrosis** (clostridial and nonclostridial) are life-threatening deep infections that involve the fascia and subcutaneous tissue (necrotizing fasciitis) and muscle (myonecrosis). These infections have the propensity to spread rapidly and cause severe systemic toxicity early in the course of infection. The mortality due to necrotizing soft tissue infections is high, particularly if there are delays in surgical or medical intervention.

1. **Microbiology**

   a. **Necrotizing fasciitis.** *Streptococcus* spp are most commonly isolated from wound cultures. Polymicrobial infections with anaerobes, enteric gram-negatives, and *Streptococcus* spp also occur.

   b. **Myonecrosis.** Clostridial myonecrosis (gas gangrene) is a severe, fulminant skeletal muscle infection caused by *Clostridium* spp. Exotoxins released by bacteria are important in the pathogenesis of clostridial myonecrosis. Nonclostridial myonecrosis is generally polymicrobial due to *Streptococcus* spp, enteric gram-negative rods (*E. coli, K. pneumoniae, Enterobacter* spp, etc.), and anaerobic bacteria.

2. **Diagnosis.** Early features include pain out of proportion to the local external findings and systemic toxicity. Crepitus may be present due to gas in soft tissues.

3. **Treatment**

   a. **Debridement.** Immediate recognition and prompt surgical exploration and debridement are critical. Frequent surveillance of the wound is essential, and repeated surgical debridement is often necessary.

   b. **Antibiotics** are chosen based on the presentation and the likely source of infection. Gram stain of intraoperative wound samples can guide initial therapy. Empiric therapy should be broad and include coverage of *Streptococcus* spp and *Staphylococcus* spp, enteric gram-negative bacteria, and anaerobes. Because clindamycin is a bacterial protein synthesis inhibitor, some practitioners add clindamycin to regimens for treatment of suspected exotoxin-producing necrotizing soft-tissue infections to attempt to reduce exotoxin production.

       c. The role of **hyperbaric oxygen** for necrotizing soft tissue infections caused by anaerobic bacteria is not clear.

IV. Urinary tract infections. The range of severity of urinary tract infections (UTIs) varies from urethritis and cystitis, which are often treated in the outpatient setting, to pyelonephritis and renal or perinephric abscess, which can produce septic shock. UTIs are the most common nosocomial infection, and cause up to 30% of gram-negative bacteremias in hospitalized patients. Fungal UTIs are discussed in **Section VIII.**

  A. Predisposing factors. Indwelling urinary catheters, neurologic or structural abnormalities of the urinary tract. and nephrolithiasis. **Prophylaxis** of UTIs in the ICU is discussed in **Chapter 12.**

  B. Microbiology. Bacteria usually enter the urinary tract via the urethra and spread to more proximal segments. Thus the same microorganisms tend to cause both upper and lower urinary tract infections. Occasionally, hematogenous seeding (especially with *S. aureus*) or spread from contiguous peritoneal infection can result in upper urinary tract infections (especially perinephric and renal abscesses). The most common organisms cultured from the urine are gram-negative rods, including *E. coli, Klebsiella, Proteus*, and sometimes *Enterobacter* spp. *Serratia* and *Pseudomonas* spp are additional causes of catheter-related infections. Gram-positive organisms, including *S. saprophyticus, Enterococcus* spp, and *S. aureus,* are sometimes involved. Urethritis can also be caused by *Chlamydia trachomatis, Neisseria gonorrhoeae, Trichomonas, Candida* spp, and herpes simplex virus (HSV).

  C. Diagnosis. Analysis of the urinary sediment for leukocytes in conjunction with urine cultures can be useful in distinguishing colonization from true infection. The urinary sediment is also helpful in determining whether the infection is in the upper or the lower urinary tract. WBC casts suggest that infection involves the kidneys or tubules. Urine cultures are essential for guiding antimicrobial therapy.

  D. Specific urinary tract infections

    1. Cystitis is infection of the bladder characterized by dysuria and frequency, cloudy or bloody urine, and localized tenderness of the urethra and suprapubic regions. More severe symptoms such as high fever, nausea, and vomiting suggest renal involvement.

    2. Acute pyelonephritis is a pyogenic infection of the renal parenchyma and pelvis. It is characterized by costophrenic angle tenderness, high fevers, shaking chills, nausea, vomiting, and diarrhea. Laboratory analysis reveals leukocytosis, pyuria with leukocyte casts, and occasional hematuria. Bacteria are often visible on Gram stain of unspun urine. Evaluation of the urinary tract should be considered because a significant proportion of pyelonephritis is associated with structural abnormalities. Treatment includes antibiotics and removal or correction of the source. Complications include papillary necrosis, impaired urine-concentrating ability, urinary obstruction, and sepsis.

    3. Renal and perinephric abscesses are uncommon and usually are due to ascending infection from the bladder and ureters. Major risk factors include nephrolithiasis, structural urinary tract abnormalities, urologic trauma or surgery, and diabetes mellitus. Most common isolates are *E. coli, Klebsiella,* and *Proteus* spp. *Candida* spp may also cause renal and perinephric abscesses. Renal and perinephric abscesses may present nonspecifically with fever, leukocytosis, and pain (flank, groin, abdomen). Urine cultures may be negative, particularly if the patient has already received antibiotics. Diagnosis can be made by abdominal ultrasound or CT scan. Treatment is drainage and antibiotics.

4. **Prostatitis** is an infrequent infection in the ICU that can occur as a result of bladder catheterization. Symptoms and signs include fevers, chills, dysuria, and an enlarged, tender, and boggy prostate. Treatment includes antibiotics and, if possible, removal of the urinary catheter.

E. **Treatment of urinary tract infections.** Prior to receiving culture results, empiric broad therapy should be initiated that cover likely organisms. Fluoro-quinolones or third- or fourth-generation cephalosporins are often used. Ceftazidime or cefepime may be selected if infection with *Pseudomonas* spp is likely. If *Enterococcus* spp is suspected, broader coverage may be obtained with ampicillin plus an aminoglycoside. Rarely, imipenem/cilastatin is used for infections that are caused by antibiotic-resistant bacteria.

V. **Intravascular catheter-related infections** can be localized to the site of insertion (site infections) or can be disseminated **(catheter-associated bloodstream infections)**. Catheters in the central circulation (central venous and pulmonary artery) are responsible for most catheter-related infections. **Risk factors** for catheter-related bloodstream infections (BSI) include total parenteral nutri-tion **(TPN)**, which increases the risk of fungal infections, and prolonged catheterization. **Fever** is the most common presenting feature, and localized signs of infection at the insertion site are often absent. Site infections or unexplained fever should prompt assessment for line infection.

A. **Microbiology.** The most common pathogens are coagulase-negative *Staphylococcus* followed by *S. aureus*. A variety of gram-negative and other gram-positive bacteria also cause catheter-related infections. *Candida* spp account for close to 10% of catheter-related BSI.

B. **Prevention** of catheter-related infections is discussed in detail in **Chapter 13.**

C. **Management**

1. **Catheter removal.** Institutional practices for management of suspected catheter-related infections vary. Some institutions/intensive care units favor replacement of catheters at a fresh site if catheter-related infection is a possibility. Others routinely change catheters over a guidewire and perform quantitative cultures. When the line has been changed over a guidewire, if blood or quantitative tip cultures are pos-itive, the rewired catheter is removed and a new line is placed at a fresh site. A strong suspicion that the catheter is the source of fever or septic complications should prompt a change in site and, at a mini-mum, blood cultures.

2. **Antibiotics.** The choice of antibiotics is dictated by the clinical situation and culture data. Empiric therapy often is started with vancomycin if there are systemic signs of infection or if preliminary blood culture results indicate gram-positive bacteremia. Often an additional agent is added to cover gram-negatives or for synergistic coverage of *Entero-coccus* spp. Further therapy should be tailored to the specific organism identified. For uncomplicated catheter-related bacteremia, antibiotics are generally continued for 7 to 14 days (14 days if *S. aureus* is isolated from the blood). Fungal infections are treated for a longer time, partic-ularly in immunocompromised hosts.

VI. **Infective endocarditis (IE).** IE is caused by microbial invasion of the endo-cardium. It most commonly involves the cardiac valves, but can also occur in the septal or mural myocardium. IE can involve native valves **(native valve endocarditis [NVE])** and prosthetic valves **(prosthetic valve endocarditis**

[PVE]). PVE that occurs within 2 months of valve replacement (early PVE) results from colonization of the valve by microbes at the time of surgery and most commonly is caused by *Staphylococcus* spp. Late PVE is similar to NVE. Microorganisms gain entry into the bloodstream via direct inoculation during procedures (GI, GU, and dental procedures, bronchoscopy, endotracheal intubation) or from a focus of existing infection such as pneumonia or dental abscess. **Acute IE** is characterized by abrupt onset and rapid progression. **Subacute IE** is characterized by insidious onset and slower progression.

A. **Predisposing factors** include abnormalities of the heart (such as those due to rheumatic heart disease and degenerative valvular lesions) and IV drug abuse. Endocarditis can occur in previously normal hearts. Intravascular devices such as central venous catheters, pacemaker wires, hemodialysis shunts, and prosthetic valves increase the chance of developing IE.

B. **Microbiology.** IE is most commonly caused by bacteria, but can be caused by fungi, viruses, and rickettsiae.

1. **Gram-positive bacteria.** *Streptococcus* spp are the most common pathogens, particularly the viridans group (such as *sanguis, mutans,* and *intermedius*). *Enterococcus* spp also cause endocarditis, particularly in elderly patients who have undergone GU procedures and in IV drug abusers. *Staphylococcus* spp, particularly *S. aureus*, often cause IE. *Staphylococcus aureus* endocarditis is often severe and is more commonly complicated by myocardial and valve ring abscesses, emboli, and metastatic lesions (such as lung, central nervous system [CNS], and splenic abscess). Identification of *Streptococcus bovis* as the causative organism should prompt a workup for a GI source such as colon cancer.

2. **Gram-negative bacteria** infrequently cause IE. IV drug abusers and patients with prosthetic valves are more susceptible. IE due to gram-negative bacteria is often severe and has an abrupt onset and high mortality. A characteristic NVE of abnormal valves is caused by a group of bacteria collectively called HACEK group of bacteria (*Haemophilus* spp, *Actinobacillus actinomycetemcomitans, Cardiobacterium hominis, Eikenella corrodens,* and *Kingella* spp) and is characterized by a subacute course, large vegetations, and frequent embolic events.

C. **Diagnosis**

1. **Physical examination** may reveal a heart murmur, petechiae, nail-bed splinter hemorrhages, retinal hemorrhages (Roth's spots), red or purple nodules on digital pads (Osler's nodes), and flat red lesions on the palms or soles (Janeway lesions).

2. **Blood cultures** are moderately sensitive for IE. Several (three or more) sets of blood cultures should be obtained within the first 24 hours if IE is suspected. Rarely, blood cultures are negative, particularly when IE is due to intracellular organisms such as rickettsiae, anaerobic bacteria, the HACEK group of bacteria, and fungi. Special media may be necessary to isolate the responsible microorganism.

3. **Echocardiography** is an important tool for diagnosing and managing IE. Transthoracic echocardiography (TTE) is far less sensitive than **transesophageal echocardiography (TEE)** for detecting vegetations, particularly in patients receiving mechanical ventilation. Echocardiography can be used to follow the progression of vegetations and to identify and follow complications such as valvular insufficiency, valve ring or myocardial abscesses, pericardial effusions, and heart failure.

D. Treatment

1. **Antibiotics.** Prolonged courses of bactericidal antibiotics are used to treat IE. For acute bacterial endocarditis, it may be necessary to begin antibiotics prior to definitive diagnosis. However, blood cultures should be obtained prior to the first dose of antibiotics.

   a. **Empiric therapy.** Sometimes treatment of subacute NVE is delayed until results of blood cultures are available.

      (1) Indications for empiric therapy

         i. Critically ill and strong suspicion of endocarditis.

         ii. Likely to have endocarditis and is to undergo cardiac surgery.

         iii. Positive blood cultures.

         iv. When the diagnosis seems certain (e.g., vegetations documented by echocardiography in the setting of fever and other clinical parameters consistent with IE).

         v. Suspected of having PVE.

      (2) Empiric initial therapy for acute NVE should include agents that are active against *Streptococcus*, *Enterococcus*, and *Staphylococcus* spp. Potential regimens include the following:

         i. Ampicillin or penicillin plus nafcillin plus aminoglycoside (gentamicin).

         ii. Vancomycin plus aminoglycoside (gentamicin). Enterococcal infection should be treated with a combination of ampicillin or vancomycin plus an aminoglycoside because ampicillin and vancomycin are only bacteriostatic for *Enterococcus* spp.

      (3) Empiric initial therapy for early or late PVE

         i. Vancomycin plus aminoglycoside (gentamicin) plus rifampin.

   b. **Subsequent antibiotic therapy** should be based on blood culture data. Determinations of minimum inhibitory and bactericidal concentrations (MIC and MBC, respectively) are extremely important in deciding the optimal regimen. Blood cultures should be obtained during therapy to verify clearance of bacteremia. Failure to clear bacteremia may indicate abscess.

2. **Surgery.** Valve replacement or valvulectomy (tricuspid) may be necessary. Indications for surgery vary depending on the valve, and include severe and refractory heart failure, valve obstruction, fungal endocarditis, prosthetic valve instability, and failure to clear bacteremia with appropriate antibiotic therapy. Surgery also may be indicated for recurrent IE, extension to the myocardium or paravalvular region, two or more embolic events, or periprosthetic leaks.

E. Complications of infective endocarditis

1. **Cardiac**

   a. **Valvular insufficiency and heart failure.** Heart failure is the most common cause of death in patients with IE.

   b. **Myocardial and paravalvular abscess.**

   c. **Heart block** may result from extension of a paravalvular abscess.

   d. **Obstruction.** Rarely, large vegetations may cause obstruction, particularly when IE is caused by fungi.

   e. **Purulent pericarditis** occurs most commonly with IE due to *Staphylococcus* spp.

2. **Extracardiac**

   a. **Immune complex disease** can damage distant organs such as the kidneys.

   b. **Embolic events** can lead to ischemia and infarction. Abscesses may occur at sites of embolization. Left-sided endocarditis predisposes

to emboli to the kidneys, brain, spleen, and heart, while right-sided endocarditis predisposes to pulmonary emboli.
  c. **Mycotic aneurysms** result from local infection of the blood vessel with dilation of the vessel. Mycotic aneurysms in the CNS can present with catastrophic subarachnoid or intracerebral hemorrhage. Mycotic aneurysms can also occur outside of the CNS.
  d. **Neurologic complications.** Toxic encephalopathy, meningitis, cerebritis, brain abscess, stroke (infarction or hemorrhage), subarachnoid or intracerebral hemorrhage.
  e. **Renal failure.**
  f. **Sepsis.**

VII. **Miscellaneous infections**
  A. **Sinusitis.** Facial trauma and the presence of nasotracheal and/or nasogastric tubes predispose ICU patients to sinusitis.
    1. **Microbiology.** Sinusitis is usually caused by gram-negative bacteria, *S. aureus,* and anaerobes.
    2. **Diagnosis** can be difficult. Many experts recommend CT scans of the face and sinuses. Needle aspiration of the sinuses may provide helpful bacteriologic data, particularly in patients who have been hospitalized for prolonged periods and may be infected with antibiotic-resistant organisms.
    3. **Treatment** is often initiated based on the clinical constellation of fever of unclear etiology, presence of nasal tubes or history of head and neck trauma, and purulent nasal discharge. Treatment includes removal of nasal tubes to allow drainage of the obstructed sinus outflow tract, nasal humidification and decongestants, and antibiotics that target likely pathogens. Surgical drainage is rarely indicated.
  B. **CNS infections**
    1. **Meningitis.** Generally, infection is limited to the subarachnoid space and cerebral ventricles and does not involve the brain parenchyma, but occasionally meningitis is complicated by brain abscess. Bacterial meningitis may result from hematogenous seeding, direct invasion from trauma or surgery, or extension of infection from a contiguous structure such as rupture of a brain or epidural abscess into the subarachnoid space.
      a. **Microbiology.** Many organisms cause meningitis. Community-acquired pathogens include *S. pneumoniae, H. influenzae, Neisseria meningitidis,* and *Listeria monocytogenes.* Meningitis caused by enteric and nonenteric gram-negative bacteria and *S. aureus* may result from trauma, neurosurgery, or bacteremia. *S. aureus* meningitis may originate from infections at other sites such as pneumonia, sinusitis, and endocarditis. Meningitis associated with CSF shunts are most often caused by *S. epidermidis.*
      b. **Diagnosis.** Collection of CSF for analysis of glucose, protein, cell count and differential, Gram stain, and bacterial culture is essential. Other specialized tests of CSF, including test for cryptococcal antigen, the Venereal Disease Research Laboratory slide test, bacterial antigen tests, and fungal smear and culture, may be indicated depending on other patient factors such as immunocompromise. In patients suspected of having cerebral edema, a CT scan of the brain should be performed prior to the lumbar puncture. Blood cultures should be obtained prior to starting antibiotics.
      c. **Treatment.** The choice of antibiotics will be determined by the clinical situation and the ability of various antibiotics to penetrate the CNS. Because host defenses are impaired in the CNS, bacterial meningitis must be treated with bactericidal antibiotics. Emergence

of penicillin-resistant community-acquired pathogens has resulted in a shift in treatment to third-generation non-antipseudomonal cephalosporins such as ceftriaxone, which penetrates the CNS well. Vancomycin is often added if there is concern about resistance to β-lactam antibiotics. *Listeria monocytogenes* meningitis should be treated with penicillin G or ampicillin, or trimethoprim/sulfamethoxazole in penicillin-allergic patients, possibly in conjunction with an aminoglycoside. Meningitis caused by gram-negative bacteria is frequently treated with a third-generation cephalosporin. If *P. aeruginosa* or other resistant gram-negative bacteria are suspected, ceftazidime, cefepime, or meropenem should be considered. Additional coverage should be added to ceftazidime if gram-positive infection is a possibility, and vancomycin should be considered if MRSA is a possibility. *Staphylococcus aureus* meningitis is usually treated with nafcillin or vancomycin in penicillin-allergic patients or if MRSA is the pathogen.

2. **Paradural abscesses include epidural and subdural abscesses.** Epidural abscesses most frequently occur in the vertebral column, while subdural abscesses usually occur in the cranium. Paradural abscesses result from trauma, neurosurgery, invasion of the paradural space (such as with epidural catheter placement), local spread from contiguous structures (such as the paranasal sinuses or paravertebral region), and hematogenous spread from distant sites. Paradural abscess can rapidly progress and can cause considerable irreversible damage to underlying neural structures. Thus, rapid diagnosis and institution of therapy are essential. Drainage of the abscess is crucial for microbiologic diagnosis as well as for treatment.

   a. **Microbiology.** Bacteria causing subdural abscesses reflect the source of infection. Infections may be caused by *S. pneumoniae, Staphylococcus* spp, *H. influenzae,* enteric gram-negatives, and anaerobes. *Staphylococcus aureus* is the most common cause of epidural abscess. Enteric gram-negatives also cause epidural abscesses, particularly in patients with urinary tract infections or following vertebral surgery.

   b. **Diagnosis.** Severe localized spinal pain is the most common presenting symptom of epidural abscess. CT scans are helpful in diagnosing and localizing subdural abscesses. Magnetic resonance imaging is the diagnostic test of choice for epidural abscesses. CT and myelography also can be helpful.

   c. **Treatment** includes antibiotics and drainage. Initial antibiotic therapy should be based on likely pathogens for the situation and then modified based on results of cultures. *Staphylococcus aureus* should be treated with nafcillin. Vancomycin or linezolid may be substituted in penicillin-allergic patients or if MRSA is the pathogen. Third- or fourth-generation cephalosporins (antipseudomonal if *P. aeruginosa* is the pathogen) are often used for gram-negative infections.

VIII. **Fungal infections.** Fungi act as opportunistic or, less commonly, as virulent pathogens and cause a variety of different syndromes ranging from superficial mucocutaneous infection to systemic infection with visceral organ involvement.

A. **Candida**

   1. **Candida spp** are the most common cause of opportunistic fungal infections in surgical and medical ICUs. The incidence of nosocomial candidal infections has increased dramatically, and *Candida* species are now among the most common organisms isolated from blood cultures.

2. **Risk factors** include treatment with broad-spectrum antibiotics, presence of indwelling devices (urinary, peritoneal, and intravascular), immunocompromise (HIV infection, transplantation, hematologic malignancy, chemotherapy, neutropenia, and burns), and TPN.

3. **Clinical manifestations**

   a. **Candiduria** may be due to infection or may reflect colonization of an indwelling urinary catheter. Candiduria should raise concerns about possible fungal balls, pyelonephritis, or candidemia.

   b. **Mucocutaneous infections** include oropharyngeal candidiasis, esophagitis, GI candidiasis, vulvovaginitis, and intertrigo.

   c. **Candidemia** is characterized by positive blood cultures, and can be associated with dissemination to visceral organs. The mortality is very high, especially with *C. glabrata*. Patients with positive blood cultures should be evaluated closely for indwelling vascular line and/or deep organ infection. Quantitative cultures of catheter tips can be performed.

   d. **Disseminated or invasive candidiasis.** Deep organ infections can result from hematogenous spread, by direct extension from contiguous sites, or by local inoculation. Diagnosis can be difficult because blood cultures are frequently negative. Positive superficial cultures (e.g., urine, sputum, and wounds) may represent colonization or contamination, and diagnostic serologic tests are not available. A high level of suspicion must be maintained in patients with the risk factors described previously. Definitive criteria for disseminated infection include positive cultures from the infected tissue or peritoneal fluid, actual invasion (histologically) of burn wounds, and endophthalmitis. Suggestive criteria include two positive blood cultures at least 24 hours apart, with one positive culture drawn at least 24 hours after the removal of vascular cannulae, and, in the right population, three or more colonized sites.

      (1) **Hepatosplenic candidiasis** is most common in patients with hematologic malignancy. The diagnosis is suggested by right upper quadrant pain, fevers, elevated alkaline phosphatase, and multiple "bull's eye" lesions on abdominal ultrasonography or CT scan, although the liver may also appear normal. Diagnosis can be confirmed by liver biopsy.

      (2) **Candidal peritonitis** results from perforation of the intestines or stomach or infection of a peritoneal dialysis catheter.

      (3) **Cardiac candidiasis** includes myocarditis, pericarditis, and endocarditis. Valvular vegetations can be quite large, and major embolic events are common and devastating.

      (4) **Renal candidiasis** arises from ascending infection from the bladder resulting in fungus balls and papillary necrosis, or from hematogenous spread resulting in pyelonephritis and abscess formation.

      (5) **Ocular candidiasis** can cause blindness.

      (6) **Other sites of disseminated candidiasis** include the CNS and the musculoskeletal system.

4. **Treatment of candidal infections.** There have been few controlled trials to define the best therapeutic modalities. Antifungal therapy should be tailored to available culture data with particular attention to the presence of fluconazole-resistant organisms.

   a. **Candiduria** can be treated with amphotericin or nystatin bladder irrigation or oral fluconazole. The choice should be guided by the organism identified (*C. glabrata* is often resistant to fluconazole) as well as the likelihood of renal involvement. Because urinary catheters often have thick fungal sediments attached, replacement of indwelling urinary catheters is also recommended.

b. **Mucocutaneous candidiasis** is initially treated with a topical agent such as nystatin, Mycostatin, clotrimazole, or ketoconazole. Systemic therapy with oral fluconazole may be indicated when patients do not respond to topical therapy.

c. **Candidemia** is treated with systemic antifungal therapy. Venous and arterial catheters should be replaced at new sites and catheter tips should be cultured. Tunneled central venous lines are often left in place unless there is failure to clear the fungemia with antibiotics. The decision to treat with fluconazole, amphotericin, or caspofungin is based on the patient's overall clinical status and the fungal isolate. *Candida glabrata* and *Candida krusei* are often resistant to fluconazole. Amphotericin and echinocandins, including caspofungin and micafungin, are options for the treatment of severe infection. In unstable patients, amphotericin or echininocandins are generally favored over fluconazole.

d. **Disseminated candidiasis** requires a combination of systemic antifungal therapy, drainage or debridement of infected areas, removal of intravascular catheters, and sometimes removal of infected valves and other foreign bodies. Although there is general consensus that *Candida* spp grown from the peritoneal cavity (i.e., not just peritoneal drains) should be treated, opinions differ with respect to whether amphotericin, echinocandins (caspofungin and microfungi), or fluconazole should be used. The same is true for hepatosplenic candidiasis. Lack of response to fluconazole is an indication to change the antifungal coverage. Severe endophthalmitis is treated with amphotericin.

B. **Aspergillus** is a cause of invasive opportunistic infection in immunocompromised ICU patients. Distinguishing colonization from infection can be difficult. Diagnosis of infection is based on serologic data, tissue histology, and cultures. Positive sputum cultures do not necessarily indicate disease and negative cultures do not rule out disease. Thus, it is helpful, although not always clinically feasible, to get pulmonary tissue for analysis.

1. **Clinical manifestations** range from localized pulmonary disease to disseminated disease.

a. **Invasive pulmonary disease** occurs in immunocompromised patients, and presents with fever and pulmonary infiltrates. Pathologic analysis reveals infarction and hemorrhage. Pulmonary thrombosis can occur when the organisms invade vessel walls. Diagnosis is made by direct analysis of pulmonary tissue. A significant proportion of patients with locally invasive disease also have disseminated disease.

b. **Dissemination** to a variety of organs occurs due to vascular invasion. Abscesses occur in the CNS, lung, liver, and myocardium. Budd-Chiari syndrome and myocardial infarctions may occur.

c. **Other pulmonary manifestations**

(1) **Aspergillomas** are fungus balls that occur in cavities in the upper lobes of the lungs, especially in bullae and occasionally in old tuberculous cavities. Patients present with cough, hemoptysis (which can be life threatening), fever, and dyspnea.

(2) **Allergic bronchopulmonary aspergillosis** causes episodic asthmatic symptoms and usually occurs in patients with chronic asthma or cystic fibrosis. Radiographic findings range from segmental infiltrates to transient nonsegmental infiltrates. Eosinophilia is present in the sputum and blood.

2. **Treatment of aspergillosis**
   a. **Disseminated disease** and **invasive pulmonary disease** are treated with IV amphotericin or voriconazole. In some cases, disseminated disease is treated with a combination of amphotericin and voriconazole. Echinocandins are also used to treat patients with invasive aspergillosis who have failed to respond to amphotericin or are intolerant of amphotericin. Surgical resection may be indicated when systemic antifungal therapy has failed.
   b. **Localized pulmonary manifestations**
      (1) **Aspergilloma.** Surgery is indicated in patients with recurrent hemoptysis. There may also be a role for corticosteroid treatment. Systemic amphotericin B does not improve outcome compared with supportive measures.
      (2) **Allergic bronchopulmonary aspergillosis** is treated with systemic corticosteroids (aerosolized steroids are not of benefit) and sometimes aerosolized antifungals. The benefits of long-term corticosteroid therapy have not been shown.

IX. **Viral infections**
   A. **Cytomegalovirus (CMV)** is an important cause of infection in immunocompromised patients. It is the most common cause of infection in solid-organ and bone marrow transplant recipients. Primary infection occurs in seronegative individuals, while secondary infection occurs when there is activation of latent infection or reinfection of a seropositive host. Primary infection in immunocompetent hosts is often asymptomatic, although, rarely, severe disease occurs. Diagnosis of CMV infection requires detection of viral components or an increase in antibodies directed to CMV.
      1. **Manifestations of CMV in immunocompromised patients**
         a. **Self-limited febrile illness** is common.
         b. **Interstitial pneumonitis.** CMV pneumonitis resulting in respiratory failure requiring mechanical ventilation has high mortality.
         c. **CMV hepatitis** is usually mild, but can be severe, particularly in liver transplant patients.
         d. **GI.** Diarrhea, GI bleeding.
         e. **Retinitis**
      2. **Treatment.** CMV infection is very difficult to treat, and infection recurs rapidly after cessation of antiviral agents. **Ganciclovir** and **foscarnet** are both used to treat CMV retinitis in AIDS patients. Ganciclovir is also given for CMV infection in organ transplant recipients. Foscarnet is used in patients with CMV who are intolerant of ganciclovir. Life-threatening CMV infection (such as CMV pneumonitis) may be treated with the combination of ganciclovir and high-dose IV CMV immunoglobulin. Administration of hyperimmune globulin to bone marrow transplant recipients with pneumonitis has resulted in improved outcome.
   B. **Herpes simplex virus (HSV) I and II**
      1. **Manifestations** of HSV infection include the following:
         a. **Mucocutaneous** and **genital** disease.
         b. **Respiratory tract infection.**
            (1) Tracheobronchitis.
            (2) HSV pneumonia generally occurring in debilitated or immunocompromised patients.
         c. **Ocular infection** such as blepharitis, conjunctivitis, keratitis, corneal ulceration, and blindness.
         d. **Esophagitis.**
         e. **Encephalitis, meningitis.**

2. **Disseminated HSV** usually occurs in patients who are extremely debilitated or immunocompromised, but occasionally occurs during pregnancy. Manifestations include necrotizing hepatitis, pneumonitis, cutaneous lesions from hematogenous spread, fever, hypotension, disseminated intravascular coagulation, and CNS involvement.

3. **Diagnosis.** Wright's and Giemsa's stains (Tzanck smear) or Papanicolaou's stain of material scraped from lesions can be helpful, but are insensitive and do not distinguish between HSV and varicella zoster virus (VZV) infection. Viral culture, histologic examination of tissue or skin biopsy, and DNA or protein staining of viral antigens are other diagnostic tests. Brain biopsy may be necessary for diagnosis of HSV encephalitis.

4. **Treatment**
   a. **Severe HSV infections,** including CNS infections, pneumonitis, and disseminated HSV, are treated with IV **acyclovir. Foscarnet** may be used to treat acyclovir-resistant HSV.
   b. **Mucosal, cutaneous, and genital infections** may be treated with **acyclovir, famciclovir,** or **valacyclovir.** Although normal hosts do not always require treatment, consideration should be given to treating critically ill or debilitated patients even if they do not fit classic criteria for immunocompromise.
   c. **Ocular infection** may be treated with topical agents such as acyclovir, and should be managed in consultation with an ophthalmologist.

C. **Varicella zoster virus (VZV)** infection may be encountered in the ICU as a primary infection (chicken pox) or reactivation infection (herpes zoster or shingles), and can cause mild to life-threatening disease.

1. **Primary VZV** infection in adults may have severe systemic effects and pulmonary involvement that causes respiratory failure. Immunocompromised patients are prone to severe systemic disease with involvement of lungs, kidneys, CNS, and liver.

2. **Herpes zoster** usually manifests as a dermatomal cutaneous infection from reactivation of VZV that has been dormant in the sensory ganglia. Rarely, reactivated herpes zoster causes CNS disease such as encephalitis and cerebral vasculitis.

3. **Treatment.** IV acyclovir is used for serious VZV infection (pneumonia, encephalitis) in immunocompromised or immunocompetent hosts.

X. **Emerging infectious diseases and bioterrorism agents.** Emerging infections are those that have newly appeared in a population or have existed previously but are rapidly increasing in incidence or geographic range. They may be categorized as newly emerging (SARS, avian influenza A), reemerging or resurging (human monkeypox, dengue), and deliberately emerging (bioterrorism agents such as anthrax). While the bacterial zoonotic pneumonias are not emerging infections, they are grouped here for convenience.

A. **Zoonotic pneumonias** (including the severe acute respiratory syndrome [**SARS**] and avian influenza A (H5N1)) are pneumonias whose etiologic agents have nonhuman reservoirs. These pneumonias are rare, and presumptive diagnoses are generally made by contact history.

1. **Microbiology. Bacteria** responsible for zoonotic pneumonias include *Chlamydia psittaci,* which causes psittacosis (from contact with parrots and their relatives), *Coxiella burnetii,* which causes Q fever (from sheep and parturient cats), and *Francisella tularensis,* which causes tularemia (from rabbit, deer, or deerfly bites). **Viral** causes of zoonotic pneumonias include the SARS-associated coronavirus (SARS-CoV), the purported etiologic agent of **SARS** and the avian influenza A

(H5N1) virus. Although overall the prognosis for patients with zoonotic infections is good, some zoonotic diseases are associated with severe complications and even death.

2. **Diagnosis.** Because zoonotic agents are difficult and can be dangerous to grow, diagnosis is often made through serologic testing. SARS may be diagnosed by viral isolation, RT-PCR or serologic testing. Additional serologic tests should be performed to exclude influenza A as well as *Legionella* spp and *F. tularensis,* which can mimic the influenza-like presentation of SARS. Avian influenza has been diagnosed by virus isolation or identification of H5-specific RNA.

3. **Treatment**

   a. **Bacterial zoonotic infections.** Extended therapy (2–5 weeks) with either doxycycline or a fluoroquinolone is recommended for zoonotic bacterial infections.

   b. **SARS.** Options are limited and treatment is primarily supportive. There are currently no recommended antiviral agents with reliable anti–SARS-CoV activity. Ribavirin and oseltamivir have been used with limited success. Other drugs that have been studied include corticosteroids, interferon-β, pegylated interferon-α, and glycyrrhizin (licorice root extract).

   c. **Avian influenza A (H5N1).** In addition to supportive therapy, oral oseltamivir (75–150 mg twice daily for 5–10 days in adults) is recommended for patients suspected to have avian influenza. The most recent isolates have been resistant to amantidine and rimantadine—these drugs have no role. Newer neuraminidase inhibitors (zanamivir and peramivir) are being studied.

B. **Bioterror agents** represent a group of bacterial and viral pathogens that can cause life-threatening syndromes in large populations. Known or suspected agents that cause acute pneumonias in this category include inhalational **anthrax, tularemia pneumonia,** and **pneumonic plague. Bioterror** agents are discussed in **Chapter 38.**

Selected References

American Thoracic Society, Infectious Diseases Society of America. Guidelines for the management of adults with hospital-acquired, ventilator-associated and healthcare-associated pneumonia. *Am J Respir Crit Care Med* 2005;171:388–416.

Cohen J, Powderly WG. *Infectious diseases.* 2nd ed. New York: Elsevier, 2004.

Darling RG, Catlett CL, Huebner KD, et al. Threats in bioterrorism. I. CDC category A agents. *Emerg Med Clin North Am* 2002;20:273–309.

David N, Gilbert RC, Moellering GM, et al. *The Sanford guide to antimicrobial therapy.* 38th ed. Vienna, VA: Antimicrobial Therapy, 2008.

Gerding DN, Muto CA, Owens RC. Treatment of *Clostridium difficile* infection. *Clin Infect Dis* 2008;46 (suppl 1):S32–S42.

Mandell LA, Wunderink RG, Anzueto A, et al. Infectious Diseases Society of America/American Thoracic Society consensus guidelines on the management of community-acquired pneumonia in adults. *Clin Infect Dis* 2007;44 (suppl 2):S27–S72.

Morens DM, Folkers GK, Fauci AS. The challenge of emerging and re-emerging infectious diseases. *Nature* 2004;430:242–249.

Mylonakis E, Calderwood SB. Infective endocarditis in adults. *N Engl J Med* 2001;345:1318–1330.

O'Grady NP, Alexander M, Dellinger EP, et al. Guidelines for the prevention of intravascular catheter-related infections. Centers for Disease Control and Prevention. *MMWR Recomm Rep* 2002;51(RR-10):1–29.

Pappas PG, Rex JH, Sobel JD, et al. Guidelines for treatment of candidiasis. *Clin Infect Dis* 2004;38:161–189.

30 Nonantibiotic Therapies for Sepsis

Anahat Dhillon and Edward Bittner

Sepsis and septic shock are important causes of morbidity and mortality in intensive care units, carrying a 28-day mortality of more than 30%. Millions of people are affected worldwide, with 1,400 patients dying everyday. The cost in patient lives, quality of life after survival, and the monetary burden all make sepsis a major health care issue. Sepsis is a spectrum of disease from a mild inflammatory response to multiple organ failure. Early detection and treatment to prevent progression of disease are crucial to possibly improving survival.

I. **Definitions**
   A. **Systemic inflammatory response syndrome (SIRS):** Clinical presentation is secondary to systemic manifestations resulting from activation of the innate immune response regardless of cause. It can be triggered by infection or noninfectious causes such as surgery, burns, pancreatitis, and so on. SIRS is diagnosed when two or more of the following criteria are met:
      1. Temperature: $>38°C$ or $<35°C$
      2. Tachycardia: heart rate >90
      3. Tachypnea: respiratory rate >20 or $Paco_2$ <30 or mechanical ventilation
      4. Leukocytosis (WBC $>12,000/\mu L$), leucopenia (WBC $<4,000/\mu L$), or $>10\%$ bands
   B. **Sepsis:** Evidence or strong suspicion of infection. The sentence and SIRS. Other supporting variables may include
      1. Elevated lactate
      2. Elevated plasma C-reactive protein
      3. Elevated procalcitonin
      4. Arterial hypotension
      5. Cardiac index >3.5 L/min/m^2
      6. Central venous oxygen saturation $>70\%$
      7. Evidence of organ dysfunction such as hypoxemia, oliguria, or hyperbilirubinemia.
   C. **Severe sepsis:** Sepsis with evidence of organ hypoperfusion or dysfunction. Evidence of early organ dysfunction include hypoxemia, oliguria, thrombocytopenia, hyperbilirubinemia, altered mental status, lactate >2, and cardiac dysfunction.
   D. **Septic shock:** Sepsis with persistent arterial hypotension despite adequate volume resuscitation.
   E. **Multiple organ dysfunction syndrome (MODS):** The dysfunction of more than one organ which requires intervention. Examples include ventilatory support for ARDS and dialysis for renal failure.

II. **Pathophysiology.** Sepsis is a heterogeneous syndrome with clinical manifestations varying between patients, underlying etiology and over time. Each response is determined by many factors, including the virulence of the organism; the size of the inoculum; and the patient's coexisting conditions, age,

and genetics. Thus, it is not surprising that the pathogenesis has been difficult to elucidate and may be protean.

A. Bacterial factors. All classes of microorganisms, including gram-positive
and gram-negative bacteria, fungi, viruses, and parasites have structural
components that interact with the host immune response. For example,
gram-negative bacteria have **endotoxin** (lipopolysaccharide, [**LPS**]), a
potent mediator of many of the clinical manifestations of gram-negative
sepsis. Gram-positive bacteria tend to liberate exotoxins, such as **toxic
shock syndrome toxin.** The importance of these substances in clinical practice is that they may not be directly neutralized by antibiotics, thus mag-
nifying the early damage of certain infections.

B. Host response

1. The host's response to infection is critical to recovery. The initiation of
   the **innate immune response** occurs with the recognition of typical
   structural components of microbes by host cells (e.g., LPS). **Toll-like
   receptors (TLR)** are host's molecules that can recognize specific bacterial structures and trigger a protean initial inflammatory cascade, and
   can be targeted for therapeutic purposes.

2. The proinflammatory response (**adaptive immunity**) is mediated by
   cytokines such as tumor necrosis factor-α (TNF-α), interleukin-6 (IL-
   6), and IL1-β. At various times after the initial proinflammatory state,
   counterregulatory cytokines and proinflammatory antagonists are
   secreted resulting in an anti-inflammatory state. A state of immuno-
   paralysis can result whereby the host has inadequate immune responses
   to microorganisms resulting in subsequent morbidity and mortality following infection.

C. Cellular injury. Failure to generate ATP during sepsis and critical illness
may in part be due to impaired delivery of oxygen to vital tissues secondary to impaired oxygenation and perfusion. In addition, **cytopathic hypoxia,**
resulting from mitochondrial dysfunction, may underlie the apparent disconnection between the cellular oxygen tension, which is usually adequate and the low ATP.

D. Genetics. Twin studies have suggested a genetic polymorphism in the
cytokine response to sepsis, which may result in differences in mortality.

E. Coagulation cascade. Inflammation is a procoagulant state. Inflammation
and coagulation are both activated during severe infection, and share
common mediators. One of them, activated protein C, has been successfully targeted for therapy (see **Section V**).

F. Epithelial and endothelial dysfunction. Epithelial cell dysfunction resulting
from the deleterious effects of the systemic inflammatory response can
result in impaired barrier function, increased permeability, and may be a
final step in the pathway to sepsis-related MODS. **Endothelial** cells play a
critical role in systemic inflammation and in maintaining a balance
between coagulation and anticoagulation. Such an imbalance may result
in the development of microvascular thrombosis leading to abnormal
microcirculation and impaired oxygen delivery to tissues. In addition,
endothelial cells play an active role in recruiting inflammatory cells to
sites of infection and inflammation.

III. Manifestations. The early signs of sepsis include tachycardia, hyperventilation, fever, and disorientation. Later signs can involve any or all organ systems. The mortality when multiple organs fail is extremely high.

A. Cardiovascular: Tachycardia and hypotension are commonly present and
may initially be due to vasodilatation and intravascular hypovolemia.

Sepsis-induced myocardial depression can occur early or late in the course, contributing to hypotension.

B. **Respiratory:** Hyperventilation is common early in sepsis. Poor oxygenation can be secondary to leaky alveolar capillaries. Acute lung injury and acute respiratory distress syndrome are common complications of severe sepsis.

C. **Renal:** Oliguric renal insufficiency can be prerenal due to hypotension, impaired perfusion, or hypovolemia. Direct damage to the kidneys can lead to acute tubular necrosis. Oliguria may progress to acute renal failure requiring renal replacement therapy.

D. **Central nervous system:** Sepsis-induced encephalopathy can range from mild confusion, delirium, and coma.

E. **Hepatic:** Cholestasis is common. Inflammatory mediators resulting in dysfunction of bile canaliculi can lead to hyperbilirubinemia. Transaminitis may be mild or severe secondary to ischemia.

F. **Metabolic:** Catecholamines inhibit insulin release and increase gluconeogenesis. Patients may be hyper- or hypoglycemic.

G. **Hematologic:** Consumptive coagulopathy, platelet sequestration, and platelet destruction are common.

IV. **Markers of sepsis.** The diagnosis of sepsis is made with a suspicion of infection and clinical signs of systemic inflammation. These signs are neither sensitive nor specific for sepsis, thus there has been a search for biochemical markers of sepsis, which would lead to earlier more definitive diagnosis. Multiple cytokines, peptides, receptors, and acute-phase reactants are being studied as possible ideal markers. Some examples of well studied, clinically available assays include

A. **C-reactive protein** is an acute-phase protein that is released from hepatic cells in response to inflammation. It is an inexpensive test that suggests the presence of inflammation. Its disadvantages include that is nonspecific, has a slow time to peak, and has no correlation with the severity of inflammation.

B. Cytokines such as **IL-6** and **IL-8** are primary host response in inflammation. They are highly sensitive markers of systemic inflammation, however the levels are highly variable, level is not correlated with degree of inflammation, and they have a short half-time in plasma. Levels of IL-6 and IL-8 may be useful to distinguish infectious versus noninfectious causes of neutropenic fever and also in onset of early sepsis in neonates.

C. **Procalcitonin (PCT)** is a propeptide of calcitonin with a longer half-life. Elevated PCT levels are highly specific for severe sepsis and onset of organ dysfunction. It is elevated in inflammatory states that are noninfectious; however, the plasma levels are not as high as in severe sepsis. Patients with levels more than 2 ng/mL are at high risk for having severe sepsis. PCT may have utility in differentiating between an infectious or noninfectious etiology of SIRS. It can also be helpful in monitoring the efficacy of treatment.

V. **Treatment.** The European Society of Intensive Care Medicine, the International Sepsis Forum, and the Society of Critical Care Medicine started the **Surviving Sepsis Campaign** to improve the diagnosis and treatment of sepsis. They have developed evidence based guidelines that are an excellent source for clinicians. The most recent guidelines are available on their Web site: www.survivingsepsis.org

The primary therapy of sepsis and septic shock is early identification and treatment of the causative agent. As such it is imperative to initiate the search for and treatment of possible sources promptly.

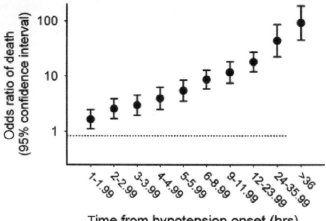

Time from hypotension onset (hrs)

FIGURE 30-1 Mortality risk (expressed as adjusted odds ratio of death) with increasing delays in initiation of effective antimicrobial therapy. Bars represent 95% confidence interval. An increased risk of death is already present by the second hour after hypotension onset (compared with the first hour after hypotension). The risk of death continues to climb, though, to >36 hours after hypotension onset. (From Kumar A, et al. Duration of hypotension before initiation of effective antimicrobial therapy is the critical determinant of survival in human septic shock. *Crit Care Med.* 2006;34: 1589-1596 with permission).

A. **Diagnosis**
  1. **Cultures.** Two sets of peripheral blood cultures should be obtained under sterile technique. If a new central line is placed, blood cultures should be drawn at the time of insertion, prior to removal of the drapes. Urine, sputum, cerebrospinal fluid, or other body fluids should be cultured as dictated by the clinical situation.
  2. **Imaging studies.** If the patient is stable, then further imaging such as CT scans should be performed to identify possible sources of infection. In an unstable patient, bedside diagnostic studies with the use of ultrasound can be helpful.
B. **Broad-spectrum intravenous (IV) antibiotics** should be started as soon as blood cultures are obtained and within 1 hour of identification of sepsis (**Fig. 30-1**). Ideally, all cultures should be obtained prior to initiation of antibiotics. However, antibiotics should not be delayed if there is a significant delay in obtaining cultures, as the mortality from sepsis increases with each hour delay in initiation of treatment. Initial antibiotic choice is dictated by the suspected origin and pathogens (see **Chapter 29**). As culture and sensitivity results become available over the next 24 to 48 hours, drugs should be tailored based on the data. Extended use of broad-spectrum antibiotics is not recommended as it may select for greater resistance.
C. **Source control.** If a *nidus* of infection is identified by imaging studies or physical examination, intervention (For example, surgical or percutaneous) must be considered. The choice of intervention is based on patient stability, resources available, and the source. For example, often abscesses are amenable to percutaneous drainage, whereas necrotizing fasciitis requires surgical debridement. The one exception to early source control is necrotizing pancreatitis where delaying surgery might be of benefit.
D. **Hemodynamic support.** Septic shock has classically been defined as a hypovolemic/distributive shock state with low vascular tone and a high cardiac

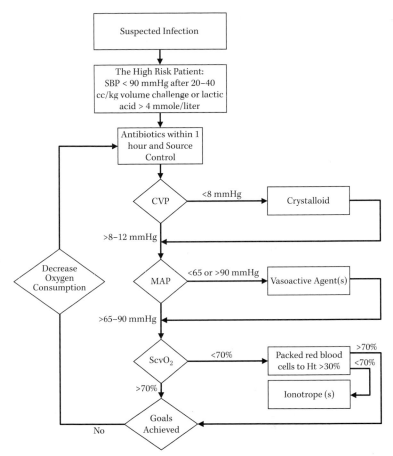

FIGURE 30-2 Algorithm for early goal directed therapy (EGDT) for management of severe sepsis/septic shock. (From Otero R, et al. Early goal-directed therapy in severe sepsis and septic shock revisited: concepts, controversies, and contemporary findings. *Chest* 2006; 130:1579–95 with permission).

output. However, it is becoming apparent that patients may have a component of toxin-mediated myocardial dysfunction as well as maldistribution of flow with peripheral vascular dysfunction leading to cellular ischemia. As such, supporting the septic patient may necessitate the use of fluids, vasopressors, and inotropes to maintain tissue perfusion.

1. **Early goal-directed therapy (Fig. 30-2).** Early optimization of hemodynamic and fluid management to balance oxygen delivery with oxygen demand is important in the management of septic patients. A recent clinical trial showed decreased mortality with early, aggressive goal-directed therapy **instituted in emergency departments.** These data have been extrapolated and many institutions have set up protocols for early therapy in all severely septic patients. The priority is to identify goals of resuscitation that indicate global and regional tissue perfusion and provide logical strategies to achieve the goals set. Since no

single marker has been shown to be an adequate or superior end point for resuscitation, a group of goals are used. These include

a. A target of **mean arterial blood pressure (MAP)** >65 mm Hg is often set as a starting point for resuscitation. This goal is varied based on the patient's baseline blood pressure. Chronically hypertensive patients often require a higher target.

b. An initial target of **central venous pressure (CVP) of 8 to 12 mm Hg** in nonventilated and 12 to 15 mm Hg in mechanically ventilated patients. Patients with noncompliant ventricles, pulmonary hypertension will sometimes require a higher CVP for adequate filling.

c. **A urine output** goal >0.5 mL/kg/h.

d. A **central venous oxygen saturation (Scvo$_2$)** of >70%. Scvo$_2$ or mixed venous oxygen saturation (Svo$_2$) are used as markers of global tissue perfusion. In patients with shock states, Svo$_2$ runs 5% to 7% lower than Svo$_2$.

e. **Serum lactate** concentration and base deficits are also used as indicators of global perfusion with the goal to normalize lactates and correct deficits.

2. **Hemodynamic management** should focus on restoration of intravascular volume and tissue perfusion.

a. **Fluids.** Patients may initially require large volumes of IV fluids to offset any third space losses. The choice of fluid used for resuscitation has not been shown to result in a significant difference in outcome. Regardless of whether crystalloids or colloids are used, administration should target a composite goal of CVP, Scvo$_2$, and urine output. If no improvement in these parameters is seen with fluid administration, rate of administration should be decreased and other therapies should be instituted. Depending on the patient's comorbidities, consideration should be given to transfusion of red blood cells to maintain hemoglobin of 10 g/dL. Hydroxyethyl starch may increase the risk of renal failure in patients with sepsis hence is not recommended in these patients.

b. **Vasopressors** may be required to maintain perfusion to vital organs. Ideally, vasopressors should be started after the hypovolemia has been corrected. However, it is often necessary to initiate vasopressor therapy early to avoid life-threatening hypotension. Vasopressor choice often depends on each individual patient's hemodynamic profile (**Chapter 6**). Generally, the initial pressors of choice are norepinephrine or dopamine. **Norepinephrine** causes less tachycardia than dopamine and provides more vasoconstrictive effects. **Epinephrine** is used as a second-line agent in patients who are poorly responsive to norepinephrine. **Vasopressin** levels in septic shock have been reported to be lower than anticipated. Thus, there has been interest in the use of low-dose vasopressin (0.01–0.04 U/min) in management of septic patients. Although the doses of vasopressin used in septic shock should be well below the doses that cause compromise of coronary or splanchnic blood flow, patients should be closely monitored for these complications. Despite the lack of high-level evidence of its benefit, vasopressin is still commonly used as an adjunct to norepinephrine.

c. **Inotropes. Dobutamine** is used when there is evidence of myocardial dysfunction as suggested by elevated filling pressures, low cardiac output, a low central venous saturation, or echocardiographic findings of low ejection fraction. Dobutamine can cause tachyarrhythmias, but is often preferred over milrinone given its shorter half-life, making it easier to titrate. A cardiac output monitor is often used in conjunction with venous saturations to titrate the inotrope.

3. **Recombinant human activated protein C (APC)** may be used to treat patients with severe sepsis. APC is an endogenous protein that is a modulator of the coagulation and inflammatory cascades associated with sepsis. A randomized control trial showed a 6% absolute mortality reduction. The benefit from therapy was greatest in patients with a high risk of death (e.g., APACHE II scores more than 25) and more than one organ failure.

   a. Many institutions have developed guidelines for the use of APC. The Massachusetts General Hospital guidelines include severe sepsis with (a) three or more SIRS criteria and (b) the presence of acute (less than 24 hours) sepsis-induced organ failure of 2 or more systems.

   b. Contraindications to APC include hypersensitivity, active internal bleeding, recent hemorrhagic stroke (within 3 months), intracranial or intraspinal surgery, evidence of cerebral herniation, intracranial neoplasm or mass lesion, presence of an epidural catheter, or trauma or surgery with an increased risk of life-threatening bleeding (**Table 30-1**).

TABLE 30-1	Contraindications to Administration of Activated Protein C (APC) in Patients with Severe Sepsis

If the patient has any of the following, they should not receive APC.
- Patients with recent surgery (within last 30 d) and *single* organ dysfunction
- APACHE II <25
- Surgery in the previous 12 h
- Thrombocytopenia ≤30,000 platelets/mm^3
- Patient requiring therapeutic doses of antithrombin agents (i.e., heparin >15,000 U/d, direct thrombin inhibitors, fondaparinux 5 mg or higher) and to treat a thrombotic condition within the previous 8 h, LMWH at a dose higher than prophylaxis within the previous 12 h
- Systemic thrombolytic therapy within the past 3 d, ASA >650 mg/d within the past 3 d, glycoprotein IIb/IIIa antagonists within the past 7 d, warfarin within the past 4 d, or clopidogrel or ticlopidine within the past 4 d
- International normalized ratio (INR) >4.5
- Evidence of postoperative bleeding
- Evidence of active and clinically significant gastrointestinal bleeding
- Central nervous system mass lesion, stroke within last 3 mo, history of AVM, cerebral aneurysm, intracranial surgery, or history of severe head trauma requiring hospitalization
- Cirrhosis (history of esophageal varices, portal hypertension, or Child's class C)
- New nephrostomy tube or evidence of a bleeding complication following a percutaneous procedure, e.g., decreasing Hb or flank hematoma after femoral line placement
- Unexplained mental status changes or neurologic exam changes in whom a CT scan has not been performed to rule out a mass lesion or CNS bleed
- End-stage disease processes in which there is not a commitment to aggressive management of the patient
- Enrolled in a clinical trial involving a molecule that targets the coagulation cascade
- Pulmonary, splenic, or live contusions following trauma
- Epidural catheter in place within 12 h of initiation of therapy with rhAPC
- Pediatric patients only with the approval of Pediatric Infectious Disease or unless treating purpura fulminans
- Patient weight exceeds 227 kg (requires adjudication for consideration of modified dosing)

   c. **Dosing.** APC is administered as a continuous IV infusion at 24 μg/kg/h for **96 hours.**

   d. **Monitoring/adverse effects/clearance.** Patients should be closely monitored for signs of bleeding, which is the major adverse effect. Plasma levels are nondetectable within 2 hours of stopping the infusion. If surgery, percutaneous procedure, or epidural catheter placement needs to be performed, APC should be stopped 2 hours prior to the procedure. APC can be restarted 1 hour after a percutaneous procedure and 12 hours after a surgical procedure, lumbar puncture, or epidural catheter removal, if adequate hemostasis has been achieved. Concomitant use of full-dose heparin and APC is contraindicated. In patients receiving renal replacement therapy, dialysis should be run without heparin if possible. If clotting occurs, lowest possible dose of heparin should be used.

4. **Corticosteroids.** The role of exogenous steroids in the treatment of sepsis remains controversial. One multicenter randomized controlled trial in patients with vasopressor-unresponsive septic shock showed a significant increase in shock reversal and reduction of mortality in patients with relative adrenal insufficiency. However, a more recent trial that included all septic patients did not show a mortality benefit but did show a faster resolution of septic shock with the use of steroids. Given the known side effects of corticosteroids, such as increased rates of infection and myopathy, and the conflicting data on mortality benefit, the use of steroids has been limited.

   a. **Patient selection:** IV hydrocortisone can be given to patients whose blood pressures are nonresponsive to fluid therapy and are on high or escalating doses of vasopressors. ACTH stimulation testing is not recommended to identify patients.

   b. **The recommended dose is 50 mg of hydrocortisone every 6 hours.** Higher dose of corticosteroids may be harmful and should not be used for the treatment of septic shock.

   c. **The duration of therapy** should be 7 days, or possibly less, and should be discontinued as soon as the patient is no longer on vasopressors. It is unclear whether patients need to be tapered off the steroids. A short duration of treatment generally does not require a taper.

5. **Other supportive therapies**

   a. **Ventilation:** Twenty to forty percent of patients with severe sepsis will develop some degree of ALI/ARDS. The use of lung **protective ventilation strategies** targeting tidal volumes of 6 cm^3/kg, plateau pressures <30 cm H$_2$O with permissive hypercapnia, and judicious fluid administration is recommended (**Chapter 20**). Consider the use of these strategies early in the resuscitation of severely septic patients. In patients who do develop acute lung injury, the routine insertion of a pulmonary artery catheter has failed to show any benefit and is thus not recommended. Additionally, if patients do not have evidence of tissue hypoperfusion, a fluid-conservative therapy is recommended as it decreases days of mechanical ventilation and ICU length of stay without increasing renal failure or mortality. All patients should be ventilated with a weaning protocol in place and should regularly undergo spontaneous breathing trials to evaluate for possible extubation.

   b. **Glucose control:** Hyperglycemia in septic shock is associated with worse outcomes, as are large swings in glucose with periods of significant hypoglycemia (**Chapter 28**). Consistent maintenance of glucose in the 110 to 150 range is currently recommended for patients with severe sepsis. This may require the use of IV insulin with hourly point of care testing. Patients on an insulin infusion should have a glucose calorie source to avoid hypoglycemia. Point of care testing of glucose should be validated with plasma glucose values when the values are extreme, as finger sticks may overestimate plasma glucose levels.

c. **Sedation** protocols with predetermined sedation goals and daily awakening are recommended as these lead to shorter duration of mechanical ventilation and length of stay in general ICU patients (see **Chapter 7**).

d. **Blood product administration:** Once tissue hypoperfusion has resolved and the patient does not have other indications for transfusion such as myocardial ischemia or acute hemorrhage, red blood cells should be transfused to target hemoglobin of 7.0 to 9.0 g/dL in adults. Erythropoietin is not recommended as treatment for sepsis-associated anemia, unless the patient has other indications for its use. Use of fresh frozen plasma and other component therapy is not recommended for use to correct laboratory evidence of coagulopathy, unless there is clinical evidence of bleeding or an invasive procedure is planned.

e. **Prophylaxis.** Septic patients should have prophylaxis for ventilator-associated pneumonia, deep vein thrombosis, and stress ulcer prophylaxis (**Chapter 13**).

f. **Goals of care:** As with all critically ill patients, the goals of care should be discussed either with the patient or the surrogate decision maker and readdressed as dictated by the clinical situation.

Selected References

Angus DC et al. Epidemiology of severe sepsis in the United States: analysis of incidence, outcome and associated costs of care. *Crit Care Med* 2001;29:1303–1310.

Annane D, Sebille V, Charpentier C, et al. Effect of treatment with low doses of hydrocortisone and fludrocortisone on mortality in patients with septic shock. *JAMA* 2002;288:862–871.

Bernard GR, Vincent JL, Laterre PF, et al. Efficacy and safety of recombinant human activated protein C for severe sepsis. *N Engl J Med* 2001;344:699–709.

Dellinger RP, Levy MM, Carlet JM, et al. Surviving Sepsis Campaign: international guidelines for management of severe sepsis and septic shock: 2008. *Crit Care Med* 2008;36:296–327.

Hotchkiss RS, Karl IE. The pathophysiology and treatment of sepsis. *N Engl J Med* 2003;348:138–150.

Kumar A, Roberts D, Wood KE, et al. Duration of hypotension before initiation of effective antimicrobial therapy is the critical determinant of survival in human septic shock. *Crit Care Med* 2006;34:1589–1596.

Otero R, Nguyen B, Huang DT, et al. Early goal-directed therapy in severe sepsis and septic shock revisited: concepts, controversies, and contemporary findings. *Chest* 2006;130:1579–1595.

Reinhart K et al. Markers of sepsis diagnosis: what is useful? *Crit Care Clin* 2006;22:503–519.

Rivers E, Nyugen B, Havstad S, et al. Early goal-directed therapy in the treatment of severe sepsis and septic shock. *N Engl J Med* 2001;345:1368–1377.

Sprung CL, Annane D, Keh D, et al. Hydrocortisone therapy for patients with septic shock. *N Engl J Med* 2008;358:111–124.

31 Stroke, Seizures, and Encephalopathy

Dorothea Strozyk and Lee Schwamm

Nontraumatic acute cerebral dysfunction can be the reason for initial hospital presentation, accompanying underlying illness, or complicated medical or perioperative management. The majority of etiologies require specific and urgent intervention, and understanding acute dysfunction of the brain is of paramount importance. Common disorders include ischemic stroke, intracerebral hemorrhage (ICH), subdural hemorrhage, subarachnoid hemorrhage (SAH), seizures, and encephalopathy (of infectious, inflammatory, hypo-/hypertensive, or toxic/metabolic origin). The neurologic examination is critical in distinguishing focal versus generalized processes and can help to identify the likely etiology.

I. **Stroke** is the acute onset of a focal neurologic deficit or disturbance in the level of arousal due to cerebral ischemia, hemorrhage, or venous occlusion. Therapy is aimed at restoring adequate cerebral blood flow and preventing secondary brain injury.

   A. **Acute ischemic stroke** is due to acute vascular occlusion. Symptoms often include sudden onset of visual loss, weakness or numbness on one side of the body, ataxia, unexplained falling, dysarthria, or aphasia. Thrombosis in situ may occur in diseased segments of small penetrating vessels (e.g., lacunar stroke) or larger arteries (e.g., atherosclerotic stenosis, arterial dissection), and emboli may be liberated from proximal sites (e.g., heart, aorta, carotid artery) to lodge in otherwise normal major cerebral arteries or their distal branches.

   1. **Lacunar strokes** tend to occur in patients with diabetes and chronic hypertension and may be clinically silent or present as pure motor hemiparesis, pure sensory loss, or a variety of well-defined syndromes (e.g., dysarthria-clumsy hand, ataxic-hemiparesis). Descending compact white matter tracts or brainstem gray matter nuclei are injured, often producing widespread and striking initial deficits. However, the prognosis for recovery with lacunar stroke is better than with large-artery territory stroke. Nevertheless, because the risk of hemorrhagic transformation in these patients is low, many centers favor the use of intravenous (IV) **thrombolysis** in all but the most clinically mild lacunar strokes. Because initial small-vessel clinical syndromes may sometimes be due to large-artery thrombosis affecting end vessels, all patients presenting with acute ischemic symptoms should undergo some form of acute neurovascular imaging to establish large-vessel patency (e.g., computed tomographic angiography, magnetic resonance angiography [MRA], ultrasound, or conventional contrast angiography [CTA]). This should not delay IV thrombolysis using recombinant **tissue plasminogen activator** (**tPA,** alteplase) in appropriate patients.

   2. **Large-artery occlusion** is divided into disorders of the anterior (internal carotid artery and branches) and posterior (vertebrobasilar arteries and branches) circulations. These strokes carry a risk of swelling and hemorrhagic transformation. The "ischemic penumbra" refers to a

region of brain with inadequate blood supply that still may be salvaged with rapid restoration of normal blood flow. Although the center of an ischemic zone (the core) may be irreversibly injured before the patient obtains medical attention, the surrounding ischemic penumbra may be saved by rapid intervention.

a. **Middle cerebral artery (MCA) occlusion** is characterized by weakness of the contralateral face and arm with hemianopia and a preference of the eyes and head toward the side of the involved hemisphere ("looking toward the lesion"). Additional findings include aphasia in dominant-hemisphere strokes, hemineglect in nondominant-hemisphere strokes (patient "ignores" the left side of the body, the surroundings, or the presence of the deficit itself), and a variable degree of leg weakness depending upon how much of the MCA stem is involved (and thus how much of the underlying white matter or basal ganglia is affected). Involvement restricted to branches of the MCA may produce fragments of this syndrome, often with sparing of leg strength.

b. **Anterior cerebral artery (ACA) occlusion** is rare, and causes isolated weakness of the lower limb. If both ACAs are affected, a generalized decrease in initiative (abulia) may also occur.

c. **Border zone** or "watershed" infarction is the result of insufficient blood flow to parts of the brain supplied by the distal territories of more than one of the major cerebral vessels. This develops most commonly in the setting of severe, sustained hypotension (e.g., cardiac arrest) or in the presence of severe atherosclerotic narrowing of one or both carotid arteries. Because the region most commonly affected is the white matter underneath the motor areas (the ACA/MCA border zone), the classic presentation is that of proximal arm/leg weakness with preservation of distal strength, the so-called person in a barrel.

d. **Posterior circulation** infarction involves the brainstem, cerebellum, thalamus, and occipital and mesial temporal lobes. As a result, patients can present with bilateral limb weakness or sensory disturbance, cranial nerve deficits (sensory and/or motor), ataxia, nausea and vomiting, visual field deficits, or decreased level of consciousness, including coma. The full-blown syndrome results from occlusion of the basilar artery trunk, with fragments of the syndrome produced by branch occlusions. Edema and mass effect from cerebellar stroke may be life threatening due to the confined space of the posterior fossa, with resulting upward or downward transtentorial herniation (see section on cerebellar hemorrhage).

3. **Conditions mimicking stroke** include seizure, migraine, toxic-metabolic derangement, and amyloid spells. Diffusion-weighted MR imaging helps to distinguish cerebral infarction from stroke mimics by identifying areas of intracellular swelling (i.e., cytotoxic edema) associated with ischemia.

a. While partial complex **seizures** may mimic stroke, especially if speech is impaired, postictal neurologic deficits (Todd's phenomena) may masquerade as any focal neurologic deficit, including weakness, sensory loss, or aphasia lasting hours to days after a seizure.

b. The aura associated with a **migraine** headache may include focal neurologic deficits such as weakness, numbness, or aphasia, and may occur in the absence of headache ("typical aura without headache"). Patients with recurrent migraine headaches are at a somewhat increased risk for true ischemic stroke. Patients who present with persistent symptoms similar in quality to their typical migrainous aura or who present with a new focal deficit accompanied by their typical aura should be evaluated for stroke.

c. **Toxic-metabolic states** such as hypo- or hyperglycemia, hyponatremia, hypoxia, or intoxication may produce focal or global neurologic deficits. Laboratory evaluation including electrolytes should be performed in all cases. Occult infections can also exacerbate deficits from old strokes and masquerade as new or recurrent stroke.

d. Patients with **amyloid angiopathy** may have transient neurologic dysfunction associated with microscopic hemorrhages that are suggestive of transient ischemic attacks (TIAs). MR imaging gradient-echo sequences, which easily identify areas of hemosiderin deposition, may suggest diagnosis of cerebral amyloid angiopathy.

4. **Important etiologies of ischemic stroke** include cardiac and arterial **thromboembolism**, intracranial and extracranial **atherosclerosis**, endocarditis, paradoxical emboli, arterial dissection, vasculitis, and inherited and acquired hypercoagulable disorders. Carotid or vertebral artery **dissection** may occur spontaneously, after trauma, or in connective tissue disease (e.g., fibromuscular dysplasia). Dissection can be recognized on axial T1 fat suppression MR imaging or angiography. **Vasculitis** may occur in primary central nervous system (CNS) disease or as part of a systemic syndrome such as systemic lupus erythematosus (SLE) or polyarteritis nodosa. **Hypercoagulability** may be due to clotting factor imbalance (protein C, protein S, antithrombin III deficiency) or autoimmunity (antiphospholipid antibodies). Sickle cell disease can also lead to focal cerebral arterial occlusion. Special attention should be given to the possibility of dissection, hypercoagulable states, autoimmune syndromes, and hemoglobinopathies when evaluating stroke in the young.

5. **Acute evaluation** for IV **thrombolysis** should be performed in all patients presenting within 3 hours of symptom onset to an appropriate facility. This includes accurate neurologic assessment, CT or MR imaging to exclude hemorrhage and early ischemic changes, laboratory exclusion of stroke mimics, hemostatic profile (platelets, prothrombin time [PT], activated partial thromboplastin time [aPTT], electrocardiogram [ECG]), and historical/imaging findings consistent with acute ischemia. If available, echo-planar MR with diffusion- and perfusion-weighted imaging or functional CT may provide further insight into vascular anatomy and tissue injury (**Fig. 31-1**). Alternatively, ultrasound may permit rapid and repeatable neurovascular assessment of the carotid bifurcation, cervical vertebral arteries, and intracranial arterial branches. Specialized centers may offer endovascular approaches to reperfusion, including intraarterial thrombolysis, mechanical thrombectomy, or angioplasty. These approaches may provide benefit beyond the 3-hour window of IV tPA, extending this window up to 8 hours in the anterior circulation, and perhaps up to 24 hours in the posterior circulation. The only drug approved for use in acute ischemic stroke remains IV tPA. Therapeutic efforts to extend the use of IV tPA beyond 3 hours have focused on targeting patients with an ischemic penumbra, that is, the region of critically hypoperfused but potentially viable tissue around an irreversibly damaged infarct core. The penumbra can be imaged as a mismatch between perfusion-weighted magnetic resonance imaging (MRI) (PWI) and diffusion-weighted MRI (DWI) and is present in up to 80% of patients within 3 hours of symptom onset,

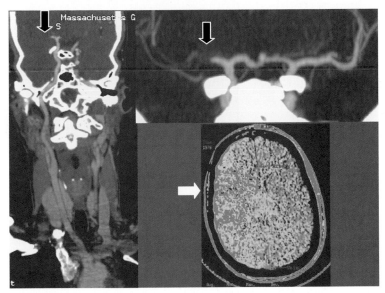

FIGURE 31-1 CT angiography three-dimensional reformatted images in a 28-year-old female demonstrating complete right MCA occlusion due to paradoxiacal embolism through a patent foramen ovale. The initial image shows a curved reformat from the aortic arch to the distal ICA bifurcation. The second image is a magnified view of the MCA stem occlusion. The third is a CT perfusion image showing abnormal perfusion to the right hemisphere in the territory of the occluded artery.

although it diminishes rapidly with time. Advanced CT techniques can also identify similar perfusion parameters as MRI, and have been used to identify mismatch in both clinical trials settings as well as clinical practice. See http://www.acutestroke.com for the Massachusetts General Hospital Acute Stroke Service protocols, and http://www.stroke-center.org for completed and active clinical trials in cerebrovascular disease.

6. **Subacute evaluation** should identify the cause and help define the risk for recurrent stroke. **Echocardiography** with agitated saline contrast injection should be performed to exclude intracardiac thrombus and to assess left ventricular size and function, left atrial size, mitral and aortic valvular disease, and right-to-left shunt. An adequate assessment for intracardiac shunt, including patent *foramen ovale* (PFO), must demonstrate full opacification of the right atrium and physiologic evidence of an increase in right atrial pressure sufficient to demonstrate shunting. **Transesophageal** studies are more sensitive to left atrial thrombus and atheromatous disease of the aortic arch. A 24-hour Holter monitor may identify paroxysmal atrial fibrillation. Particularly in young patients, the cause of the stroke should be vigorously pursued, including evaluation for inherited or acquired hypercoagulable syndromes.

7. **TIAs** are traditionally considered to be sudden, focal neurologic deficits that last less than 24 hours and are believed to be of vascular origin (**Fig. 31-2**). This definition is falling out of favor because ischemic

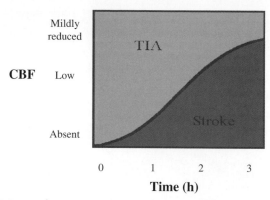

FIGURE 31-2 Graphic representation of cerebral ischemia as a function of both the degree of cerebral blood flow reduction and the duration of ischemia. Relatively mild reductions in blood flow can be tolerated for hours without progression to infarction, whereas steep reductions are poorly tolerated even for less than 1 hour.

symptoms lasting more than several hours almost always are associated with evidence of infarction on advanced imaging techniques (diffusion-weighted imaging [DWI]), and occasionally symptoms lasting only a few minutes also have imaging that demonstrates infarction. Therefore, even transient symptoms consistent with ischemic injury should be evaluated as potential ischemic stroke. Recent data suggest that 5% of TIAs are followed by a stroke within 48 hours, and 10% of patients with a TIA will have a stroke within 3 months. Urgent evaluation of TIAs is imperative for assessing cerebral arterial patency, identifying risk factors for recurrent ischemia, and initiating treatment(s) that can reduce the risk of subsequent stroke.

8. **Acute treatment.** If the time of onset is clearly established to be less than 3 hours and cranial CT excludes intracranial hemorrhage or well-established stroke, all patients with a significant nonresolving deficit and the clinical diagnosis of ischemic stroke are potential candidates for **IV tPA.** A 0.9-mg/kg (maximum 90 mg) dose is infused over 60 minutes with 10% of the total dose administered as an initial IV bolus over 1 minute. Contraindications to IV tPA are summarized in **Table 31-1.** Following IV tPA, no aspirin, heparin, or warfarin should be given for 24 hours. Patients with severe strokes (National Institutes of Health Stroke Scale [NIHSS] >20; **Table 31-2**) have a higher rate of hemorrhage after tPA; however, many centers favor treatment of these patients, given their otherwise unfavorable prognosis. Proximal artery occlusions are less likely to recanalize with IV tPA and are more likely to produce severe clinical deficits.

a. **Mechanical clot retrieval** devices for acute stroke therapy are approved by the Food and Drug Administration for use within 8 hours of symptom onset. Selection of candidates is based on identifying a large-vessel occlusion amenable for treatment with the device within 8 hours since symptom onset. Those likely to benefit are patients with a significant neurological deficit where the irreversible core ischemia in approximately less than one third of the MCA territory or less than 100 cm^3 (**Fig. 31-3**).

T A B L E 31-1	MGH Inclusion and Exclusion Criteria for Administering Intravenous Tissue Plasminogen Activator to Adult Patients with Acute Ischemic Stroke

Inclusion Criteria
- A significant neurologic deficit expected to result in long-term disability
- Noncontrast CT scan showing no hemorrhage or well-established new infarct
- Acute ischemic stroke symptoms with the patient last known well, clearly defined, less than **3 h** before rt-PA will be given

Contraindications
- SBP greater than 185 or DBP greater than 110 mm Hg (despite measures to reduce it)
- CT findings (intracranial hemorrhage, subarachnoid hemorrhage, or major infarct signs)
- Platelets less than 100,000, PTT greater than 40 s after heparin use, or PT greater than 15 or INR greater than 1.7, or known bleeding diathesis
- Recent surgery/trauma (less than 15 d)
- Seizure at onset (with postictal impairments)
- Active internal bleeding (less than 22 d)
- Recent intracranial or spinal surgery, head trauma, or stroke (less than 3 mo)
- History of intracranial hemorrhage or brain aneurysm or vascular malformation or brain tumor
- Suspicion of subarachnoid hemorrhage

Warnings (conditions that might lead to unfavorable outcomes)
- Stroke severity too mild
- Rapid improvement
- Stroke severity—too severe (e.g., NIHSS greater than 22) [Many centers do not exclude patients based on an increased NIHSS alone]
- Glucose less than 50 or greater than 400 mg/dL
- Life expectancy less than 1 y or severe comorbid illness or CMO on admission
- Increased risk of bleeding
  - Subacute bacterial endocarditis
  - Hemostatic defects including those secondary to severe hepatic or renal disease
  - Diabetic hemorrhage retinopathy, or other hemorrhagic ophthalmic conditions
  - Septic thrombophlebitis or occluded AV cannula at seriously infected site
  - Patients currently receiving oral anticoagulants, e.g., warfarin sodium
- Increased risk of bleeding due to pregnancy
- Advanced age (increased risk of bleeding)
- Documented left heart thrombus

From the Massachusetts General Hospital Acute Stroke Services (www.acutestroke.com).
CT, computed tomography; NIHSS, National Institutes of Health Stroke Scale; INR, International Normalized Ratio; tPA, tissue plasminogen activator; CMO, comfort measures only.

    b. Intraarterial thrombolytic (tPA, urokinase) administration can be considered for patients with confirmed large-artery occlusion (by CTA, MRA, or angiography) who are past the 3-hour IV tPA window or ineligible for IV tPA according to national recommendations or locally developed protocols. Doses of up to 1.25 million units of urokinase or up to 22 mg of intraarterial tPA have been used in conjunction with mechanical clot disruption to recanalize proximal arteries and restore function.

    c. Continuous IV **unfractionated heparin,** although without proven benefit in acute stroke, is sometimes used in patients ineligible for thrombolysis and can be considered in patients with basilar

National Institutes of Health Stroke Scale (NIHSS)

TABLE 31-2

NIH Stroke Scale Item (with Abbreviated Scoring Instructions)	Scoring Definitions	Score (0–42)
1a. **Loss of consciousness**	0 = Alert and responsive 1 = Arousable to minor stimulation 2 = Arousable only to painful stimuli 3 = Reflex responses or unarousable	
1b. **Questions**—Ask patient's age and month. Must be exact.	0 = Both correct 1 = One correct (or dysarthria, intubated, foreign language) 2 = Neither correct	
1c. **Commands**—Open/close eyes, grip and release nonparetic hand (other 1 step commands or mimic OK).	0 = Both correct (OK if impaired by weakness) 1 = One correct 2 = Neither correct	
2. **Best gaze**—Horizontal eye movement by voluntary or Doll's eyes.	0 = Normal 1 = Partial gaze palsy, abnl gaze in 1 or both eyes 2 = Forced eye deviation or total paresis which cannot be overcome by Doll's	
3. **Visual field**—Use visual threat if necessary. If monocular, score field of good eye.	0 = Normal 1 = Partial hemianopia, quadrantonopia, extinction 2 = Complete hemianopia 3 = Bilateral hemianopia or blindness	
4. **Facial palsy**—If stuporous, check symmetry of grimace to pain.	0 = Normal 1 = Minor paralysis, flat NLF, asymm smile 2 = Partial paralysis (lower face) 3 = Complete paralysis (upper & lower face)	
5. **Motor arm**—Arms outstretched 90 degrees (sitting) or 45 degrees (supine) for 10 s. Encourage best effort. Score both arms separately.	0 = No drift × 10 s 1 = Drift but doesn't hit bed 2 = Some antigravity effort, but can't sustain 3 = No antigravity effort, but even minimal mvt counts 4 = No movement at all X = unable to assess due to amputation, fusion, fracture, etc.	L R
6. **Motor leg**—Raise leg to 30 degrees supine × 5 s. Score both legs separately.	0 = No drift × 5 s 1 = Drift but doesn't hit bed 2 = Some antigravity effort, but can't sustain 3 = No antigravity effort, but even minimal mvt counts 4 = No movement at all X = Unable to assess due to amputation, fusion, fracture, etc.	L R

NIH Stroke Scale Item (with Abbreviated Scoring Instructions)	Scoring Definitions	Score (0–42)
7. **Limb ataxia**—check finger-nose-finger; heel-shin-knee; and score only if out of proportion to paralysis.	0 = No ataxia (or aphasic, hemiplegic) 1 = Ataxia in upper or lower extremity 2 = Ataxia in upper *and* lower extremity X = Unable to assess due to amputation, fusion, fracture, etc.	L R
8. **Sensory**—use safety pin. Check grimace or withdrawal if stuporous. Score only stroke related losses.	0 = Normal 1 = Mild-mod unilateral loss but pt aware of touch (or aphasic, confused) 2 = Total loss, pt unaware of touch. Coma, bilateral loss	
9. **Best language**—Describe picture, name objects, read sentences. May use repeating, writing, stereognosis.	0 = Normal 1 = Mild-mod aphasia; (difficult but partly comprehensible) 2 = Severe aphasia; (almost no info exchanged) 3 = Mute, global aphasia, coma. No 1 step commands	
10. **Dysarthria**—Read list of words.	0 = Normal 1 = Mild-mod; slurred but intelligible 2 = Severe; unintelligible or mute X = Intubation or mech barrier	
11. **Extinction/neglect**—Simultaneously touch patient on both hands, show fingers in both visual fields, ask about deficit, left hand.	0 = Normal (visual loss alone) 1 = Neglects or extinguishes to double simult stimulation in any modality (visual, auditory, sensory, spatial, body parts) 2 = Profound neglect in more than one modality	

Adapted NIHSS scoring instructions from www.ninds.nih.gov/doctors/NIH_Stroke_Scale.pdf. Brott T, Adams HP Jr, Olinger CP, et al. Measurements of acute cerebral infarction: a clinical examination scale. *Stroke* 1989;20:864–870.

stenosis, internal carotid or extradural vertebral artery dissection, fluctuating deficits, or symptomatic critical carotid stenosis without large MCA infarct. This use must be balanced against the risks of hemorrhagic complications. The aPTT should be monitored every 6 hours and the heparin dose adjusted accordingly. Because of high variability in individual heparin and aPTT assays, the aPTT should be maintained in the desired numerical range based on the levels associated with achieving therapeutic anticoagulation (equivalent to 0.3–0.7 IU/mL by factor Xa inhibition), rather than a simple ratio of 1.5 to 2.5 times control. Initial heparin bolus may raise the risk of hemorrhage and is deferred except in fluctuating deficits or acute basilar thrombosis. While chronic anticoagulation reduces the risk

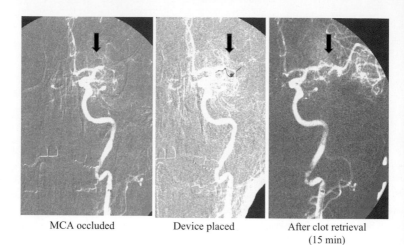

MCA occluded   Device placed   After clot retrieval
(15 min)

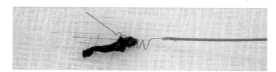

FIGURE 31-3 Serial angiographic images showing occlusion of the left middle cerebral artery, deployment of a clot retrieval device, and restoration of vessel patency. An example of residual thrombus is displayed below. The patient made a full recovery and was discharged several days

of recurrent stroke in patients with atrial fibrillation, in patients with large infarcts, initiation is often deferred for days to weeks to minimize the risk of hemorrhagic transformation. Any patient who experiences a clinical deterioration on heparin must be imaged immediately to rule out **hemorrhagic transformation.**

    d. **Antiplatelet therapy** should be considered for patients who do not qualify for thrombolytic therapy. **Aspirin** in doses ranging from 160 to 1,300 mg daily may benefit patients with **acute stroke** for whom thrombolytics or anticoagulants are not indicated. Other antiplatelet agents such as IV **abciximab** or **eptifibatide** are being studied in acute ischemic stroke. Daily doses of aspirin commonly prescribed for secondary stroke prophylaxis range from 50 to 325 mg, with guidelines for coronary event prevention recommending a minimum dose of 75 mg daily. Combination aspirin (25 mg) plus extended-release **dipyridamole** (200 mg) has been shown to be superior to aspirin alone for secondary prophylaxis. **Clopidogrel,** another antiplatelet agent, is also useful for reducing the risk of recurrent vascular events. Dual antiplatelet therapy is currently not recommended for secondary stroke prophylaxis because of increased risk of major bleeding complications.

    e. Urgent **carotid revascularization** may be indicated in cases of stroke in which there is a critical degree of carotid stenosis, a small distal infarction, and a large territory of vulnerable brain. Revascularization of larger strokes may be associated with acute reperfusion injury and should be delayed by weeks to months.

   f. In some patients with stenosis of major vessels, **pharmacologically induced hypertension** with **phenylephrine** may improve neurologic function acutely and rescue viable brain tissue, perhaps due to penumbral salvage. Early studies suggest that induced hypertension is safe in patients without cardiac comorbidities, such as angina or congestive heart failure. Newly approved devices that create a partial aortic obstruction and augment cerebral perfusion through increased collateral blood flow are under investigation for their potential efficacy in acute stroke.

9. **Subacute treatment.** Hypovolemia and hyponatremia should be avoided, and intravascular volume should be maintained with isotonic solutions. **Fever** should be aggressively controlled because even mild hyperthermia worsens outcome. Swelling is maximal at 2 to 5 days after stroke onset, and standard increased intracranial pressure (ICP) management should be initiated (see **Chapters 10** and **36**). In massive hemispheric or cerebellar infarction, decompressive surgery can be life saving and may improve outcome.

B. **Primary intracerebral hemorrhage (ICH).** The broad differential diagnosis for intracranial bleeding includes ICH, epidural and subdural hemorrhage, SAH (described subsequently), venous sinus thrombosis (also described subsequently), and, rarely, isolated intraventricular hemorrhage. These can often be distinguished initially by noncontrast CT scan, though more advanced imaging (to be discussed) may be required. The most common locations for ICH are basal ganglia, thalamus, cerebral white matter, pons, and cortical lobar surface, but 8% to 10% of incidents occur in cerebellum. **Long-standing hypertension** is the most common cause (75%), although other etiologies are recognized, such as aneurysm, trauma, vascular malformations, amyloid angiopathy, coagulopathies, neoplasms, sympathomimetic drugs, septic emboli, and vasculitis. Metastases, especially adenocarcinoma and melanoma, may present with ICH or swelling. ICH as a primary process should be differentiated from hemorrhagic transformation of ischemic infarction, in which a bland ischemic stroke develops petechial bleeding or turns into a space-occupying hematoma.

   1. **Clinical syndromes.** ICH often presents with headache, nausea, vomiting, and focal neurologic signs similar to those seen in ischemic strokes. The evolution of symptoms may occur more slowly than in ischemic stroke or may cause an acute, devastating picture. As a rule, patients with ICH present with systolic hypertension. In patients who were normotensive at baseline, this usually resolves over the first week; in chronic hypertensive patients, aggressive, multiple-drug treatment is often required to control blood pressure. In contrast to most cortical hemorrhages, the progression to death from cerebellar hemorrhage may be rapid.

      a. **Supratentorial** ICH presents with symptoms referable to the site of bleeding. With rebleeding or development of vasogenic edema or hydrocephalus, there is often worsening of symptoms with decline in arousal. Transtentorial herniation is the mode of death in massive hemorrhage.

      b. **Midline infratentorial** hemorrhage produces only dysequilibrium on standing, walking, and sometimes sitting. Romberg sign cannot be assessed because balance is already impaired with eyes open. If gait is not tested, this lesion may not be detected until other cerebellar signs emerge secondary to brain swelling. **Lateral cerebellar hemispheric** lesions produce symptoms ipsilateral to the lesion. Patients complain of limb incoordination and demonstrate ataxia with falling toward the side of lesion, dysmetria (overshoot) on finger-nose-finger testing, dysdiadokinesia (inaccuracy on rapid alternating movements), intentional tremor (exaggerated on approaching the target), and nystagmus (worse looking toward lesion). Speech may be dysarthric (slurred) or explosive.

2. **Acute evaluation** of patients with suspected ICH consists of brain imaging; both CT and MR are very sensitive. In addition, toxicology screen, PT, aPTT, and platelets should be checked and signs of occult malignancy excluded. Hemorrhage volume correlates with outcome, and can be estimated easily in cubic centimeters on unenhanced head CT using the "ABC/2" method, where A is the greatest diameter of the hemorrhage on a single slice, B is the hemorrhage diameter perpendicular to A on the same slice, and C is the approximate number of axial CT slices revealing hemorrhage multiplied by slice thickness in centimeters. Thirty-day mortality for patients with a parenchymal hemorrhage volume of greater than 60 cm^3 on their initial CT and a Glasgow Coma Scale (GCS) score of 8 or less is 90%, and for those with a volume of less than 30 cm^3 and a GCS score of 9 or greater it is 20%. The FUNC score is a recently validated clinical assessment tool that predicts, at hospital admission, functional independence at 90 days, and is available for use to clinicians (http://www.massgeneral.org/stopstroke/funcCalculator.aspx). **Subacute evaluation** should identify the etiology by imaging and history. MR imaging with susceptibility may identify areas of prior occult cortical hemorrhage and suggest a diagnosis of amyloid angiopathy in patients with lobar ICH. Repeat MR in 3 to 6 weeks may also detect lesions (e.g., tumor) masked by acute hemorrhage. Rarely, aneurysmal hemorrhage may result in primarily parenchymal hematoma, mimicking ICH. Conventional contrast angiography or CTA is indicated in any suspicious case. Prognosis is based on clinical presentation and imaging findings. Patients with cerebellar lesions less than 2 cm in diameter or with self-limited cerebellar signs usually do well, those with 3-cm lesions or progressive drowsiness do poorly without intervention, and 20% have lesions greater than 3 cm and a poor prognosis regardless of treatment. Prognosis in patients with cortical ICH is also related to hematoma size. It should be noted, however, that the most common cause of death in large ICH is withdrawal of supportive care, and the prognosis for large ICH with extended rehabilitation is less clear.

3. **Acute treatment** consists largely of supportive care, blood pressure control, reversal of coagulopathy, and ICP monitoring or surgical intervention in selected cases. To correct elevated PT, **vitamin K,** 10 mg infused at 1 mg/min, should be given IV, accompanied by rapid transfusion of fresh frozen plasma (FFP); **protamine** is used for elevated aPTT. Platelets should be provided to patients with platelet counts less than 100,000; patients who have uremic or pharmacologic (e.g., aspirin) platelet dysfunction may benefit from **desmopressin.** Reduction of systolic blood pressure to a target blood pressure of 160/90 is important to prevent rebleeding; If SBP is >200 mm Hg or MAP is >150 mm Hg, aggressive reduction of blood pressure with continuous IV infusion, with frequent blood pressure monitoring every 5 minutes is advised. If SBP is >180 mm Hg or MAP is >130 mm Hg and there is evidence of or

suspicion of elevated ICP, then consider monitoring ICP and reducing blood pressure using intermittent or continuous IV medications to keep cerebral perfusion pressure >60 to 80 mm Hg. Any clinical deterioration in association with reduction of BP should prompt reconsideration of ongoing BP management strategy. β-Blockers such as **labetalol** are preferred for blood pressure control, given their additional benefit of being antiarrhythmic; conversely, nitrates may paradoxically increase ICP by dilating the cerebral vasculature. IV calcium channel blockers such as **nicardipine** may be useful if further reduction in blood pressure is needed. **Neurosurgical consultation** should be obtained early, especially in cerebellar hemorrhage of diameter 2 cm or greater. Resection of lobar or basal ganglia ICH can be life saving. Surgical methods include open craniotomy and stereotactic drainage. Intraventricular tPA may also improve outcome in patients with intraventricular extension of the ICH. Recombinant activated **factor VIIa** has recently been reported to reduce hematoma expansion following ICH, but has failed to reduce death or severe disability at 90 days. Although failing to demonstrate clinical benefit, the trials of recombinant activated factor VIIa have suggested possible venues for further investigation. **Obstructive or communicating hydrocephalus** may develop, and usually requires external ventricular drainage, although it may not need permanent ventricular shunting (**Fig. 31-4**). Corticosteroids do not appear to be of benefit in ICH unless there is further deterioration due to vasogenic edema. **Anticonvulsant therapy** is indicated in cases with seizure, where the hematoma extends to the cortex, or when the consequence of a seizure itself would be deleterious (e.g., refractory ICP, coagulopathy, unstable fractures).

4. When **ICH** is suspected **in patients who received thrombolysis for acute stroke,** a head CT should be obtained immediately, along with neurosurgical and hematologic consultation, PT, aPTT, complete blood count (CBC), and D-dimer and fibrinogen concentrations. Treatment of verified symptomatic hematoma includes use of 2 U of **FFP** to replete factors V and VII, 20 U of **cryoprecipitate** to replete fibrinogen, and 6 U of **platelets.** Patients treated with heparin should receive **protamine** IV push, 1 mg per each 100 units of unfractionated heparin given in the preceding 4 hours. If an anticoagulant dose of low-molecular-weight heparin had been used, the maximum dose of protamine (50 mg) should be given. The foregoing laboratory values should be repeated every hour for the next 4 hours until bleeding is brought under control. If these measures fail to control bleeding, **aminocaproic acid,** 5 g IV over 1 hour, may be given.

C. **Cerebral venous thrombosis (CVT)** most commonly occurs in the sagittal, transverse, or straight sinus (often called venous sinus thrombosis), although the clot may extend into the vein of Galen or the internal jugular vein. Smaller, cortical venous thromboses can also occur, as can cavernous sinus thrombosis. CVT may occur in the setting of infection, tumor, trauma, hypovolemia, coagulation disorders, systemic inflammatory diseases, oral contraceptive use, pregnancy, and the puerperium. Despite a thorough diagnostic evaluation, nearly 25% of cases will be deemed idiopathic.

1. The **clinical syndrome** includes signs of increased ICP such as headache, nausea, and vomiting, often more pronounced after prolonged recumbency. Focal neurologic signs or seizures may be seen in the setting of vasogenic edema or venous infarction. Without recanalization, altered

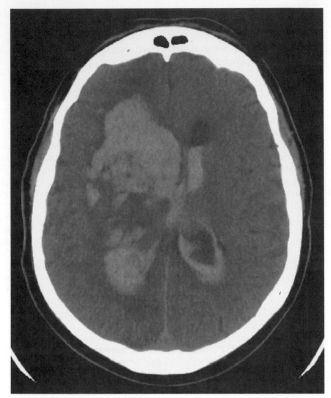

FIGURE 31-4 Axial image from an unenhanced CT of the brain showing a large right intracerebral hemorrhage with extension into the lateral ventricles and early obstructive hydrocephalus requiring ventriculostomy.

sensorium can progress to coma. If the diagnosis is not considered, it is often overlooked until venous hemorrhage has occurred.

2. **Acute evaluation** relies on an imaging. CT with contrast may demonstrate filling defects in the superior sagittal sinus and torcula ("empty delta" sign) in up to 30% of patients, parenchymal abnormalities suggestive of deranged venous drainage in up to 60% of patients, small ventricles from increased ICP, or contrast enhancement of the falx and tentorium from venous hypertension. CT or MR venography provides enhanced sensitivity. Transfemoral angiography is diagnostic if MR is inconclusive. Lumbar puncture may demonstrate an elevated opening pressure, increased protein and red cells, and mild pleocytosis.

3. **Acute treatment** is effective if initiated early, but prognosis for recovery worsens significantly without treatment. Continuous IV unfractionated **heparin** titrated to aPTT of 60 to 80 should be given and maintained until the patient stabilizes or improves. Heparin should be given even in the presence of hemorrhage. In certain cases of extensive

thrombosis or rapid deterioration in patient condition, transvenous thrombolysis with locally injected chemical thrombolytic or mechanical clot disruption should be considered at experienced centers. Measures to control ICP elevation and prophylaxis for seizures must be undertaken, and factors that exacerbate clotting (e.g., dehydration) must be avoided.

D. Subarachnoid hemorrhage (SAH) may be traumatic or nontraumatic. Nontraumatic SAH is caused most commonly by the **rupture of a cerebral aneurysm.** The majority of aneurysms arise from the carotid artery circulation, most commonly the ACA and less frequently the posterior communicating artery or the MCA. Posterior circulation aneurysms commonly arise from the basilar tip or may also result from intradural vertebral dissections with pseudoaneurysm formation and rupture. Aneurysms may exist on a congenital basis, arise in the setting of atherosclerosis, or more rarely occur due to infection (mycotic) or emboli. Rupture of cerebral aneurysms releases blood into the subarachnoid space and causes up to 30% mortality in the first 24 hours. The primary brain injury may be anything from minimal to lethal, and abrupt loss of consciousness at onset is characteristic. Rebleeding of untreated aneurysms occurs in up to 30% of patients in the first 28 days, with 70% mortality. Hypotension, aspiration pneumonia, neurogenic pulmonary edema, seizures, obstructive hydrocephalus, or ischemia due to vasospasm may produce secondary brain injury. Serial examination and brain imaging can identify symptoms suggestive of most of these complications, but separate techniques are necessary to distinguish vasospasm.

1. **Clinical syndromes.** The "worst headache of my life" complaint should raise suspicion of SAH. Nausea, vomiting, altered sensorium, and focal cranial nerve defects (especially third-nerve palsy) are associated with SAH. A warning headache may occur due to a sentinel bleed in which blood may be confined to the aneurysm wall without true SAH. Clinical grading predicts outcome (**Table 31-3**) and risk of vasospasm (**Table 31-4**).

2. **Acute evaluation. CT scan** is the best initial test for SAH, and will detect SAH in approximately 95% of cases. Lumbar puncture should be performed in cases where SAH is suspected and CT is negative. Xanthochromia is a helpful sign of old blood products in the CSF, but it takes at least 4 hours to develop. Angiography should be performed

TABLE 31-3	Classification of Patients with Intracranial Aneurysms According to Surgical Risk (Hunt and Hess Classification System)
Grade	**Characteristics**
I	Asymptomatic or minimal headache and slight nuchal rigidity
II	Moderate to severe headache, nuchal rigidity, no neurologic deficit other than cranial nerve palsy
III	Drowsiness, confusion, mild focal deficit
IV	Stupor, moderate to severe hemiparesis, possibly early decerebrate rigidity, vegetative disturbances
V	Deep coma, decerebrate rigidity, moribund

In the original classification, one grade was added if major concurrent health problems were present such as lung, heart, liver, or kidney comorbities. In current practice, many centers do not add a grade for medical comorbidities.

urgently if SAH is suspected. A small proportion of SAH cases will have normal angiography. Follow-up imaging is needed in most cases, and attention should be given to base-of-skull arteriovenous fistulas and aneurysms compressed by hematoma. MR or CTA may also reveal aneurysms and may help with surgical planning. With improved surgical and anesthetic techniques, early aneurysm localization with angiography and early definitive aneurysm repair have greatly improved outcome. Concerns that angiography itself might lead to aneurysmal rebleeding have proven unwarranted.

3. **Subsequent evaluation.** Transfemoral angiography remains the gold standard for documenting vasospasm; however, it is invasive and carries some risk. **Vasospasm** may develop at any time, but is most frequent between days 4 and 14 post rupture. Many centers perform **serial transcranial Doppler ultrasound** to detect presymptomatic narrowing of cerebral vessels at the base of the brain. Risk of clinically significant vasospasm can be predicted by classifying the presence of focal collections of blood on the CT scan in the area around the circle of Willis arteries (Fisher groups 1–4; see **Table 31-4**). This method was first described by CM Fisher and colleagues using unscaled measurements based off hard copy printed films obtained at 24 hours post SAH but prior to surgery. In the modern era of early surgical intervention for ruptured aneurysms, the findings on the initial CT may be less reliable, and the exact clot thickness required for each group is subject to interpretation.

4. **Acute treatment** consists of definitive obliteration of the culprit aneurysm (clipping or endovascular therapy) and prevention of delayed ischemic deficits. Systolic arterial blood pressure should be strictly controlled (<140 mm Hg) until the aneurysm is secured. Surgery, endovascular therapy, or both are performed urgently; intervention choice is based on aneurysm location, anatomy, patient comorbidities, surgical and endovascular risk, and operator experience. A calcium channel antagonist, **nimodipine,** 60 mg orally every 4 hours given for 21 days, reduces ischemic symptoms from 33% to 22%. In addition, **magnesium**

TABLE 31-4	Classification of Subarachnoid Hemorrhage According to Risk of Vasospasm (Fisher Group Classification System)
Group[a]	**Characteristics of Subarachnoid Hemorrhage on Computed Tomography Scan**
1	No detectable subarachnoid blood, or trace diffuse blood
2	Diffuse blood with clot less than 3×5[b] mm (in axial plane) and less than 1 mm in vertical layer
3	Blood clot greater than 3×5 mm (in axial plane) or greater than 1 mm in vertical layer
4	Intracerebral or intraventricular blood with no detectable subarachnoid or only minimal diffuse subarachnoid blood

[a]The Fisher system does not refer to progressive grades of vasospasm risk, but rather to distinct groups. Only Group 3 (and not Group 4) was associated with a risk of severe symptomatic vasospasm (>95%). Patients with focal clot in basal cisterns plus intracerebral hemorrhage would still be Group 3.
[b]This method was first described using unscaled measurements based off hard copy printed films obtained at 24 hours post SAH but prior to surgery. In the modern era of early surgical intervention for ruptured aneurysms, the findings on the initial CT may be less reliable, and the exact clot thickness required for each group is subject to interpretation.

sulfate continuous infusion started within 72 hours after aneurysmal SAH has been shown to reduce delayed ischemic complications by 34%. Barring all contraindications for magnesium therapy, the infusion is started after the aneurysm is secured and continued for 14 days at levels of 3 to 4.5 meq/L as tolerated. Further therapy is focused on maximizing cerebral blood flow and oxygen utilization to minimize the clinical sequelae of vasospasm. This is generally accomplished by creating a hyperdynamic state with induced hypertension, hypervolemia, and optimal oxygen-carrying capacity. Release of natriuretic factors causes **cerebral salt wasting** and subsequent volume loss, with resultant serum hypo-osmolarity and urine hyperosmolarity. The **treatment for cerebral salt wasting is volume repletion** with IV saline, either normal saline (0.9%) or **hypertonic saline** solutions. Volume restriction, which would be appropriate for syndrome of inappropriate antidiuretic hormone (ADH) secretion (SIADH), should be avoided because it leads rapidly to hypovolemia, hypotension, and decreased blood flow distal to areas of vasospasm. Oral NaCl tablets and mineralocorticoid administration (**fludrocortisone,** 0.1 mg orally twice a day) may also be useful. **Albumin** (250 mL of 5% albumin every 6–8 hours) is often used in addition to normal saline to keep central venous pressures at 8 to 12 mm Hg. It has been the practice for patients with Fisher group 3 hemorrhage or evidence of vasospasm to be given blood transfusions to maintain a hemoglobin concentration of at least 9.0 g/dL; the intention is to support an optimal balance of oxygen-carrying capacity and blood viscosity in areas with compromised cerebral perfusion. Recent studies in other clinical scenarios have raised some question about the relative benefit of transfusion. Induced hypertension with an α-adrenergic agonist such as **phenylephrine** is safe and effective at reversing ischemic symptoms due to decreased cerebral blood flow in patients with vasospasm. The hypercatecholaminergic state following SAH can trigger the development of a stunned myocardium and acute heart failure; this condition, although usually fully reversible, can result in several days of marked global cardiac hypokinesis. When combined with the need for induced hypertension, this requires in some patients invasive hemodynamic monitoring and inotropic support with agents such as **norepinephrine** or **dobutamine.** In refractory vasospasm or in patients who cannot tolerate induced hypertension, intraarterial vasodilators such as **nicardipine** or the use of **balloon angioplasty** may alleviate cerebral ischemia. In spite of an increased risk for complications, they have become a mainstay of therapy, because of their ability to reduce major ischemic events. **Intraarterial milrinone,** a phosphodiesterase inhibitor, combines vasodilating and inotropic properties, and can be infused in the involved cerebral territories followed by continuous IV infusion. Milrinone has not yet been studied widely, but shows initial promising results in increasing vessel diameter with preservation of blood pressure. Newer, multimodal intracerebral monitors, including brain tissue oxygenation and cerebral microdialysis catheters, may provide early warning signs of vasospasm and help to guide appropriate therapy. Evidence for prophylactic anticonvulsant therapy is limited, but it may be helpful in the first 2 weeks, especially in those patients in whom seizure would be deleterious, such as patients with markedly increased ICP. No benefit from corticosteroids has been demonstrated in patients with SAH.

II. Seizures may occur in more than 10% of patients during their ICU stay. Repeated tonic-clonic seizures may be easily recognized and they must be treated early; uncontrolled generalized motor seizures that persist for more than 60 minutes are associated with significant increases in neuronal injury and mortality. Conversely, nonconvulsive seizures are often undetected; up to 8% of comatose patients *with no outward evidence of seizure* have been found to have ongoing nonconvulsive seizures. While single seizures should prompt a search for etiology and subsequent correction of inciting conditions and/or seizure prophylaxis, **status epilepticus** (continuous seizure lasting longer than 5 minutes, or more than one seizure without restoration of appropriate mental status) is a medical emergency. **Table 31-5** summarizes common causes of seizures in the ICU.

TABLE 31-5	Common Etiologies of Seizures in the Intensive Care Unit

Neurologic Pathology
Neurovascular
   Ischemic or hemorrhagic stroke
   Vascular malformation
Tumor
   Primary
   Metastatic
Infection
   Abscess
   Meningitis
   Encephalitis
Inflammatory disease
   Vasculitis
   Acute disseminated encephalomyelitis
Trauma
Primary epilepsy
Inherited central nervous system metabolic disturbance

Complications of Critical Illness
Hypoxia
Drug/substance toxicity
Drug/substance withdrawals
   Anticonvulsants
   Barbiturates
   Benzodiazepines
   Alcohol
Fever (febrile seizures)
Infection
Metabolic abnormalities
   Hyponatremia
   Hypocalcemia
   Hypophosphatemia
   Hypoglycemia
   Renal/hepatic dysfunction
Surgical manipulation (craniotomy)

Adapted from Varelas PN, Mirski MA. Seizures in the adult intensive care unit. *J Neurosurg Anesthesiol* 2001;13:163–175.

A. **Clinical syndrome.** Seizures may be categorized into multiple subtypes. The most relevant in the ICU are generalized tonic-clonic, partial complex, and an unremitting form of either (status epilepticus). In **generalized tonic-clonic seizures,** patients present with stiffening, followed by limb jerking and impaired consciousness, often accompanied by hyperdynamic vital signs. Seizures with subtle motor manifestations may go unrecognized in critically ill patients; careful observation of a patient may reveal subtle but evident rhythmic limb or facial movements indicative of seizure. **Partial complex seizures** produce a decrease in responsiveness without a complete loss of consciousness. They may be accompanied by stereotypic limb movements (e.g., chewing, blinking, swallowing), but not rhythmic limb jerking.

B. Other conditions mimicking seizure include benign entities (myoclonus, fasciculations, tremor, spasticity) and potentially dangerous entities (brainstem ischemia, rigors, metabolic encephalopathy). For example, sudden onset of bilateral arm and leg posturing coupled with impaired eye movements is often seen in acute basilar artery occlusion. When in doubt, neurologic consultation and electroencephalogram (EEG) should be requested. For detection of ongoing subclinical seizures, long-term video-EEG monitoring may be of benefit, and should be considered in critically ill patients with unexplained alterations in level of consciousness.

C. **Acute evaluation** consists in confirming the diagnosis and identifying potential causes. In many cases, EEG is not required due to obvious motor signs. All patients should undergo laboratory screen including CBC, electrolytes, blood urea nitrogen (BUN), creatinine, glucose, Ca, Mg, PO_4, liver function tests (including NH_3), anticonvulsant medications levels, blood and urine toxicology screen, and, when indicated, pregnancy test and arterial blood gases. CT scan and lumbar puncture may be necessary to establish the underlying diagnosis once seizures are controlled. Physical examination should look for signs of occult head trauma, substance abuse, fever, meningismus, and diabetes. Always check for Medical Alert bracelets or wallet information, and try to contact relatives or neighbors to determine prior medical and seizure history. Nonconvulsive status epilepticus can only be diagnosed by EEG. An EEG can also document triphasic waveforms suggestive of metabolic encephalopathy. Long-acting muscle relaxants in the absence of EEG monitoring have **no role** in the initial management of uncontrolled seizures, except in patients who cannot otherwise be adequately ventilated.

D. **Acute treatment** consists in safely aborting seizures as early as possible with the appropriate degree of intervention. Most patients require no intervention and will spontaneously recover after one seizure. Some patients require **benzodiazepines** and **phenytoin** without intubation, while some extreme cases may require **pentobarbital** anesthesia. Management by defined protocol is the best method for assuring that patients are treated promptly, and a thorough evaluation must be completed as soon as the patient is stabilized. A standard protocol approach is outlined in **Table 31-6.**

E. Proper **phenytoin drug maintenance** dosing can be confirmed by sending phenytoin levels 20 minutes after the loading dose in patients who are still seizing. When treating status epilepticus, aim for uncorrected levels of 20 to 30 µg/mL. Once seizures are controlled, phenytoin maintenance dosing is 300 to 400 mg/d, with a target serum level of 10 to 20 µg/mL. Because phenytoin is largely albumin bound and renally excreted, **correction for hypoalbuminemia** or acute renal failure is necessary once the acute episode

TABLE 31-6   Protocol for Treating Status Epilepticus

0–2 min   Assess basic life support
- Start supplemental oxygen; monitor O_2 saturation
- Initiate seizure precautions (e.g., padding bed rails)
- Obtain seizure history
- Look for evidence of head trauma or toxic ingestion/injection
- Send urine and blood toxicology, electrolytes, blood urea nitrogen, creatinine, glucose, Ca, Mg, osmolarity, anticonvulsant drug levels
- Consider prophylactic therapy (e.g., phenytoin)

2–5 min   **If the initial seizure has not stopped, or has stopped and restarted**
- Give 2 mg IV **lorazepam,** every 2 min, up to 0.1 mg/kg
- If lorazepam is not immediately available, diazepam 10–20 mg or midazolam 2–5 mg can be substituted
- Start **phenytoin** 20 mg/kg IV load at $\geq$50 mg/min
- Phenytoin IV can cause bradycardia, hypotension, and full-blown cardiovascular collapse, and therefore must be given in a monitored setting
- In a patient with epilepsy presumed on phenytoin, give 10 mg/kg while awaiting drug levels
- Fosphenytoin can be substituted for phenytoin at a dose of 20 mg phenytoin equivalents (PE)/kg IV at $\leq$150 mg PE/min
- Begin IV normal saline, give **thiamine** 100 mg IV and **dextrose** 25–50 g IV if blood glucose is <60 mg/100 dL
- Treat fever with acetaminophen and ice packs
- Consider intubation to maintain airway patency
- Check arterial blood gas

6–30 min
- Monitor electrocardiogram, airway; check blood pressure every 60 s
- Repeat benzodiazepines every 15 min for continued motor seizures during phenytoin load
- Determine presumptive pathophysiologic mechanism

31–50 min
- Give **phenobarbital** 10–20 mg/kg IV at $\leq$70 mg/min
- Many patients require endotracheal intubation and mechanical ventilation by this point in the protocol
- Call for urgent continuous EEG monitoring and obtain expert consultation

>50 min
- Give **pentobarbital** 3–5 mg/kg IV to induce burst suppression; in most adults, pentobarbital bolus 400 mg over 15 min then 100 mg every 15–30 min until burst suppression appears is reasonably well tolerated, followed by an infusion at 0.3–9.0 mg/kg/h to maintain burst suppression
  - Alternative agents include the following:
    Midazolam drip (may be preferable if blood pressure is unstable) 0.2 mg/kg slow IV push, followed by 0.1–2.0 mg/kg/h to stop electrographic and clinical seizures; or
    Propofol 2-mg/kg load and 2–10 mg/kg/h to stop clinical and electrographic seizures or maintain burst suppression on EEG
    Valproate 15-mg/kg IV load may be useful as an adjunctive agent.
- For all infusions, decrease the infusion periodically to check the EEG pattern that is being suppressed; if electrocerebral silence ("flatline") occurs, always decrease the dose until bursts are seen again
- Prepare an infusion of α-agonist (e.g., phenylephrine) for treatment of anticipated hypotension

EEG, electroencephalogram; IV, intravenous.

is controlled: phenytoin (corrected) = phenytoin(measured)/[(0.2 × albumin) + 0.1] for low albumin, and phenytoin (corrected) = phenytoin (measured)/[(0.1 × albumin) + 0.1] for low albumin and acute renal failure. Recently, the FDA has approved levetiracetam IV for use as an adjunctive therapy in the treatment of partial-onset seizures in adults with epilepsy. IV levetiracetam is an alternative for patients when oral administration is temporarily unavailable. Though not approved in status epilepticus, some centers include IV levetiracetam in their status treatment protocol.

III. Encephalopathy

A. Toxic-metabolic injury to the CNS is a frequent and reversible cause of impaired cognition in the ICU, but always remains a diagnosis of exclusion. Frequent causes include medication effects; perturbations in electrolyte, water, glucose, or urea homeostasis; acute renal or hepatic failure; sleep disturbances; and psychiatric disturbances. Treatment is supportive, with removal of the offending agent when possible. Hyperammonemia with or without signs of liver abnormality can cause profound encephalopathy and increased ICP, and often responds to oral **lactulose** and reduction of nitrogen (protein) intake. Wernicke's encephalopathy, secondary to thiamine deficiency (usually in alcoholics, and occasionally in persons on severe diet regimens or other rapid reduction in nutrition), presents with ataxia, eye movement paralysis, nystagmus, apathy, or confusion. Treatment includes **thiamine** 100 mg IV, which should be continued daily for at least 5 days.

B. Hypertensive encephalopathy is due to sustained, severe hypertension or relative hypertension with impaired autoregulation. Early, reversible symptoms are likely due to blood–brain barrier disruption and vasogenic edema; with sustained hypertension, cerebral hemorrhage and irreversible injury may occur. Because acute elevations in blood pressure may be seen commonly in many types of brain injury in which antihypertensive therapy could be deleterious (e.g., ischemic stroke, traumatic brain injury), accurate diagnosis is essential. Clinical manifestations range from headache and visual scotoma to confusion, seizures, and coma. The likelihood of recovery depends on the extent of injury prior to treatment. **Head CT** is insensitive and may reveal bilateral posterior-predominant subcortical hypodensity. **MR** imaging reveals T2 and apparent diffusion coefficient hyperintensity with a posterior predilection, which may also involve diffuse subcortical white matter, cortical gray matter, and cerebellum; gradient-echo sequences often reveal microscopic petechial hemorrhages. Management of hypertensive crisis is outlined in **Chapter 6.** Most patients with hypertensive encephalopathy have underlying chronic hypertension. This shifts upward the range of pressures at which cerebrovascular autoregulation occurs.

C. Infectious/inflammatory

1. The most treatable **viral encephalitis** (and second most common after HIV) is due to acute **herpes simplex** infection. Patients present with headaches, fever, seizure, or cognitive impairments. Early in the course, there is a CSF lymphocytosis (5–500 cells/mm^3) with normal glucose and mild increases in protein, followed by hemorrhagic necrosis with bloody CSF. The EEG shows characteristic bursts of periodic high-voltage slow waves, and MR imaging reveals temporal and inferior frontal lobe involvement. CSF polymerase chain reaction (PCR) is extremely sensitive, although false negatives can occur, especially in the setting of very high CSF leukocytosis. Because therapy with **acyclovir** (10 mg/kg every 8 hours) reduces mortality and morbidity, it should be instituted in any suggestive case. Other forms of viral encephalitis, including those due to human herpes viruses 6 and 7, Epstein-Barr virus, cytomegalovirus, and varicella zoster virus, may respond to specific antiviral treatments. Encephalitis due to arboviruses (arthropod-borne viruses) such as eastern equine, California, and St. Louis encephalitis, do not respond to acyclovir but can present in a similar manner. West Nile encephalitis commonly presents with paraparesis in addition to headache, fever, and encephalopathy. Vasogenic edema, seizures, and increased ICP may occur in all of these disorders, and patients require close monitoring in an ICU setting.

2. **Bacterial meningitis** must be diagnosed and treated rapidly, although in the early hours it may be clinically indistinguishable from viral meningoencephalitis. Acute onset of headache, meningeal signs (neck stiffness, photophobia), fever, and altered sensorium should suggest the diagnosis of acute bacterial meningitis. Etiology, diagnosis, and treatment of meningitis are outlined in Chapter 29.

3. **Acute disseminated encephalomyelitis (ADEM) and acute hemorrhagic leukoencephalitis (AHL).** Often preceded by a routine viral illness or mycoplasma pneumonia, these infections present with cerebral demyelination (ADEM) or hemorrhage (AHL) and **malignant cerebral edema.** Initial presentations have variable localizing signs, but encephalopathy, stupor, and coma ensue rapidly. Early brain MR can reveal characteristic demyelination, edema, and/or widespread petechial hemorrhage, with markedly increased CSF protein concentration. High-dose IV **methylprednisolone** and supportive care should be provided. ADEM has a better prognosis than AHL.

4. **Other infectious agents and inflammatory conditions.** Granulomatous diseases such as sarcoidosis as well as fungal, mycobacterial, and protein infectious (prion) agents can also affect the CNS and lead to encephalopathy. Characteristic imaging or CSF analysis may be helpful, but tissue biopsy is often required to diagnose these more uncommon etiologies.

Selected References

Albers GW, Amarenco P, Easton JD, et al. Antithrombotic and thrombolytic therapy for ischemic stroke: the Seventh ACCP Conference on Antithrombotic and Thrombolytic Therapy. *Chest* 2004;126:483S–512S.

Bousser MG. Cerebral venous thrombosis: diagnosis and management. *J Neurol* 2000;247:252–258.

Broderick J, Connolly S, Feldmann E, et al. Guidelines for the management of spontaneous intracerebral hemorrhage in adults: 2007 update: a guideline from the American Heart Association/American Stroke Association Stroke Council, High Blood Pressure Research Council, and the Quality of Care and Outcomes in Research Interdisciplinary Working Group. *Stroke* 2007;38:2001–2023.

Davis SM, Donnan GA, Parsons MW, et al. Effects of alteplase beyond 3 hours after stroke in the Echoplanar Imaging Thrombolytic Evaluation Trial (EPITHET): a placebo-controlled randomised trial. *Lancet Neurol* 2008;7:299–309.

de Gans J, van de Beek D. Dexamethasone in adults with bacterial meningitis. *N Engl J Med* 2002;347:1549–1556.

Fisher CM, Kistler JP, Davis JM. Relation of cerebral vasospasm to subarachnoid hemorrhage visualized by computerized tomographic scanning. *Neurosurgery* 1980;6:1–9.

Johnston SC, Gress DR, Browner WS, et al. Short-term prognosis after emergency department diagnosis of TIA. *JAMA* 2000;284:2901–2906.

Kidwell CS, Alger JR, Saver JL. Beyond mismatch: evolving paradigms in imaging the ischemic penumbra with multimodal magnetic resonance imaging. *Stroke* 2003;34:2729–2735.

Mayberg MR, Batjer HH, Dacey R, et al. Guidelines for the management of aneurysmal sub-arachnoid hemorrhage. A statement for healthcare professionals from a special writing group of the Stroke Council, American Heart Association. *Stroke* 1994;25:2315–2328.

Rordorf G, Koroshetz WJ, Ezzeddine MA, et al. A pilot study of drug-induced hypertension for treatment of acute stroke. *Neurology* 2001;56:1210–1213.

Rost NS, Smith EE, Chang Y, et al. Prediction of functional outcome in patients with primary intracerebral hemorrhage. The FUNC score. *Stroke* 2008;39:7.

Shneker BF, Fountain NB. Assessment of acute morbidity and mortality in nonconvulsive sta-tus epilepticus. *Neurology* 2003;61:1066–1073.

van Gijn J, Rinkel GJ. Subarachnoid haemorrhage: diagnosis, causes and management. *Brain* 2001;124:249–278.

Varelas PN, Mirski MA. Seizures in the adult intensive care unit. *J Neurosurg Anesthesiol* 2001;13:163–175.

32

Acute Weakness

David Greer and Edward George

I. Introduction

A. **Acute weakness in the intensive care unit (ICU)** can be caused by diseases affecting the **central nervous system (CNS)**, the **peripheral nervous system**, or **muscles**. A **careful history** can often elucidate the underlying cause and cue the correct workup. This should include recent neurologic symptoms, injuries, current medications, alcohol or illicit drug use, travel, potential envenomations or neurotoxin exposures, and accompanying sensory or autonomic symptoms.

B. Focal or lateralizing signs on examination should suggest a CNS cause, including a cerebrovascular event (ischemic or hemorrhagic), focal abscess or encephalitis, traumatic brain injury, or brainstem process.

C. Injury to the **brainstem** may cause symmetric weakness in the extremities, and the key to the examination is a careful cranial nerve examination (pupillary reactions, corneal responses, eye movements). Central pontine myelinolysis also causes symmetric weakness, with prominent eye movement abnormalities. Brainstem processes commonly cause a depressed level of consciousness.

D. Injury to the cervical **spinal cord** initially causes a flaccid quadriparesis, areflexia, and a sensory level loss depending on the level and extent of the injury. Later, hyperreflexia, urinary and bowel retention develop.

E. As a rule, **myopathic disorders** cause weakness primarily of proximal muscles, with relative sparing of deep tendon reflexes (DTRs) and sensation. **Neuropathic disorders** cause more distal weakness, loss of sensation, dysautonomia, and depressed DTRs. In the ICU setting, critical illness neuropathy and myopathy often coexist. Diseases of the neuromuscular junction often affect the respiratory muscles early, and involve the cranial musculature (especially eye movements) and proximal (limb-girdle) muscles.

F. **Laboratory and instrumental evaluation** should include a complete blood count with eosinophil count, erythrocyte sedimentation rate to aid in the diagnosis of vasculitis or myositis, liver function tests, blood urea nitrogen, creatinine, urinalysis, electrolytes, calcium, magnesium, phosphorus, and creatine phosphokinase (CPK). Other useful tests in specific instances may include a serum lactate level and antibody testing for an underlying connective tissue disorder (e.g., SLE or RA) or inflammatory disorder (e.g., myasthenia gravis or Guillain-Barré syndrome [GBS]). Patients with respiratory symptoms should have chest radiography, which may reveal, in addition to intrinsic lung disease, a potential cause for weakness (e.g., thymic enlargement with myasthenia gravis, lung mass with paraneoplastic disease, etc.). A lumbar puncture should be performed if GBS is considered. Electromyography with nerve conduction studies (EMG/NCS) may be needed to help establish a diagnosis, with nerve and/or muscle biopsy occasionally required.

II. CNS causes

A. Stroke, either ischemic or hemorrhagic, is described in **Chapter 31.** The **sudden onset of neurologic symptoms and signs** prompts an immediate evaluation. The level of consciousness may be affected, depending on the size and location of the stroke (e.g., brainstem or ventricular system). The initial steps in the workup, after stabilization of the patient, include neuroimaging. Noncontrast computed tomography (CT) should be performed to exclude an intracranial hemorrhage, and then CT angiography and CT perfusion if needed.

B. Primary brainstem processes, in addition to ischemic or hemorrhagic stroke, can include **central pontine myelinolysis.** This occurs after rapid correction of a hypo-osmolar state (typically hyponatremia) that has been present for at least 48 hours. Patients have an impaired level of consciousness, ranging from confusion to coma. Paresis involves the upper extremities more than the lower extremities, and sixth nerve palsies and rigidity are common. Other ocular abnormalities include miotic or mydriatic pupils, conjugate gaze palsies, and ocular bobbing. The purported cause for the abnormal response in the pons is that oligodendrocytes in the pons are located close to the highly vascularized gray matter, causing it to be particularly susceptible to damage from vasogenic edema and leakage of myelinotoxic substances from the vessel. Extrapontine myelinolysis can also occur, and other areas of brain that may be affected include the midbrain, basal ganglia, white matter of the folia cerebelli, and the deep layers of the cerebral cortex and adjacent white matter. The diagnosis is made typically by magnetic resonance imaging (MRI). EMG/NCS are normal. There is no specific treatment, and prognosis is poor for extensive lesions.

C. Encephalitis or abscess should be considered in patients with fever, confusion, meningismus, focal neurologic signs, or seizures. Therapy is directed at the causative agent (bacterial, viral, or fungal). Surgical treatment is warranted for large, loculated lesions or those refractory to medical (antibiotic) therapy.

III. Myopathy

A. Acutely, myopathic disorders cause **proximal** greater than distal weakness, with preserved DTRs and sensation. Chronically, patients may develop atrophy and distal weakness as well. Causes include steroid use, alcoholism, immobility, connective tissue disorders (polymyositis, dermatomyositis), infection (trichinosis), toxic (extended paralytic use, neuroleptics, heavy metal/toxin exposure), and metabolic (hyper- or hypokalemia) factors. EMG/NCS and muscle biopsy are often indicated to establish a diagnosis.

B. Critical illness myopathy occurs in the setting of sepsis, neuromuscular blockade, and corticosteroid use. Neuropathic features include abnormal fiber size, atrophy, angulated fibers, internalized nuclei, rimmed vacuoles, fatty degeneration, fibrosis, and single-fiber necrosis. Variations include **thick-filament myopathy,** seen in patients who have received **corticosteroids** for severe asthma or organ transplantation, with or without concomitant **neuromuscular blocking agents,** and necrotizing myopathy, often distinguished by a markedly elevated serum CPK. No specific therapies for these different myopathies have been found to be helpful, other than removing the causative agent(s) as early as possible. Muscle biopsy should be considered to rule out an inflammatory myopathy. **Critical illness myopathy** may be differentiated from **critical illness polyneuropathy** (CIP) on the basis of clinical presentation, as CIP demonstrates proximal and distal impairment as well as loss of DTRs. An additional method of differentiation between myopathy and polyneuropathy may be made on the basis of the nature of progression and duration of symptoms. CIP is often self-limiting, and recovery is relatively rapid and complete. However, critical illness myopathy is frequently more severe with regard to symptoms and duration. It can involve a prolonged recovery phase, with patients still experiencing marked physiologic compromise and diminished quality of life as long as 1 year after the initial presentation. EMG/NCS and muscle biopsy may be required for a definitive diagnosis. Of course, CIP and myopathy can coexist in the same patient, creating a mixed picture with a prognosis dependent on the degree of muscle and nerve injury.

C. **Acute rhabdomyolysis** occurs with traumatic crush injuries, drug overdose, toxin exposure, severe metabolic abnormalities, and infections. Patients have swollen, tender muscles, with localized or diffuse weakness. There is breakdown of skeletal muscle, with leakage of its intracellular contents, causing secondary organ damage. The serum **CPK** is highly elevated, and there may be leukocytosis, hyperkalemia, hyperuricemia, hypo- or hypercalcemia, hyperphosphatemia, lactic acidosis, thrombocytopenia, and disseminated intravascular coagulation. Management should be directed toward hydration, with a goal of urine output in excess of 2 mL/kg body weight. To minimize renal compromise associated with myoglobinuria, the urine is alkalinized by the addition of sodium bicarbonate to intravenous (IV) fluids, with a target urine pH greater than 6.5 in the setting of serum CPK concentrations greater than 5,000 to 6,000 U/L. Threshold for treatment can be lower in the setting of acidemia, hypovolemia, and/or underlying renal disease. Controlling renal failure (which may require temporary hemodialysis) and correcting metabolic abnormalities and DIC are primary goals of the therapeutic plan.

D. **Neuroleptic malignant syndrome** is a rare disorder that occurs in the setting of neuroleptic use (but also may be seen with atypical neuroleptics, metoclopramide, and selective serotonin-reuptake inhibitors). It presents with severe muscle rigidity, hyperthermia, and autonomic dysfunction. Patients commonly have leukocytosis and elevated CPK. It is felt to be caused by sudden and profound dopamine blockade, and young, dehydrated male patients are particularly susceptible. Treatment consists in discontinuing the offending agent, providing hydration, using antipyretic measures, and administering bromocriptine (2.5–7.5 mg three times a day) and dantrolene (1–10 mg/kg IV or in divided oral doses of 50–600 mg/d).

IV. **Neuropathy** can be axonal or demyelinating. Causes of neuropathy observed in the ICU include **CIP, GBS,** metabolic disorders (diabetes, porphyria, hypophosphatemia, alcoholism), **vitamin B$_{12}$ deficiency, infections** (Lyme disease), **endocrine disorders** (hypothyroidism), and toxins (diphtheria, arsenic, thallium, shellfish poisoning). Focal neuropathies can occur with trauma. Common radiculopathy syndromes are listed in **Table 32-1.**

A. **Critical illness polyneuropathy (CIP)** typically occurs in older patients who are severely ill, often with sepsis. It is a self-limited process, often with a good recovery if the underlying critical condition(s) can be treated. Additional risk factors include the duration of mechanical ventilation, hyperosmolality, parenteral nutrition, the use of nondepolarizing neuromuscular blocking agents, and the severity of illness on admission. The clinical examination is significant for motor and sensory system involvement, with a flaccid tetraparesis and muscle atrophy. DTRs are commonly reduced. EMG/NCS reveal a distal axonal sensorimotor polyneuropathy,

TABLE
32-1

Common Radiculopathy Syndromes

Disc	Root	Pain/Dysesthesias	Sensory Loss	Weakness	Reflex Loss
C4–5	C5	Neck, shoulder, upper arm	Shoulder	Deltoid, biceps, infraspinatus	Biceps
C5–6	C6	Neck, shoulder, lateral arm, radial forearm, thumb, index finger	Lateral arm, radial forearm, thumb, index finger	Biceps, brachioradialis, supinator	Biceps, brachioradialis
C6–7	C7	Neck, lateral arm, ring through index finger	Radial forearm, index and middle finger	Triceps, extensor carpi ulnaris	Triceps
C7–T1	C8	Ulnar forearm and hand	Ulnar half or ring finger, little finger	Intrinsic hand muscles, wrist extensors, flexor digitorum profundus	Finger flexion
L3–4	L4	Anterior thigh, inner shin	Anteromedial thigh and shin, inner foot	Quadriceps	Patella
L4–5	L5	Lateral thigh and calf, dorsum of foot, great toe	Lateral calf and great toe	Extensor hallicus longus, ± foot dorsiflexion, inversion and eversion	None
L5–S1	S1	Back of thigh, lateral posterior calf, lateral foot	Posterolateral calf, lateral and sole of foot, smaller toes	Gastrocnemius ± foot eversion	Achilles

with fibrillations and positive sharp waves in the proximal and distal muscles, with relative sparing of the facial muscles. Biopsy reveals predominantly axonal degeneration and denervation atrophy of both proximal and distal muscles. Succinylcholine should not be given to patients with CIP because of the risk of developing hyperkalemic cardiac arrest. Treatment consists of supportive care, treatment of the underlying conditions, and prolonged physical therapy.

B. **Guillain-Barré** syndrome ([GBS] acute inflammatory demyelinating polyneuropathy) is an acute/subacute demyelinating inflammatory neuropathy with a number of variants, including motor-sensory GBS, pure motor GBS, Miller Fisher variant (MFS), bulbar variant, and primary axonal GBS. The incidence is 1 to 2 per 100,000 adults. It is frequently precipitated by an infectious illness, including infection with *Campylobacter jejuni,* cytomegalovirus, and herpes simplex virus, as well as upper respiratory tract infections. It can also be induced by surgery and immunizations. The process consists in complement activation triggering myelin destruction in the peripheral nervous system. Axonal involvement is seen in 15% of cases, most typically with *Campylobacter* infection, and carries a much worse prognosis for complete recovery.

1. **The clinical presentation** is of migratory symmetric weakness, sensory dysesthesias, and hyporeflexia. MFS presents with ataxia, ophthalmoplegia, and hyporeflexia, without significant appendicular weakness.

2. **Evaluation** includes cerebrospinal fluid (**CSF**) analysis and EMG/NCS. The CSF reveals elevated protein with normal cell counts (albuminocytologic dissociation), but the protein may be normal in the first week. If a marked pleocytosis (>20 cells) is present, an evaluation for HIV and Lyme disease should be undertaken. Characteristic findings on EMG/NCS include motor nerve conduction block, prolonged distal conduction, and slowing of nerve conduction. An important early finding is prolongation, dispersion, or absence of F waves, indicative of root demyelination. Antibody testing is also performed to distinguish the different variants of GBS. Neuroimaging is not considered useful in straightforward cases of GBS, but can show nerve root enhancement on contrast-enhanced spine MRI.

3. **Management** should place emphasis on supportive care of the complications, particularly **respiratory failure** and **autonomic dysfunction**. Indications for intubation include a vital capacity of less 15 mL/kg and a maximum negative inspiratory pressure of less than 30 mm Hg, as well as the clinical appearance of a tiring patient. Patients with early cranial nerve dysfunction are more susceptible to aspiration and dysautonomia. Performance of bedside pulmonary function tests may be difficult in patients with significant facial weakness due to the decreased ability to form a good seal. **Early tracheostomy** should be considered in patients with severe weakness, especially including the bulbar musculature. Extubation attempts should be delayed in patients with ongoing dysautonomia because the stress of weaning can cause dramatic fluctuations in blood pressure as well as cardiac dysrhythmias. Dysautonomia typically consists of rapid, wide fluctuations in blood pressure, but other causes of hypotension in GBS patients include sepsis, pulmonary embolus, venous pooling, and electrolyte disturbances. Patients tend to be hypersensitive to both vasopressor medications as well as IV antihypertensive medications, and hypotension is best treated with fluid boluses and Trendelenburg position. The ICU physician should be alert to the concept of simple patience during

a period of dysautonomia, as they are typically short-lived and self-limited. Vasoactive medications should be used in small doses, and the choice of agent should take into consideration its half-life. Dysrhythmias are generally of minor significance, but sinus bradycardia, sinus arrest, and atrioventricular block can occur; tachydysrhythmias, such as supraventricular tachycardia and ventricular tachycardia, may occur in the setting of tracheal intubation or suctioning. Complete heart block is treated with a temporary pacemaker. Other important features of management include pain control (often responsive to neuropathic pain agents, nonsteroidal anti-inflammatory drugs, and narcotics), deep vein thrombosis prophylaxis, and splinting to prevent contractures.

4. **Specific therapies** for GBS include **plasma exchange** and **intravenous immunoglobulin (IVIg)**. Relative contraindications to treatment with plasma exchange include sepsis, myocardial infarction within 6 months, marked dysautonomia, and active bleeding. Side effects include vasovagal reactions, hypovolemia, anaphylaxis, hemolysis, hematoma formation, hypocalcemia, thrombocytopenia, hypothermia, and hypokalemia. Standard therapy consists of five exchanges each of 2 to 4 L over 90 to 120 minutes with 5% albumin repletion, over alternating days. IVIg does not require placement of a central venous catheter, is less expensive than plasma exchange, and does not produce hemodynamic instability. Side effects include aseptic meningitis, anaphylaxis (especially in IgA-deficient patients), acute renal failure, and thromboembolic events (including ischemic stroke). Some studies have suggested a higher relapse rate with IVIg compared with plasma exchange. The dose of IVIg is 0.4 g/kg/d for 5 days. Corticosteroids have no benefit in the treatment of GBS.

V. **Neuromuscular junction.** Transmission of neural impulses can be affected by myasthenic syndromes, botulism, hypermagnesemia, organophosphate poisoning, nerve agents (e.g., sarin), and prolonged effects of paralytic agents.

A. **Myasthenia gravis** is an autoimmune disease with antibodies directed against the acetylcholine receptor (in approximately 80% of cases), leading to destruction/simplification of the synaptic cleft. Its prevalence is 14 per 100,000 adults. It occurs in individuals of all ages, with a peak in women in the third and fourth decades and in men in the sixth and seventh decades. Typically, symptoms increase in severity within the first 3 years of onset and are punctuated by spontaneous, brief remissions. Common presenting signs include ophthalmoparesis, ptosis, jaw weakness, proximal limb weakness, and progressive respiratory failure. **Myasthenic crisis** presents as a dramatic worsening, particularly of respiratory symptoms, often triggered by a viral infection, surgery, childbirth, or an exacerbating medication. Bulbar function should be assessed early to determine the need for elective intubation. **Cholinergic crisis** can also present with respiratory decompensation, and occurs with overmedication with cholinergic agents. Symptoms include excessive salivation, thick bronchial secretions, muscle fasciculations, abdominal cramping, diarrhea, and miosis (myasthenic patients typically have mydriasis).

B. **Diagnosis** of myasthenia gravis is by EMG/NCS, antibody testing, and the **edrophonium test,** which must be performed in an ICU or emergency department setting. Markers of improvement include an increase in sustained upward gaze, ptosis, or dynamometry of a muscle or muscle group in an extremity. The dose is 1 mL of edrophonium in a 10-mg/mL solution.

One-tenth of a milliliter (1 mg) is given as a test dose, waiting 30 seconds for excessive muscarinic effects. The remainder is then given over 1 minute. Edrophonium has a rapid onset (30 seconds) and short duration of action (2–20 minutes). The test is considered positive if there is unequivocal improvement in an objectively weak muscle. Atropine, 0.5 mg IV, should be given if abdominal cramps, bronchospasm, vomiting, or bradycardia occurs. If the bradycardia persists and is accompanied by hypotension, an additional 1 mg of atropine should be given. Edrophonium can also be given if the differential between myasthenic and cholinergic crisis is considered, although in a smaller dose (1 mg); patients without myasthenia may be unchanged or worsened by the test.

C. **EMG/NCS testing** should be performed after discontinuation of anticholinesterase medications for 12 hours. Surface electrodes are used for repetitive stimulation at a rate of 2 to 5 Hz before and after maximal voluntary contraction of the tested muscle. An abnormal result is defined as a 15% or greater reduction in the compound muscle action potential (CMAP) amplitude between the first and fourth responses with supramaximal stimulation. Single-fiber EMG has emerged as a highly sensitive and specific test for MG as well, but requires technical expertise. Antibody testing, in addition to the acetylcholine receptor antibody, should also include antimuscle-specific kinase (MuSK) antibody.

D. All patients with myasthenia should have a chest CT or MRI performed to detect the presence of a **thymoma** or enlargement of the thymus gland. If a thymoma is detected, it is an absolute indication for removal unless the patient is considered a poor surgical candidate. Patients undergoing thymectomy should undergo preoperative plasma exchange. Removal of the thymus in myasthenic patients may lead to remission in a significant number.

E. **Treatment** of myasthenia gravis involves stabilization of the patient, especially from a respiratory standpoint. ICU monitoring should be considered for patients with respiratory symptoms, and bedside PFTs are notoriously poor indicators for the need for mechanical ventilation; these patients can experience a rapid deterioration. When the vital capacity has fallen to less than 15 mL/kg or is less than 25% of the predicted value, respiratory failure should be considered to be imminent. Specific therapies include **immunomodulation** and **anticholinesterase agents.** Plasma exchange standard therapy is five exchanges each of 2 to 4 L over 90 to 120 minutes with 5% albumin repletion over alternating days. The IVIg dose is 0.4 g/kg/d for 5 days. **Corticosteroids** are typically initiated during the acute setting, but their benefit is typically delayed by several days, and may be associated with some clinical worsening, and thus should not be used as the sole therapy. **Pyridostigmine** may also be used in the acute setting, but its use is tempered by respiratory side effects, such as increasing bronchial secretions, thus limiting its use in nonintubated patients.

F. Medications that can worsen myasthenic symptoms include antibiotics (clindamycin, aminoglycosides, tetracycline, gentamycin, bacitracin, trimethoprim-sulfamethoxazole), hormones (corticotropin, thyroid hormone, oral contraceptives), cardiovascular agents (quinidine, propranolol, procainamide, practolol, lidocaine, verapamil, nifedipine, diltiazem), psychotropic agents (chlorpromazine, promazine, phenelzine, lithium, diazepam), anticonvulsants (phenytoin, trimethadione, carbamazepine), paralytics, and miscellaneous agents (penicillamine, chloroquine).

G. The **differential diagnosis** for myasthenia gravis should include Lambert-Eaton myasthenic syndrome, which may be the initial presentation of an

TABLE 32-2	Comparative Features of Guillain-Barré Syndrome and Myasthenia Gravis	
	GBS	**MG**
Ascending weakness	+++	−
Abnormal ocular movements	− (can be seen in Miller Fisher variant)	+++
Sensory manifestations	+++	=
Pain	+++ (especially back pain)	−
Dysautonomia	+++	−
Hyporeflexia	+++	±
Specific antibody testing	+++	+++
Responsive to steroids	−	+++
Immune mediated	+++	+++
EMG/NCS	Conduction block Loss of F and H waves	↓response on repetitive stim. Single fiber EMG diagnostic

EMG, electromyography; GBS, Guillain-Barré syndrome; MG, myasthenia gravis; NCS, nerve conduction studies.

occult malignancy, congenital myasthenic syndromes, Graves disease, botulism, progressive external ophthalmoplegia, and intracranial mass lesions. Lambert-Eaton syndrome is a paraneoplastic syndrome affecting the presynaptic release of acetylcholine. In contrast to myasthenia gravis, autonomic and sensory symptoms are seen with this disorder, and the EMG reveals an incremental *improvement* with higher-frequency repetitive stimulation. Comparative features for myasthenia gravis and Guillain-Barré syndrome are listed in **Table 32-2**.

Selected References

Berrouschot J, Baumann I, Kalischewski P, et al. Therapy of myasthenic crisis. *Crit Care Med* 1997;25:1228–1235.

Cosi V, Versino M. Guillain-Barré syndrome. *Neurol Sci* 2006;27:S47–S51.

De Jonghe B, Sharshar T, Lefaucher JP, et al. Paresis acquired in the intensive care unit: a prospective multicenter study. *JAMA* 2002;288:2859–2867.

Deem S, Lee CM, Curtis JR. Acquired neuromuscular disorders in the intensive care unit. *Am J Respir Crit Care Med* 2003;168:735–739.

Dhand UK. Clinical approach to the weak patient in the intensive care unit. *Respir Care* 2006;51:1024–1040.

Fulgham JR, Wijdicks EFM. Guillain-Barré syndrome. *Crit Care Clin* 1997;13:1–15.

Grand'Maison F. Methods of testing neuromuscular transmission in the intensive care unit. *Can J Neurol Sci* 1998;25:S36–S39.

Greer DM. Intensive care management of neurological emergencies. In: Layon AJ, ed. *A textbook of neurointensive care*. Philadelphia: WB Saunders, 2004:397–436.

Herridge MS, Cheung AM, Tansey CM, et al. One-year outcomes in survivors of the acute respiratory distress syndrome. *N Engl J Med* 2003;348:683–693.

Hughes RA, Cornblath DR. Guillain-Barré syndrome. *Lancet* 2005;366:1653–1666.

Hund E. Neurological complications of sepsis: critical illness polyneuropathy and myopathy. *J Neurol* 2001;248:929–934.

Jani-Acsadi A, Lisak RP. Myastenic crisis: guidelines for prevention and treatment. *J Neurol Sci* 2007;261:127–133.

Lampl C, Yazdi K. Central pontine myelinolysis. *Eur Neurol* 2002;47:3–10.

Latronico N, Peli E, Botteri M. Critical illness myopathy and neuropathy. *Curr Opin Crit Care* 2005;11:126–132.

Pandit L, Agrawal A. Neuromuscular disorders in critical illness. *Clin Neurol Neurosurg* 2006;108:621–627.

Pelonero AL, Levenson JL, Pandurangi AK. Neuroleptic malignant syndrome: a review. *Psychiatr Serv* 1998;49:1163–1172.

Van der Meché FGA, Van Doorn PA, Meulstee J, et al. Diagnostic and classification criteria for the Guillain-Barré syndrome. *Eur Neurol* 2001;45:133–139.

Vassilakopoulos T, Petrof BJ. Ventilator-induced diaphragmatic dysfunction. *Am J Respir Crit Care Med* 2004;169:336–341.

Drug Overdose, Poisoning, and Adverse Drug Reactions

Susan Wilcox and Richard Pino

I. Introduction

  A. Drug overdose and poisoning are frequently cared for in the ICU. Although an overdose of prescription or nonprescription drugs might poison, that is, injure or kill cells, in this chapter the term "poisoning" will be reserved for compounds not used for therapy. Drug overdose and poisoning might be iatrogenic (e.g., coagulopathy secondary to warfarin during adjustment), secondary to intentional (e.g., suicide attempt) or unintentional (e.g., a child taking his or her grandparent's digitalis) ingestion of a drug, due to an animal bite (e.g., rattlesnake), the result of inhalation (e.g., carbon monoxide), or a result of substance abuse (e.g., cocaine).

  B. Initial treatment and stabilization might include giving cardiopulmonary support, administering an antidote, beginning the elimination of an ingested drug by gastrointestinal decontamination with activated charcoal, and initiating correction of acid–base alterations. The intensivist needs to understand the sequelae of each drug taken in overdose.

  C. In view of the large number of drugs and poisonous substances, the physician should be familiar with reference resources in each institution and the telephone number of the area **poison control center.** Hospitals often have readily available texts and online drug and toxicology information.

  D. Each overdose should be approached in a systematic manner to determine the following:

  1. The substance(s) taken.
  2. The last dose of the drug and its dosing frequency.
  3. The reason for the medication.
  4. Other medications usually taken.
  5. Coexisting disease.
  6. The effects of the overdose, for example, hypotension, respiratory failure, or life-threatening dysrhythmias.
  7. Whether the effects of the drug can be reversed or the drug can be eliminated without further harm to the patient.

II. Overdose and adverse effects of prescription and nonprescription drugs

  A. Acetaminophen (APAP) is the most commonly overdosed medication in the world and a leading cause of hepatic failure. While many ingestions are intentional, overdoses may also occur in patients who are seeking analgesia or using acetaminophen chronically. Alcoholism, malnutrition, and use of certain medications can lower the toxic threshold of chronic APAP ingestion. Because of the largely preventable severe toxicity of missed APAP overdose, a high index of suspicion should be maintained in all ingestion patients or patients with unexplained transaminitis.

  1. Most APAP is metabolized by glucuronization and sulfation to inactive compounds. Less than 10% is converted by a cytochrome P-450 mixed-function oxidase to N-acetyl-p-benzoquinoneimine (NAPQI), which has a half-life of nanoseconds. If NAPQI is not neutralized by conjuga-

tion with glutathione, it injures the bilipid layer of the hepatocyte. APAP overdose (7.5 g for adult, 150 mg/kg for children) overwhelms the hepatic glutathione stores, resulting in cell death.

2. **Baseline and daily laboratory tests** include prothrombin time (PT), alanine leucine aminotransferase (ALT), aspartate serine transferase (AST), and bilirubin.

3. **Treatment** is the enteral administration of **N-acetylcysteine (NAC)**. NAC serves as a glutathione substitute, enhances glutathione synthesis, and increases the amount of APAP that is conjugated by sulfation. If the elapsed time after APAP ingestion is 4 hours or less or additional overdosed drugs are suspected, activated charcoal is given and an APAP level is drawn. The serum APAP level is then plotted on a nomogram as a function of time after ingestion. The nomogram has three lines indicating lower limits for possible, probable, and high-risk groups. Individuals who have APAP levels above the possible line are treated with an NAC loading dose of 140 mg/kg orally diluted in a fruit juice or carbonated beverage. Because of its objectionable taste, it is often administered via a gastric lavage or nasotracheal tube. Aggressive antiemetic therapy may be needed when the elapsed time is 8 hours or longer; the initial loading dose is given prior to obtaining an APAP level. Additional doses are 70 mg/kg every 4 hours for 17 doses or until the APAP levels are in the nontoxic range. Doses are repeated when a patient vomits an NAC dose within 1 hour of administration. An IV form of the drug is available. Dosing is 150 mg/kg over 15 minutes, followed by 50 mg/kg infused over 4 hours, then 100 mg/kg over 16 hours. This drug has a high incidence of anaphylactoid reactions (**Section VIII.B**).

4. **Severe hepatotoxicity** secondary to the overdose of APAP is indicated by an ALT or AST greater than 1,000 IU/L. This hepatotoxicity may progress to fulminant hepatic failure and eventually lead to liver transplantation or death secondary to sepsis, cerebral edema, hepatorenal syndrome, and metabolic acidosis (72–96 hours). There is complete resolution of hepatic dysfunction (4–14 days) in survivors.

B. **Antipsychotic agents** are derived from several classes of compounds in addition to the classic phenothiazines. They are used for the treatment of acute and chronic psychiatric disease, the control of acute agitation (**haloperidol** and **quetiapine**), the treatment of migraine headaches, as antiemetics (e.g., **droperidol,** promethazine, prochlorperazine) and as prokinetics (e.g., **metoclopramide**).

1. **Toxic manifestations** of antipsychotics include seizures, hypotension, cardiac conduction delays manifested by prolonged QT interval on the electrocardiogram (ECG) , ventricular dysrhythmias, especially *torsades de pointes*, extrapyramidal symptoms, and the neuroleptic malignant syndrome (NMS). The judicious use of intravenous (IV) haloperidol in the ICU is not usually associated with any of these. However, because of its long half-life, prolonged sedation may occur, especially in the elderly, after sequential escalated doses.

2. **Treatment** of antipsychotic overdose is supportive. Gastrointestinal decontamination is employed.

   a. **Seizures** can be treated initially with benzodiazepines, progressing to barbiturate therapy if needed. As for any patient with seizures, other causes (e.g., hypoxemia, cerebral hemorrhage, embolic disease, other drugs, etc) should be ruled out.

   b. **Hypotension** can be treated with phenylephrine or norepinephrine. Epinephrine in lower doses and dopamine may further decrease blood pressure secondary to unopposed β_2-receptor stimulation. The α effects of dopamine might not be present secondary to the reduction in postsynaptic norepinephrine stores.

   c. **Magnesium** is first-line therapy for torsades de pointes.

   d. **Physostigmine** (1–2 mg IV for adults, 0.2 mg/kg for children) with repeated doses as needed every 0.5 to 1.5 hours is used for the treatment of an anticholinergic syndrome.

   e. **Dystonic reactions** can be treated with diphenhydramine (25–50 mg).

3. **Neuroleptic malignant syndrome (NMS)** is a relatively rare life-threatening reaction to antipsychotics within 24 to 72 hours after administration. It is characterized by an altered mental status (which may initially be attributed to a treatment failure) prior to the development of fever, muscle rigidity, and autonomic dysfunction.

   a. **Fever** occurs from an imbalance of dopamine in the hypothalamus, which causes a change in the mechanisms for temperature homeostasis, and centrally mediated muscle rigidity. This is in contrast to the accelerated calcium-associated skeletal muscle metabolism in **malignant hyperthermia (MH)** in **Section VI**. The onset of NMS is slower, with less severe symptoms than with MH. The postoperative patient usually has a common reason (e.g., atelectasis, wound infection) for an increase in temperature before MH and NMS are considered. NMS has been seen after the use of prochlorperazine and promethazine as an antiemetic and should be considered as a source of fever in an ICU patient receiving haloperidol, metoclopramide, or droperidol. Initial treatment is the discontinuation of the drug in question and cardiopulmonary support followed by cooling.

   b. **Dantrolene** (initial IV dose of 1–2.5 mg/kg every 6 hours, followed by 100–300 g orally [PO] per day or 1 mg IV/kg every 6 hours for 24–72 hours) is used to control skeletal muscle rigidity and hypermetabolism. At these doses, there is profound muscle weakness, which might necessitate intubation and mechanical ventilation. The mannitol in dantrolene will create a brisk diuresis as treatment for myoglobin-induced renal failure secondary to rhabdomyolysis.

   c. **Bromocriptine** (2.5 mg thrice daily), a dopamine agonist, is given to offset the action of the antipsychotic on the dopamine receptor.

   d. **Amantidine** (100–200 mg enterally, twice a day) and **levodopa/carbidopa** (25/250 enterally four times a day) have also been used.

   e. Laboratory studies include creatinine phosphokinase (CPK) levels, urinary myoglobin, and electrolytes.

C. **β-Blockers** inhibit the pathway of G-protein → cyclic adenosine monophosphate (cAMP) production → myocyte protein kinase → calcium release → excitation–contraction coupling. The more lipid-soluble β-blockers (e.g., propranolol, metoprolol, and labetalol) also have a membrane-stabilizing function. These agents are used to decrease myocardial contractility, the automaticity of pacemaker cells, and the conduction velocity through the atrioventricular (AV) node. β-Blockers are divided into β_1 and β_2 classes based on actions at *therapeutic* doses. With therapeutic doses in susceptible patients or with increased drug levels of a β-selective agent, both β_1 and β_2 effects can be present [e.g., bronchospasm (β_2 blockade) induced with esmolol (β_1)].

1. **Lipophilic β-blockers** are metabolized by the liver, with their bioavailability increased in hepatic disease or by inhibitors of hepatic enzymes such as cimetidine and erythromycin. Nonlipophilic β-blockers are eliminated by the kidney. Renal insufficiency or the use of drugs affecting renal perfusion, for example, nonsteroidal anti-inflammatory drugs (NSAIDs), increases blood levels. Most patients with β-blocker toxicity have symptoms within 4 hours and resolution within 72 hours. The toxic effects of sotalol may not be noticed for several days after ingestion because of its long half-life.

2. **Hypotension** secondary to decreased myocardial contractility can occur even in the absence of severe bradycardia. **Bradydysrhythmias** (sinus, junctional rhythm, AV block, and idioventricular rhythm), widening of the QRS complex, the QT interval, and the asystole have been associated with β-blocker toxicity, especially for the lipophilic agents. Lipophilic β-blocker overdose has been associated with **central nervous system (CNS)** symptoms ranging from a decreased level of consciousness to seizures and coma.

3. **Electrocardiography** is essential in the diagnosis of β-blocker toxicity. Digitalis and calcium channel blocker toxicity (see later discussion) should be considered because these drugs are often given with β-blockers to control heart rates. As for any patient with neurologic symptoms, electrolytes and serum glucose should be checked. Computed tomography of the head is useful to eliminate the possibility of an intracranial process (e.g., neoplasm, hematoma, aneurysm) as a basis for these symptoms.

4. **The initial treatment** of β-blocker toxicity is cardiopulmonary support, gastrointestinal decontamination with activated charcoal, and correction of hypoglycemia, with electrolytes as needed.

   a. **Glucagon** is the pharmacologic agent of choice because the myocardial receptor for glucagon is not affected by β-antagonists. The increase in cAMP via stimulation of adenylate cyclase by glucagon increases myocardial contractility and heart rate, thereby overcoming the effects of the β-blockade. The initial dose of glucagon is 50 to 150 μg/kg (up to a total dose of 10 mg if needed) followed by an infusion of 0.07 mg/kg.

   b. **Epinephrine** is the β-agonist of choice. Atropine and pacing are not usually effective except for sotalol.

   c. **Sotalol-induced dysrhythmias** can be treated with overdrive pacing in addition to lidocaine and magnesium.

D. **Calcium channel antagonists** comprise one of the largest leading classes of antihypertensives and antidysrhythmics. The antihypertensive effect is through inhibiting the influx of extracellular calcium through slow voltage–gated slow membrane channels in vascular smooth muscle. This is the sole action of the dihydropyridine family (nifedipine, amlodipine, and felodipine). Myocardial depression may also occur in some compromised individuals and in overdose secondary to the effects on atrial and ventricular myocytes.

   1. **Calcium channel antagonists** are highly protein bound, with variable bioavailability and half-lives. Metabolism is hepatic. Verapamil and diltiazem are converted to active metabolites. They are also potent inhibitors of microsomal metabolizing enzymes and may increase the concentration of drugs that are metabolized by this pathway, for example, phenytoin and theophylline. Conversely, the elimination of calcium channel antagonists is decreased by inhibitors of these hepatic enzymes, for example, erythromycin.

2. **Bradycardia, conduction defects** (e.g., asystole, idioventricular rhythms, bundle-branch blocks), and **hypotension** are the hallmarks of verapamil and diltiazem toxicity. Overdose of the dihydropyridines results in hypotension with reflex tachycardia. A common finding with excess of calcium channel blocker is an **ileus** in a patient who had been tolerating enteral nutrition. Other symptoms are related to hypotension (e.g., stroke, lethargy, coma).

3. **Treatment** initially consists of cardiovascular support. **Calcium chloride** (1 g) or **calcium gluconate** (3 g) is repeated as needed until the blood pressure rises, the heart rate increases, or there is no effect after four to five administrations. As with β-blockade overdose, **glucagon** administration (see **Section II.C.4.a**) might be effective.

   a. **Cardiac pacing and vasopressor inotropes** (norepinephrine, dopamine) should be considered if the heart rate and/or blood pressure do not respond to the former treatments.

   b. **Nonabsorbed drug** should be removed via gastrointestinal decontamination with activated charcoal. This might require several doses because many of the calcium channel antagonists are usually taken in extended-release forms.

E. **Digoxin** is still frequently used for ventricular rate control in atrial fibrillation and atrial flutter. Because of a narrow therapeutic window, renal dysfunction, and changes in bioavailability secondary to drug interactions, mild digitalis toxicity is relatively uncommon. Through the inhibition of the Na^+/K^+-ATPase, pump cardiac myocytes gain intracellular Ca^{2+}—it is a positive inotrope especially in the failing heart. Digitalis has a chronotropic effects by several mechanisms. An increase in CNS vagal tone decreases the rate of sinoatrial (SA) node depolarization and prolongs the refractory period of the bundle of His. With the exception of the SA node, the increase of Na^+ increases phase 4 depolarization and increases excitability as well as delayed afterpotentials.

1. **Digoxin** is eliminated by renal clearance after an enterohepatic circulation. **Digitoxin** is cleared by hepatic metabolism. The therapeutic index is narrow, and plasma levels can be affected by several factors. The addition of quinidine, amiodarone, or verapamil to a therapeutic regimen will significantly increase established digoxin levels. Increased levels may result from antibiotic administration through decreased metabolism when gastrointestinal flora are reduced. Hypokalemia, hypocalcemia, and hypomagnesemia will increase the sensitivity of the myocardium to digitalis.

2. **Initial symptoms** of toxicity are **gastrointestinal:** anorexia, nausea, and vomiting. Toxicity may not be readily diagnosed because these symptoms may stem from a variety of causes other than digitalis. **Dysrhythmias,** especially in patients with compromised hearts, are more common indicators of toxicity when other reasons have been excluded. Almost any rhythm or conduction disturbance may be manifested but premature ventricular contractions (PVCs), first-degree AV block, and atrial fibrillation are common. A characteristic ST depression is seen on the ECG.

3. **Treatment** of digoxin toxicity can be difficult. It is poorly dialyzed. **Atropine and/or cardiac pacing** is effective for treating bradydysrhythmias. The administration of **magnesium, lidocaine, or phenytoin** will often treat ectopy. With a significant overdose, the inhibition of the Na^+/K^+-ATPase will result in significant hyperkalemia, which may be refractory to most treatments. Hyperkalemia in the setting of digitalis

should not be treated with calcium gluconate, due to the largely theoretical and rarely reported concern for potentiating lethal arrhythmias. This will eventually result in a loss of total body potassium that must be repleted when the overdose is treated. The most effective method of digoxin overdose treatment is the removal of free digitalis by Fab fragments **of antidigitalis immunoglobulin G (IgG) (Digibind)** that enhances clearance from the circulation by renal elimination and accelerates removal from tissues. The dose of Digibind is calculated from a formula based on the body load of digitalis. This calculation requires a digoxin level that may not be available. It is simpler to administer Digibind (40 mg/vial) until the dysrhythmias are effectively treated or until the maximum dose of 800 mg (20 vials) is reached. Digoxin levels, although elevated, will reflect both the drug bound to the Fab fragments and the unbound drug.

F. **Lithium** is a treatment for bipolar disease. Toxicity may be the result of a suicide attempt, increased levels during chronic treatment, or increased levels after the new administration of a thiazide diuretic or placement on a low-sodium diet. Gastrointestinal absorption is rapid, the element is distributed in whole-body water, and there is renal elimination with significant reabsorption. The half-life of lithium is 30 hours.

1. **Serious toxicity** is present at serum lithium levels of 2.5 to 3.5 mEq/L, with life-threatening complications at levels higher than 3.5 mEq/L. A change in renal function that permits increased resorption of lithium in the proximal convoluted tubule (e.g., hypovolemia, hyponatremia, NSAIDs) will increase serum lithium levels. Nephrogenic diabetes insipidus is the most common toxicity seen. Dysrhythmias and circulatory collapse have been reported.

2. **Treatment** is gastrointestinal decontamination if an intentional overdose is suspected. Half-normal saline (0.45%) should initially be given to restore euvolemia because the patient usually has a high serum osmolality. The administration of a thiazide diuretic or amiloride may help to control the polyuria. Hemodialysis is required for a life-threatening lithium overdose.

G. **Salicylates. Acetylsalicylic acid (ASA, aspirin)** is the most commonly used salicylate and has traditionally been the agent of salicylate overdose. ASA overdose has decreased because of child-proof containers, the awareness of **Reye's syndrome,** and the use of nonsalicylate analgesics. **Methylsalicylate** is found in topical formulations used to treat musculoskeletal pain and in oil of wintergreen. Chronic use on excoriated skin may result in salicylism. **Bismuth subsalicylate** is found in antidiarrheal preparations.

1. **ASA is absorbed** in ionized form in the stomach and in enteric form in the distal small intestine. Hydrolysis of ASA to salicylic acid with elimination by renal filtration and excretion is the major metabolic pathway. There are several secondary metabolic pathways for salicylic acid. In severe overdose, these pathways become overwhelmed and the elimination half-life of salicylic acid is prolonged up to 30 hours. A toxic salicylate concentration is greater than 30 mg/dL. Initially, hyperventilation, via direct CNS stimulation by the drug, produces a respiratory alkalosis. Bicarbonate is renally excreted and hypokalemia ensues in a compensatory fashion. An anion-gap metabolic acidosis occurs secondary to the uncoupling of oxidative phosphorylation and inhibition of the tricarboxylic acid cycle in the liver. Patients may be agitated and have tinnitus. Hyperglycemia or hypoglycemia may be present. Often, hypernatremia with dehydration exists that is related

to a large insensible loss with hyperventilation. Uncommon events are pulmonary edema, coma, hyperpyrexia, and gastrointestinal bleeding.

2. **Laboratory tests** include plasma salicylate levels until the peak level is obtained, electrolytes, blood urea nitrogen (BUN), creatinine, glucose, liver function tests, and arterial blood gas tensions and pH as needed.

3. **Initial treatment** is gastrointestinal decontamination with activated charcoal; cardiovascular and respiratory support; replacement of electrolytes, glucose, and fluids; and alkalinization of the urine to "ion trap" salicylic acid and prevent reabsorption by the proximal convoluted tubules. Hemodialysis should be considered when there is renal dysfunction or when salicylate levels are higher than 80 mg/dL.

H. **Tricyclic antidepressant (TCA)** toxicity is the most common cause of prescription-related drug deaths, and usually occurs within 24 hours of ingestion. The onset of toxic symptoms occurs within hours. In general, TCAs decrease the neuronal reuptake of epinephrine and norepinephrine by inhibiting fast sodium channels and blocking cholinergic, histamine, and γ-aminobutyric acid (GABA) channels. **Trazodone** does not block the reuptake of norepinephrine, but does block adrenergic receptors. **Amoxapine** blocks dopamine receptors.

1. TCAs are quickly absorbed from the gastrointestinal tract and are rapidly distributed to tissue sites. Elimination is by hepatic hydroxylation and demethylation. The enzymes responsible for hydroxylation are saturated at high concentrations of substrate, resulting in a prolonged elimination. TCAs have half-lives of 8 to 30 hours in therapeutic concentrations, which may be prolonged to 81 hours in an overdose.

2. **Initial signs of TCA toxicity** are anticholinergic: tachycardia, hyperthermia, ileus, mydriasis, urinary retention, dry mucous membranes and skin, and altered mental status.

   a. **Manifestations of serious TCA toxicity** are dysrhythmias, hypotension, respiratory depression, pulmonary edema, self-limited seizures, and coma. Life-threatening toxicity is present with serum concentrations of greater than 1 μg/mL, with fatality at greater than 3 μg/mL.

   b. **The ECG** in an overdose usually demonstrates a sinus tachycardia with a first-degree AV block, nonspecific intraventricular conduction delay (secondary to an inhibition of phase 0 depolarization), and rightward axis. Classic findings that increase concern are a QRS of greater than 100, a rightward axis for the terminal 40 ms of the QRS, and a prominent R wave with an R/S ratio of greater than 0.7 in lead AVR, although the predictive utility of these findings is not clear in the literature. An atrial electrocardiogram with an esophageal lead might be useful for distinguishing this pattern from ventricular tachycardia, which is also common with TCA overdose.

   c. **Hypotension** is caused by decreased myocardial contractility (due to blockade of the fast sodium channels), depletion of norepinephrine reserves in neurons, and vasodilation (due to α blockade). The usual cause of death is refractive hypotension.

   d. **Treatment** consists of initial gastrointestinal decontamination with activated charcoal and cardiopulmonary support, as needed. Refractive hypotension should be treated by repletion of intravascular volume and administration of norepinephrine. Administration of sodium bicarbonate also effectively treats TCA cardiotoxicity, either through the alkalinization of the blood (to pH 7.5) or through supplementing Na^+, but not by drug trapping, because there is minimal renal elimination. Class 1a and 1c antiarrhythmics are not recommended, as they may worsen sodium channel blockade. Additionally, phenytoin has been associated with arrhythmias and is not generally recommended for cardiac conduction abnormalities or seizures.

  I. **Serotonin syndrome** may occur with intentional overdose, therapeutic drug use, or pharmacologic interactions with serotonergic medications. The syndrome is characterized by **alterations in mental status, neuromuscular abnormalities, and autonomic instability.**

1. Hospitalized patients may be exposed to numerous serotonergic medications, such as **SSRIs, MAOIs, meperidine, and other analgesics, antiemetics, valproate, and linezolid.**

2. The clinical presentation of serotonin syndrome may range from mild symptoms of diarrhea, hypertension, and anxiety, to high fevers over 40°C, muscle rigidity, and coma. **Hyperreflexia and clonus** are typical of the syndrome, although muscular rigidity may obscure these findings. Hyperthermia develops from muscular activity. There are no laboratory studies specific for serotonin syndrome, and diagnosis is based on history and physical examination. However, patients may demonstrate metabolic acidosis, rhabdomyolysis, elevated AST and creatinine, or disseminated intravascular coagulopathy. A high clinical suspicion must be maintained, or the diagnosis will be overlooked.

3. **Treatment** begins with supportive care. Mild cases can be treated with removal of the offending medications, IV fluids, and benzodiazepines. Moderate and severe cases should additionally have vital signs corrected aggressively, including active cooling measures as needed, and be treated with 5-HT_{2A} antagonists. **Cyproheptadine** 12 mg followed by 2 mg every 2 hours as symptoms continue is a recommended dosing regimen. Patients with very high fevers should be given nondepolarizing neuromuscular paralysis and intubated promptly. Antipyretic medications are of no benefit, as hyperthermia does not originate from the hypothalamus. Physical restraints may worsen the syndrome by encouraging further isometric muscle contractions.

III. **Alcohols**
  A. **Ethanol (EtOH)** is the most extensively used nonprescription drug. It is also present in a variety of cough and cold preparations, mouthwashes, and perfumes.

1. **Ethanol is absorbed** from all levels of the gastrointestinal tract, but primarily in the stomach and small intestine, with blood levels achieved within 60 minutes of ingestion. It is initially metabolized to acetaldehyde by alcohol dehydrogenase in the liver. A cytochrome P-450–dependent pathway is used for less than 10% of metabolism, but is increased in chronic drinkers. Acetaldehyde is metabolized to acetate via acetaldehyde dehydrogenase. Ethanol elimination may be as low as 12 mg%/h in nondrinkers to 50 mg%/h in chronic alcoholics. The blood alcohol level will reflect the peak amount of ethanol ingested.

2. **The effects of ethanol intoxication** depend on whether there is chronic or acute use and the amount ingested. The standard values for blood alcohol levels are only valid for the nondependent person.
    a. **Acute intoxication** in the "nonalcoholic" may be manifested by euphoria to total circulatory and respiratory collapse. A frequent cause of morbidity is hypoxemia secondary to **aspiration** of gastric

contents after loss of airway reflexes. **Dehydration** may be present from an ethanol-induced depression of antidiuretic hormone. A "holiday heart" syndrome of **atrial fibrillation** or **flutter** associated with ethanol use in nonalcoholics that corrects with cessation of use is well known.

b. **Chronic intoxication** is a spectrum of comorbid conditions. Many patients have no symptoms other than an increased tolerance for ethanol. Malnutrition, peptic ulcer disease, bone marrow suppression, and immunosuppression may be subtle. Pulmonary complications secondary to concomitant tobacco and ethanol use are common. More severe forms of chronic ethanol intoxication include cardiomyopathy, dysrhythmias, Wernicke's encephalopathy, Korsakoff's psychosis, cerebella ataxia, ketoacidosis, hepatic cirrhosis, and gastrointestinal hemorrhage.

3. **Treatment** of the EtOH-intoxicated patient in the ICU is initially focused on the reason for admission (e.g., subdural hematoma, aspiration, musculoskeletal trauma, coingestion) in addition to cardiopulmonary support.

a. **Other causes for altered mental status** (e.g., sepsis, encephalopathy, hypoglycemia, or head trauma) should be ruled out. The emergence of focal neurologic signs should prompt a detailed workup (e.g., the beginning of an acute subdural hematoma might not be evident on an admission computed tomography but be evident several hours later).

b. **Fluid losses** secondary to alcohol-induced diuresis, decreased oral intake, and vomiting need to be repleted. Cardiovascular support will depend on the level of intravascular volume depletion and degree of cardiomyopathy.

c. Attention to **pulmonary function** and secretion clearance is important in view of the high probability of pulmonary dysfunction secondary to smoking. Although antibiotic coverage for aspiration of community-acquired flora is usually not needed, empiric administration of a broad-spectrum antibiotic (e.g., ampicillin/sulbactam) may be prudent in the initial stages of treatment if malnutrition or immunosuppression is suspected.

d. **Vitamin therapy** with thiamine and folate and repletion of electrolytes should be initiated. Alcoholic ketoacidosis requires volume resuscitation and glucose administration in a manner similar to resuscitation for diabetic ketoacidosis.

e. **The altered coagulation profile** of patients with cirrhosis, including the thrombocytopenia of splenomegaly, does not require treatment unless there is a clinical indication. Bleeding esophageal varices may require endoscopic or surgical intervention.

4. **EtOH withdrawal** is often seen following elective surgery or an emergent admission. Symptoms include anxiety, tremors, irritability, hypertension, and hallucinations that generally peak approximately 24 hours after cessation of EtOH but may appear within 10 hours. These symptoms might easily be attributed to a mild postoperative effect of drugs or disorientation in a "pleasantly confused" elderly patient.

a. **Denial** and underestimation of one's EtOH daily consumption is commonplace. Clearly, some elderly patients who have had "one glass of wine a night" for years will exhibit signs of withdrawal. A tactful and nonjudgmental approach often elicits a more accurate history in such situations.

    b. Tonic-clonic seizures may occur within 48 hours after a decrease in EtOH use.

    c. Delirium tremens (DT) is a life-threatening syndrome marked by autonomic instability (hypertension, tachycardia, hyperpyrexia, tremors, and diaphoresis) that may be present 3 to 5 days following the cessation of EtOH.

  5. Benzodiazepines, through their binding the GABA receptors, are cross-tolerant with EtOH. All benzodiazepines have been used with success. IV or EtOH **diazepam** or **lorazepam** can be administered on a dosage schedule that is appropriate for the patient's age, size, and physical condition. The long activity of diazepam secondary to its active metabolite nordiazepam should be considered in subsequent dosing schedules.

    a. For the treatment of seizures and severe DTs, the IV route is used with escalating doses.

    b. Tracheal intubation and mechanical ventilation may be required if respiratory depression occurs due to the needed high doses of benzodiazepines.

    c. Immediately following a seizure, an arterial blood gas measurement will usually exhibit metabolic acidosis with a pH sometimes lower than 7.0. Measurement is not indicated in this setting because the acidosis will spontaneously correct after the seizure.

  6. Haloperidol is useful for the psychotic reactions accompanied by ethanol withdrawal. It can be given IV beginning at 1 mg, with doubling of the dose after each intervention. Because of the long half-life, prolonged sedation, but without respiratory depression, may occur after sequential administrations. The QT segment on the ECG should be checked for prolongation during haloperidol treatment (see **Chapter 19**).

B. Methanol (MtOH) (wood alcohol) is a commonly used solvent. It is often ingested after synthesis in home distilleries (i.e., "moonshine") or by alcoholics seeking any form of alcohol. Peak levels are reached within 90 minutes of ingestion. The fatal dose may be as little as 60 mL. The majority of the MtOH is initially converted by alcohol dehydrogenase to formaldehyde, followed by oxidation by several enzymes to formic acid.

  1. Signs and symptoms include blurred vision/blindness, gastrointestinal reactions (nausea, vomiting, severe abdominal pain, diarrhea), a severe anion-gap metabolic acidosis, a large osmolal gap (increased osmolality not accounted for by glucose, sodium, or BUN), and respiratory depression.

  2. Treatment of MtOH poisoning, in addition to cardiopulmonary support, is the administration of **IV EtOH** to achieve a blood level of 100 mg%. Start with a loading dose of 0.6 g/kg followed by 66 to 154 mg/kg depending on the past ethanol use pattern of the patient. The EtOH will compete with MtOH for metabolism by alcohol dehydrogenase and reduce the production of formaldehyde. **Hemodialysis** is initiated to remove nonmetabolized MtOH. **Fomepizole,** an inhibitor of alcohol dehydrogenase that is used for the treatment of ethylene glycol toxicity (see later discussion), is also efficacious in treating MtOH ingestion.

C. Ethylene glycol, commonly used as antifreeze and also found in other solvents, is usually lethal after an ingestion of 100 mL, if not treated swiftly. Like EtOH and MtOH, ethylene glycol is initially metabolized by alcohol dehydrogenase. Subsequent metabolic products are lactic acid, aldehydes, glycolate, and oxalic acid.

1. **Intoxication** is marked by a severe anion-gap metabolic acidosis, a large osmolal gap, and tissue damage secondary to the deposition of oxalate crystals. Oxalate crystals may also been seen in the urine, which assists in diagnosis. Hypocalcemia results from the chelation of calcium by the oxalate. Patients may be admitted in coma and have seizures, neuromuscular dysfunction secondary to hypocalcemia (myoclonic activity, loss of deep tendon reflexes, tetany), acute renal failure, and congestive heart failure and pulmonary edema (both related to deposition of oxalate).

2. **Treatment** of ethylene glycol toxicity includes cardiopulmonary support, treatment of the metabolic acidosis, IV EtOH administration as for MtOH poisoning (see prior discussion), and hemodialysis. **Fomepizole** (Antizol) is a competitive inhibitor of alcohol dehydrogenase that treats ethylene glycol poisoning and prevents renal injury by limiting the formation of toxic metabolites. The initial dose is 15 mg/kg, followed by 10 mg/kg every 12 hours for four doses, and then 15 mg/kg every 12 hours (all given as infusions over 30 minutes) until the ethylene glycol levels are less than 20 mg/dL.

D. **Isopropyl alcohol** is found in rubbing alcohol, skin lotions, and cleaning products.

1. **Intoxication** occurs approximately 30 minutes after ingestion. Isopropopanol metabolizes to acetone, and can lead to hypotension, respiratory depression, abdominal pain, and GI bleeding. Patients usually develop an osmolal gap, but no anion gap.

2. **Treatment** is supportive care with IV fluids, vasopressors, and respiratory support, as needed. Patients with significant refractory hypotension may require hemodialysis.

IV. Substance abuse

A. **Amphetamine and cocaine intoxications** can be the primary reason for admission, or comorbidities of trauma. **Amphetamines** are indirect sympathomimetics that increase postsynaptic catecholamines by inhibiting the presynaptic uptake and storage of catecholamines as well as their destruction by oxidase. **Cocaine** works in a similar fashion, and also binds to the dopamine-reuptake transporter. Both have been associated with seizures, intracerebral hemorrhage, ischemic strokes, hypertension, tachycardia, myocardial ischemia and infarctions, dysrhythmias, hyperpyrexia, rhabdomyolysis, acute renal failure, disseminated intravascular coagulation, and pulmonary edema. Pulmonary edema may occur several days after drug use, and initially appears as acute respiratory distress with hypoxemia followed by a noncardiogenic pulmonary edema. Treatment is supportive care for the organ systems involved and aggressive control of hyperpyrexia, if present. Unopposed β-blockade should be avoided because it worsens outcome. Hyperadrenergic symptoms can be treated with benzodiazepine administration.

B. **Barbiturates** are used to treat seizure disorders, induce general anesthesia, and produce conscious sedation in children. They are a source of substance abuse and have been implicated in suicides. Coingestion of other substances must be considered. These highly lipid-soluble drugs are absorbed rapidly from the gastrointestinal tract and rapidly distributed to the brain. Barbiturates are oxidized by enzymes in the smooth endoplasmic reticulum of hepatocytes and are cleared to a variable extent by the kidney. Induction of the oxidative enzymes may increase elimination of compounds metabolized by the same pathways and also produce tolerance to barbiturates.

1. **Severe acute barbiturate overdose** is manifested by coma, hypoventilation, hypothermia, and hypotension (secondary to cardiovascular depression).

2. **Treatment** includes cardiopulmonary support and the removal of barbiturate by alkaline diuresis and gastrointestinal decontamination with activated charcoal. Neurologic status is assessed with frequent physical examinations, computed tomography to determine the presence of focal lesions, and lumbar puncture to rule out meningitis. An **isoelectric electroencephalogram** may indicate suppression of neuronal activity by the barbiturate rather than brain death.

C. **Benzodiazepines** have sedative, anxiolytic, anticonvulsant, and hypnotic actions and high abuse potential. They enhance the binding of GABA to its receptor and potentiate neuronal inhibition through hyperpolarization of the plasma membrane.

1. Oral formulations are easily absorbed from the gastrointestinal tract and appear in the systemic circulation within 30 minutes. The metabolism of all benzodiazepines is by hepatic cytochrome P-450 with transformation to secondary products and conjugation to inactive compounds that are cleared by the kidney. The metabolite of diazepam desmethyldiazepam has a long half-life and retains the affinity for the GABA receptor and have half-lives greatly exceeding those of their parent compounds. As for other drugs that use the cytochrome P-450 pathway, their metabolism can be increased by increased age, hepatic disease, and inducers (e.g., EtOH, barbiturates) or decreased by inhibitors (e.g., cimetidine, erythromycin). Toxicity, manifested by profound sedation to the point of requiring an invasive and expensive neurologic investigation, may be seen if the initial dose is not decreased after a few days, especially for elderly patients.

2. **The toxicity** of benzodiazepines taken in overdose is minimal due to a high therapeutic index. Patients will exhibit CNS depression marked by drowsiness, stupor, or ataxia. Coma, respiratory depression, and death are rare. If co-ingested with EtOH, barbiturates, TCAs, or antipsychotics, however, the safety margin of benzodiazepines is markedly diminished. Profound CNS depression, cardiovascular instability, and respiratory failure may be present. Lorazepam given through a continuous IV infusion has the additional toxicity associated with its vehicle, propylene glycol. Propylene glycol may lead to metabolic acidosis, renal failure, seizures, arrhythmias, and CNS depression. Patients receiving infusions of more than 1 mg/kg/d should be monitored for the development of an osmolar gap. An osmolar gap of ≥ 10 is a predictor of propylene glycol toxicity.

3. **Treatment** is supportive after gastrointestinal decontamination with activated charcoal. **Flumazenil** is a benzodiazepine antagonist that will reverse the effects of an overdose. The dose is 0.5 to 5 mg IV. Because the half-life is almost 1 hour, redosing after 1 to 2 hours is required to prevent resedation. Seizures from co-ingested drugs (e.g., TCAs, EtOH) may occur when flumazenil use reverses the therapeutic effects of the benzodiazepine.

D. **Opioid overdose** in the ICU is often iatrogenic. Manifestations include somnolence, decreased respiratory drive with hypercarbia, and, rarely, apnea. Symptoms are treated by temporarily stopping or reducing the source of the opiate, administering naloxone in 40-μg increments to reverse the respiratory depression without compromising pain control, and providing ventilatory support as needed.

1. Patients admitted to the ICU after illicit use of opioids may have had respiratory depression reversed by naloxone or nalmefene in the emergency department, need further monitoring for respiratory depression and continued treatment with naloxone, have a requirement for mechanical ventilation, or need treatment for an overdose of co-ingested substances.

2. **Heroin** may cause the rapid onset of noncardiogenic pulmonary edema, similar to neurogenic pulmonary edema. This can occur several days after heroin use and is often initially diagnosed as acute respiratory distress syndrome (ARDS). Resolution follows ventilatory support with positive end-expiratory pressure and appropriate diuresis.

3. **Withdrawal** of therapeutic or abused opiates is often associated with an abrupt increase in sympathetic output. Agitation, severe hypertension, tachycardia, and pulmonary edema may result. α-2-Adrenergic blockade with **clonidine** (0.1–0.3 mg/d, by mouth or by a weekly patch) will relieve some of the symptoms. Benzodiazepines can be used treat anxiety and concomitant ethanol withdrawal. **Early consultation** with specialists in substance abuse facilitates continuity of treatment.

E. **Designer drugs** are "recreational" drugs that are produced through small modifications of the chemical structure of a variety of compounds. Because of these structural changes, the drugs may fall outside current classifications of illicit compounds. The designer drugs used in a community and their precise effects vary, but are usually well known to law enforcement agencies and emergency room personnel. Treatment is usually supportive. In particular, **Ecstasy** (MDMA) causes a feeling of euphoria in patients, but can lead to hyperpyrexia, likely related to overexertion with inadequate fluid intake, rhabdomyolysis, serotonin syndrome, multiorgan failure, and sudden death. Additionally, some patients will consume large volumes of free water in an effort to prevent hyperthermia, occasionally leading to hyponatremia, and even cerebral edema. These patients should be treated with fluid restrictions unless significantly symptomatic, in which case they may warrant hypertonic saline. All other patients with a more classic presentation require aggressive fluid repletion, and β-blockers can be used to decrease sympathetic tone. Some severely hyperthermic patients may warrant active cooling and dantrolene.

V. Poisonings

A. **Carbon monoxide (CO)** is a common cause of poisoning because CO is undetectable and ubiquitous whenever there is incomplete oxidation of propane, natural gas, kerosene, and gasoline. It is a frequent prehospital cause of death following smoke inhalation (see Chapter 35). An unappreciated source is through the metabolism of methylene chloride that is inhaled or absorbed from commercial paint products. CO binds to any heme protein and cuproprotein with an affinity greater than that of oxygen.

1. Mild symptoms include headache and nausea. The signs and symptoms of more serious exposures may reflect tissue hypoxia and reperfusion injury: ataxia, dyspnea, myocardial ischemic, dysrhythmias, hypotension, lactic acidosis, seizures, and coma. The diagnosis is made on clinical suspicion and the level of arterial or venous carboxyhemoglobin (COHg) measured spectrophotometrically with a co-oximeter. Because oxyhemoglobin and COHg absorb light at the same wavelength, pulse oximetry cannot be used as an indicator of CO poisoning. The delayed onset of a wide range of neuropsychiatric symptoms (parkinsonism, dementia, personality changes, psychosis, incontinence) may occur

3 to 240 days after exposure to CO, with a 1-year recovery of 50% to 75%. Advanced age may be one risk factor. There are no predictive laboratory or clinical tests for this syndrome.

2. **Treatment** of CO poisoning is 100% O_2 to compete with CO bound to hemoglobin. The half-life of CO is 2 to 7 hours. This is reduced to an average of 90 minutes with 100% O_2 via face mask, 60 minutes by endotracheal administration, and 23 minutes with hyperbaric O_2 (HBO) at 2.8 to 3 atmospheres absolute (2,128–2,280 mm Hg) (see also Chapter 35).

B. **Cyanide**-containing compounds are widely used in industry and found in many synthetic compounds, insecticides, and cleaning solutions. It can be released from many burning plastics during structure fires (see Chapter 37) and from the metabolism of sodium nitroprusside when used in high doses, for prolonged periods, and in patients with hepatorenal insufficiency.

1. **Symptoms** of mild cyanide toxicity include lethargy, confusion, agitation, increasing tachycardia, tachyphylaxis, and lactic acidosis. In the appropriate clinical scenario, lactate levels have been considered one of the best markers for cyanide toxicity because cyanide levels are usually not readily available. The difference between the arterial and mixed venous oxygen saturation pressure increases to more than 70% because tissues cannot utilize oxygen. Severe poisoning produces coma, seizures, cardiac collapse, and respiratory failure.

2. **Treatment** is gastrointestinal decontamination with activated charcoal used for ingested cyanide compounds. **Sodium nitrite** (300 mg IV over >5 minutes in a volume of 100 mL of 5% dextrose) can be administered. Rapid administration of sodium nitrite will cause hypotension. The nitrite reacts with hemoglobin to form methemoglobin. The cyanide complexed to cytochrome oxidase will then form methemoglobin–cyanide, thereby restoring active enzyme. In severe toxicity, inhaled **amyl nitrite** has been used as quick source of nitrite. In patients with suspected concomitant carboxyhemoglobinemia, such as a victim of a fire, nitrites are not recommended, as development of methemoglobinemia will further decrease oxygen-carrying capacity. The sodium thiosulfate may be given as directed. Recent data have suggested that **hydroxocobalamin** may also be effective in the treatment of cyanide toxicity in smoke inhalation patients. Subsequent treatment with **sodium thiosulfate** (12.5 g) leads to the formation of thiocyanate that can be removed by the kidney. If needed, additional half doses of sodium nitrite and sodium thiosulfate can be given.

VI. **Malignant Hyperthermia (MH)** is an inherited hypermetabolic state caused by the inability of skeletal muscle sarcoplasmic reticulum to reuptake calcium after exposure to volatile anesthetics or succinylcholine. The precise pathophysiologic mechanism of MH is not known. It usually occurs immediately after induction of anesthesia, especially if succinylcholine is administered, or at some time during the anesthetic. MH can also occur several hours into the postoperative period.

A. **Signs** of MH reflect its hypermetabolic state: Severe hypercarbia that is difficult to correct with increased ventilation, metabolic acidosis, tachycardia, and a temperature increase of 1°C to 2°C every 5 minutes. Initially, signs of MH may be considered mild and mistaken for atelectasis or infection. The true extent of hypercarbia and metabolic acidosis is best measured in a sample of central venous blood, which may reveal a partial dioxide pressure of 90 mm Hg in contrast to an arterial partial carbon dioxide pressure of 60 mm Hg. Hyperkalemia, hypertension, hypercalcemia, CK increasing to 20,000 U or more within the first 12 to 24 hours, and myoglobinuria are also seen. Dysrhythmias stem from the hypercarbia and the combined metabolic and respiratory acidosis. Disseminated intravascular coagulation may occur due to the release of tissue thromboplastin from damaged muscle tissue.

B. **Initial treatment** of MH hinges on the administration of **dantrolene** to inhibit the release of calcium from the sarcoplasmic reticulum and decrease the intracellular calcium concentration. The initial dose is 2.5 mg/kg with doses repeated until the hypercarbia, heart rate, temperature, and acidosis resolve. A total initial dose greater than the recommended maximum of 10 mg/kg is sometimes required. A dose of 1 mg/kg IV or orally can be repeated every 6 hours for 48 to 72 hours to prevent the recrudescence of MH.

1. **Metabolic acidosis** requires treatment with sodium bicarbonate if respiratory compensation is inadequate.
2. **Persistent dysrhythmias** are controlled with procainamide.
3. **Hyperthermia** can be treated with external cold packs and gastric and rectal lavage with cold saline.
4. **Myoglobinuria** is initially treated with the mannitol that is admixed with the dantrolene (each ampoule of dantrolene [20 mg] contains 3 mg of mannitol).
5. **Hypokalemia and hypocalcemia** are common after treatment of the crisis.

C. Therapy for MH is often begun prior to the knowledge of CK and blood gas measurements. **In the face of a normal value** or an incomplete clinical picture, the use of dantrolene should be discontinued because it can produce muscle weakness so severe that mechanical ventilation will be required.

VII. **Propofol infusion syndrome** is associated with propofol infusion rates of more than 4 mg/kg/h for more than 48 hours. Patients develop metabolic acidosis, rhabdomyolysis, hepatomegaly, bradycardia, asystole, or death, thought to be attributable to a defect in the mitochondrial respiratory chain.

A. **Early markers** of the syndrome include an anion-gap acidosis and an elevated lactate, as well as the development of a Brugada pattern on ECG.

B. **Treatment** begins with stopping the propofol infusion and providing hemodynamic support. The syndrome may be reversible in the early phases, but is often refractory to conventional cardiopulmonary support measures. Hemodialysis or hemofiltration is the most effective treatment for this syndrome and should be initiated early.

VIII. **Anaphylaxis and anaphylactoid reactions**

A. **Anaphylaxis** is a life-threatening immunologic response to an antigenic stimulus usually within a few minutes after exposure.

1. **Common drugs** known to cause anaphylaxis in susceptible individuals are thiobarbiturates, penicillins, cephalosporins, protamine in patients receiving NPH insulin, and IV contrast dye for radiology procedures. Many patients have a known anaphylaxis to bee stings and foods such as shellfish, peanuts, soybeans, and eggs. Simplistically, following an initial sensitization, some individuals synthesize high titers of immunoglobulin E (IgE). On reexposure, the antigen binds to specific IgEs on the surfaces of mast cells and basophils, initiating activation of the cells. A rapid, massive release of mediators of the immune response (e.g., histamine, prostaglandins, leukotrienes, kinins) subsequently occurs.

2. **Signs and symptoms.** The "classic" cutaneous manifestations of urticaria and flushing may not be evident prior to life-threatening symptoms of respiratory distress, hypotension, hypovolemia, pulmonary hypertension, and dysrhythmias.

3. **Treatment** for a severe reaction includes endotracheal intubation before airway edema becomes severe, rapid infusion of crystalloid to replete the lost intravascular volume (liters will be needed), and the parenteral administration of epinephrine (begin with 300–500 μg IV).

   a. **Epinephrine** will increase blood pressure through effects on vascular tone (α_1) and augmentation of cardiac output (β_1), will inhibit the release of mediators (β_2), and is a potent bronchodilator (β_2). Bronchodilation can be maintained with an infusion of epinephrine titrated to effect (>1–2 μg/min) with the caveat that lower doses (0.5–1 μg/min) may cause vasodilatation through β_2 activity on vascular smooth muscle.

   b. **Secondary treatment** includes the blockade of H_1 and H_2 receptors with **diphenhydramine** (0.5–1.0 mg/kg, IV) and the administration of **corticosteroids** (1–2 g of methylprednisolone) to further inhibit the immune response.

   c. **Subsequent management** includes immunologic testing as needed and the standard intensive care management of resolving respiratory and cardiovascular sequelae of the anaphylaxis and resuscitation. The choice of invasive monitors will depend on the comorbidity and severity of the reaction in a given patient.

B. **Anaphylactoid reactions,** in contrast to anaphylaxis, do not involve presensitized IgE. Anaphylactoid reactions may involve the IgG- or complement-mediated release of immunologic mediators or be the result of an idiosyncratic interaction of the drug with mast cells or basophils.

   1. Many drugs that may cause anaphylaxis in some individuals will cause an anaphylactoid reaction in others (thiobarbiturates, protamine).

   2. **Mild anaphylactoid reactions** caused by drug-induced histamine release produce transient hypotension, flushing, and urticaria. Such reactions are frequently noted with atracurium (but not *cis*-atracurium), *d*-tubocurarine, morphine, and vancomycin. These are easily treated with crystalloid administration, low doses of ephedrine, and time.

   3. **Severe anaphylactoid reactions** are clinically indistinguishable from anaphylaxis and are treated in the same manner.

IX. **Nerve agent toxicity.** The treatment of injury secondary to nerve agents employed as chemical weapons is a daunting task due to multiple logistical, psychological, and medical issues. Tabun, sarin, and soman are colorless and odorless fluorinated cyanide-containing volatile organophosphates (GX agents). VX agents are sulfur-containing organophosphates that are more persistent liquids. These compounds bind covalently to the enzymatic site of acetylcholinesterase (AChE). This bond becomes stronger with time (called "aging"). Soman ages AChE within minutes of contact. Exposure to these agents results in a rapid accumulation of acetylcholine at nicotinic and muscarinic receptors within *seconds*. Only synthesis of AChE corrects the depletion. Activation of neuromuscular nicotinic receptors result in a depolarizing blockade with progression to a complete blockade and respiratory arrest. In the CNS, confusion, convulsions, and coma will occur. Muscarinic stimulation leads to bradycardia with likely asystole, bronchorrhea, bronchoconstriction, excessive salivation, urination, lacrimation, and diarrhea.

A. **Protection of health care providers** is a prerequisite to patient care. Protective gear that will specifically isolate the wearer from exposure to the chemical agent must be utilized prior to entering environment where further exposure is possible or treating someone who has not been adequately decontaminated by established protocols.

B. Initial treatment is the administration muscarinic agonists, pralidoxime chloride (2-PAM), and anticonvulsants.

1. **Muscarinic blockers**

   a. **Atropine.** The dose of atropine for controlling toxic symptoms is 10 to 20 mg during the first 3 hours after exposure. The starting dose is 2 mg IV for adults and 0.02 mg/kg IV for children. To fully antagonize the muscarinic activity, the patient is basically put into an anticholinergic overdose that may require up to 50 mg/24 hours to achieve.

   b. **Scopolamine** (0.25 mg IV initially, then intramuscularly [IM] every 4–6 hours) may limit the anticholinergic effect.

2. **Benzodiapines** are freely used for sedation and for their anticonvulsive properties.

3. **2-PAM** (1–2 g IM; children 15–25 mg/kg IM) and obidoxime (used in some countries) are reactivators of AchE by competing with the generation of the covalent bond between the toxin and the active site of the enzyme.

C. Definitive hospital care. Most individuals who are exposed to high concentrations of chemical agents will die before treatment. Patients who reach definitive care are those who have been minimally exposed to chemical agents or who have received an initial antidote and supportive care.

1. **Medical treatment** will continue as described previously. Analgesia, sedation, and supportive care for multisystem organ involvement are required.

2. **Evaluation of concurrent trauma** is essential. Patients may be triaged to an intensive care unit before a standard trauma workup has been performed.

3. **Symptoms of other injuries** may be absent or difficult to assess. For example, a recovering patient may have abdominal pain from a perforated viscus that is masked by pain secondary to 2-PAM or the effects of the AChE inhibitor. Depth of sedation may be difficult to ascertain with atropine-induced miosis.

4. **Logistics** of medical supply are important. In the scenario of a mass casualty requiring mechanical ventilation, there may be insufficient equipment such as ventilators and bronchoscopes. Critical care will be provided outside of the intensive care unit. Similarly, intensivists will necessarily provide emergency medical care as needed.

Selected References

Arroliga AC, Shehab N, McCarthy K, Gonzales JP. Relationship of continuous infusion lorazepam to serum propylene glycol concentration in critically ill adults. *Crit Care Med* 2004;32:1709–1714.

Ben Abraham R, Rudick V, Weinbroum AA. Practical guidelines for acute care of victims of bioterrorism: conventional injuries and concomitant nerve agent intoxication. *Anesthesiology* 2002;97:989–1004.

Borron SW, Baud FJ, Barriot P, Imbert M, Bismuth C. Prospective study of hydroxocobalamin for acute cyanide poisoning in smoke inhalation. *Ann Emerg Med* 2007;49:794–801.

Boyer EW, Shannon M. The serotonin syndrome. *N Eng J Med* 2005;352:1112–1120.

Brent J, McMartin K, Phillips S, et al. Fomepazole for the treatment of ethylene glycol poisoning. *N Engl J Med* 1999;340:832–838.

Brent J, McMartin K, Phillips S, et al. Fomipazole for the treatment of methanol poisoning. *N Engl J Med* 2001;344:424–429.

Buckley NA, Chevalier S, et al. The limited utility of electrocardiography variables used to predict arrhythmia in psychotropic drug overdose. *Crit Care* 2003;7:R101–R107.

Callaham M, Schumaker H, Pentel P. Phenytoin prophylaxis of cardiotoxicity in experimental amitriptyline poisoning. *J Pharmacol Exp Ther* 1988;245:216–220.

Chen JY, Liu PY, Chen JH, Lin LJ. Safety of transvenous temporary cardiac pacing in patients with accidental digoxin overdose and symptomatic bradycardia. *Cardiology* 2004;102: 152–155.

Ernst A, Zibrak JD. Carbon monoxide poisoning. *N Engl J Med* 1998;339:1603–1608.

Gold BS, Dart RC, Barish RA. Bites of venomous snakes. *N Engl J Med* 2002;347:347–356.

Gyamlani GG, Parikh CR. Acetaminophen toxicity: suicidal vs. accidental. *Crit Care* 2002;6:155–159.

Hall AP, Henry JA. Acute toxic effects of "Ecstasy" (MDMA) and related compounds: overview of pathophysiology and clinical management. *Br J Anaesth* 2006;96:678–685.

Kam PC, Cardone D. Propofol infusion syndrome. *Anaesthesia* 2007;62:690–670.

Kenar L, Karayilanoglu AT. Prehospital management and medical intervention after a chemical attack. *Emerg Med J* 2004;21:84–88.

Larach MG, Brandom BW, Allen GC, Gronert GA, Lehman EB. Cardiac arrests and deaths associated with malignant hyperthermia in North America from 1987 to 2006: a report from the North American Malignant Hyperthermia Registry of the Malignant Hyperthermia Association of the United States. *Anesthesiology* 2008;108:603–611.

Liebelt EL, Francis PD, Woolf AD. ECG lead a VR versus QRS interval in predicting seizures and arrhythmias in acute tricyclic antidepressant toxicity. *Ann Emerg Med* 1995;26: 195–201.

Lundquist P, Rammer L, Sorbo B. The role of hydrogen cyanide and carbon monoxide in fire casualties: a prospective study. *Forensic Sci Int* 1989;43:9–14.

Mowry JB, Furbee RB, Chyka PA. Poisoning. In: Chernow B, ed. *The pharmacologic approach to the critically ill patient*. 3rd ed. Baltimore: Williams & Wilkins, 1994:975–1008.

Schiodt FV, Rochling FA, Casey DL, Lee WM. Acetaminophen toxicity in an urban county hospital. *N Engl J Med* 1997;337:1112–1117.

Shannon MW, Borron SW, Burns M. *Haddad and Winchester's clinical management of poisoning and drug overdose*. 4th ed. Philadelphia: WB Saunders, 2007.

Van Deusen SK, Birkhahn RH, Gaeta TJ. Treatment of hyperkalemia in a patient with unrecognized digitalis toxicity. *J Toxicol Clin Toxicol* 2003;41:373–376.

34

Adult and Pediatric Resuscitation

Arthur Tokarczyk and Richard Pino

I. **Overview.** The intensivist needs to be well versed in advanced cardiopulmonary resuscitation (CPR), not only to administer care in the ICU, but also to assist throughout the hospital. The algorithms and protocols presented here are based on the American Heart Association 2005 Guidelines for cardiopulmonary resuscitation. Formal training with routine recertification is essential to maintenance of skills. In addition to competence in resuscitation, the responsibilities of the intensivist include personnel and resource management that involves clear and deliberate communication and delegation of responsibilities in a crisis.

II. **Cardiac arrest**
   A. **Initial response** to a cardiac arrest can be quite rapid in the hospital setting. In the ICU, because of continuous ECG monitoring, the frequent use of arterial blood pressure determinations, and the optimal nurse-to-patient ratios, abnormalities in the circulation and dysrhythmias are identified immediately.
   B. **Etiologies.** Cardiac arrest in adults may be due to a number of causes, both from intrinsic cardiopulmonary problems to metabolic and anatomic abnormalities.
   1. Myocardial infarction
   2. Pericardial tamponade
   3. Pulmonary embolus
   4. Tension pneumothorax
   5. Hypoxemia
   6. Acid–base derangements
   7. Hypovolemia
   8. Hypothermia
   9. Electrolyte abnormalities, including potassium, calcium, and magnesium
   10. Adverse drug events
   C. **Pathophysiology.** A cascade of events begins with the systemic hypoperfusion caused by cardiac arrest. Initially, hypoxemia leads to anaerobic metabolism and acidosis. This leads to systemic vasodilation, pulmonary vasoconstriction, and insensitivity to catecholamines. With resuscitation after a period of hypoxia, the different organs are susceptible to reperfusion injury.

III. **Adult resuscitation**
   A. **Basic Life Support (BLS) primary survey and Advanced Cardiac Life Support (ACLS) secondary survey.** ACLS relies on **proper BLS assessment and care**, including high-quality **CPR** and defibrillation, as appropriate. In addition to the initial survey, ACLS achieves definitive treatment by adding drug therapy and advanced airway management. In ventricular fibrillation (VF) arrest, immediate intervention with CPR and defibrillation have been

shown to increase the chances of survival to discharge, while advanced interventions such as advanced airway management and pharmacologic interventions have not been shown to improve survival to discharge.

1. **Airway.** The patient may or may not already have a secured airway. Otherwise, the airway patency needs to be initially assessed with a head tilt-chin lift maneuver, jaw thrust, or artificial airway. The patient should be evaluated for spontaneous ventilation, using the algorithm—**look** rise and fall of the chest, **listen** for exhalation, and **feel** for airflow.

2. **Breathing (also see Chapter 4).** In the absence of adequate ventilation, the rescuer will initiate **two breaths** via bag-valve mask ventilation with 100% oxygen. At this point, breaths should be evaluated and maintained at a rate of **10 to 12 breaths/min**, or alternating with compressions in a **30:2 ratio**. If appropriate rise and fall of the chest is not achieved, then the airway should be repositioned and examined for a foreign body. Additionally, **a definitive airway may be placed as long as it does not interfere** with other resuscitative efforts, and it should be done by the most experienced person. Proper placement of the endotracheal tube is confirmed with end-tidal CO_2 measurement (usually with a colorimetric CO_2 indicator) and auscultation of the chest. In the event of inability to obtain intravenous access, a number of medications may be administered through the ETT, limited to epinephrine, atropine, naloxone, vasopressin, and lidocaine. The dose is typically 2 to 2.5 times the intravenous dose, diluted in 5 to 10 mL of water or saline.

3. **Circulation.** Evaluation of appropriate circulation should involve palpation of the **carotid pulse for at least 5, but not more than 10, seconds.** If no definite pulse is palpated, then chest compressions are begun at a rate of 100 compressions/min, alternating with ventilation in a 30:2 ratio. In the event of advanced airway placement, compressions continue at 100/min without stopping for ventilation at 10 to 12 breaths/min. **Compressions** should be performed with the rescuer's hands on the sternum at the level of the nipple, depressing the chest 1.5 to 2 in and allowing the chest to completely recoil after each compression. Adequacy of compressions may be assessed by palpating a pulse or observing the pressure using invasive arterial pressure monitoring. Furthermore, the patient should be placed onto a hard surface to facilitate the quality of compressions. Return of spontaneous circulatory flow should be revaluated after every five cycles, or 2 minutes. After successful return to a perfusing rhythm, chest compressions must continue for an additional 2 minutes.

4. **Defibrillation,** with CPR, forms the basis of successful adult resuscitation for VF, with the attention focused on minimal interruption of other interventions. As time progresses, the likelihood of a return of spontaneous circulation (ROSC) decreases. The successful utilization of **automated external defibrillators (AEDs)** has resulted in the training of additional responders, such as police, fire personnel, security guard, airline attendants, and so on. AEDs are available in many public areas, and include adhesive electrode pads for both delivery of shock and sensing of the rhythm. Since the AEDs only advise to the appropriateness of defibrillation, they are also manually triggered. In light of evidence supporting minimizing interruption of chest compressions, the current recommendation is for a single shock between cycles of CPR and the palpation for a pulse after an additional 2 minutes of chest compressions. This is to minimize any delays in coronary perfusion, despite ROSC.

a. **Biphasic waveform defibrillators** have been replacing monophasic defibrillators. They utilize a positive current in one direction then reversed in the opposite direction. Unless there is documentation of previous successful defibrillations, other known energy levels, for example, 200 J, are recommended for the first shock, with additional shocks at the same or higher dose. As mentioned above, CPR should continue through the charging, and it is the responsibility of the operator to make sure that all personnel are "cleared," or not in contact with the patient, during defibrillation.

b. **Monophasic waveform defibrillators** supply a shock in a single direction. These have been replaced by biphasic defibrillators in most institutions.

5. **Diagnosis and cardioversion of dysrhythmias.** Although the most common nonperfusing waveforms are VF and ventricular tachycardia (VT), instability may be also due to bradycardia and supraventricular tachycardia (SVT). A useful diagnostic and therapeutic tool is **adenosine** that has the ability to reveal underlying atrial rhythms (**Fig. 34-1**) and possibly convert an SVT to sinus rhythm. This diagnosis is complex, differentiating a wide-complex SVT from VT, and thus should not be used in the event of VT. A more sensitive method for diagnosing the atrial activity is the **atrial electrogram.** If the patient is not dependent on atrial pacing and has intraoperatively placed atrial pacing wires, these can be connected to a precordial lead and monitored temporar-

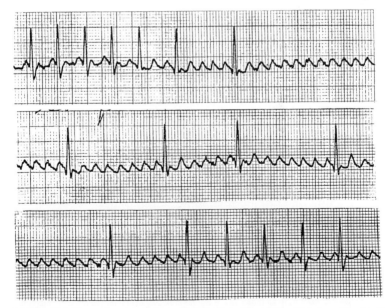

FIGURE 34-1 Diagnosis of a rhythm with adenosine. The initial ventricular response of 180 beats/min disappears after atrioventricular conduction is inhibited by adenosine, revealing an underlying rhythm of atrial flutter (300 beats/min, *top*), followed by a 6 to 8:1 block (*middle*), then a 2 to 3:1 block of atrial flutter with a ventricular rate of 120 beats/min.

ily. Additionally, a **transesophageal pacer** can be utilized to obtain the atrial electrogram (**Fig. 34-2**). If this is not immediately available, then a transvenous pacing wire can be passed through a No. 4 endotracheal tube for the same purpose. Typically, for synchronized cardioversion of a paroxysmal SVT (PSVT), the operator should choose a lower initial dose, such as 50 J (**Fig. 34-3**). With more resistant rhythms, such as **atrial fibrillation (AF) and atrial flutter,** an initial dose of 100 J may be indicated. For hemodynamically stable VT, an initial cardioversion at 100 J is warranted. In all dysrhythmias, the responder must be cognizant of the precipitating causes of the abnormality.

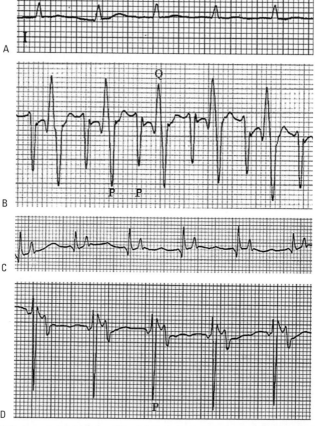

FIGURE 34-2 Suspected atrial flutter with a 2:1 block. **A.** Standard lead I of the ECG: The flutter waves are not distinct. **B.** Atrial electrogram obtained through an esophageal lead, showing an atrial rate of 300 beats/min with P waves (P) and Q waves (Q) easily seen. The polarity of the P wave is inverted because of the positioning of the esophageal probe. **C.** After treatment with amiodarone and cardioversion, normal sinus rhythm is seen on the standard ECG and the atrial electrogram **(D).**

6. **Pacing** involves pharmacologic and electronic choices for symptomatic bradycardia. Initial pharmacologic treatment for bradycardia, such as atropine, are often effective, but lack precision in heart rate control and are not universally efficacious. Atropine should not be used in Mobitz type II second-degree block or complete heart block (**Chapter 19**), in which case pacing should be attempted. Transcutaneous pacing if often the most feasible method of control with sedation required for patient comfort.

7. **Intravenous access** is important for effective medication administration, although **it should not interfere with prompt initiation of CPR** and delivery of shocks due to a stronger support with evidence. Central circulation access is ideal for resuscitation medications, as circulation time is greatly accelerated over peripheral access. It should be noted that the drawback of central access is that it may not be feasible during active resuscitation or compressions. Upper extremity veins are well suited for peripheral access, while intraosseous cannulation is also safe and effective in the absence of peripheral access. Many patients will have additional central access, including hemodialysis ports, portacaths, and peripherally inserted central catheters (PICC).

8. **Medications** are used to treat hypotension, myocardial ischemia, and dysrhythmias (additional information on the medications listed in this section may be found in the **Appendix**). For treatment of dysrhythmias, current guidelines recommend attempts at CPR and defibrillation, if necessary, before medical therapy. A few critical drugs may be given via the endotracheal tube (naloxone, atropine, vasopressin, epinephrine, and lidocaine) if IV access is not present. The dose is typically 2 to 2.5 times that of the IV dose diluted in 5 to 10 mL of saline or sterile water.

    a. **Adenosine** is an endogenous purine nucleotide with an extremely short half-life of 5 seconds. It is useful for its ability to slow atrioventricular (AV) nodal conduction to convert SVT to a sinus rhythm. Because it exerts its primary effect on the AV node, it is not useful for ventricular dysrhythmias or atrial fibrillation/flutter (**Fig. 34-1**). In fact, the more common transient vasodilatation may manifest as hypotension if given inappropriately during VT. Other adverse effects may include angina, bronchospasm, and dysrhythmias. For peripheral intravenous administration, an initial dose of 6 mg should be given rapidly with a fluid flush. If this is nondiagnostic or ineffective, the dose can be increased to 12 mg for

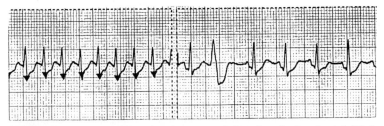

FIGURE 34-3 Synchronous cardioversion of a supraventricular tachycardia. Arrowheads (left) indicate synchrony of the defibrillator with the patient's rate (300 beats/min) prior to cardioversion (right) to a rate of 140 beats/min that was followed with pharmacologic therapy.

successive doses, although other, longer-duration agents may be required for recurrent PSVT. With central venous administration, the dose is reduced by half; the initial dose should be 3 mg, followed by 6 mg as needed. [**PALS:** 0.1 mg/kg; repeat dose 0.2 mg/kg; maximum dose 12 mg.]

b. **Amiodarone** (also see **Chapter 19**) is a versatile antiarrhythmic agent with effects on sodium, potassium, and calcium channels, as well as α- and β-adrenergic blocking properties. Indications include unstable VT, defibrillation with VF, rate control of VT, conversion of AF to sinus rhythm, ventricular rate control with atrial arrhythmias unresponsive to digitalis and due to accessory pathways, and as adjunctive treatment to cardioversion for SVT and atrial tachycardia. Typical acute side effects include hypotension, bradycardia, and QT-interval prolongation. **Dosing for unstable VT and VF** is **300 mg** in 20 to 30 mL saline or D_5W, given rapidly. For more stable dysrhythmias, such as AF with rapid ventricular response, the initial dose is 150 mg over 10 minutes, followed by an infusion of 1 mg/min for 6 hours, and 0.5 mg/min, with a maximum daily dose of 2 g. [**PALS:** loading dose 5 mg/kg; maximum dose 15 mg/kg/d.]

c. **Atropine** (also see **Chapter 19**) is an anticholinergic agent that reverses hemodynamically significant bradycardia or AV block. However, atropine is not suitable for treatment of Mobitz type II heart block or complete heart block, in which case pacing should be initiated. Dosing for symptomatic bradycardia is 0.5 mg, repeated every 3 to 5 minutes to a maximum dose of 0.04 mg/kg. For asystole, dosing is a 1-mg bolus, repeated every 3 to 5 minutes if needed; full vagal blockade is possible at 3 mg. [**PALS:** 0.02 mg/kg, minimum 0.1 mg, maximum dose 0.5 mg in child, 1 mg in adult.]

d. **β-Blocking agents** (also see **Chapter 19**). The utility of β-blockers in ACLS is limited to rate control in patients with preserved ventricular function and narrow complex tachycardias from a reentry SVT or automatic focus that is not controlled with vagal maneuvers or adenosine. These agents can be used for heart rate control in AF and atrial flutter. Typical side effects include hypotension, bradycardia, possible exacerbation of reactive airway disease, and AV conduction delays. Contraindications include second- or third-degree heart blocks, hypotension, acute or severe congestive heart failure, and pre-excitation syndrome such as Wolf-Parkinson-White (WPW). **Esmolol** is a very short-acting $β_1$-blocker, with a half-life of approximately 5 minutes. It is administered as a 0.5 mg/kg IV bolus (over 1 minute), with a 4-minute infusion of 0.05 mg/kg/min. A repeat dose of 0.5 mg/kg IV can be given, with an infusion of 0.1 mg/kg/min, up to 0.3 mg/kg/min. **Metoprolol** is another selective $β_1$-blocker, and it is given as a 5 mg IV bolus at 5-minute intervals. **Propranolol** is a nonselective β-blocker ($β_1$ and $β_2$), given as a IV bolus of 1 to 2 mg at 2-minute intervals, and has a slightly longer duration of action than metoprolol.

e. **Calcium chloride** is used specifically for treatment of symptomatic hypocalcemia, symptomatic hyperkalemia, magnesium intoxication, or reversal of calcium channel blocker toxicity. When given as calcium chloride, doses of 200 to 1,000 mg IV, over 5 minutes, are given as needed. [**PALS:** 2.7 mg/kg to 5.0 mg/kg IV, over 5 minutes.]

f. **Dopamine** is a δ, α- and β-adrenergic receptor agonist (also see **Chapter 6**). Although not frequently used in ACLS, dopamine can be used to increase heart rate in the event of bradycardia refractory to atropine treatment, and to increase vascular tone to raise the blood pressure and end-organ perfusion. Most common side effects include tachyarrhythmias. The initial dose should be started low (150 μg/min, or 2–3 μg/kg/min) and titrated to desired result or limited by adverse effects.

g. **Epinephrine** continues to be the primary pharmacologic agent in cardiac arrest due to its α-adrenergic effects in increasing coronary and cerebral perfusion. The limitation of efficacy lies in β-adrenergic activation by increasing myocardial oxygen demands, ischemia, and myocardial toxicity. Even though it is a mainstay of treatment, this is no good evidence that demonstrates an improvement in survival to discharge after cardiac arrest. High-dose epinephrine was supported by early ROSC and survival reports, but several randomized trials have failed to show any benefit with escalating doses in cardiac arrest. Theoretically, a higher dose may be justified in β-blocker or calcium channel blocker overdose. Dosing for intravenous administration is 1 mg (10 mL of a 1:10,000 solution) every 3 to 5 minutes during cardiac arrest. Epinephrine can be given via the endotracheal route at 2 to 2.5 mg per dose, until IV/IO access is established. [**PALS**: bradycardia, 0.01 mg/kg; pulseless arrest, 0.01 mg/kg.]

h. **Ibutilide** is an antiarrhythmic agent that is utilized to convert or control AF and flutter by prolonging the action potential and refractory period of cardiac tissue. In patients with normal cardiac function, it is used to convert AF or atrial flutter of duration less than 48 hours, and for rate control in AF or atrial flutter in patients unresponsive to β-blockers or calcium channel blockers. Additionally, it is useful for cardioversion of AF or AD in patients with pre-excitation syndrome (WPW). The most common side effects of ibutilide are ventricular arrhythmias, requiring continuous monitoring for 6 hours after dosing. Additionally, it carries minor incidence of hypotension and bradycardia. It is contraindicated with prolonged QTc >440 ms. Dosing is based on weight; for patients more than 60 kg, the intravenous dose of 1 mg is administered over 10 minutes, with an additional 1 mg IV dose given similarly in 10 minutes, if necessary. For patients less than 60 kg, the initial dose should be 0.01 mg/kg, administered as above.

i. **Isoproterenol** is a nonselective β-agonist that is no longer recommended in the ACLS algorithms. It may be considered for symptomatic bradycardia unresponsive to epinephrine and dopamine in the period until a pacemaker is available.

j. **Lidocaine** is a local anesthetic that has been relegated as an alternative to amiodarone as an adjunct to defibrillation and prevention of VF after myocardial infarction. This change in status over the years is due to randomized controlled trials showing inferior rates of ROSC and higher rates of asystole. Dosing is 1 to 1.5 mg/kg IV, with additional doses at 0.5 to 0.75 mg/kg IV push, at 5- to 10-minute intervals. [**PALS**: 20 μg/kg.]

k. **Magnesium** is a cofactor in many enzyme reactions, and hypomagnesemia can worsen hypokalemia in addition to inducing VT. The utility of magnesium as therapy is based on two observational studies in treating *torsades de pointes*. Adverse effects include hypotension and bradycardia. Emergent administration is 1 to 2 g diluted in 10 mL D_5W over 5 to 20 minutes. [**PALS:** 20 to 50 mg/kg, maximum 2 g.]

l. **Procainamide** is useful for conversion of AF and atrial flutter to sinus rhythm, controlling rapid ventricular response in SVT, and converting wide complex tachycardia. It has largely been replaced by amiodarone. Dosing is begun with an infusion of 20 to 30 mg/min for a total loading dose of 17 mg/kg or until arrhythmia is terminated, the patient has nausea, there is hypotension, or the QRS widens by 50%. A maintenance infusion should be maintained at 1 to 4 mg/min. Procainamide administration should be followed with serum levels of procainamide and *N*-acetylprocainamide, the active metabolite.

m. **Sodium bicarbonate** is not recommended for routine use in most cardiac arrests due to harmful effects, including paradoxical worsening of intracellular acidosis. The exceptions include treatment of hyperkalemia, tricyclic antidepressant, and phenobarbital overdose. Bicarbonate may be considered in severe metabolic acidosis unresponsive to standard ACLS treatments. The initial bicarbonate dose is 1 mEq/Kg IV, with repeat doses of 0.5 mEq/kg administered at 10-minute intervals. [**PALS:** 1 mEq/kg.]

n. **Sotalol** is a class III antiarrhythmic agent with nonselective β-blocking properties. Similar to ibutilide, it is used in patients with preserved ventricular function and monomorphic VT, AF with rapid ventricular response, atrial flutter, and pre-excitation syndrome such as WPW. Most common side effects include bradycardia, arrhythmias, including *torsades de pointes*, and hypotension. IV dosing is 1 to 1.5 mg/kg administered at a rate of 10 mg/min. The required slow rate of infusion is a limiting factor in emergent situations.

o. **Vasopressin** is a noradrenergic vasoconstrictor and antidiuretic hormone analogue. It is useful as an alternative to epinephrine during treatment of VF and requires less frequent dosing due to a longer half-life. Although retrospective data indicate a possible survival benefit in patients with asystole, randomized controlled trials fail to display any advantage over epinephrine in regard to ROSC, early survival, or survival to discharge. Dosing is 40 U intravenously, replacing the first or second dose of epinephrine.

p. **Verapamil and diltiazem** are calcium channel blockers that slow AV nodal conduction and increase refractoriness, with depressant effects on myocardial contractility. They are used for reentry SVT unresponsive to adenosine or vagal maneuvers and rate control in AF and atrial flutter. Because of their vasodilator and negative inotropic effects, side effects include hypotension, worsening of congestive heart failure, bradycardia, and exacerbation of accessory pathways in WPW syndrome. Verapamil dosing is initially 2.5 to 5 mg IV over 2 minutes, with repeat doses 5 to 10 mg given every 15 to 30 minutes up to 20 mg. Diltiazem dosing is 0.25 mg/kg (20 mg), followed by a repeat dose of 0.35 mg/kg (25 mg). Diltiazem can also be infused at a rate of 5 to 15 mg/h, titrated to heart rate. In the event of significant hypotension due to calcium channel blocker use, calcium chloride 500 to 1,000 mg is recommended.

Ventricular Fibrillation/Pulseless Ventricular Tachycardia

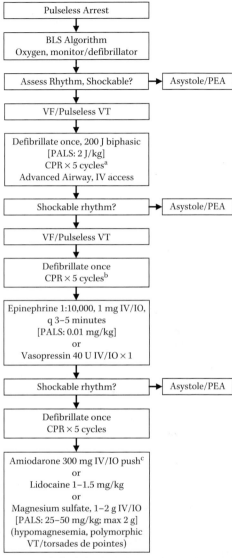

FIGURE 34-4 Algorithm for ventricular fibrillation and pulseless ventricular tachycardia. BLS, basic life support; CPR, cardiopulmonary resuscitation; IO, intraosseous; IV, intravenous; PALS, pediatric advanced life support; PEA, pulseless electrical activity; q, every; VF, ventricular fibrillation; VT, ventricular tachycardia.

aIn order to minimize lapses in CPR, compressions should be continued during defibrillator charging.

bOne cycle of CPR should follow the last successful defibrillation.

cAmiodarone bolus should be administered in 20–30 mL saline or D_5W. This is followed by an infusion of 1 mg/min for 6 hours and then 0.5 mg/min thereafter. An additional dose of 150 mg IV can be readministered for recurrence of VF or pulseless VT.

Asystole/PEA

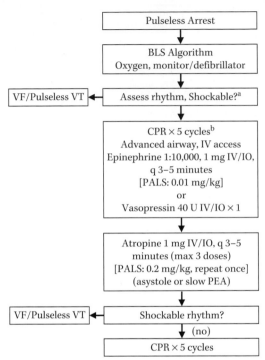

FIGURE 34-5 Algorithm for ventricular asystole and PEA. BLS, basic life support; VF, ventricular fibrillation; BLS, basic life support; CPR, cardiopulmonary resuscitation; IO, intraosseous; IV, intravenous; PALS, pediatric advanced life support; PEA, pulseless electrical activity; q, every; VF, ventricular fibrillation; VT, ventricular tachycardia.

[a]If rhythm is unclear and could be VF, then treat as shockable rhythm/VF.

[b]After determination of nonshockable rhythm, a cause should be considered for treatment:

   Hypovolemia (give volume resuscitation)
   Hypoxemia (start oxygen)
   Hypokalemia (give potassium)
   Hyperkalemia (insulin/glucose, calcium, bicarbonate)
   Bicarbonate appropriate acidosis (bicarbonate)
   Tension pneumothorax (thoracostomy)
   Cardiac tamponade (pericardiocentesis)
   Drug overdose (specific treatment)

9. **Specific ACLS algorithms**
   a. VF/pulseless VT (**Fig. 34-4**)
   b. Asystole/PEA (**Fig. 34-5**)
   c. Unstable tachycardia (**Fig. 34-6**)
   d. Stable tachycardia (**Fig. 34-7**)
   e. Bradycardia (**Fig. 34-8**)

Unstable Tachycardia

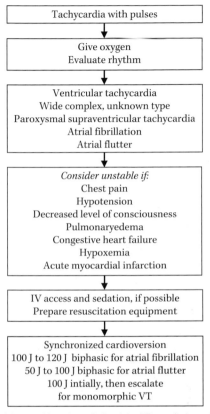

Tachycardia with pulses

↓

Give oxygen
Evaluate rhythm

↓

Ventricular tachycardia
Wide complex, unknown type
Paroxysmal supraventricular tachycardia
Atrial fibrillation
Atrial flutter

↓

Consider unstable if:
Chest pain
Hypotension
Decreased level of consciousness
Pulmonaryedema
Congestive heart failure
Hypoxemia
Acute myocardial infarction

↓

IV access and sedation, if possible
Prepare resuscitation equipment

↓

Synchronized cardioversion
100 J to 120 J biphasic for atrial fibrillation
50 J to 100 J biphasic for atrial flutter
100 J intially, then escalate
for monomorphic VT

FIGURE 34-6 Protocol for unstable tachycardia in adults. VT, ventricular tachycardia.

10. **Direct cardiac compression with open chest** is an option for patients with penetrating chest trauma, pericardial tamponade, chest wall deformity, or any recent chest surgery. This allows for direct assessment and compression of the myocardium and direct defibrillation with internal paddles starting at 5 to 10 J.

11. **Termination of CPR** is warranted after a prolonged, competent trial of CPR and ACLS. The likelihood of survival to discharge becomes exceedingly small in the absence of ROSC after a prolonged BLS and ACLS interval of 15 to 20 minutes. Although there is a paucity of significant data, intermittent ROSC may delay the termination of resuscitative efforts. The circumstances and decision to terminate efforts should be documented.

12. **Unique situations in resuscitation**
    a. **Do not resuscitate (DNR)** orders are advance directives that express the patient's wishes in the event resuscitation is an option. These

Narrow complex
↓
Vagal maneuvers
↓
Adenosine → Conversion to sinus rhythm
↓
Diagnosis of rhythm without conversion
↓

Wide complex of unknown type
↓
Esophageal lead
↓
Clinical information
↓

Ventricular tachycardia
├─ Normorphic VT → Cardioversion
└─ Polymorphic VT
   ├─ Normal baseline Q-T
   └─ Long baseline Q-T

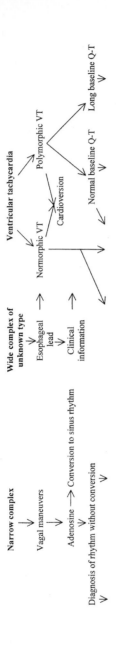

Atrial fibrillation / Atrial flutter	Supraventricular tachycardia			Ventricular tachycardia			
	Rhythm	EF ≥ 40%	EF < 40%	EF ≥ 40%	EF < 40%	EF ≥ 40%	Consider torsades
Rate control Diltiazem β-blocker Digoxin	*Junctional*	Amiodarone β-blocker Diltiazem/verapamil	Amiodarone	*Preferred:* Procainamide Sotalol *Acceptable:* Amiodarone Lidocaine	Amiodarone (150 mg) or lidocaine (0.5–0.75 mg/kg) Synchronized cardioversion	Treat ischemia Correct electrolytes *One of the following:* β-blocker Lidocaine Amiodarone Procainamide Sotalol	Correct electrolytes *One of the following:* Magnesium Overdrive pacing Isoproterenol Phenytoin Lidocaine
Rate control/conversion Amiodarone Procainamide	*Paroxysmal*	Diltiazem/verapamil β-blocker Digoxin DC cardioversion Consider: procainamide, amiodarone, sotalol	Amiodarone Digoxin Diltiazem				
Conversion DC cardioversion Ibutilide	*Ectopic or multifocal atrial*	Diltiazem/verapamil β-blocker Amiodarone	Amiodarone Diltiazem				

FIGURE 34-7 Protocol for stable tachycardia in adults. DC, direct current; EF, ejection fraction; VT, ventricular tachycardia.

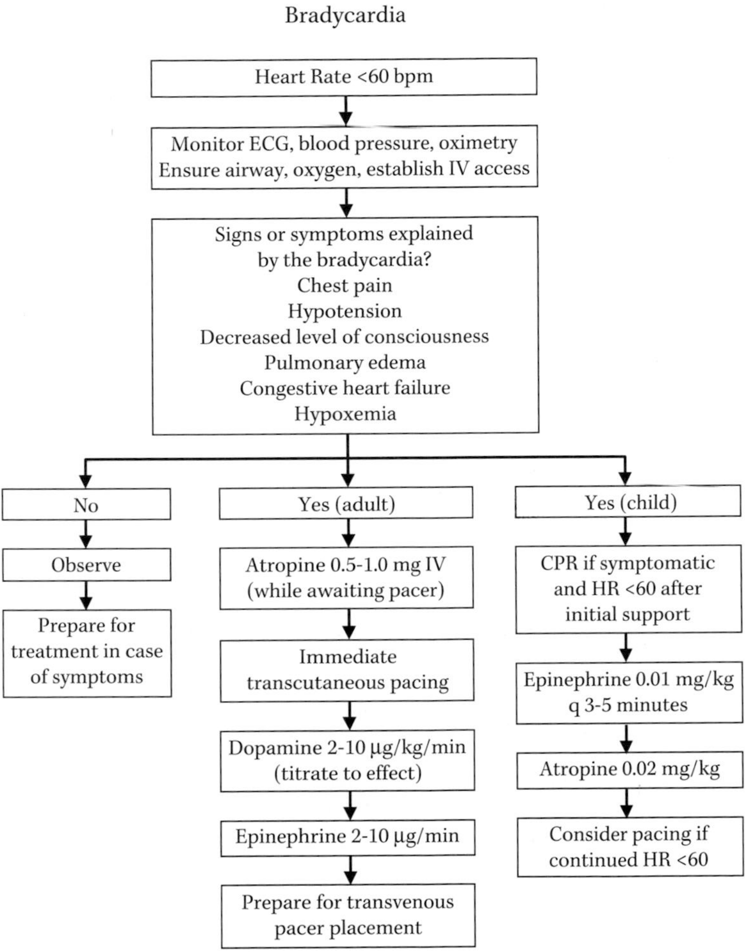

Bradycardia

FIGURE 34-8 Bradycardia algorithm. CPR, cardiopulmonary resuscitation; ECG, electrocardiogram; HR, heart rate; IV, intravenous; q, every.

orders are not automatically modified or suspended in the perioperative period, but instead each situation needs to be carefully addressed. This includes the patient's desire for perioperative resuscitation, limits of perioperative resuscitation, and reinstatement of the original DNR orders. The intensivist may be asked to respond to arrests and incubate outside the intensive care unit. In those situations, the patient's code status should be determined, as the responder is ethically and legally bound to follow the patient's directives.

IV. Pediatric resuscitation

A. Basic life support. In the most recent 2005 AHA guidelines, the rules for BLS sequences have been simplified, with only minor modifications to the age categories of the pediatric patient. The **neonatal** period includes newborns up to hospital discharge, while **infants** are less than 1 year. Additionally, for the layperson, a child is categorized as up to 8 years, while for the health care provider this age is extended to adolescence, or even 18 years. Cardiac arrests in the pediatric population are most commonly due to **hypoxemia** from respiratory arrest or airway obstruction. For all victims of sudden collapse, the health care provider should "phone first," while for victims of likely asphyxiation or witnessed arrest the lone health care provider should administer five cycles of CPR before initiating EMS. Additional updates and differences for the pediatric population are provided for health care providers.

1. **Airway** (see also **Chapter 4**). The pediatric airway management is quite similar to that of an adult, with few changes to accommodate anatomical differences. In order to clear the airway, infants should receive back slaps and chest thrust in lieu of abdominal thrusts, due to the risk of gastrointestinal and hepatic injury. The rescuer needs to be cognizant of airway obstruction due to overzealous head tilt-chin lift maneuvers.

2. **Breathing.** Administration of the ventilations need to be slow, in order to prevent gastric distention, and with sufficient volume, in order to cause rise and fall of the chest. The rate is **12 to 20 breaths/min**, increased to **40 to 60 for the neonate**. With an advanced airway, the rate of breathing for the child and infant changes to **8 to 10 breaths/min** without pausing compressions, just like an adult.

3. **Circulation.** The recommendation for assessment of pulses in the infant is to check the femoral or brachial pulses, due to the difficulty in palpating the neck. The **ratio of compressions to breaths in single-rescuer CPR is the same as that of the adult (30:2)**. The **rate** of compressions is also 100/min for children and infants, and the **depth** should be approximately one-third the depth of the chest. For the child, the compression location is lower half of the sternum, avoiding the xiphoid process. For children, the heel of one hand is used while two to three fingers are used for infants. In the case of two rescuers, the infant should receive compressions with the hands encircling the chest and thumbs depressing the chest at the nipple line. The exception is for two-person compressions, in which the compression to breath ratio is 15:2. Lastly, the neonate should receive 90 compressions and 30 breaths/min, avoiding simultaneous compressions and ventilations.

B. Pediatric advanced life support. The management of pediatric resuscitation has a few differences from adult resuscitation, including predominating etiologies and presenting causes. Anatomic differences in size and physiologic differences warrant adjustments in drug and defibrillator administration.

1. **Intubation.** Sizing of an endotracheal tube is more variable in pediatric patients, and for neonates and infants a 3.0-, 3.5-, or 4.0-mm-inner diameter (ID) endotracheal tube is often sufficient. In older children, the rule-of-thumb formula used is based on age: uncuffed tube size in millimeters-ID = 4 + (age/4). When choosing a cuffed tube, the approximate size should be 0.5 mm smaller than an uncuffed tube. In the absence of intravenous access, lidocaine, epinephrine, atropine,

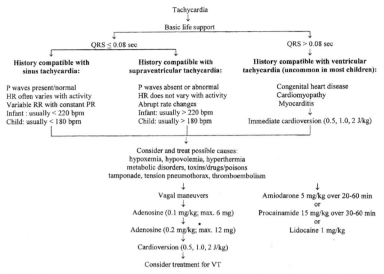

FIGURE 34-9 Protocol for tachycardia in children. HR, heart rate; VT, ventricular tachycardia.

and naloxone may be administered via the endotracheal route in the pediatric patient.

2. **Cardioversion and defibrillation.** For infants less than 10 kg, the smaller infant paddles should be used, and the standard adult paddles (8–10 cm) are used for children more than 10 kg. Although the ideal energy doses are not known, the dose for patients more than 40 kg should be 150 J, while initial dose for patients less than 40 kg should be 2 J/kg. This may be increased to 4 J/kg if the lower dose is ineffective. Defibrillation is still the definitive treatment for VF, and carries a higher survival rate than for adults. The dose for cardioversion is much lower at 0.2 J/kg for initial attempts with subsequent doses elevated up to 1 J/kg, if necessary.

3. **Intravenous access.** Central venous access provides for secure long-term access, although early intravenous or intraosseous access is essential. With cardiac arrest, intraosseous access is recommended in the absence of established intravenous access. The endotracheal route may be utilized for select medications mentioned earlier. Once the pediatric patient is stabilized, alternate intravenous access should be obtained to allow removal of intraosseous access.

4. **Medication** is most often based upon weight, and these have been illustrated in the medication section earlier.

5. **Specific ACLS algorithms** are similar to those used in adults, with the exception of drug and defibrillation dosages. Included are the algorithms for several situations:
   a. PALS pulseless arrest (**Fig. 34-4**)
   b. PALS asystole/PEA (**Fig. 34-5**)
   c. PALS bradycardia (**Fig. 34-8**)
   d. PALS tachycardia (**Fig. 34-9**)

Selected References

American Heart Association in collaboration with International Liaison Committee on Resuscitation. Guidelines 2005 for cardiopulmonary resuscitation and emergency cardiovascular care. *Circulation* 2000;112(suppl):I1–I211.

Bella BS, Alvarado JP, Myklebust H, et al. Quality of cardiopulmonary resuscitation during in-hospital cardiac arrest. *JAMA* 2005;293:305–310.

Eisenberg MS, Mengert TJ. Cardiac resuscitation. *N Engl J Med* 2001;344:1304–1313.

Martens PR, Russell JK, Wolcke B, et al. Optimal response to cardiac arrest study: defibrillation waveform effects. *Resuscitation* 2001;49:233–243.

Niemann JT, Stratton SJ, Cruz B, Lewis RJ. Endotracheal drug administration during out-of-hospital resuscitation: where are the survivors? *Resuscitation* 2002;53:153–157.

Wik L, Hansen TB, Fylling F, et al. Delaying defibrillation to give basic cardiopulmonary resuscitation to patients with out-of-hospital ventricular fibrillation: a randomized trial. *JAMA* 2003;289:1389–1395.

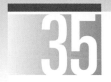

Transfusion Medicine

Jeffrey Ustin and Hasan Alam

I. **Indications for transfusion therapy.** Blood component transfusion is usually performed because of decreased production, increased utilization/destruction or loss, or dysfunction of a specific blood component (red cells, platelets, or coagulation factors).

A. **Anemia**

1. **Red cell mass.** The primary reason for transfusion is to maintain oxygen-carrying capacity to the tissues by the normal mass of red blood cells. Healthy individuals or individuals with chronic anemia can usually tolerate a hematocrit (Hct) of 20% to 25%, assuming normal intravascular volume. The Hct assumes red blood cell normocytosis and appropriate hemoglobin (Hgb) content. A patient with hypochromic normocytic anemia may have an Hct within normal range but a decreased oxygen-carrying capacity. For this reason, **many institutions use Hgb (g/dL) in lieu of Hct (%)** as an indicator of red blood cell mass. Modern techniques assay total red cell Hgb and the red blood cell count to calculate the Hct instead of measuring the packed cell volume by centrifugation.

2. If a patient is anemic, the etiology should be clarified. It may be **secondary to decreased production** (marrow suppression), **increased loss** (hemorrhage), or **destruction** (hemolysis).

3. Anemia in critically ill adults is common, but the Hgb level that should prompt red blood cell transfusion is controversial. Results from a large, controlled study of critically ill patients suggested that a "restrictive" transfusion policy (i.e., maintaining a Hgb level of 7–9 g/dL) improved hospital survival when compared with a more traditional transfusion regimen (i.e., maintaining Hgb at 10–12 g/dL).

4. Estimating the volume of blood to transfuse can be calculated as follows:

$$\text{Volume to transfuse} = (\text{Hct}_{\text{desired}} - \text{Hct}_{\text{present}}) \times \text{BV}/\text{Hct}_{\text{transfused blood}}$$

where BV is blood volume, which may be estimated at 70 mL/kg ideal weight in male adults and 65 mL/kg in female adults.

B. **Thrombocytopenia.** Spontaneous bleeding is unusual with platelet counts more than 5,000 to 10,000 μL, but in the immediate postoperative period counts more than 50,000 are preferable. Thrombocytopenia is due to decreased bone marrow production (e.g., chemotherapy, tumor infiltration, and alcoholism) or increased utilization or destruction (e.g., hypersplenism; idiopathic thrombocytopenic purpura; and drug effects such as with heparin, histamine-2 blockers, and ticarcillin). It is also seen with massive blood transfusion.

II. **Blood typing and cross-matching**

A. **Donor blood** and **recipient blood** are typed in the red cell surface **ABO** and **Rh systems** and screened for antibodies to other cell antigens. **Cross-matching** involves directly mixing the patient's plasma with the donor's red cells to establish that hemolysis does not occur from any undetected antibodies. An individual's red cells have A, B, AB, or no surface antigens. If a person's red cells are lacking either surface antigen A or B, then antibodies will be produced against it. A person who is type B will have anti-A antibodies in the serum, and a type O individual, that is, a person having neither A nor B surface antigens will have circulating anti-A and anti-B antibodies. Consequently, a person who is type AB will not have antibodies to either A or B and can receive red blood cells from a person of any blood type. Type O blood has neither A nor B surface antigens, and a person with this blood type is a universal red cell donor and can donate blood cells to persons of any other blood type.

B. **Rh surface antigens** are either present (Rh-positive) or absent (Rh-negative). Individuals who are Rh-negative will develop antibodies to the Rh factor when exposed to Rh-positive blood. This is not a problem with the initial exposure, but hemolysis will occur due to the circulating antibodies with subsequent exposures. This can be a particular problem during pregnancy. The anti-Rh antibodies are immunoglobulin (IgG) and freely cross the placenta. In Rh-negative mothers who have developed Rh antibodies, these antibodies are transmitted to the fetus. If the fetus is Rh-positive, massive hemolysis will occur, termed hemolytic disease of the newborn. **Rh-immune globulin,** an Rh-blocking antibody, prevents the Rh-negative patient from developing anti-Rh antibodies. Rh-immune globulin is routinely administered to Rh-negative women pregnant with Rh-positive fetuses and should be given to Rh-negative individuals who receive Rh-positive blood, especially women of childbearing age. The recommendation is one dose (approximately 300 μg/vial) for every 15 mL of Rh-positive blood transfused.

III. Blood component therapy
A. Whole blood
   1. Whole blood has been largely replaced by component therapy because of storage impediments and no demonstrable superiority of the former. The exceptions may be for children younger than 2 years undergoing complicated cardiovascular surgery, exchange transfusions, where whole blood may have an outcome benefit in reduced transfusions, and during warfare. Overall, component therapy is far more efficient and practical for transfusion.
   2. Whole blood must be ABO and Rh identical.
B. Red blood cells
   1. 1 U of packed red blood cells (pRBCs, volume approximately 250 mL) will usually raise the Hb of a euvolemic adult by 1 g/dL once equilibration has taken place.
   2. **pRBCs** must be ABO compatible (**Table 35-1**). If an emergency blood transfusion is needed, type-specific (ABO) red cells can usually be obtained within minutes if the patient's blood type is known. If type-specific blood is unavailable, type O Rh-negative red cells should be transfused. Type-specific blood should be substituted as soon as possible to minimize the amount of type O plasma (containing anti-A and anti-B antibodies) transfused.
C. Platelets
   1. 1 U of random donor platelets increases the platelet count by 5,000 to 10,000 μL. If thrombocytopenia is due to increased destruction (e.g., due to development of antiplatelet antibodies), platelet transfusions will be less efficacious. A posttransfusion platelet count drawn 10 minutes after completion of platelet transfusion confirms platelet

T A B L E 35-1	Transfusion Compatibility					
	Donor					
Recipient	**A**	**B**	**0**	**AB**	**Rh+**	**Rh−**
1. Red Blood Cells						
A	X		X			
B		X	X			
0			X			
AB	X	X	X	X		
Rh+					X	X
Rh−						X
2. Fresh Frozen Plasma						
A	X			X		
B		X		X		
0	X	X	X	X		
AB				X		
Rh+					X	X
Rh−					X	X

Compatible transfusions are marked by X.

refractoriness if the count fails to increase by 5,000 μL per random donor unit transfused.

2. **ABO-compatible platelets** are not required for transfusion, although they may provide a better response as measured by the posttransfusion platelet count. **Single-donor platelets** are obtained from one individual by platelet pheresis; 1 U is equivalent to approximately six random donor units. Single-donor platelets may be used to reduce exposure to multiple donors or in cases of poor response to random donor platelets where destruction is suspected. In cases where alloimmunization causes platelet refractoriness, **HLA-matched platelets** may be required for effective platelet transfusion. **Rh-negative women** of childbearing age should receive Rh-negative platelets if possible because some RBCs are transfused with platelets. If this is impossible, Rh-immune globulin may be administered.

D. **Fresh frozen plasma (FFP)** in a dose of 10 to 15 mL/kg will generally increase plasma coagulation factors to 30% of normal.
   1. Factors V and VIII are most labile and quickly become depleted in thawed FFP. Fibrinogen levels increase by 1 mg/mL of plasma transfused. Acute reversal of warfarin requires only 5 to 8 mL/kg of FFP.
   2. ABO-compatible FFP transfusion (**Table 35-1**) is required, but Rh-negative patients may receive Rh-positive FFP.
   3. 6 U of platelets contain the equivalent of 1 U of FFP.
   4. Volume expansion in itself should not be an indication for FFP transfusion.

E. **Cryoprecipitate** is the material formed from thawing FFP at 1°C to 6°C.
   1. Each unit of cryoprecipitate contains a minimum of 80 IU of factor VIII and approximately 200 to 300 mg of fibrinogen. It also contains factor XIII, von Willebrand's factor, and fibronectin.
   2. **Indications for cryoprecipitate** include hypofibrinogenemia, von Willebrand's disease, hemophilia A (when factor VIII is unavailable), and

preparation of fibrin glue. The dose of cryoprecipitate is **I U per 7 to 10 kg,** which **raises the plasma fibrinogen by approximately 50 mg/dL** in a patient without massive bleeding.

3. ABO compatibility is not required for transfusion of cryoprecipitate, but it is preferred because of the presence of 10 to 20 mL of plasma per unit.

F. **Factor concentrates.** Individual coagulation factors are available for patients with discrete factor deficiencies. These may be derived from pooled human plasma or synthesized by recombinant gene technology.

1. **Activated recombinant factor VII (rFVIIa)** was originally developed to control bleeding in patients with hemophilia A or B who had developed circulating inhibitors to factors VIII and IX. Subsequently, **rFVIIa** has been used to treat hemorrhage related to trauma; severe postpartum disseminated intravascular coagulation (DIC); and perioperative bleeding associated with prostatectomy, spinal fusion, or cardiac surgery. **rFVIIa** may work by complexing with a tissue factor after endothelial injury and subsequent stimulation of the coagulation cascade. Its half-life is approximately 2 hours, and only 20 to 40 μg/kg may be needed to reverse a coagulopathy. There is an increasing number of reports in the literature of thromboembolic complications in patients that are treated with this agent. In addition, it is an expensive drug. Based on the most current literature, there is a **very limited role for factor VIIa in massively bleeding patients.** It should be considered only in carefully selected patients who have diffuse coagulopathy (as opposed to surgically correctable source of hemorrhage), if they fail to respond to conventional component therapy, and its administration should be governed by an institutional protocol.

G. **Technical considerations**

1. **Compatible infusions.** Blood products should not be infused with 5% dextrose solutions, which will cause hemolysis, or with lactated Ringer's (LR), which contains calcium and may induce clot formation. Sodium chloride 0.9%, albumin 5%, and FFP are all compatible with pRBC.

2. **Blood filters** (80 μm) should be used for all blood components except platelets to remove debris and microaggregates. **Leukocyte filters** may be used to remove white blood cells to prevent transmission of cytomegalovirus in the immunocompromised, to prevent alloimmunization to foreign leukocyte antigens, and to diminish the incidence of febrile reactions. **Platelets** should be transfused through a 170-μm blood filter.

IV. **Volume expanders.** For the composition and general characteristics of various fluid solutions, see **Chapter 7.** There is ongoing controversy as to which is superior for resuscitation and maintenance of the critical patient.

A. **Colloids**

1. **Albumin.** Under normal circumstances, administered albumin has an intravascular half-life of 10 to 15 days. The wisdom of routine infusion of albumin for volume repletion in critically ill patients has been called into question by a Cochrane group meta-analysis and one large randomized trial (the *SAFE* trial) demonstrating no difference in outcome when albumin was compared to crystalloid resuscitation. A **higher mortality** may actually occur with the use of albumin for resuscitation of traumatic brain injury patients (**Chapter 9**). Although not supported by specific evidence, the use of albumin seems sensible in individual situations, such as to continue resuscitation of the patient with a **temporarily open abdomen,** who requires operative closure in 24 to 48 hours.

In such a patient, having a reduced edema of the abdominal wall will greatly facilitate surgical closure, which may prevent infection and hasten recovery.

2. **Hydroxyethyl starch (HES)** is available in the United States as a high-molecular-weight 6% preparation in either 0.9% sodium chloride or LR solution. HES is stored in the reticuloendothelial cells of the liver for a prolonged time. Amylase excretion by the kidneys is diminished by attachment to HES, which may result in an elevated serum amylase for several days after HES infusion, which should not be confused with pancreatitis. HES may affect coagulation by decreasing factor VIII levels (a prolonged PTT can be seen). Although in stable adults, HES infusions (up to 1.5 L) have not been associated with clinically significant bleeding, in a coagulopathic patient these products should be used with great caution or not at all. In addition, recent data have indicated significant **nephrotoxicity of HES in patients with septic shock**. Although these findings have not been investigated in other categories of patients, they suggest caution with these products in all critically ill patients. Anaphylactoid reactions are rare.

B. **Crystalloids** are available in multiple formulations (see **Chapter 7**). Hypotonic solutions are typically chosen as maintenance IV fluids, while normal saline or LR are used as a basic resuscitation fluid. **Hypertonic saline** is used in treatment of traumatic brain injury (see **Chapter 10**) and occasionally as a resuscitation fluid.

C. **Immunomodulatory effects of resuscitation fluids** can be seen for both crystalloids and colloids. It has been demonstrated that crystalloid fluids can cause an increased oxidative burst as well as apoptosis and changes in gene regulation. Similar effects are seen with HES but not with albumin.

V. Pharmacologic therapy

A. **Erythropoietin** increases red cell mass by stimulating proliferation and development of the erythroid precursor cells. It has been used to correct anemia in patients with chronic renal failure, and to increase red cell mass prior to preoperative autologous donation. A recent controlled trial of weekly erythropoietin in critically ill patients demonstrated no difference in the rate or quantity of blood transfusion and a minimal increase in Hct (dosing regimen was 40,000 U subcutaneously [SQ] weekly for 3 weeks, and patients also received supplemental iron 150 mg elemental per day in a liquid enteral formulation). There was a significant increase in the rate of thrombotic events unless the patient was receiving heparin. At this time, the routine use of erythropoietin is not indicated in the critically ill. A less clear-cut use for erythropoietin may be in the severely anemic patient who refuses blood transfusion. In addition to iron, folate supplementation is also recommended for patients taking erythropoietin. Initial recommended doses in renal patients range from 50 to 100 IU/kg IV or SQ three times a week.

B. **Granulocyte colony-stimulating factor (GCSF) and granulocyte-macrophage colony-stimulating factor (GMCSF)** are myeloid growth factors useful for shortening the duration of neutropenia induced by chemotherapy. GCSF is specific for neutrophils, and GMCSF increases production of neutrophils, macrophages, and eosinophils. Administration of these drugs enhances both neutrophil count and function. As such, they are frequently used for the treatment of febrile neutropenia. Treatment results in an initial brief decrease in the neutrophil count (due to endothelial adherence), then a rapid (usually after 24 hours) sustained leukocytosis that is dose dependent. Recommended doses are GCSF 5 μg/kg/day or GMCSF 250 μg/m^2/day until absolute neutrophil count is more than 10,000 mm^3.

C. Other drugs used to enhance hemostasis are discussed in **Chapter 26.**

VI. Blood conservation and salvage techniques. Blood transfusion of critically ill patients is common, with approximately 40% of patients being transfused during an ICU stay. Those patients who are older and stay longer in the ICU are more likely to receive a transfusion. Recent research focusing on possible deleterious effects of homologous blood transfusion in critically ill patients has sparked an interest in techniques to diminish or eliminate the need for blood transfusion.

A. Phlebotomy losses from critically ill patients can be significant, ranging from 40 to almost 400 mL/d, with higher losses in surgical units versus medical units. Patients with more severe illnesses and a greater number of dysfunctional organs suffer higher phlebotomy losses due to a greater number of blood draws. Techniques demonstrated to reduce phlebotomy losses include (a) a "closed" system of blood sampling where the initial aspirated blood is reinjected into the patient instead of discarded, (b) use of small-volume phlebotomy tubes, and (c) "point-of-care" testing at the bedside, which frequently requires less blood than the clinical laboratory. Finally, the presence of both arterial and central venous catheters in critically ill patients is correlated with higher phlebotomy losses, suggesting another reason to repeatedly evaluate the need for such catheters with respect to hemodynamic monitoring or medication/nutritional support administration.

B. Surgical drain salvage devices allow the reinfusion of shed blood. Most commonly used in patients with blood collected from chest tubes, these are useful for reducing homologous transfusions in the immediate postoperative period. Use of these devices requires skilled nursing for proper administration and sterile technique. They are contraindicated in conditions where the drained cavity is infected. A potential danger is hyperkalemia from reinfusion of hemolyzed cells, which is occasionally life threatening.

VII. Complications of blood transfusion therapy
A. Transfusion reactions

1. **Acute hemolytic transfusion reactions** are estimated to occur in 1 in 250,000 transfusions, and are usually due to clerical errors. Symptoms include anxiety, agitation, chest pain, flank pain, headache, dyspnea, and chills. Nonspecific signs include fever, hypotension, unexplained bleeding, and hemoglobinuria. **Table 35-2** describes the steps to be taken if a transfusion reaction is suspected.

2. **Nonhemolytic transfusion reactions** are usually due to antibodies against donor white cells or plasma proteins. These patients may complain of anxiety, pruritus, or mild dyspnea. Signs include fever, flushing, hives, tachycardia, and mild hypotension. The transfusion should be stopped and a hemolytic transfusion reaction ruled out (see prior discussion).
   a. If the reaction is only urticaria or hives, the transfusion should be slowed, and antihistamines (**diphenhydramine,** 25–50 mg IV) and glucocorticoids (**hydrocortisone,** 50–100 mg IV) may be administered.
   b. In patients with known febrile or allergic transfusion reactions, leukocyte-poor red cells (leukocytes removed by filtration or centrifugation) may be given and the patient pretreated with antipyretics (**acetaminophen,** 650 mg) and an antihistamine.

TABLE 35-2	Treatment of Suspected Acute Hemolytic Transfusion Reaction

1. Stop transfusion
2. Send remaining donor blood and fresh patient sample to blood bank for re–cross-match
3. Send patient sample to laboratory for free hemoglobin, haptoglobin, Coombs' test, DIC screen
4. Treat hypotension with fluids and/or vasopressors as necessary
5. Consider use of corticosteroids
6. Consider measures to preserve renal function and maintain brisk urine output (intravenous fluid, furosemide, mannitol)
7. Monitor patient for DIC

DIC, disseminated intravascular coagulation.

    c. Anaphylactic reactions occur rarely and may be more common in patients with an IgA deficiency. These reactions are usually due to plasma protein reactions. Patients with a history of transfusion anaphylaxis should only be transfused with washed red cells (plasma free).

B. Metabolic complications of blood transfusions

    1. Potassium (K^+) concentration changes are common with rapid blood transfusion, but seldom of clinical importance. With storage, red cells leak K^+ into the extracellular storage fluid. This is rapidly corrected with transfusion and replenishment of erythrocyte energy stores.

    2. Calcium is bound by citrate, which is used as an anticoagulant in stored blood products. Rapid transfusion (1 U of packed red blood cells in 5 minutes) may decrease the ionized calcium level. An equal volume of an FFP transfusion is more likely to cause citrate toxicity compared with packed RBCs because citrate tends to concentrate in plasma during blood processing. Usually, the decreased ionized calcium level is transient because the citrate is rapidly metabolized by the liver. Severe hypocalcemia, manifested as hypotension, QT-segment prolongation on the electrocardiogram, and narrowed pulse pressure may occur in patients who are hypothermic, who have impaired liver function, or who have decreased hepatic blood flow. Ionized calcium levels should be monitored during rapid transfusions, and calcium replaced intravenously with calcium gluconate (30 mg/kg) or calcium chloride (10 mg/kg), if signs or symptoms of hypocalcemia are present.

    3. Acid–base status. Although banked blood is acidic due to citrate anticoagulant and accumulated red cell metabolite, the actual acid load to the patient is minimal. Acidosis in the face of severe blood loss is more likely due to hypoperfusion and will improve with volume resuscitation. Alkalosis (from metabolism of citrate to bicarbonate) is common following massive blood transfusion.

C. Infectious complications of blood transfusions have been markedly reduced due to improved testing of donated blood. Recent changes to U.S. blood bank screening for viral pathogens include addition of specific nucleic acid testing of small pooled donated samples to enhance detection of hepatitis C virus (HCV) and human immunodeficiency virus (HIV) before serologic antibody conversion has occurred. Pooled products (e.g., cryoprecipitate) have an increased risk of infection proportional to the number of donors.

1. **Hepatitis B.** The current risk of HBV transmission is estimated to be 1 in 220,000 U transfused. Although the majority of infections are asymptomatic, with approximately 35% of infected individuals demonstrating acute disease, approximately 1% to 10% become chronically infected with potentially significant long-term morbidity.

2. **Hepatitis C.** The risk of transfusion-related HCV is approximately 1 in 1,935,000 U. Risks of HCV infection are more serious than those with HBV, however, because 85% of patients suffer chronic infection, 20% develop cirrhosis, and 1% to 5% of infections cause hepatocellular carcinoma.

3. **HIV.** Because of improved screening and testing, the risk of transfusion-associated HIV has been estimated to be approximately 1 in 2.1 million units transfused in the United States.

4. **Cytomegalovirus (CMV).** The prevalence of antibodies to CMV in the general population is approximately 70% by adulthood. The incidence of transfusion-associated CMV infection in previously noninfected patients is quite high. CMV infection in healthy individuals is usually asymptomatic, but immunosuppressed patients, such as those who have received bone marrow or stem cell transplantation, are at high risk for serious complications, including death. Prevention of CMV infection in high-risk individuals who are exposed to cellular blood elements through transfusion is extremely important. Thus, the American Association of Blood Banks recommends that either CMV-seronegative or leukoreduced blood be administered to transplant recipients who are CMV-negative and to patients undergoing chemotherapy with severe neutropenia an expected consequence.

5. **West Nile virus.** Infection was first documented in the western hemisphere in 1999 in New York City. Now it is a seasonal epidemic causing febrile and neurological illnesses including meningoencephalitis, aseptic meningitis, and acute flaccid paralysis. Transfusion transmission was first documented in 2002 and screening is done in high epidemic regions. The current risk in these areas is estimated at 1 in 1 million units transfused.

6. **Bacterial infections.** Exclusion of donors with evidence of infectious disease and the storage of blood at 4°C reduces the risk of transmitted bacterial infection. However, the necessity of room-temperature storage of platelets to maintain functional integrity creates an ideal medium for bacterial growth. Infection rates for platelets are estimated at 1 in 1,000 to 2,000 U, with an estimated 15% to 25% of infected transfusions causing severe sepsis. Organisms likely to infect platelet concentrates include *Staphylococcus aureus*, coagulase-negative *Staphylococcus*, and diphtheroids. Red blood cells are much less likely to become contaminated with bacteria, but the most commonly cultured organism is *Yersinia enterocolitica,* and the mortality rate from transfusion-acquired sepsis is a striking 60%.

D. **Transfusion-related acute lung injury (TRALI)** is a syndrome of severe hypoxemia, dyspnea, and pulmonary edema, often accompanied by fever and hypotension, which is associated with blood transfusion. The pathophysiology is incompletely understood; possible mechanisms of injury include (a) donor blood containing WBC antibodies to recipient WBC antigens resulting in granulocyte or lymphocyte activation and subsequent pulmonary endothelial injury and (b) donor blood containing biologically active lipids, which similarly activate granulocytes. Symptom onset is usually within a few hours of receiving a blood transfusion, and the clinical findings fulfill criteria for acute lung injury/acute respiratory distress syndrome (see **Chapter 20**). Incidence of TRALI is estimated at 1 to 2 in 5,000 transfusions. Any transfused product that contains plasma may cause TRALI, but the most commonly reported causative products are pRBCs, FFP, and whole blood. Mortality from TRALI is approximately 5%. Treatment is the same as for other forms of acute lung injury and frequently requires mechanical ventilation. Resolution is often rapid given the initial severe oxygenation impairment. Most patients show dramatic clinical improvement within 48 hours and radiographic clearing of edema within a few days.

VIII. Massive transfusions (see Appendix 35-1)

A. **Massive transfusion** is arbitrarily defined as the administration of at least 8 to 10 U of blood transfused within a 12-hour period.

1. Transfusion of 10 to 12 U of red blood cells can cause a 50% drop in the platelet count and produce a **dilutional thrombocytopenia** that can result in diffuse oozing and failure to form clot.

2. The normal human body has tremendous reserves of clotting factors, and adequate hemostasis generally occurs with a plasma clotting factor concentration as low as 30% of normal. There is an approximate 10% decrease in clotting factor concentration for each 500 mL of replaced blood loss. Small quantities of the stable clotting factors also are present in the plasma of each unit of red cells transfused. Bleeding from factor deficiency during a massive transfusion is usually due to diminished levels of fibrinogen and labile factors (V, VIII, and IX). Bleeding from hypofibrinogenemia is unusual unless the fibrinogen level is less than 75 mg/dL. Labile clotting factors are administered in the form of FFP.

3. **Additional complications of massive transfusion** include hypothermia from the rapid infusion of blood, citrate toxicity (**Section VII.B.2**), and dysrhythmias secondary to hypocalcemia and hypomagnesemia. If ongoing bleeding is present, hypotension and metabolic acidemia are to be expected. Hypotension may also be a result of ischemic- or septic-mediated myocardial depression.

4. **Once bleeding has begun from** a dilutional **coagulopathy** and thrombocytopenia, **it can be very difficult to control.** Therefore, it is recommended that 1 U of FFP be administered for every 1 to 2 U of pRBCs. Additionally, 6 U of platelets should be administered for every 10 U of pRBCs. Careful attention must be paid to the use of cell saver units of blood. Like banked blood, these are nearly devoid of clotting factors and must be included in the transfusion count.

5. In addition to transfusion of appropriate blood products, the strategy for massive transfusion includes **maintaining intravascular volume,** administering **calcium** as needed to offset the effects of citrate, and the use of **vasopressors with inotropic properties** as a *temporizing* measure to maintain systemic arterial pressure until euvolemia has been established. A monitor of cardiac output or filling may be useful in the acute phase of bleeding. Ongoing surgical bleeding is an indication for operative correction. Antifibrinolytic agents (see **Chapter 26**) may be considered and employed if fibrinolysis is contributing to bleeding. Frequent laboratory measures of coagulation status are indicated because these parameters change rapidly in the setting of massive hemorrhage and transfusion. Finally, **direct communication with the blood bank** is fundamental to expedite component preparation.

6. Unfortunately, there are no good markers to determine when further transfusion is futile.

APPENDIX 35-1
Abridged Massive Transfusion Protocol of the Massachusetts General Hospital Trauma Service

1. The protocol can be initiated at any time during the trauma patient's hospitalization, including prior to arrival to MGH
2. Appropriate candidates include
   a. Any patient with an initial blood loss of at least 40% of blood volume, or in whom it is judged that at least 10 U of blood replacement is immediately required
   b. Any patient with a continuing hemorrhage of at least 250 ml/h
   c. Any patient, when clinical judgment is made such that blood loss as identified in "A" and "B" is imminent
3. Once the decision is made to initiate this protocol, the appropriate physician needs to
   a. Notify the blood bank with the age and gender of the patient
   b. Ensure that a blood bank sample is obtained
4. The blood bank fellow is available to assist in decision-making.
5. RBC selection
   a. At least 4 U of emergency-release, uncross-matched group O negative pRBCs will be released for all Rh-negative or Rh-unknown patients.
   b. All patients will receive Rh-negative cells as long as inventory is adequate. An effort will be made to provide Rh-negative cells to females age less than 50. The blood bank will decide to switch the patient to Rh-positive RBCs based on the available inventory and the anticipated requirement.
   c. Group O RBCs will be used until the patient's blood group is known after which the patient will be switched to group-specific RBCs.
6. Blood components requests
   After the initial assessment, if >10 total units are expected to be needed, the clinical team should request:
   a. 10 pRBCs
   b. 10 FFPs
   c. 1 dose of platelets
7. It is *essential* that the clinical team communicates to the blood bank when the patient is being moved to a different ward.
8. Laboratory monitoring for ongoing blood support in cases requiring >10 U of RBCs:
   a. Transfusion support should be individualized for each patient.
   b. The following general guidelines apply:
      1. Check Hb, platelet count, INR, and fibrinogen after each blood volume lost/infused.
      2. Include the number of "cell saver" units in the tally of pRBCs.
      3. Target a ratio of 2 pRBCs to 1 FFP during the course of acute bleeding.
      4. Anticipate fibrinolysis and treat with antifibrinolytics if there is ongoing diffuse bleeding.
      5. Verify that the INR is <2 and fibrinogen >100. Values outside these ranges may indicate systemic fibrinogenolysis, DIC, or hemodilution.
      6. In the absence of platelet transfusion, anticipate a halving of the platelet count with each blood volume resuscitation. Transfuse platelets to maintain an anticipated platelet count >50,000 µl.
      7. A stat AST or ALT can be used to document shock liver (values >800), which is an independent indication for antifibrinolytic therapy.
   c. Monitor and treat abnormalities of ionized Ca^{2+}, K^+, pH, and temperature.
9. Not all massively injured patients can be saved. The decision to withdraw support for the massively injured patient should be made by consensus of the treating team.

Selected References

American Society of Anesthesiologists Task Force on Blood Component Therapy. Practice guidelines for perioperative blood transfusion and adjuvant therapies. *Anesthesiology* 2006;105:198–208.

Boehlen F, Morales MA, Fontana P, et al. Prolonged treatment of massive postpartum haemorrhage with recombinant factor VIIa; case report and review of the literature. *BJOG* 2004;111:284–287.

Boffard KD, Riou B, Warren B, et al. Recombinant factor VIIa as adjunctive therapy for bleeding control in severely injured trauma patients: two parallel randomized, placebo-controlled, double-blind clinical trials. *J Trauma* 2005;59:8–18.

Cochrane Injuries Group Albumin Reviewers. Human albumin administration in critically ill patients: systematic review of randomized controlled trials. *BMJ* 1998;317:235–340.

Corwin HL, Gettinger A, Fabian TC, et al. Efficacy and safety of epoetin alfa in critically ill patients. *N Eng J Med* 2002;357:965–976.

Dutton RP, Hess JR, Scalea TM. Recombinant factor VIIa for control of hemorrhage: early experience in critically ill trauma patients. *J Clin Anesth* 2003;15:184–188.

Fowler RA, Berenson M. Blood conservation in the intensive care unit. *Crit Care Med* 2003; 31(suppl):S715–S720.

Goodnough LT. Risks of blood transfusion. *Crit Care Med* 2003;31(suppl):S678–S686.

Gunter OL, Au BK, Isbell JM, et al. Optimizing outcomes in damage control resuscitation: identifying blood product ratios associated with improved survival. *J Trauma* 2008;65: 527–534.

Hebert PC, Wells G, Blajchman MA, et al. A multicenter, randomized, controlled clinical trial of transfusion requirements in critical care. *N Engl J Med* 1999;340:409–417.

Hess JR, Holcomb JB. Transfusion practice in military trauma. *Transfus Med* 2008;18(3): 143–150.

Holcomb JB, Wade CE, Michalek JE, et al. Increased plasma and platelet to red blood cell ratios improves outcome in 466 massively transfused civilian trauma patients. *Ann Surg* 2008;248:447–458.

Lake CL, Moore RA, eds. *Blood: hemostasis, transfusion, and alternatives in the perioperative period.* New York: Raven Press, 1995.

O'Connell NM, Perry DJ, Hodgson AJ, et al. Recombinant FVIIa in the management of uncontrolled hemorrhage. *Transfusion* 2003;43:1711–1716.

Spinella PC, Perkins JG, Grathwohl KW, et al. Effect of plasma and red blood cell transfusions on survival in patients with combat related traumatic injuries. *J Trauma* 2008;64:S69–S78.

Stainsby D, MacLennan S, Thomas D, et al. Guidelines on the management of massive blood loss. *Br J Hem* 2006;135:634.

The SAFE Study Investigators. A comparison of albumin and saline for fluid resuscitation in the intensive care unit. *N Engl J Med* 2004;350:2247–2256.

The SAFE Study Investigators. Saline or albumin for fluid resuscitation in patients with traumatic brain injury. *N Engl J Med* 2007;357:874–884.

Neurological Trauma

Sherry Chou and Marc de Moya

I. Head injury

A. Epidemiology. Traumatic brain injury (TBI) is the most common cause of death and morbidity associated with blunt trauma. More than half a million patients sustain TBI in the United States each year. Of them, approximately one-seventh is pronounced dead upon arrival in the emergency department. For severe head injuries, the mortality is 30%, with the incidence of significant disability reaching up to 95%. TBI is also a leading cause of death and disability in the military theater.

B. Mechanisms

1. **Blunt.** The most common causes of blunt TBI are motor vehicle collisions (MVC) and falls. Younger patients are more likely affected by MVC and older patients are more likely to sustain falls. MVC are often associated with large changes in velocity, which lead to shearing forces and rapid deceleration injury. This will often lead to direct injury (coup) and opposite side injury (contracoup).

2. **Penetrating.** Gunshot wounds are the most common type of penetrating TBI. They produce direct injury secondary to the transmission of kinetic energy and cavitation.

C. Clinical classification. The Glasgow Coma Score (GCS, **Table 36-1**) divides the clinical examination into three categories: verbal, eye opening, and motor. The score ranges from 3 to 15.

1. **Mild injury: GCS 14 to 15.** There may have been loss of consciousness, but it is usually brief (<5 minutes). These patients may have associated intracranial pathology despite the high GCS that warrants 24-hour observation.

2. **Moderate injury: GCS 9 to 13.** These patients require close monitoring and may necessitate more invasive therapies.

3. **Severe injury: GCS ≤8.** These patients suffer the highest morbidity and mortality and will require intensive care monitoring.

D. Initial assessment

1. **History.** Understanding the mechanism of injury, the changes in velocity endured, and the medical history of the patient are important factors in determining associated injuries, comorbidities, and prognosis. Additional information about the behavior of the patient initially at the scene concerning seizure activity, mental status, ability to move extremities, and time of insult.

2. **Physical examination.** The initial hospital examination should focus on the following:

   a. **Vital signs.** Look for evidence of a **Cushing response:** hypertension associated with bradycardia and changes in respiratory pattern. These are signs of brainstem herniation. Dysrhythmias may occur with intracranial hemorrhage, and a variety of respiratory pattern changes may occur: bradypnea, tachypnea, Cheyne-Stokes, apnea. These respiratory patterns are associated with hypo- or hyperventi-

TABLE 36-1	Glasgow Coma Score	
Category	**Score**	

Category	Score
Best Motor Response	
Obeys commands	6
Localizes	5
Withdraws from pain	4
Abnormal flexion	3
Abnormal extension	2
None	1
Verbal Response	
Oriented	5
Confused	4
Inappropriate words	3
Incomprehensible sounds	2
None	1
Eye Opening	
Spontaneously	4
To speech	3
To pain	2
None	1

Note: Highest score is 15 and lowest possible score is 3. Score may be limited by intubation or paralysis, which is denoted by adding all possible scores and adding 1 plus T or P.

lation. Profound hypotension is rarely associated with isolated head injuries in the acute setting, rather, it is usually found in the setting of other associated injuries (neurogenic or hemorrhagic shock).

   b. **Inspection/palpation:** Periorbital ecchymosis (raccoon eyes) or retroauricular ecchymosis (battle signs), otorrhea, rhinorrhea, and blood from the auditory canal are associated with basal skull fractures. Depressed skull fractures, lacerations, and maxillary instability may also be associated with significant intracranial injury. Of note, scalp lacerations may be a source of significant blood loss.

3. **Imaging**
   a. **Computed tomography (CT)** scan is the first-line imaging modality used to further classify TBI. The Marshall Classification System for diffuse axonal injury is used for prognostic and research purposes. CT scans have enabled practitioners to categorize brain injury according to the presence of blood. **Without the use of intravenous (IV) contrast,** one can identify fresh blood in the subdural, epidural, subarachnoid, intraparenchymal, or intraventricular regions. Diffuse axonal injury occurs with shear injury and may show diffuse small petechial hemorrhages on CT. With the addition of IV contrast, CT angiograms are possible to evaluate the cerebrovascular system for evidence of associated vascular injuries.
   b. **Magnetic resonance imaging (MRI)** provides more detailed information about the parenchyma; however, it does little to change management during the acute phase. MRI may provide additional

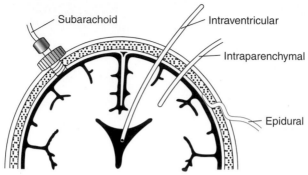

FIGURE 36-1 Illustration of four different methods for transducing ICP. From Lee KR, Hoff JT. Intracranial pressure. In: Youmans JR, ed. *Neurological surgery.* 4th ed. Philadelphia: WB Saunders, 1996:505. permission.

prognostic information by showing areas of tissue death versus tissue edema. **MR angiography** (MRA) is an additional method for evaluating the cerebrovascular system.

E. Monitoring

1. **Intracranial pressure (ICP)** monitors most commonly used are intraparenchymal or intraventricular catheters, but other types are available (**Fig. 36-1**).

   a. **Indications.** Brain Trauma Foundation guidelines provide level II recommendations that all patients with a GCS ≤ 8 with an abnormal CT scan (hematomas, contusions, swelling, herniation, or compressed basal cisterns) should have their ICP monitored. A level III recommendation is made for those patients with a GCS ≤ 8 and a normal CT, if minimum two of the following conditions are met: age >40, unilateral or bilateral posturing, or systolic blood pressure <90 mm Hg.

   b. **Interpretation** of ICP measurement. **An ICP more than 20 mm Hg is considered abnormal** and must prompt close evaluation of the patient. The ICP can be used to help guide therapy and to measure the effects of the therapies. ICP elevation is usually a result of mass effect because of the particular relationship between the contents of the cranial vault (a fixed volume) and the contents of the cranium (brain, blood, CSF), also known as the Monro-Kellie doctrine. In order to maintain a constant pressure, as one component increases, the others must decrease in volume. As the brain parenchyma swells, cerebrospinal fluid (CSF) is minimized and the blood flow may become eliminated.

   c. **Pressure** waves (**Fig. 36-2**) are rhythmic variations in the ICP tracing.

   d. **Brain herniation** is the end result of the summed pressures in the cranial vault. When the intracranial compartments reach certain elevated pressures, the brain matter will shift and cause secondary compression of other central nervous system (CNS) structures. This may result in the Cushing response (bradycardia and hypertension).

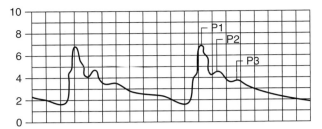

FIGURE 36-2 Morphology of the intracranial pressure waveform in the setting of normal ICP and compliance. Variation is found with each cardiac and respiratory cycle. P1, P2, and P3 are cardiac pulsations. The increments of measure are in mm Hg. From Lee KR, Hoff JT. Intracranial pressure. In: Youmans JR, ed. *Neurological surgery.* 4th ed. Philadelphia: WB Saunders, 1996:497. need permission.

(1) **Uncal herniation** usually involves the displacement of the medial edge of the uncus and the hippocampal gyrus medially and over the ipsilateral edge of the tentorium, causing compression of the midbrain. The ipsilateral or contralateral third nerve may be stretched or compressed causing a dilated pupil and third nerve palsy. Patients may present acutely with asymmetrical pupils (anisocoria). This may progress to marked papillary dilation and contralateral hemiparesis. In some instances, uncal herniation causes midline shift of the brainstem and compression of the contralateral cerebral peduncle onto the contralateral edge of the tentorium, or Kernohan's notch. This will cause a paradoxical weakness of hemiplegia ipsilateral to the cranial lesion.

(2) **Subfalcine herniation** occurs most commonly when the cingulate gyrus of the frontal lobe is pushed under the falx cerebri following mass effect from an ipsilateral lesion. Compression of the anterior cerebral artery (ACA) between cingulate gyrus and the falx cerebri may occur causing ipsilateral or contralateral ACA infarction. Clinical signs of increased tone or paresis in the contralateral leg may be present.

(3) **Central transtentorial herniation** is the displacement of the basal nuclei and cerebral hemispheres downward while the diencephalons and adjacent midbrain are pushed through the tentorial notch. This is usually as a result of a lesion at the vertex or the frontal–occipital poles. Often they initially present with impairment of vertical gaze and bilateral extensor posturing.

(4) **Upward cerebellar herniation** is an uncommon injury marked by upward herniation of the vermis and cerebellar hemispheres through the tentorial opening, usually due to infratentorial space-occupying lesions.

(5) **Tonsilar herniation of the cerebellum** is the downward displacement of cerebellar tonsils through the foramen magnum, typically resulting from mass effect in the posterior fossa. Symptoms include neck stiffness, cardiac rhythm and hemodynamic disturbances, respiratory depression, apnea, and may rapidly lead to death.

e. **Hydrocephalus.** Communicating hydrocephalus is usually due to the presence of blood, which causes an obstruction of CSF flow in the subarachnoid space and impaired absorption of the CSF through the arachnoid villi. Noncommunicating hydrocephalus often is caused by an obstruction of CSF flow at the fourth ventricle, cerebral aqueduct, third ventricle, or interventricular foramen by clotted blood or compression.

2. Brain oxygenation/perfusion

   a. Tissue oxygenation. The delivery of oxygen to the brain depends upon several factors. The amount of oxygen delivered and/or extracted from the brain can be monitored. These can be measured by direct brain tissue oxygen monitors or indirectly by continuous jugular venous bulb saturation measurements. Both techniques have significant limitations. Brain tissue oxygen monitors can only measure oxygen saturation in the small amount of tissue around the probe insertion site. Jugular venous bulb saturation measurements do not reflect regional focal brain hypoxia. Some have advocated these as endpoints of resuscitation with 50% as a cutoff for O_2 saturation and 15 mm Hg as a cutoff for direct tissue measurements.

   b. Cerebral perfusion pressure (CPP) is the difference between the mean arterial pressure and the ICP, measured in mm Hg. Current data support maintaining CPP $\geq$60 mm Hg in patients with TBI. CPP can be maintained by lowering ICP or by elevation of MAP using vasopressors in a euvolemic patient. There is controversy in the literature concerning using CPP-directed therapies, but this is currently the standard of care.

F. Management

1. Surgical decompression

   a. CSF drainage. Ventriculostomies can be placed to therapeutically drain some of the CSF while monitoring the ICP. This may be particularly helpful in the face of intraventricular bleeds that may cause a noncommunicating hydrocephalus. There is up to a 6% to 10% risk of infection.

   b. Craniotomy/craniectomy. The indications to surgically evacuate a hematoma vary between the types of hematomas.

   (1) Epidural hematoma (EDH): >30 cm^3 regardless of the GCS. Those with <30 cm^3 EDH with $\leq$1.5 cm thickness and <0.5 cm midline shift with GCS >8 without focal deficits may be watched closely by examination and/or serial head CT scans.

   (2) Subdural hematoma (SDH): >10 mm in size or >5 mm midline shift should be evacuated regardless of GCS. Those with GCS <9, with SDH <10 mm, and <5 mm midline shift whose GCS has decreased by two points since the time of initial monitoring or anisocoria or ICP >20 mm Hg should be considered for surgical evacuation.

   (3) Traumatic **intraparenchymal** bleeds. Those with parenchymal mass lesions and signs of progressive neurological deterioration referable to a lesion, medically refractory intracranial hypertension (ICH), or sign of mass effect on CT scan should be treated operatively. GCS 6 to 8 with frontal or temporal contusions >20 cm^3 with >5 mm midline shift and/or cisternal compression on CT scan, and patients with any lesion >50 cm^3 should have operative intervention. The operative treatment here is decompressive hemicraniectomy and duraplasty, which creates more space for brain to swell outward and thus controls intracranial pressure.

2. **ICP management**
    a. **Osmotic agents** function by shifting fluid out of the intracellular and interstitial spaces to the intravascular space. They may also have anti-inflammatory or other protective mechanisms.
        (1) **Mannitol** is generally used when the ICP is sustained >20 mm Hg for more than 10 minutes. The dose **is 0.5 to 1.0 g/kg** every **4 to 6 hours.** This must be done in patients who are euvolemic. **Osmotic gap >10,** a serum **Na >160 mEq,** or **serum osmolarity >320 mOsm** are general endpoints in addition to the decreasing ICP. Osmotic gap is the difference between measured serum osmolality and calculated serum osmolality. Osmotic gap >10 indicates continued presence of mannitol in the patients' serum, and additional doses of mannitol are less effective in this situation. Potential risks associated with mannitol include hypovolemia, renal failure, and worsening of cerebral edema due to migration of mannitol into areas of damaged brain. Mannitol use for ICP control may become less effective over time.
        (2) **Hypertonic saline.** These solutions can be used in a variety of ways. **3% NaCl,** 125 to 250 cm^3 bolus, every 6 hours or a continuous infusion at 0.5 to 1.0 cm^3/kg/h is targeted to the desired ICP. **23.4% NaCl,** 30 cm^3 bolus over 30 minutes (every 4–6 hours) is another effective method to decrease ICP. Small randomized studies have suggested that bolus use of hypertonic saline may be more effective in ICP control in patients with head trauma. The hypertonic saline solutions carry the potential risks of central pontine myelinolysis, seizures, congestive heart failure, hypokalemia, hyperchloremic acidosis, coagulopathy, phlebitis, and renal failure. It should be withheld when the serum Na is >160 mEq/L.
    b. **Loop diuretics** (10–20 mg of **furosemide** IV every 4–6 hours) may be useful for subacute treatment of ICH.
    c. **Head elevation 30 to 45** degrees above horizontal should be performed on all patients at risk of ICH. Other positional measures include **avoiding head rotation,** which may partially obstruct venous drainage, and making sure cervical collars are not too restrictive.
    d. **Adequate sedation and analgesia.** Short-acting narcotics and sedatives, that is, IV morphine sulfate or fentanyl and propofol must be instituted to ensure patient comfort and a lower ICP.
    e. **Metabolic therapy**
        (1) **Barbiturates** exert their ICP lowering effect via several mechanisms including decreasing cerebral metabolic rate for oxygen (CMRO$_2$), reducing cerebral blood volume and cerebral blood flow, and inhibiting free radical peroxidation.
            i. **Pentobarbital** is the most common barbiturate used. Pentobarbital use at 10 mg/kg IV bolus over 30 minutes, followed by 5 mg/kg IV bolus every hour for 3 hours and then a maintenance infusion of 1 mg/kg/h to maintain serum pentobarbital level at 3 to 4 mg/dL. This regimen has been shown to improve ICP control in a randomized trial of patients with severe head injury.
            ii. **Thiopental** is a less studied barbiturate most commonly used as premedication for intubation in patients at risk for elevated ICP. 250 mg IV bolus of thiopental may reduce ICP for 15 to 20 minutes.

(2) **Barbiturate adverse effects** include hypotension, myocardial depression, vasodilatation, ileus, temperature dysregulation, and a higher propensity for infection. Patients receiving induced coma therapy with pentobarbital require adequate volume resuscitation, and often require vasopressor and inotropic support. Barbiturate use is associated with higher incidence of pneumonia, hepatic dysfunction, and sepsis syndrome.

f. **Hypothermia.** Lowering brain temperature may lower ICP by decreasing cerebral metabolism and altering cerebral blood flow. Small studies of mild-to-moderate hypothermia (temperature 33°C–36°C) in head injury have demonstrated improved ICP control, decreased $CMRO_2$, and improved coupling between cerebral blood flow and $CMRO_2$. The effect on neurologic outcome from hypothermia is inconclusive. As a result, induced hypothermia has not been widely accepted as standard treatment in TBIs. It is a treatment option for elevated ICP following neurotrauma.

(1) **Potential complications** include coagulopathy, hypotension, bradycardia, and increased susceptibility to infection. Induced hypothermia is contraindicated in patients with uncontrolled bleeding.

g. **Corticosteroids**

(1) Steroids use has **no role in trauma induced ICP elevation.**

(2) Consistent benefit of steroid use has only been shown in patients with ICP elevation from severe vasogenic edema due to rapidly expanding intracranial neoplasm. In the setting of cerebral edema associated with intracranial **neoplasms,** dexamethasone up to 10 mg IV every 4 hours may reduce cerebral edema and improve neurologic function.

(3) Empiric steroid use in patients with **bacterial meningitis** has been associated with improved outcome whether or not there was ICP elevation.

3. Compartment syndrome of the thorax/abdomen

a. **Positive end-expiratory pressure (PEEP)** has been associated with ICP elevation. The presumed mechanism is through pressure transmission to mediastinal structures, which causes impaired cerebral venous outflow. Although the correlation between PEEP and ICP is not seen in all patients, PEEP increase should be performed carefully, and ICP be monitored closely in those patients with elevated ICP.

b. **Increased intra-abdominal pressures (IAP)** have been associated with ICP elevation in patients with severe head trauma. A "multiple compartments syndrome" (abdomen and cranium) should be considered in post-trauma patients with refractory ICP elevation. Decompressive laparotomy has been reported as an effective treatment of refractory ICP elevation in trauma patients with associated intra-abdominal hypertension (bladder pressure >20 mm Hg).

4. **Systemic considerations**

a. **Cerebral perfusion** and **blood pressure.** Prehospital hypotension is associated with poor outcome in TBI. Systemic hypotension may lead to decreased CPP and exacerbate secondary brain injury. The decreased CPP may be exaggerated in TBI secondary to impaired cerebral autoregulation that normally protects patients from cerebral hypoperfusion.

b. **Systemic hypoxia** may cause decreased oxygen delivery to the brain leading to secondary brain injuries. The optimal arterial blood oxygen saturation to maintain cerebral oxygenation has not been established. In treating patients with head injury and particularly those with elevated ICP, we recommend that the clinician aggressively maintain normal oxygenation (SpO_2 >93%).

c. **Ventilation.** Optimal ventilation should maintain a $PaCO_2$ of 35 to 40 mm Hg. Brief use of hyperventilation to decrease ICP is effective, but maintaining constant hyperventilation worsens neurologic outcomes. These poor outcomes may be related to the vasoconstriction that occurs with hyperventilation and associated $PaCO_2$ <30 mm Hg.

d. **Treat hyperthermia.** Detrimental effects of hyperthermia in CNS injuries include increasing cerebral metabolic demand, elevating ICP, and lowering seizure threshold. Hyperthermia should be treated aggressively in all patients with severe neurological injuries. Treatment options include antipyretic medications such as acetaminophen, surface-cooling devices, endovascular-cooling devices, and shivering control. Many medications used in association with head injury (anticonvulsants and antibiotics, for example) may induce hyperthermia as a secondary effect. These medications should be avoided or changed in patients with refractory hyperthermia.

e. **Treat hyperglycemia.** Small studies have suggested association between hyperglycemia and worse neurological outcome in patients with different types of severe neurological injuries. Whether treatment of hyperglycemia improves overall neurological outcome in neurotrauma remains to be established. Studies using brain microdialysis catheters have demonstrated critical levels of cerebral hypoglycemia follow systemic hypoglycemia. Hypoglycemia should be avoided in treatment of hyperglycemia in patients with severe neurological injuries. A reasonable goal is a blood glucose concentration of 120 to 150 mg/dL.

f. **Secondary prophylaxis.** Patients with severe traumatic head injuries are in the highest risk categories for developing thromboembolic complications, stress-induced gastric ulcers, and nosocomial pneumonia. All patients with severe head trauma are recommended to receive sequential compression devices for mechanical **thromboembolism** prophylaxis, unless there is a contraindication (e.g., limb ischemia or burn injury). All neurotrauma patients are recommended to receive dose-adjusted unfractionated heparin or low-molecular-weight heparin for chemoprophylaxis as soon as systemic and brain hemorrhages stabilize. Early initiation of **enteral nutrition,** gastric pH elevation with use of histamine-II or proton pump inhibitors, and avoidance of unnecessary corticosteroid use are effective prophylaxes for stress-induced gastric ulcers in this patient population. **Head elevation,** oral decontamination (e.g., daily oral chlorhexidine use), and early weaning from ventilator are effective methods to decrease risk for nosocomial pneumonia in patients with traumatic head injury.

g. **Seizure prophylaxis** after TBI has been shown to decrease the incidence of seizure incidence for the first 7 days following head injury, though seizures were not associated with worse outcome. Based on this study, neurotrauma patients have routinely received anticonvulsants for 7 days. Certain traumatic injuries such as SDH and hemorrhagic cerebral contusions (particularly those located in the temporal lobes) are associated with a higher incidence of seizure, and these patients may have an indication for longer use of anticonvulsants. There are no clinical data to support the use or disuse of anticonvulsants in special subpopulations of neuro-trauma patients. The incidence of subclinical nonconvulsive status epilepticus in comatose patients with brain injuries is **as high as 30%**. Routine electroencephalography (EEG) evaluation and/or 24-hour continuous EEG monitoring may be indicated in high-risk patients with traumatic head injury who are comatose. Patients who have developed clinical seizures at the time of head trauma or following head trauma should remain on a full dose of anticonvulsants for a longer duration.

II. ICU management of traumatic spinal cord injuries

A. The incidence of traumatic spinal cord injury (SCI) in United States is approximately 11,000 new cases per year, or 40 new cases per 1 million people. Approximately 450,000 people are living with SCI in the United States. The average age of traumatic SCI is 31.8 years. The male-to-female ratio is 4:1. Traumatic SCI most often presents with incomplete tetraplegia (31%) or complete paraplegia (27%).

B. Initial assessment

1. Spine immobilization

a. Transport. Any patient with suspected traumatic SCI should be transported using spine immobilization, which includes rigid cervical collar, lateral support devices, and tape or straps to secure all devices to a hard backboard. In the event of emesis, the backboard can be rapidly turned 90 degrees to minimize aspiration. The patient must remain immobilized with the spine in neutral position, and **log-rolling** techniques must be used for moving patients with potential traumatic SCI.

2. Clinical assessment

a. The goal of the initial assessment of a traumatic SCI is to **prevent a secondary injury** due to movement of an unstable spine, hypoxia, and hemodynamic compromise. Airway security, oxygenation, hemodynamic stability, and search for potentially life-threatening concomitant injuries should be the first line of clinical assessment.

b. Respiratory compromise occurs acutely in 67% of traumatic SCI patients, and includes aspiration pneumonia, atelectasis, and, later, infectious pneumonia and respiratory failure (22.6%). Signs of impending respiratory failure include increasing respiratory rate, increasing work of breathing, and worsening need for supplemental oxygen.

c. Cardiovascular patients with high SCI may present with bradycardia, hypotension, temperature dysregulation, dysautonomia, respiratory insufficiency, and/or neurogenic shock.

(1) Neurogenic shock from SCI presents with hypotension, bradycardia, and hypothermia. Acute treatment for neurogenic shock should include aggressive fluid resuscitation with crystalloids and vasopressor therapy. α-Agonists such as **phenylephrine** can be added for treatment of low peripheral vascular resistance from functional sympathetectomy. β_1-Agonists may be necessary for severe bradycardia.

(2) Hypotension has been associated with secondary neurologic injury in SCI, and should be avoided. Maintaining spinal cord perfusion by maintaining MAP >85 mm Hg for 7 days may be helpful.

| TABLE 36-2 | American Spinal Injury Association (ASIA) Impairment Scale and Definitions |

Impairment Category	Classification	Description
A	Complete	No residual motor or sensory function in the sacral segments S4-5
B	Incomplete	Sensory but not motor function is preserved below the neurological level (including sacral segments S4–S5)
C	Incomplete	Motor function is preserved below the neurological level, and more than half of key muscles below the neurological level have a muscle grade less than 3
D	Incomplete	Motor function is preserved below the neurological level, and at least half of key muscles below the neurological level have a muscle grade of 3 or more
E	Normal	Motor and sensory functions are normal

Definitions	
Neurologic level of injury	The most caudal level at which both motor and sensory functions are intact
Motor level	The most caudal level at which muscle group is graded 3/5 or greater, with more cephalad segments graded normal (5/5) strength
Sensory level	The most caudal dermatome to have normal sensation for both pinprick and light touch on both sides
Skeletal level	The level at which, by radiologic examination, the greatest vertebral damage is found

(3) **Autonomic dysfunction** such as bradycardia and neurogenic shock is common in cervical level injuries. Autonomic dysreflexia may also occur, but this requires intact spinal reflexes and do not occur until patients have emerged from spinal shock.

d. Assess the degree of impairment. The American Spinal Injury Association (ASIA) impairment scale is used by many large centers and clinical trials to quantify degree of neurological impairment in SCI. **Table 36-2** summarizes the categories of ASIA impairment scale. **Table 36-3** summarizes the motor functions of spinal cord levels and associated reflexes.

C. **Clinical signs and symptoms of traumatic SCI**

1. **Complete spinal cord transection syndrome.** Patients with complete spinal cord transection lose all motor functions and all modalities of sensation as well as all reflexes at or below the level of spinal cord lesion. This syndrome is acutely associated with **spinal shock,** where the victims develop flaccid paralysis with complete absence of reflex and autonomic activity below the level of injury, including bowel and bladder function. In some instances, spinal reflexes above the level of transection may also be depressed. Spinal shock occurs in minutes after complete cord transection and may last days to weeks. Once spinal shock resolves, patients with complete spinal cord transection develop hyperreflexia and spastic paralysis below the level of SCI.

TABLE 36-3	Motor Functions by Spinal Cord Levels	
Spinal Segment	**Motor Function**	**Reflex Arc**
C3-4	Elevate (shrug) shoulder	
C3-5	Diaphragmatic movement	
C1–C6	Neck flexors	
C1–T1	Neck extensors	
C5-6	Arm abduction and elevation, elbow flexion	Brachioradialis and pectoralis reflexes
C6–C8	Elbow extension, forearm supination, wrist and finger extension, and forearm pronation	Biceps and triceps reflexes
C7–T1	Wrist flexion, movement of small muscles of the hand	Finger flexor reflex
T1–T6	Intercostal muscles	
T7–L1	Abdominal muscles	Abdominal reflexes
L1–L3	Hip flexion	Cremasteric reflex
L2–L4	Knee extension and thigh adduction	Patellar reflex and adductor's reflex
L4-5, S1	Foot dorsiflexion, toe extension	
L5, S1-2	Knee flexion	
L5, S1-2	Foot plantar flexion and toe flexion	Ankle jerk (Achilles) reflex
S1–S3	Anal sphincter muscle tone	Anal wink reflex

2. **Brown-Séquard syndrome.** This is the syndrome of **hemisection of spinal cord.** Loss of position and vibration sense occurs below the level of SCI on the same side, and loss of pinprick and temperature sensation occurs on the opposite side of the cord injury. Upper motor neuron type muscle weakness occurs on the same side as the spinal cord lesion. At the level of the SCI, there is a band of loss of all sensory modalities on the same side as the lesion.

3. **Central cord syndrome** is the most common SCI syndrome and accounts for approximately 9% of traumatic SCI. Central cord syndrome presents with arm greater than leg weakness and area of cape-like anesthesia involving the shoulders and arms. This syndrome occurs with trauma typically in older people with cervical spondylosis, but may occur in younger patients, and is thought to be a hyperextension injury leading to spinal cord edema. This syndrome usually has a better prognosis than other types of SCI syndromes.

4. **Anterior spinal cord syndrome** typically occurs secondary to occlusion of the anterior spinal artery. The patient is paralyzed to varying degrees below the level of the vascular SCI, with complete loss of pain and temperature sensation but preservation of touch, vibration, and joint position sensation.

5. *Tabes dorsalis* **syndrome** occurs due to injury to the posterior spinal cord causing ataxia due to vibration and joint position sensory loss. Injuries to the lumbosacral roots cause abnormal bowel, bladder and sexual function, as well as lancinating pain, which characterize this syndrome.

6. *Cauda equina* **syndrome.** The cauda equine is composed of lumbosacral nerve roots in the thecal sac below the termination of the spinal cord.

Traumatic injury to this area produces symptoms of nerve root compression and pain, as well as prominent symptoms of bowel, bladder, and sexual dysfunction. Injuries at this spinal level cannot cause upper motor neuron pattern muscle weakness.

D. Urgent radiographic assessment is important to determine the extent of traumatic SCI. Radiographic studies in patients with potential traumatic SCI should include, at the minimum, anteroposterior and lateral plain radiographs of the entire spine. However, CT scan of the spine with sagittal and coronal reformatting is more sensitive for spine fractures, and has become standard of care in some trauma centers, replacing plain radiographs.

1. Evaluation of cervical spine injury when a CT scan is not available should include anteroposterior and lateral plain radiographs of the cervical spine to include C7–T1 junction and an open-mouth view to assess odontoid process (C2) or C1 fracture and dislocation.

2. Full evaluation of the spine should be carried out because multilevel spinal fractures occur in 5% to 30% of traumatic SCI may occur at noncontiguous levels. First and second rib fractures are associated with cervical spine injury, especially at C6-7 level.

3. MRI is helpful in diagnosing spinal cord abnormalities, ruptured disks, EDH, or ligamentous injuries associated with traumatic SCI.

4. **CT angiography** is helpful for evaluation of associated vascular injuries in the carotid and vertebral arteries. Patients with cervical spine dislocations, fractures through foramen transversarium in the cervical spine, and base of skull fractures are at higher risk for suffering associated vertebral and carotid artery traumatic dissections. Screening criteria for blunt trauma are shown in **Table 36-4**. These injuries often are associated with TBI and bleeding. The use of systemic anticoagulation needs to be weighed against the risk of increasing the intracranial bleeding. In general, once the bleeding has stabilized on subsequent CT scans, it is reasonable to consider anticoagulation for a significant cerebrovascular injury.

a. **Treatment options**

(1) **Minimal intimal injury:** Observe and repeat imaging in 7 days.

TABLE 36-4	Screening Criteria Guideline for Blunt Cerebrovascular Injury

Neurologic
- Evidence of CVA or TIA
- Horner's syndrome
- Neurologic examination not explained by brain imaging

Anatomic
- Skull base fractures (foramen lacerum)
- Seat belt sign
- Soft tissue injury of the neck (swelling or altered MS)
- Severe cervical hyperextension/rotation/hyperflexion
- Cervical bruit in pt <50 y
- Cervical spine fractures

Statistic-based
- Diffuse axonal injury
- LeFort II/III fractures

(2) >25% of lumen affected/pseudoaneurysm/thrombosis
    i. If surgically accessible: Repair, if not accessible consider anticoagulation.
    ii. High risk for bleeding: Consider aspirin.
    iii. Low risk for bleeding: IV heparin goal PTT 50 to 60 seconds.
(3) Active extravasation: Consider embolization.

E. Cervical spine clearance
  1. Awake, nonintoxicated, and asymptomatic patients (no pain, no neurological or distracting injuries) do not need radiographic evaluation.
  2. Awake, nonintoxicated patients with normal neurological function and C-spine radiographic studies but *with neck pain* can be further evaluated with dynamic flexion/extension radiographs or MRI of the C-spine within 48 hours of injury.
  3. In obtunded patients with prehospital cervical spine immobilization and normal cervical spine MRI, cervical spine immobility may be safely discontinued.
  4. Multidetector CT scans are being used at MGH and at other centers for clearance of the obtunded patient. Removal of the cervical collar should be a priority. Published data from MGH and others have demonstrated a 20% incidence of complications associated with hard cervical collars. Our current protocol for cervical spine clearance in obtunded patients includes
    a. Normal CT scan from base of skull to T1 demonstrates no fractures, normal alignment (normal lordosis), no evidence of prevertebral swelling, no subluxations, normal intervebral disk spaces, and atlantoaxial space. This must be read as normal by the attending radiologist and the trauma attending staff. If the CT is normal by the above criteria, the cervical collar may be removed.
    b. Abnormal CT scan using the above criteria warrants an MRI to evaluate the major ligaments. If the MRI shows that the ligaments are intact, the collar may be removed. If the MRI shows evidence of ligament injury, the collar remains.
  5. Those with radiographic evidence of bone or ligamentous injury require evaluation by orthopedic or neurosurgical service.

F. Therapeutic interventions
  1. Corticosteroids. IV **methylprednisolone** given **within 8 hours of acute SCI at 30 mg/kg bolus and 5.4 mg/kg/h infusion for 23 hours** may improve neurologic recovery at 6 weeks, 6 months, and 1 year. Concerns about the adequacy of the methodologies used to reach these results are such that several professional societies no longer recommend the use of high-dose methylprednisolone for acute SCI.
  2. Spine stabilization
    a. Spinal fractures presenting with misalignment and cord compression require reduction of the misalignment. Closed reduction is an option for cervical spine injuries.
    b. Presence of associated disk herniation should be evaluated and treated, as this could cause increased cord impingement and further neurologic deterioration.
    c. Contraindications to cervical traction include atlantooccipital dislocation or similar ligamentous disruptions, comminuted skull fractures, extensive scalp lacerations, or the need for emergency craniotomy.
    d. Currently, there is no conclusive evidence supporting the benefit of early versus late surgery. Indications for emergent surgical treatment include progressive neurologic deterioration, expanding

EDH, spinal cord edema, or infarction. Selected patients with incomplete SCI have been reported to have improved neurologic recovery if early decompression is performed within 8 hours.

e. Penetrating spinal injuries may be associated with CSF leak and infection, but rarely lead to spinal instability. Operative treatment is often not warranted as removal of penetrating foreign body, or debridement, is associated with lower risk of infection or enhanced neurologic recovery.

G. Nutritional support

1. Acute SCI is associated with a catabolic state which may lead to complications such as muscle wasting, poor wound healing, increased infection risk, and development of pressure ulcers. Full-caloric, high-nitrogen nutritional support is recommended for all SCI patients.

2. **Adynamic ileus** is a prominent feature of SCI. Patients will require aggressive bowel regimens and potentially promotility agents to prevent ileus and secondary malnutrition.

3. SCI patients are at high risk for **peptic ulcer formation** secondary to acute illness, respiratory failure, and steroid use. Early stress ulcer prophylaxis with antihistaminic agents or proton pump inhibitors and enteral nutrition support is essential.

H. Prevention of venous thromboembolism (VTE)

1. The incidence of thromboembolic complications in traumatic SCI is as high as 60%, and the risk is highest during the first 2 weeks after SCI. Patients should be placed on mechanical prophylaxis with sequential compression devices unless there is a contraindication. Chemoprophylaxis with dose-adjusted unfractionated or low-molecular-weight heparin significantly decreases the incidence of thromboembolism and should be initiated as early as possible.

2. **Inferior vena cava (IVC) filters** may be considered for SCI patients with thromboembolic complication. Current data do not suggest a benefit in placing IVC filters for primary prevention of pulmonary embolism.

III. Determination of brain death
A. Definitions

1. The Uniform Determination of Death Act states "An individual who has sustained either irreversible cessation of circulatory and respiratory functions, or irreversible cessation of all functions of the entire brain, including the brainstem, is dead. A determination of death must be made in accordance with accepted medical standards."

2. **There is no federally mandated definition of brain death in United States.** Brain death determination guidelines are formulated locally at individual institutions. Guidelines and recommendations in this chapter are adapted from the Massachusetts General Hospital protocol for brain death determination, and may differ from those used in other institutions.

3. **Brain death is a clinical diagnosis** based on clinical criteria. It must be understood as no different from a diagnosis of death made by other criteria.

4. The most common diagnoses leading to brain death are cerebrovascular events, severe head injuries, and global ischemic insult to brain from hypoxia, and/or hypoperfusion.

5. Guidelines outlined in this chapter address brain death determination in an adult population (age 18 and above). Brain death determination in pediatric population is different and readers should refer to those specific guidelines.

B. Prerequisites

1. The proximate cause of catastrophic and irreversible CNS dysfunction must be known, along with clinical and neuroimaging evidence supporting the diagnosis of an irreversible CNS catastrophe.

2. Clinician must exclude all medical conditions that may potentially confound the clinician's ability to perform clinical assessment of brain death. Potential confounding medical conditions may include severe electrolyte and acid–base disturbance, endocrine disturbance, profound hypoglycemia, diffuse denervation such as seen in Guillain-Barré syndrome, and so on.

3. Toxicology screening must demonstrate barbiturate level less than 10 μg/mL or absent barbiturate level, and no evidence of drug intoxication or poisoning.

4. Pharmacologic neuromuscular blockade must be absent.

5. Patient must have a core temperature of 36.5°C (96.8°F) or greater.

6. If any of the above prerequisites are not met in a patient suspected to have irreversible neurological injury, clinicians should consider the use of ancillary tests for determination of brain death.

C. Clinical examination

1. **Coma** is defined as unresponsiveness with no cerebrally mediated, purposeful motor response to noxious stimuli in any location. Noxious stimuli utilized for this determination may include nasal tickle with cotton swab, application of supraorbital and nail bed pressure. Cerebrally mediated motor responses may include grimace to noxious stimuli, movement of the limb away from noxious stimuli, and cerebrally mediated reflexive motor responses such as decorticate posturing to noxious stimuli.

2. **Brainstem reflexes.** Brain death determination requires the complete absence of all brainstem functions. We recommend the following methods for assessing brainstem reflexes:

   a. **Pupillary light reflex.** In a darkened examination room, carefully apply and sustain light to each eye individually and observe for any pupillary size change. Chronic postsurgical pupillary changes may impair a clinician's ability to determine brainstem function, and ancillary test may be considered.

   b. **Oculocephalic (OCP) response.** Also known as the "doll's eye reflex," the normal OCP response is characterized by horizontal or vertical eye movement in the direction opposite to rapid head turn. Absence of eye movement to head turn demonstrates a lack of OCP response.

   c. **Vestibuloocular reflex (cold-calorics).** In patients with unstable cervical spine or unknown spinal stability, OCP response cannot be assessed with head turning. The vestibule-ocular reflex in this case can be tested using 30 to 50 mL ice water irrigation of the tympanic membranes. A normal brainstem response would be tonic horizontal eye movement toward the side of ice water irrigation, with possible fast-phase nystagmus in the direction opposite from side of ice water instillation. Each tympanic membrane should be tested separately, with 5 to 10 minutes time lapse in between tests to allow return to normal temperature prior to repeat examination. Complete absence of eye movement demonstrates the lack of this brainstem reflex.

   d. **Corneal response.** Presence of normal corneal response depends on sensory input from cornea via cranial nerve V, intact reflex arc through the brainstem, and intact motor output through cranial nerve VII. To test this response, gently stroke the cornea on each side with a cotton swab, and observe for reflexive blinking motion of the corresponding eye. Facial myokymias may result from denervation of facial muscles and should not be interpreted as a positive corneal response.

e. **Cough response** can be tested by stimulating the tracheal–bronchial tree with a suctioning catheter. Normal response would be presence of cough response.

f. **Gag response** can be tested by stimulation of the posterior pharynx using a tongue depressor or cotton swab, and observe the movement of palate and uvula.

3. Certain non–cerebrally mediated reflexes may remain intact and visible in a patient who has irreversible lost all cerebral functions. These clinical phenomena are consistent with the diagnosis of brain death and include

a. Spontaneous reflexive motor movements from a spinal reflex arc. These movements may include spontaneous triple flexion of lower extremities (stereotypic hip and knee flexion and toe extension), Babinski's reflex, and presence of deep tendon reflexes.

b. Truncal posturing, which may involve shoulder elevation and adduction, neck extension, back arching with associated intercostals muscle expansion, and respiration-like movements, are spinal reflexes and are consistent with a diagnosis of brain death. Certain patients with irreversible brain damage may demonstrate the "*Lazarus sign*," characterized by spontaneous abduction or adduction of an extremity, raising of the torso, head turning, and back arching, often in synchrony with external stimulation such as ventilator-delivered breaths.

c. Autonomic responses such as sweating and blushing.

4. **Apnea test.** The apnea test is often the final step in clinical determination of brain death after all other prerequisites listed above have been fulfilled. The time of completion of an apnea test confirming apnea is documented time of death of the patient. Apnea test must be performed meticulously and stopped if patient develops hemodynamic instability, oxygen desaturation, or cardiac arrhythmias. We recommend the following steps in conducting an apnea test:

a. Prior to beginning the apnea test, ensure that the patient has core temperature of 36.5°C (97°F) or greater, systolic blood pressure of 90 mm Hg or greater (vasopressor can be used), arterial partial pressure of carbon dioxide of 40 mm Hg or greater, and a normal arterial blood pH (7.35–7.45). If the patient has central diabetes insipidus, it should be corrected with vasopressin use, and patient should have even to positive fluid balance 6 hours prior to apnea test.

b. Preoxygenate the patient with 100% Fio_2 for 5 to 10 minutes. Send arterial blood gas immediately prior to starting apnea test to determine baseline $Paco_2$.

c. Begin the apnea test by disconnecting patient from the ventilator while leaving a catheter in the endotracheal tube to deliver supplemental oxygen at 8 to 10 L/min.

d. Observe the chest wall carefully for any movements resembling respiratory effort. This may be done by both visual observation and by palpation with examiner's hands over the patient's chest. Chest wall movements due to cardiac pulsations may be distinguished from respiratory efforts by correlating these movements with patient's electrocardiogram. It is generally recommended that a respirator not be used to detect efforts of respiration in an apnea test as artifacts such as cardiac pulsations or movement of fluid inside ventilator tubing may cause false-positive findings. If a respiratory effort is observed, apnea is not confirmed and apnea test should be stopped.

e. If no respiratory efforts are observed, send arterial blood gases at 5, 8, and 10 minutes from initiation of apnea test. An increase of $Paco_2$ by 20 mm Hg at 8 minutes from apnea test baseline and a decrease in arterial pH by 0.02 per minute of apnea (final pH of less than 7.3 if the initial arterial pH is greater than 7.4) confirm apnea and support the diagnosis of death by brain criteria. Otherwise, apnea is *not* confirmed even if no respiratory effort was observed.

f. If patient develops clinical instability requiring cessation of apnea test prior to 8-minute time window, draw a blood gas immediately prior to resuming mechanical ventilation. If patient has shown no signs of respiratory effort and his/her blood gas meets criteria as stated in the prior step, apnea is confirmed and the result is supportive of the diagnosis of brain death.

5. **Pitfalls.** Certain clinical conditions may interfere and confound clinical determination of brain death and require an ancillary test. These conditions may include

a. Severe facial trauma.

b. Pre-existing pupillary abnormalities (such as a postsurgical pupil).

c. Persistence of certain sedative drugs in patient's serum. Medications of concern may include tricycles antidepressants, anticholinergics, neuromuscular blockade agents, benzodiazepines, and narcotics, and so on.

d. Persistent metabolic derangement such as uremia and hyperammonemia.

e. Prior history of sleep apnea and/or prior pulmonary disease leading to chronic CO_2 retention.

6. **Ancillary tests in brain death determination.** When brain death is suspected but the clinical determination is either not feasible or confounded by other medical conditions, ancillary tests could be used to confirm a total and irreversible loss of brain function. In these situations, the time of interpretation of these confirmatory test-showing results consistent with brain death would be documented as the time of death.

a. **Conventional angiography.** Standard four-vessel diagnostic cerebral angiography showing absence of intracranial arterial filling of contrast at the level of carotid bifurcation or circle of Willis is consistent with brain death.

b. **Technetium-99 m nuclear cerebral scintigraphy** measures cerebral perfusion using radiolabeled isotope. The isotope should be injected within 30 minutes of its reconstitution, and images acquired at 30 and 60 minutes and 2 hours post contrast injection. Complete absence of brain radioisotope uptake supports the diagnosis of brain death.

c. **Electroencephalography (EEG).** A standard 16-channel EEG adherent to minimal technical criteria can be used to confirm brain death. The patient must have a core body temperature of 90°F or above, have complete absence of electrocerebral activity for at least 30 consecutive minutes, and show no change of EEG pattern to external stimulation. The EEG interpretation must be confirmed by a neurologist prior to declaration of brain death by EEG confirmation.

d. **Transcranial Doppler ultrasound (TCD).** Small systolic peaks in early systole with absent diastolic flow or reverberating flow on TCD in a patient who had known prior TCD results may support the diagnosis of greatly increased intracranial pressure and thereby brain death. Absence of TCD signal alone is not sufficient for confirmation of brain death as up to 10% of patients do not have adequate temporal bone window for TCD insonation. TCD is not a preferred modality for confirmation of brain death due to its operator-dependent variability and lack in specificity.

   e. **Somatosensory-evoked potentials (SSEP)** study of bilateral median nerve stimulation adhering to minimal technical criteria demonstrating bilateral absence of N20-P22 response may also be used to support the diagnosis of brain death.

7. **Organ donation.** Immediate involvement of local organ bank organizations can significantly improve donation rates. A clear plan must be discussed with organ bank representatives prior to approaching the family.

   a. **Donation after brain death**
      (1) Allows a greater number of organs to be recovered given the ability to minimize warm ischemic time.
      (2) The patient is brought to the OR and all organs are cooled prior to stopping circulation. They are then quickly infused with cold preservation fluid.

   b. **Donation after cardiac death (DCD)**
      (1) The patient is in an irreversible state of significant neurologic compromise but is not brain dead.
      (2) The patient must also have significant hemodynamic compromise, such that removal from the ventilator and hemodynamic support would cause imminent death.
      (3) The patient is usually brought to the OR where life support is removed and the patient's condition deteriorates to the point that death is pronounced.
      (4) At the time of death, the patient is immediately cooled and the organs are harvested. The longer warm ischemia time limits the number of viable organs that can be successfully transplanted.

   c. **Techniques to improve organ donation rates**
      (1) Contact organ bank as soon as it becomes evident that a patient may have a devastating neurologic event.
      (2) Health care practitioners should resist the temptation to introduce the topic of organ donation and focus on the condition of the patient, ensuring that all medical questions are addressed with the family.
      (3) Communicate the condition of the patient to the organ bank and allow the third party to discuss organ donation possibilities with the patient's family if appropriate.

Selected References

American Academy of Pediatrics Task Force on Brain Death in Children. Report of special task force. Guidelines for the determination of brain death in children. *Pediatrics* 1987;80(2): 298–300.

American College of Surgeons, Committee on Trauma. Spine and spinal cord trauma. In: *Advanced trauma life support program for doctors; ATLS.* 8th ed. Chicago: American College of Surgeons, 1997;215–242.

Bracken MB, Shepard MJ, Collins WF, et al. A randomized, controlled trail of methylprednisolone or naloxone in the treatment of acute spinal-cord injury. Results of the Second National Acute Spinal Cord Injury Study. *N Engl J Med* 1990;322:1405–1411.

Brain Trauma Foundation. Treatment guidelines for severe traumatic brain injury 2007. Available online: http://www.braintrauma.org/site/PageServer?pagename=Guidelines

Kirshblum SC et al. Spinal cord injury medicine. 1. Etiology, classification, and acute medical management. *Arch Phys Med Rehabil* 2002;83(3 suppl 1):S50–S57, S90–S98.

Layon AJ. Ethical issues in the neurointensive care unit. In: Layon AJ, Friedman WA, eds. *Textbook of neurointensive care*. Philadelphia: Saunders, 2004:833–841.

Libenson MH. Diseases of the spinal cord. In: Feske SM, ed. *Office practice of neurology*. Philadelphia: Churchill Livingstone, 2003:520–547.

Narayan R, Polvishock J, Wilberger J, eds. *Neurotrauma*. New York: McGraw-Hill, 1996.

Practice parameters for determining brain death in adults (summary statement). The quality standards subcommittee of the American Academy of Neurology. *Neurology* 1995;45(5): 1012–1014.

Vale FL, Burns J, Jackson AB, et al. Combined medical and surgical treatment after acute spinal cord injury: results of a prospective pilot study to assess the merits of aggressive medical resuscitation and blood pressure management. *J Neurosurg* 1997;87:239–246.

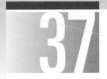

The Burned Patient

Nicolas Melo and Rob Sheridan

I. Introduction
   A. Dramatic improvements in the care, survival, and quality of life of burn injury victims have evolved over the past several decades. The removal of deep wounds and achievement of immediate biologic closure helps to attenuate the inevitable development of wound sepsis. To support a patient with a serious burn through the physiologic trial of staged wound closure requires sophisticated critical care, many aspects unique to the **burn unit**. This chapter presents these techniques in a concise format.
   B. **The role of intensive care in management of burns** is to bring a patient from a tragic injury to the optimal outcome—full reintegration into family, community, and productive work.
   C. **Overall management strategy.** Patients with large burns typically present with a deep wound, associated with pain, impending sepsis, and potentially progressive multiorgan dysfunction. Immediate needs must be met, but a specific overall plan of care must also be generated. An organized plan of care can be viewed as having four phases (**Table 37-1**). The **initial evaluation and resuscitation phase,** from the first through third day, requires that aggressive fluid resuscitation be performed while the patient is thoroughly evaluated for other injuries and comorbidities. The second phase involves **initial wound excision and biologic closure,** which is the primary focus to profoundly changes the natural history of the disease. Typically, a series of staged operations are completed during the first few days after injury. The third phase, **definitive wound closure,** involves removal of temporary wound dressings with definitive covers, in addition to closure and acute reconstruction of areas of high complexity and small surface area, such as the face and hand. The final stage of care is **rehabilitation.** Although rehabilitation begins early, it becomes more involved toward the end of the acute hospital stay.

II. Physiologic implications of burn injury
   A. **Predictable physiologic changes.** Successfully resuscitated burn patients manifest a sequence of predictable physiologic changes (**Table 37-2**). Anticipation of these changes is possible:
      1. **Early ebb phase and later hyperdynamic phase.** The ebb phase relates to a period of hours to a day after injury in which there is a relative hypodynamic state, which requires aggressive critical support in the resuscitation period. The flow phase relates to the subsequent predictable development of high cardiac output, reduced peripheral vascular tone, fever, and muscle catabolism that become particularly exaggerated in patients with large burns.
      2. **Physiology of the resuscitation period.** A unique feature of the burn patient is massive diffuse capillary leak, believed to be secondary to wound-released inflammatory mediators that result in the extravasation of fluids, electrolytes, and even moderate-sized colloid molecules. A

TABLE 37-1	Phases of Burn Care	
Phase	**Objectives**	**Time Period**
Initial evaluation and resuscitation	Accurate fluid resuscitation and through evaluation	0–72 h
Initial wound excision and biologic closure	Exactly identify and remove all full-thickness wounds and achieve biologic closure	Days 1–7
Definitive wound closure	Replace temporary with definitive covers and close small complex wounds	Days 7–Week 6
Rehabilitation, reconstruction, and reintegration	Initially to maintain range and reduce edema, subsequently to strengthen and facilitate return to home, work, school	Day 1 through discharge

guide to volume resuscitation of the burned patient is described in **Section IV**.

3. **Postresuscitation physiology**. In an adequately resuscitated burn patient, volume requirements abruptly decline 18 to 24 hours after injury, as the diffuse capillary leak predictably abates. Subsequently, a diffuse inflammatory state evolves that is characterized by a hyperdynamic circulation, fever, and massive protein catabolism. Release of inflammatory mediators, catecholamines, and the counter regulatory hormones cortisol and glucagons attempt to balance the flood of bacteria and their by-products from the wound. In addition, a compromised gastrointestinal and epithelial barrier, nerve damage, and infection compound these changes.

B. **Physiologic support**. The metabolic stress associated with a large burn is enormous. Because of a lack of homeostatic barrier associated with the loss of an intact skin barrier, support requires ensuring accurate fluid repletion, control of environmental temperature, prompt removal of nonviable tissue with physiologic wound closure, support of the gastrointestinal barrier, and proper management of pain and anxiety. A critical component is support of **body temperature**. Burn patients have vast evaporative water and energy losses if they are maintained in the typical cool, dry air

TABLE 37-2	Predictable Physiologic Changes in Burn Patients	
Period	**Physiologic Changes**	**Clinical Implications**
Resuscitation period (day 0–3)	Massive capillary leak	Closely monitor fluid resuscitation
Postresuscitation period (day 3 until 95% wound definitive wound closure)	Hyperdynamic and catabolic state with high risk of infection	Remove and close wounds to avoid sepsis; nutritional support is essential
Recovery period (95% wound closure until 1 y after injury)	Continued catabolic state and risk of nonwound septic events	Accurate nutritional support essential; anticipate and treat complications

of a hospital. Burn units and operating rooms need to be engineered to maintain high ambient temperatures and humidity to avoid hypothermia.

III. **Initial evaluation.** The initial management of a seriously burned patient is usually not completed prior to arrival in the intensive care unit. All of these patients should be approached as potential polytrauma patients. The evaluation follows the primary and secondary survey format of Advanced Trauma Life Support (ATLS).

A. **The primary survey** encompasses the first few seconds and minutes of the initial evaluation of the burn patient. Points of emphasis include

1. **Airway evaluation and protection** (see also **Chapter 4**). The security of the airway must be established, realizing that **progressive mucosal edema** can compromise airway patency over the first few postinjury hours. This is especially true of young children, as airway resistance varies inversely with the fourth power of the airway radius. In evaluation of the airway, anticipatory swelling of the tongue, face, eyes, neck, and oropharynx needs to be kept in mind. The presence of soot and foreign bodies in the airway should lean the practitioner toward intubation of the trachea. The mechanism of injury is also important in the decision-making process of managing the airway, as thermal or electrical burns, or the inhalation of toxic substances, such as carbon monoxide, may lead to intubation. It is important to discuss the care of the patient with a surgeon specialized in treating burn patients, and together deciding if observation or intubation is appropriate. Endotracheal intubation should be performed immediately if progressive airway edema is suspected. Facial and airway edema makes the burn patient's airway among the most challenging to intubate. The method of intubation must be carefully selected, and expert help should be summoned whenever possible. The method of intubation depends on the stage after the burn injury, and whether airway swelling has started to be a significant issue or not. If the intubation is done prophylactically, performing it through a **direct laryngoscopy** is sensible, if there are no other contraindications. If the airway is already swollen, or it appears to be some difficulty anticipated, an awake fiberoptic intubation should be considered. When difficulty to intubating is foreseen, it is very important to have a surgeon present who is skilled to perform rapidly a cricothyroidotomy. Once the intubation is successfully carried out, it is critical to secure the endotracheal tube properly, since inadvertent extubation in the patient with a burned, swollen face and a difficult airway is potentially lethal. A harness system using umbilical ties is recommended.

2. **Vascular access and initial fluid support.** Reliable and secure vascular access is essential. This usually requires central venous access, although the placement of central lines is most safely performed after immediate postburn hypovolemia has been corrected.

3. **Multiple trauma issues.** All of these patients must be approached as a polytrauma patient, since other injuries are common (**Chapter 9**).

B. **Burn-specific secondary survey.** In parallel with the trauma secondary survey, a number of burn-specific issues must be considered during the initial evaluation (**Table 37-3**).

1. **History.** The initial evaluation is the best time to elicit important points of medical history and mechanism of injury. These data should be actively sought from emergency personnel and family members, since access to these individuals and their information often is transient. Important points include time of injury, details of the injury mechanism, initial neurologic status, extrication time, and tetanus immune status.

TABLE 37-3   Important Aspects of the Burn-Specific Secondary Survey

System	Important Additional Considerations
History	1. Important points include the mechanism of injury, closed space exposure, extrication time, delay in seeking attention, fluid given during transport, and prior illnesses and injuries
Head & neck	1. The globes should be examined and corneal epithelium stained with fluorescein before adnexal swelling makes examination difficult. Adnexal swelling provides excellent coverage and protection of the globe during the first days after injury. Tarsorrhaphy is virtually never indicated acutely 2. Corneal epithelial loss can be overt, giving a clouded appearance to the cornea, but is more often subtle, requiring fluorescein staining for documentation. Topical ophthalmic antibiotics constitute optimal initial treatment
Cardiac	1. The cardiac rhythm should be monitored for 24–72 h in those with electrical injury and particular caution exercised with those with a history of myocardial infarction
Pulmonary	1. Ensure inflating pressures are less than 40 cmH_2O by performing chest escharotomies when needed
Vascular	1. The perfusion of burned extremities should be vigilantly monitored by serial examinations. One should not wait until flow in named vessels is compromised to decompress the extremity 2. Fasciotomy is indicated after electrical or deep thermal injury when distal flow is compromised. Clinically worrisome extremities should be decompressed regardless of compartment pressure readings
Abdomen	1. Nasogastric tubes should be in place and their function verified, particularly prior to air transport in unpressurized helicopters 2. An inappropriate resuscitative volume requirement may be a sign of an occult intra-abdominal injury 3. Torso escharotomies may be required to facilitate ventilation in the presence of deep circumferential abdominal wall burns
Genitourinary	1. It is important to ensure that the foreskin is reduced over the bladder catheter after insertion, as progressive swelling may otherwise result in paraphimosis
Neurologic	1. An early neurologic evaluation is important, as the patient's sensorium is often progressively compromised by medication or hemodynamic instability during the hours after injury
Extremities	1. The need for escharotomy usually becomes evident during the early hours of resuscitation. Many escharotomies can be delayed until transport has been enabled if transport times will not extend beyond 6 h postinjury
Wound	1. Wounds, although often underestimated in depth and overestimated in size on initial examination, should be evaluated for size, depth, and the presence of circumferential components
Laboratory	1. Arterial blood gas analysis is important when airway compromise or inhalation injury is present 2. A normal admission carboxyhemoglobin concentration does not eliminate the possibility of a significant exposure as the half-life of carboxyhemoglobin is 30–40 min in those effectively ventilated with 100% oxygen 3. Urinalysis for occult blood should be sent in those with deep thermal or electrical injuries

Adapted from Sheridan RL, Tompkins RG. In: Greenfield LJ, et al, eds. *Surgery: scientific principles and practice.* Philadelphia: J.B. Lippincott Co, 1996.

2. **Burn-specific systematic physical examination.** Burn and trauma patients require a comprehensive physical assessment at the time of their initial admission. Several aspects of this physical assessment are unique to burn patients.

   a. **Head, eyes, ears, nose, and throat.** Pressure on the burned occiput should be avoided. The globes should be inspected prior to the development of massive adnexal edema that can severely limit an adequate examination. A clouded cornea is usually indicative of a serious burn, and any suspicion of any level of eye injury warrants a complete ophthalmologic examination. More subtle injuries are detectable after fluorescein staining. Adnexal burns are noted, but acute tarsorrhaphy is virtually never indicated. For burns of the ear, pressure is avoided on the burned auricle and topical mafenide acetate is applied. Finally, signs of inhalation injury, such as carbonaceous debris and singed vibrissae are noted on examination of the nose and throat. Devices used to secure the nasogastric and endotracheal tubes are adjusted so that they do not apply pressure on the nasal septum.

   b. **Neurologic.** Imaging of the head and axial spine may be indicated depending on the mechanism of injury. In paralyzed or obtunded patients, it is important to make sure there is no pressure on peripheral nerves so that neuropathies are avoided. Those burned in structural fires should be assessed for carbon monoxide exposure by history, neurologic examination, and carboxyhemoglobin level, since selected patients with significant exposures may benefit from hyperbaric treatment.

   c. **The neck.** Injury to the cervical spine is of particular concern in high-voltage injuries. Extremely deep circumferential neck burns may require escharotomy to facilitate normal venous drainage of the head.

   d. **The chest** should be assessed for compliance and deep eschar should be sectioned if it interferes with ventilation. Escharotomy is best done bilaterally if needed, along the anterolateral portion of the chest wall. The presence of bilateral breath sounds should be verified.

   e. **Cardiovascular system.** Most patients initially are hypovolemic and respond favorably to volume administration. Occasionally, patients with massive burns will have an element of primary myocardial dysfunction. These patients, identified with invasive monitoring, will benefit from the administration of β-adrenergic agonists such as dobutamine.

   f. **Genitourinary system.** In males, foreskin retracted over the glans should be reduced after catheterization of the bladder so that progressive edema does not result in acute paraphimosis. Occasionally, a deeply burned foreskin must be sectioned to permit bladder catheterization.

   g. **Musculoskeletal system.** Burned extremities must be assessed for other trauma and monitored for adequacy of perfusion. It can sometimes be difficult to identify fractures in this setting, so liberal use of radiography is appropriate. Fractured and burned extremities are initially stabilized with external splints. Progressive edema during resuscitation can result in the late development of compartment syndrome and profound limb ischemia, secondary to swelling within circumferential eschar or inelastic muscle compartments. Extremity perfusion should be monitored throughout the resuscitation

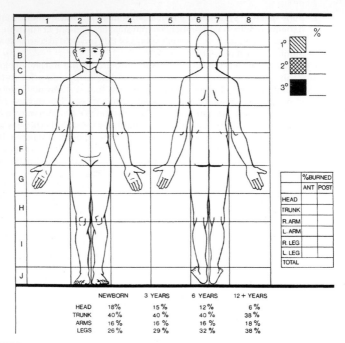

		NEWBORN	3 YEARS	6 YEARS	12 + YEARS
	HEAD	18%	15 %	12%	6 %
	TRUNK	40%	40 %	40%	38 %
	ARMS	16 %	16 %	16 %	18 %
	LEGS	26 %	29 %	32 %	38 %

FIGURE 37-1 Example of one of a number of age-specific burn diagrams available to facilitate accurate estimation of the extent of a burn, compensating for anthropometric differences between age groups.

period. Escharotomies should be performed at any hint of inadequate perfusion.

3. **Initial wound evaluation and management.** Wounds are assessed for extent, using a Lund-Browder or other burn diagram (**Fig. 37-1**), depth, using the practiced examiner's eye, and the presence of circumferential components, which may require decompression to assure adequate perfusion.

4. **Laboratory and radiographs.** Little laboratory evaluation is required beyond routine electrolyte and hematologic testing except for carboxyhemoglobin and arterial blood gas determinations in the proper clinical setting. Chest radiographs are appropriate to ensure proper placement of endotracheal tubes, resuscitative cannulas, and the absence of chest trauma. Inhalation injuries rarely cause early radiographic changes. The mechanism of injury will dictate the need for other radiographs.

5. **Possibility of abuse.** All patients should be screened for abuse as the injury mechanism. Approximately 20% of burns in young children are reported to state authorities for investigation, but abuse occurs in all age groups. Often this determination is not made until the patient has been admitted into ICU. The entire team must consider this possibility and file any suspicious case with appropriate state agencies. Careful and complete documentation of the circumstances and physical characteristics of the injury is essential. Photographic documentation is ideal.

IV. Resuscitation
   A. **Physiology of the immediate postburn period.** In the first hour after an extensive burn, patients experience little derangement in intravascular volume. As wound-released mediators are absorbed, and as stress- and pain-triggered hormonal release occurs, a diffuse loss of capillary integrity occurs that results in the extravasation of fluids, electrolytes, and even moderate-sized colloid molecules. For reasons yet unknown, this leak abates between 18 and 24 hours later in those successfully resuscitated. An increased leak can be seen in those whose resuscitations are delayed, thought due to the systemic release of reactive oxygen species formed upon reperfusion of marginally perfused tissues.
   B. **Formulas** have been developed over the past 40 years that attempt to predict resuscitation volume requirements. The multiple variables that impact resuscitation requirements render all such formulas inherently inaccurate. No two injuries are exactly alike, and no formula has yet been developed that accurately predicts volume requirements in all patients. Several formulas are widely used to determine initial infusion rates and to roughly guide resuscitation efforts. One such consensus formula is the modified Brooke, which is summarized in **Table 37-4**.
   C. **Monitoring.** Inaccurate volume administration is associated with substantial morbidity. Burn resuscitations must be guided by hourly reevaluation of resuscitation endpoints, which are summarized in **Table 37-5**. A simple and effective parameter to guide resuscitation after burns is **the urine output**, but other resuscitation endpoints, including acid–base status, mixed venous oxygen saturation, are often used as for the resuscitation of other unstable trauma patients (see **Chapter 9**).

TABLE 37-4	The Modified Brooke Formula

First 24 h
Adults and children >10 kg:
   Ringer's lactate: 2–4 cm^3/kg/%burn/24 h (first half in first 8 h)
   Colloid: none
Children ≤10 kg:
   Ringer's lactate: 2–3 cm^3/kg/%burn/24 h (first half in first 8 h)
   Ringer's lactate with 5% dextrose: 4 cm^3/kg/h
   Colloid: none

Second 24 h
All patients:
   Crystalloid: To maintain urine output. If silver nitrate is used, sodium leeching will mandate continued isotonic crystalloid. If other topical is used, free water requirement is significant. Serum sodium should be monitored closely. Nutritional support should begin, ideally by the enteral route
   Colloid: (5% albumin in Ringer's lactate):
      0%–30% burn: none
      30%–50% burn: 0.3 cm^3/kg/%burn/24 h
      50%–70% burn: 0.4 cm^3/kg/%burn/24 h
      >70% burn: 0.5 cm^3/kg/%burn/24 h

Adapted from Sheridan RL, Tompkins RG. Burns. In: Greenfield LJ, et al, eds. *Surgery: scientific principles and practice.* Philadelphia: J.B. Lippincott Co, 1996.

D. Recognition and management of resuscitation problems. The volume of infusate required by patients with large injuries can be enormous. It is essential to promptly recognize when resuscitation is not proceeding as it should, and what to do if this is found to be the case. At any point during resuscitation, the total 24-hour volume can be predicted based on the known volume infused so far and the current rate of infusion. If this number exceeds 6 mL/kg/% burn/24 hours, it is likely that the resuscitation is not proceeding optimally. At this point, one can consider further administration of colloids, or the placement of a pulmonary artery catheter to gather additional information (**Chapter 1**).

V. **Neurologic issues** that must be commonly addressed are pain and anxiety management, the exposed globe, and peripheral neuropathies.
   A. **Uncontrolled pain and anxiety** have adverse physiologic as well as psychological consequences. Both can contribute to the development of posttraumatic stress syndrome.
      1. Inadequate pain management may occur because of the extraordinary opiate doses often required to adequately address pain in the seriously burned patient.
      2. The opiate tolerance that rapidly develops in patients with large open wounds can be remarkable. Despite this, addiction is rare; opiate requirements rapidly decrease after wound closure. The best way to manage pain in burn patients is with prompt biologic closure of their wounds.
      3. Successful management is greatly aided by an organized pharmacological guideline supplemented with nonpharmacological measures (**Chapter 7**).
   B. **Ocular exposure.** Commonly, progressive contraction of the burned eyelids and periocular skin results in exposure of the globe. This results in desiccation of the globe, followed by keratitis, ulceration, and globe-threatening infection. Frequent lubrication of the exposed globe with hourly application of ocular lubricants and surgically releasing the eyelid release in those who do not rapidly respond help prevent these sequelae.
   C. **Peripheral neuropathies** can be seen in burn patients because of direct thermal damage to peripheral nerves, or because of one of the many metabolic derangements that these patients can suffer. Many peripheral neu-

TABLE 37-5	Age-Specific Resuscitation Endpoints
Endpoint	**Target**
Sensorium	Comfortable, arousable
Urine output	Infants: 1–2 cm³/kg/h Children: 0.5–1 cm³/kg/h All others: 0.5 cm³/kg/h
Base deficit	Less than 2
Systolic pressure	Infants: 60–70 mm Hg Children: 70–90 + (twice age in years) mm Hg Adolescents and adults: 90–120 mm Hg

Adapted from Sheridan RL, Tompkins RG. Burns. In: Greenfield LJ, et al, eds. *Surgery: scientific principles and practice.* Philadelphia: J.B. Lippincott Co, 1996.

ropathies can be avoided. Diligent monitoring of extremity perfusion will avoid the morbidity of constricting eschar and missed compartment syndromes. Proper application of well-fitting splints will avoid pressure-induced neuropathies. Careful positioning of deeply sedated or anesthetized patients will avoid traction and pressure injuries.

VI. Pulmonary issues

A. **Airway.** Secure placement of the endotracheal tube should be regularly verified. If inhalational injury is a concern, the patients can be extubated after the fiberoptic evaluation of the airway and confirmation by an experienced burn physician that the airway injury is in a stable or improving phase. If the airway injury is not the major concern, but the patient requires continued debridements in the operating room, or the dressing changes are very painful, the ICU physicians may decide to maintain the endotracheal intubation for the duration of treatment, and evaluate for possible tracheostomy.

B. **Inhalation injury**

1. **Diagnosis of inhalation injury.** Inhalation injury is a clinical diagnosis based on a history of closed spaced exposure, and presence of singed nasal vibrissae and carbonaceous sputum. **Fiberoptic bronchoscopy** facilitates diagnosis in equivocal cases and may help document laryngeal edema. Such information is useful when making decisions regarding preemptive intubation for evolving upper airway edema. When the airway edema seems to have decreased, it is important to evaluate before proceeding with extubation with a fiberoptic scope, as it may decrease the risk of reintubations.

2. **Clinical consequences and management.** Five events with major clinical implications occur predictably in patients with inhalation injury.

   a. **Acute upper airway obstruction** is anticipated and managed with endotracheal intubation.

   b. **Bronchospasm** from aerosolized irritants is a common occurrence during the first 24 to 48 hours, particularly in young children. This is managed with inhaled β_2-adrenergic agonists (**Chapter 21**). Some children will require intravenous bronchodilators such as terbutaline or low-dose epinephrine infusions and occasionally steroids. Ventilatory strategies should be designed to minimize auto-PEEP.

   c. **Small airway obstruction** occurs as necrotic endobronchial debris sloughs and complicates clearance of secretions. Small endotracheal tubes can become suddenly occluded, and it is important to be prepared to evaluate and respond to a sudden patient's respiratory deterioration. Therapeutic bronchoscopy facilitates clearance of the airways.

   d. **Pulmonary infection** develops in 30% to 50% of patients. Differentiating between pneumonia and tracheobronchitis (purulent infection of the denuded tracheobronchial tree) is often difficult, but generally of little clinical consequence. A patient with newly purulent sputum, fever, and impaired gas exchange should be treated; the antibiotic coverage is adjusted according to the results of sputum Gram stain and culture. Secretion clearance is a particularly important component of management, because inhalation injury to bronchial mucosa greatly impairs mucociliary clearance.

   e. **Respiratory failure** is common in those sustaining inhalation injury, and is managed as outlined in **Chapters 5** and **20**.

3. **Carbon monoxide (CO) exposure** is common in patients injured in structural fires. Many are obtunded from a combination of CO, anoxia, and hypotension. **Hyperbaric oxygen** has been proposed as a means of improving the prognosis of those suffering serious CO exposures, but its use remains controversial.

   a. **Physiology.** Carbon monoxide avidly binds and inactivates heme-containing enzymes, particularly hemoglobin and the cytochromes. The formation of carboxyhemoglobin results in an acute physiologic anemia, much like an isovolemic hemodilution. As a carboxyhemoglobin concentration of 50% is physiologically similar to a 50% isovolemic hemodilution, the routine occurrence of unconsciousness at this level of carboxyhemoglobin makes it clear that other mechanisms are involved in the pathophysiology of CO injury. It is likely that CO binding to the cytochrome system in the mitochondria, interfering with oxygen utilization is more toxic than CO binding to hemoglobin. For unknown reasons, between 5% and 20% of patients with serious CO exposures have been reported to develop delayed neurologic sequelae.

   b. **Management options.** These patients can be managed with 100% isobaric oxygen or with hyperbaric oxygen. If serious exposure has occurred, manifested by overt neurologic impairment or a high carboxyhemoglobin level, then hyperbaric oxygen treatment is probably warranted if it can be administered safely.

   c. **Hyperbaric oxygen (HBO) treatment** regimens vary, but an exposure to 3 atmospheres for 90 minutes, with three 10-minute "air breaks" is typical. An air break refers to the breathing of pressurized room air rather than pressurized oxygen, which decreases the incidence of seizures from oxygen toxicity. Because treatment is generally in a monoplace chamber, unstable patients are suboptimal candidates. Other relative contraindications are wheezing or air trapping, which increases the risk of pneumothorax, and high fever, which increases the risk of seizures. Prior to placement in the chamber, endotracheal tube balloons should be filled with saline to avoid balloon compression and associated air leaks. Upper body central venous cannulation should be avoided, if possible, to reduce the chance of a pneumothorax that may enlarge suddenly during decompression. Myringotomies are required in intubated patients.

   d. **Cyanide exposure** is often detectable in patients extricated from structural fires, but is rarely of the severity to justify the risk of treatment with amyl nitrate and sodium thiosulfate.

VII. Gastrointestinal issues

   A. **Ulcer prophylaxis.** Until the routine use of prophylactic therapies, burn patients had a virulent ulcer diathesis ("Curling's ulcer") that was a common cause of death. Ulceration is believed to be secondary to periods of reduced splanchnic flow. At present, it is advisable to treat most patients with serious burns with empirical histamine receptor blockers and/or proton pump inhibitors (see **Chapter 27**). While it is unclear when to stop prophylactic therapy, most would agree that patients with closed wounds who are tolerating tube feedings are at low enough risk that this therapy can be stopped.

   B. **Nutritional support.** Burn patients have predictable and protracted needs for supplemental protein and caloric support, which needs to be accurate, since both under- and overfeeding have adverse sequelae (see **Chapter 11**).

TABLE 37-6	Common Topical Antimicrobial Agents
Silver sulfadiazine	Painless on application, fair to poor eschar penetration, no metabolic side effects, broad antibacterial spectrum
Mafenide acetate	Painful on application, excellent eschar penetration, carbonic anhydrase inhibitor, broad antibacterial spectrum
0.5% Silver nitrate	Painless on application, poor eschar penetration, leeches electrolytes, broad spectrum (including fungi)

1. **Routes and timing.** Continuous tube feedings are ideal and usually successful. Tube feedings are begun at a low rate during resuscitation. Initially, a sump nasogastric tube is used so that gastric residuals can be used to help determine tolerance of the feedings. Parenteral nutrition is used if tube feedings are not tolerated. Highly catabolic burn patients tolerate prolonged periods of fasting very poorly.

2. **Nutritional targets** in severely injured burned patients remain controversial. The many formulas propagated to predict these requirements vary widely in their predictions. The current consensus is that protein needs are approximately 2.5 g/kg/d, and caloric needs are between 1.5 and 1.7 times the calculated basal metabolic rate, or 1.3 to 1.5 times the measured resting energy expenditure.

3. **Monitoring.** Substrate support needs to be titrated to nutritional endpoints during a lengthy burn hospitalization if the complications of over- or underfeeding are to be avoided. Regular physical examination, quality of wound healing, nitrogen balance, and indirect calorimetry are all useful in this regard. The combination of a highly catabolic state, the critical need to heal extensive wounds, and the length of time that support is required make monitoring and adjustment of nutritional support particularly important in patients with extensive burns.

VIII. **Infectious disease issues**

   A. **Wound topical care.** The best way of avoiding wound sepsis is through prompt excision and successful closure of deep wounds. Topical agents are an adjunct in this regard, slowing the inevitable occurrence of wound sepsis in deep wounds and minimizing desiccation and colonization of healing wounds. There are several agents in wide general use, the most common itemized in **Table 37-6.**

   B. **Antibiotic use.** Burn physiology includes the routine occurrence of moderate fever, which is not necessarily a sign of infection. When unexpected fever occurs, a complete physical assessment is done; wounds are inspected for evidence of sepsis; directed labs and radiographs are taken; and cultures of blood, urine, and sputum are sent. If the patient appears unstable, empirical broad-spectrum coverage is reasonable pending return of culture data (see **Chapters 12** and **29**). If no infectious focus is identified, antibiotics should be stopped. It is critically important that deteriorating burn patients be compulsively evaluated for occult foci of infection to allow prompt treatment prior to the development of systemic sepsis.

   C. **Infection control (Chapter 13).** Patients referred from other facilities often harbor highly resistant bacterial species. Proper infection control practices are of particular importance to avoid cross contamination of vulnerable patients with these organisms. Universal precautions and compulsive hand washing are essential components of practice.

System	Complication
Neurologic	1. Delirium 2. Seizures 3. Peripheral nerve injuries 4. Delayed peripheral nerve and spinal cord deficits
Otologic	1. Auricular chondritis 2. Sinusitis and otitis media
Ophthalmic	1. Ectropia 2. Corneal ulceration 3. Symblepharon
Renal	1. Early acute renal failure 2. Late renal failure secondary to sepsis, multiorgan failure, and nephrotoxic agents.
Adrenal	1. Acute adrenal insufficiency
Cardiovascular	1. Endocarditis and suppurative thrombophlebitis
Pulmonary	1. Carbon monoxide intoxication. 2. Pneumonia 3. Acute respiratory distress syndrome (ARDS)
Hematologic	1. Neutropenia, thrombocytopenia, DIC
Gastrointestinal	1. Hepatic dysfunction, acalculous cholecystitis 2. Pancreatitis 3. Gastroduodenal ulceration 4. Intestinal ischemia
Genitourinary	1. Urinary tract infections
Musculoskeletal	1. Burned exposed bone 2. Fractured and burned extremities 3. Heterotopic ossification
Soft tissue	1. Hypertrophic scar formation

Adapted from Sheridan RL, Tompkins RG. Burns. In: Greenfield LJ, et al, eds. *Surgery: scientific principles and practice.* Philadelphia: J.B. Lippincott Co, 1996.

- **D. Recognition and management of burn complications.** Successful management requires that a predictable series of complications (see **Table 37-7**), mostly infectious, be successfully treated as the wound is progressively closed. Compulsive attention to changes in clinical status will facilitate early detection and successful intervention.

IX. Rehabilitation efforts in the burn ICU

- **A. Physical and occupational therapists** play important roles in the burn ICU. Initially, twice-daily passive ranging of all joints and static antideformity positioning is begun to prevent the development of contractures.
- **B. Perioperative therapy.** Physical and occupational therapists should be informed of the sequence of planned operations and the modifications of therapy plans that these imply. Therapists should be encouraged to range

patients under anesthesia in conjunction with planned operations and to fabricate custom face molds and splints in the operating room, particularly in children who often poorly tolerate these activities when awake.

X. **Intraoperative support** is detailed in **Chapter 33** of the *Clinical Anesthesia Procedures of the Massachusetts General Hospital.* Here, we wish to emphasize the critical importance of continuity of care between the burn unit and the operating room teams. In our burn service, several members of the burn team work both in the ICU and in the operating room.

XI. **Special considerations**
   A. **Electrical injury**
      1. Patients exposed to low and intermediate voltages may have severe local wounds, but rarely suffer systemic consequences.
      2. Those exposed to high voltages commonly suffer compartment syndromes, myocardial injury, fractures of the long bones and axial spine, and release of free pigment in the plasma that may cause renal failure if not promptly cleared.
      3. Those suffering high-voltage injuries should receive cardiac monitoring, radiographic clearance of the spine, and examination of the urine for myoglobin. Fluid resuscitation initially is based on burn size, but this generally does not correlate well with deep tissue injury, so resuscitation need to be closely monitored and adjusted. Muscle compartments at risk should be closely monitored by serial physical examinations—they should be decompressed in the operating room when an evolving compartment syndrome is suspected. Wounds are debrided and closed with a combination of skin grafts and flaps.
   B. **Tar injury**
      1. Numerous thermoplastic road materials are the source of occupational injury. They are highly viscous and heated to between 300°F and 700°F.
      2. The wounds should be immediately cooled by tap water irrigation. Resuscitation is based on burn size, and monitored. Wounds are dressed in a lipophilic solvent and then debrided, excised, and grafted. The underlying wounds are generally quite deep.
   C. **Cold injury**
      1. Soft-tissue necrosis from cold injury is often managed in the burn unit. Wound care is conservative until the extent of irreversible soft-tissue necrosis is apparent; this often requires several weeks if not months. When definitely demarcated, surgical debridement, excision, and reconstruction or closure is carried out, if needed, with lesser injuries often healing without need for surgery.
      2. Cold-injured patients may manifest all the problems of systemic **hypothermia** when they present, and should be managed accordingly.
   D. **Chemical injury**
      1. Patients can be exposed to thousands of chemicals, which are often heated. It is important to consider the thermal, local chemical, and systemic chemical effects.
      2. Liberal consultation with **poison control information centers** (see **Chapter 33**) for guidance regarding systemic effects is extremely useful. Most agents can be washed off with tap water.
         a. **Alkaline substances** may take longer than the traditional 30 minutes. When the soapy feel that these alkalis typically impart to the gloved finger is gone, or when litmus paper applied to the wound shows a neutral pH, irrigation can be stopped.

      b. Concentrated **hydrofluoric acid** exposure will cause dangerous hypocalcemia, and subeschar injection of 10% calcium gluconate and emergent wound excision may be appropriate.

      c. **Elemental metals** should be covered with oil, and **white phosphorus** should be covered in saline to prevent secondary ignition.

E. Toxic epidermal necrolysis (TENS)

    1. TENS is a diffuse process of unknown pathophysiology in which epidermal–dermal bonding is acutely compromised. Patients commonly present with a drug exposure preceding the illness and have both a cutaneous and visceral wound.

    2. This disease is similar in presentation to a total-body *second*-degree burn. With good wound care, most patients will heal the cutaneous wound without the need for surgery. Involvement of the aerodigestive tract mucosa may lead to sepsis and organ failures, particularly if septic complications are not promptly recognized and treated.

F. Purpura fulminans

    1. Purpura fulminans is a complication of meningococcal sepsis in which extensive soft-tissue necrosis, and commonly organ failures, occurs. It is believed to be secondary to a transient hypercoagulable state that occurs early in the primary septicemic event.

    2. These patients often present with sepsis-associated organ failures and extensive deep wounds. Both should be managed concurrently, since the wounds are prone to infection if not promptly excised and closed.

	Possible Conflicting Priorities in Patients Who Suffered Contemporaneous Burns and Trauma
Area of Conflict	**Consensus Resolution**
Neurologic	
Patients with burns and head injuries must have cerebral edema controlled during resuscitation; pressure monitors increase risk of infection	A very tightly controlled resuscitation with short-term placement of indicated pressure monitors with antibiotic coverage
Chest	
Patients with blunt chest injuries and overlying burns may require chest tubes through burned areas with risk of empyema, and difficulty closing the tract	Use a long subcutaneous tunnel to decrease trouble closing the tract and remove tubes as soon as possible to decrease empyema risk
Abdomen	
Blunt abdominal injuries may be hard to detect if there is an overlying burn. There is a high incidence of wound dehiscence operating through a burned abdominal wall	Liberal use of imaging to detect occult injuries and routine use of retention sutures after laparotomy
Orthopedic	
Optimal management of a fracture may be compromised by an overlying burn	Most such extremities are best managed with prompt excision and grafting of the wound with external fracture fixation

TABLE 37-8

G. **Soft-tissue infections** (See also **Chapter 29**)
   1. Patients with soft-tissue infections share many characteristics of burn patients.
   2. These patients need to go directly to the operating room. Operative goals are exposure of the infection so that its anatomic extent can be accurately described and its microbiology determined by culture, Gram stain, and biopsy. Debridement under general anesthesia is repeated until infection is controlled, and the wounds are then closed or grafted. Broad-spectrum, and then focused, antibiotics are important adjuncts.
H. **The burned polytrauma patient.** Burn care priorities frequently conflict with orthopedic, neurosurgical, and other priorities. Thoughtful resolution these differences is an important part of successful management (**Table 37-8**). These situations commonly require a great deal of judgment and liberal consultation.

Selected References

Goldstein AM, Weber JM, Sheridan RL. Femoral venous catheterization is safe in burned children: an analysis of 224 catheters. *J Pediatrics* 1997;3:442–446.

Prelack K, Cunningham J, Sheridan RL, Tompkins RG. Energy provided and protein provisions for thermally injured children revisited: an outcome-based approach for determining requirements. *J Burn Care Rehabil* 1997;10:177–182.

Rabban JT, Blair JA, Rosen CL, Adler JN, Sheridan RL. Mechanisms of pediatric electrical injury. New implications for product safety and injury prevention. *Arch Pediatr Adolesc Med.* 1997;151:696–700

Sheridan RL, Gagnon SW, Tompkins RG, et al. The burn unit as a resource for the management of acute nonburn conditions in children. *J Burn Care Rehabil* 1995;16:62–64.

Sheridan RL, Hinson M, Blanquierre M, et al. Development of a pediatric burn pain and anxiety management program. *J Burn Care Rehabil* 1997;18:455–459.

Sheridan RL, Hurford WE, Kacmarek RM, et al. Inhaled nitric oxide in burn patients with respiratory failure. *J Trauma* 1997;42:641–646.

Sheridan RL, Prelack K, Cunningham JJ. Physiologic hypoalbuminemia is well tolerated by severely burned children. *J Trauma* 1997;43:448–452.

Sheridan RL, Weber JM, Benjamin J, et al. Control of methicillin resistant *Staphylococcus aureus* in a pediatric burn unit. *Am J Infect Control* 1994;22:340–345.

Disaster Preparedness in the ICU

Todd Seigel and Edward George

I. **Introduction.** Since the 1970s, the **incident command system (ICS)** has been the organizing structure for the management of **mass casualty incidents (MCIs)**. The MCI response includes four main components: search and rescue, triage and initial stabilization, definitive care, and evacuation. In preparing for an MCI, every ICU should be able to accurately assess its technical and logistical capabilities, and reliably communicate these to the chain of command. In preparing for a large influx of critically ill patients who may require prolonged ICU courses, ICU staff must appreciate the nature and degree of care for injuries most commonly encountered in MCIs such as burns, blast injury, and illness or injury from biological, nuclear, or chemical agents.

II. **ICU organization during MCIs**
   A. **Organization of the ICU** in the event of a disaster can be modeled after the ICS that is implemented throughout the hospital. Development of a command structure within the ICU should focus not only on executing function within the unit, but integration of the ICU with other critical care units and the overall hospital response. **The ICU leader** can be a senior administrator, nursing or medical director, and is responsible for providing control and direction of the ICU for the duration of the event. This includes providing updates on the situation to staff and receiving status updates from other ICU leaders. In addition, the ICU leader will select other staff to operate in leadership positions to complement personnel assigned to similar roles at different levels of the institution's response plan. A simplified schema of the leadership structure during MCIs is shown in **Table 38-1**.
   B. **The approach to disaster management in the ICU** should focus on the role of the ICU within the hospital response as well as maximizing the capabilities of available resources.
      1. **Physical capacity** needs to be assessed and maximized. Patients who are in the ICU prior to the MCI may need to be retriaged with anticipation of the approaching surge. Any patients who can be moved out of the ICU should be expeditiously transferred. In addition, some hospitals may have the contingencies for converting units not normally used for critical care to ICU space. This may include the post-anesthesia care unit (PACU) and stepdown units.
      2. **Triage** to the ICU is crucial, as is coordination with the **emergency department (ED)**. Based on available resources, some patients (such as stable mechanically ventilated patients) may not need ED evaluation and therefore be transported directly from the field to the ICU. Triage will be impacted by available space, staffing ratios, as well as patient injury. Appropriate ICU triage should focus only on patients with survivable insults. In addition, patients who may otherwise merit critical care may not be appropriate for the ICU during times of mass casualty. This includes patients with large surface area burns, recurrent cardiac

TABLE 38-1	Leadership Roles During a Mass Casualty Incident
Position	**Role**
Public information officer	• Manages all internal hospital communication pertinent to the ICU • May work with other hospital personnel for key media briefings
Liaison officer	• Acts as an intermediary between ICUs and between ICUs and the ED • Handles communication with state and federal agencies
Safety officer	• Advises the ICU team regarding the management of hazardous conditions • In the event of biological, chemical or radiological disaster, coordinates with experts for specialized response • Organizes distribution of protective equipment
Security officer	• Implements access control procedures, including ICU lockdown • In the event of criminal action, collects evidence for law enforcement officials.
Medical officer	• Oversees general operations of clinical care • Ensures adequate physician staffing
Logistics chief	• Oversees the provision of resources needed for continuous operations,
Operations chief	• Oversees the patient flow process from triage through discharge • Manages patient data • Prepares for failure of traditional registration or computer systems

arrest, severe neurologic insult, and patients at extremes of age. Conversely, triage criteria cannot be so stringent that care is withheld from patients solely in the interest of resource preservation.

3. **Decontamination** may need to be addressed within the ICU, and appropriate hospital safety officer should be involved in creating a decontamination area for staff of each critical care unit. Allocation of space may also be a consideration; depending on the incident, **negative-pressure isolation** or potential for burn care may impact triage decisions. Mass casualty triage focused on stringent **rationing of resources** based on patient acuity and potential for survival are fundamental in the field and in the ED, but may not be appropriate for the ICU.

4. **Human resources and staff scheduling.** Contact lists should be updated and disseminated. In addition, foresight must be used in scheduling such that all available personnel are not activated immediately upon recognition of the disaster. Staff fatigue and potential injury should be anticipated, and scheduling should focus both on the immediate response and staged relief staffing.

5. **Resource allocation** is crucial in disaster management. In addition to institutional space and human resources, consideration must be

given to special equipment or personnel that is required for appropriate management. This includes potentially fixed resources such as ventilators, capacity for negative-pressure isolation, and personal protective equipment. Accurate assessment of resources and needs enables prediction of potential challenges.

a. **Effective administration of critical care** can be particularly challenging in the setting of an MCI. Medical care should focus primarily on critical interventions that are deemed to improve survival and that can be implemented without significant cost or special equipment. Fundamental aspects to critical care should include mechanical ventilation, hemodynamic support and monitoring, and specific antibiotics or antidotes required for biological or chemical attacks.

b. **Specialized personnel,** such as radiation safety officials and infectious disease experts, should be notified as soon as possible if they are needed. In addition, laboratory personnel should be notified in the event of biological threats.

c. **Preparation for loss of infrastructure** should be made in case standard computer technology becomes unavailable or ineffective. Specific **plans for tracking patient data** should be managed with the operations officer. In addition, initial information on the scope of the disaster may be limited or inaccurate, and planning decisions must be made with this in mind. **Familiarity with the hospital disaster plan** and the scope of the incident may assist with ICU management, as well as integration of the ICU within the institutional, local, and federal responses.

III. Specific injuries

A. **Blast injury** is a general term for the harmful effects produced by the sudden changes in environmental pressure secondary to an explosion. In the United States, blast injuries are predominantly caused by industrial accidents rather than intentional bombings. Blast injuries can be categorized as primary, secondary, or tertiary. General considerations in the triage of patients with blast injury are dependent on types of injury sustained from the explosion, location of the explosion, and the type of energy that caused the explosion.

1. **Primary blast injuries** occur as a direct result of the passing shock wave generated by the explosion. Peak pressures are magnified in denser media, such as underwater. Exposure to a blast wave can cause rupture of gas-filled cavities, and this is a common feature in all of these injuries. Explosions in closed areas result in a reflection of the shock wave that can lead to greater magnitude of injury. Incidence of primary blast injury is up to four times greater when the blast occurs in a closed space.

   a. **Tympanic membrane** is the most common site of primary blast injury. Rupture of the membrane can occur with pressure as low as 2 psi.

   b. **Lung** injury is the second most common site of primary blast injury. The threshold for injury is approximately 15 psi.

      (1) Acute pressure changes in the lung cause alveolar edema and hemorrhage, leading to lung contusion.

      (2) Pneumo- and hemothoraces are also possible; the former may be unrecognized until exacerbated by positive pressure ventilation.

      (3) Disruption of the interface between alveolar walls pulmonary vasculature can also create air emboli that manifest as neurologic or cardiac dysfunction.

   c. **Bowel** injuries may include serosal tears or bowel perforation. Bowel injuries require peak pressures that are not commonly seen in air explosions, and may be more common in water explosions.

2. **Secondary blast injuries** are injuries sustained by flying debris during an explosion.

3. **Tertiary blast injuries** are blunt injuries sustained when the patient is thrust against a stationary object. A 70-kg adult subject to peak overpressure of 15 psi experiences an instantaneous acceleration approximately 14 times the force of gravity. The potential for both secondary and tertiary blast injury is high, and these account for the majority of injuries in a most explosions.

4. **Miscellaneous blast injuries** include exposure to dust and chemicals related to the explosion, including chemical and thermal burns. The source of energy used for the explosion may contribute to morbidity of these patients, and may merit special attention if the source is chemical, nuclear, or radiologic (see below).

B. **Burn injuries** in the event of an MCI are likely to be associated with other injuries, such as blast or, less commonly, chemical agents, or significant radiation exposure **(see below)**. In the setting of MCIs, burn patients are likely to present in large numbers. Effective triage should be employed in these situations. The specific management of burn patients is otherwise not different from the general burn care, as outlined in **Chapter 37**.

C. **Biological weapons** are microorganisms or derivatives of microorganisms implemented to intentionally cause harm. This includes bacteria, viruses, and bacterial toxins. Biological weapons are particularly insidious agents as they can be deployed undetected by sight or smell. In addition, the size of bacteria allows them to easily inoculate the lower respiratory tract by inhalation, the most efficient way to cause widespread harm. Unlike chemical weapons (see below), detection of an attack with biological agents is likely to be delayed, as initial symptoms of exposure are generally nonspecific and may resemble other endemic diseases. Once exposed, onset of symptoms may not occur for days to weeks, and exposed patients are likely be separated by time and space. Illness caused by biological agents is generally transmissible, and appropriate precautions must be taken by health care personnel to minimize the potential of exposure and cross-contamination. In general, due to delayed patient presentation, mass decontamination is not required. Removal of clothing and cleansing with soap and water removes >99% of infectious organisms. Health care provider protection is critical; in addition to standard precautions, airborne transmission should be assumed and strict respiratory precautions should be implemented. The Center for Disease Control (CDC) and the National Institute of Health (NIH) may be useful resources for consultation. Antibiotic treatment guidelines are listed in **Table 38-2**. The following Web sites may be useful as resources for the most current information:

- http://sis.nlm.nih.gov/enviro/biologicalwarfare.html
- http://www.bt.cdc.gov/

1. **Smallpox** is the clinical syndrome caused by variola virus, a large DNA orthopoxvirus. The World Health Organization declared smallpox eradicated in 1979 after an extensive vaccine campaign. However, stocks of the virus remain in both the United States and Russia. The transmission of the virus is predominantly via inhaled droplets after prolonged close contact. Once contracted, typical incubation period is approximately 12 to 14 days. Prodromal symptoms of variola infection are nonspecific and include fever, nausea, headache, and backache. As the prodromal illness resolves, lesions erupt in the palate, oral mucosa, and tongue. Over the course of 24 to 36 hours, these lesions

TABLE 38.2	Antibiotic Treatment Guidelines for Biological Weapons	
Agent	**Condition**	**Treatment Options**
Anthrax	Cutaneous anthrax or postexposure prophylaxis	Amoxicillin 500 mg PO TID *Treatment duration is for 60 d*
	Inhalational anthrax	Ciprofloxacin 400 mg IV every 12 h Doxycycline 100 mg IV every 12 h *Treatment duration is for 60 d*
Plague	Active disease	Ciprofloxacin 400 mg IV every12 h Doxycycline 100 mg IV every 12 h Chloramphenicol 25 mg/kg IV every 6 h Streptomycin 1 g IM BID Gentamycin 5 mg/kg IV daily *Treatment duration is 10 d*
	Postexposure or mass casualty setting	Ciprofloxacin 500 mg orally every 12 h Doxycycline 100 mg orally every 12 h *Treatment duration is 10 d for active disease, 7 d for prophylaxis*
Tularemia	Active disease	Identical to treatment for plague except treatment duration is 14 d

Table adapted from Antibiotic guidelines for anthrax, plague and tularemia. In: *Harwood-Nuss' clinical practice of emergency medicine.* 4th ed. Lippincott, 2005, *with permission.*

give way to a macular rash that typically begins on the face and moves toward the extremities. Overall **mortality rate of smallpox is approximately 30%.** The administration of the vaccine within 4 days of exposure significantly attenuates clinical illness. The vaccine is stockpiled by the CDC and can be obtained within 24 hours. Information can be found on the CDC Web site http://www.bt.cdc.gov/agent/smallpox.

2. **Anthrax** is the common name for the diseases cause by *Bacillus anthracis*, a spore-forming gram-positive rod. Human disease occurs from direct inoculation with anthrax spores; exposure can be cutaneous, inhaled, or ingested. It cannot be transmitted directly from person to person. Vaccines for anthrax exist, however, they must be administered well is advance of exposure to be effective.

    a. **Cutaneous** anthrax accounts for approximately 95% of human anthrax cases. Two to five days after skin exposure, a painless boil-like lesion develops. Eventually, the boil lesion degenerates into an ulcer, and ultimately, to a black eschar. In 10% to 20% of the cases, septicemia and subsequent death can occur. Initiation of oral antibiotics upon recognition of the eschar can minimize the potential of septicemia from cutaneous disease.

    b. **Inhalational** anthrax is caused from aerosolized spores. The mortality of inhaled anthrax is nearly 100%, though data from the recent United States outbreak in 2001 suggest a lower mortality rate. Because of high morbidity and ease of dissemination, inhalational anthrax is the most likely form of the disease to be encountered in a terrorist attack. After an incubation period of 1 to 6 days, the clinical prodrome of malaise, fever, and cough develop; chest imaging at this stage will demonstrate mediastinal lymphadenopathy as opposed to frank pulmonary infiltrates. Early administration of antibiotics (see **Table 38-2**) can attenuate the disease, but are unlikely to be helpful by the time the diagnosis is suspected. Antibiotic prophylaxis should be initiated for anyone with potential exposure to anthrax spores.

c. **Gastrointestinal** (GI) anthrax occurs after the ingestion of spores or infected meat. Lesions similar to those of cutaneous anthrax develop within the GI tract and act as a portal of entry for bacteria. Abdominal pain, nausea, vomiting, and hematochezia are common symptoms; symptoms can progress to bacteremia and death if untreated, though the mortality rate is estimated at approximately 30%; antibiotic selection parallels that of inhalational disease.

d. **Decontamination.** While the bacteria cannot be spread between people, spores can survive for long periods in the environment. Decontamination of skin can be successfully achieved with thorough washing with antimicrobial soap; patient clothing and other articles should be appropriately disposed. Health care workers should wear disposable personal protective equipment as well as respiratory masks with the ability to filter particles of approximately 1 μm. Patients who succumb to anthrax are prime vectors for spore transmission and need to be kept on strict isolation; cremation is the method of choice for ensuring decontamination.

3. **The plague** describes the clinical manifestations of infection with *Yersinia pestis*, a gram-negative bacillus. *Yersinia pestis* is a zoonotic intracellular pathogen predominantly found in rodents. It is directly transmitted to humans by fleas. Like anthrax, the bacteria can also be aerosolized and cause respiratory collapse.

a. **Bubonic plague** is caused by direct bloodstream inoculation with *Yersinia* via the flea vector. After an incubation period of 2 to 10 days, the nodes become swollen and inflamed, resulting in the characteristic "buboes" from which the disease derives its name. Bacterial propagation can result in rapid septicemia, disseminated intravascular coagulation (DIC), and ultimate death. Untreated, mortality approaches 100%, though unlike anthrax, *Yersinia* septicemia can be attenuated with **appropriate antibiotics** (see **Table 38-2**), reducing mortality to less than 15%.

b. **Pneumonic plague** results from inhalational exposure of the bacteria. After a brief incubation period, symptoms of fever malaise give way to cough and hemoptysis. This form of the plague is almost uniformly fatal. Respiratory droplet precautions should be employed, and all potentially exposed to the disease should receive antimicrobial prophylaxis.

4. **Botulism** refers to the toxin-mediated paralysis caused by *Clostridium botulinum*, an anaerobic, spore-forming gram-positive bacillus. Clinical disease is caused exclusively by the bacterial toxin; clostridial spores are not pathogenic. Among the most lethal known substances known (LD_{50} of 1 μg/kg), the botulinum toxin inhibits the release of acetylcholine at presynaptic nerve terminals. Decreased acetylcholine throughout the nervous system results in flaccid paralysis. Generally, clinical disease results from either ingestion of contaminated food or inoculation of a wound with *C. botulinum*. Human-to-human transmission does not occur.

a. **Ingestion** of *C. botulinum* or preformed botulinum toxin will result in a similar clinical disease. Initial symptoms are predominantly GI related, and include abdominal pain, bloating, nausea, and vomiting. Symptoms can occur early as 4 hours after ingestion, but can be delayed as long as 10 days. Neurologic deficits usually begin with bulbar symptoms such as dysarthria and dysphagia, and progress to flaccid paralysis.

b. **Wound botulism** refers to botulism that occurs after a cutaneous wound becomes superinfected with *C. botulinum*. Bacterial proliferation and toxin production occur to produce clinical disease. Compared to ingestion of the bacteria, symptoms occur over a longer time period. GI symptoms are absent.

c. **Inhalational and waterborne transmission** of the disease is possible, and may be the most likely method employed in events of mass casualty. Waterborne transmission is less likely as water treatment processes inactivate the botulinum toxin.

d. **Diagnosis and treatment** of botulism is challenging, and index of suspicion for the disease must remain high. Goals of initial therapy are to eliminate potential bacterial infection and inactivate the bacterial toxin. Treatment is otherwise supportive. At present, there are assays under development for toxin detection, but these are not readily clinically available. In the early stages of the disease, particularly those cases with GI involvement, gastric lavage and decontamination may be helpful. Magnesium cathartics should be avoided, as they can exacerbate neuromuscular blockade. **Penicillin G** is the first-line therapy for clostridial infection, and should also be implemented. **Botulinum antitoxin** is the only definitive treatment for botulism, and can be obtained by contacting the CDC or state health department. The antitoxin is the most effective if administered in the first 24 hours and only limits symptom progression; it does not reverse symptoms present prior to its administration.

5. **Tularemia** is caused by *Francisella tularensis*, a gram-negative coccobacillus. Though it is endemic in most of the United States, the incidence of tularemia throughout the 1990s declined to approximately 1 per million. It is highly infective and easy to aerosolize, making it is a desirable as a potential biological weapon. Tularemia has several classic clinical syndromes, ulceroglandular and typhoidal being the most common. Incubation period of the disease is approximately 2 weeks, though most clinical symptoms occur in 3 to 5 days. Symptoms are nonspecific and include fever, malaise, anorexia, and cough. Ulceroglandular tularemia, the most common form of the disease, produces painful, suppurative lymph nodes and may mimic infection with *Y. pestis*. Tularemia is responsive to antibiotic therapy, and while it can produce incapacitating infection in the host, it is rarely fatal. The microbiology laboratory should be notified in the event of a potential tularemia outbreak, as *F. tularensis* requires specific media for growth. Unlike other potential biologic weapons, the bacteria does not require any specific measures for decontamination; standard precautions are sufficient.

6. **Hemorrhagic viral illnesses,** such as Hanta, Ebola, and Marburg, are RNA viruses that may be aerosolized to produce mass casualty. Depending on the specific virus, the potential for human-to-human transmission is high, and strict respiratory precautions should be maintained. The initial symptoms of these viral illnesses resemble

those of other viral illnesses, but result in capillary permeability, hemorrhage, coagulation abnormalities. Petechial rash usually also develops. The syndrome can progress to multiorgan system failure and death; the mortality rate for Ebola virus is greater that 90%. Treatment for these illnesses is purely symptomatic.

D. **Chemical warfare** is the use of chemicals to intentionally cause mass harm. The last known use of chemical warfare was in the Tokyo subway attacks in the mid-1990s. Because of the abrupt and often incapacitating symptoms of chemical weapons, the presentation and general management of mass exposure to chemical warfare differ from that of biological warfare. Victims of chemical agents will present for evaluation in large numbers, rather than in clusters. In addition, unlike biological attacks, mass decontamination is crucial for limiting the spread and morbidity of the outbreak. Should chemical warfare be suspected, a decontamination area should be established outside the treatment area. Removal of exposed clothing eliminates the majority of the danger of transmission, though health care personnel with close exposure to victims should use standard precautions, as well as a chemical-resistant suit with positive-pressure, self-contained breathing units. Skin can be decontaminated with water and 0.5% hypochlorite solution. Once patients have been grossly decontaminated, history should focus on time and duration of the exposure. The CDC has guidelines for evaluating potential chemical hazards that may be reviewed at http://www.cdc.gov/nceh/demil/guidelines.htm. Chemical warfare agents can be divided grossly into lethal and nonlethal agents, though lethal agents may be more likely to be implemented in a terrorist incident. Lethal agents can be divided into chemical choking agents, vesicants, nerve agents, and systemic asphyxiants, or "blood agents."

 1. **Chemical choking agents.** In general, these agents act as pulmonary irritants by combining with lung water to create **hydrochloric acid** and **oxygen free radicals**. Subsequent inflammation and cellular destruction result in acute pulmonary edema and respiratory failure. The gases are denser than air, and depending on the method and location of release may impact victims more severely in low-lying geographical areas or who are closest to the ground. Even at low concentrations, **chlorine** has a characteristic yellow-green color and has the odor of bleach. **Phosgene** is colorless, but has an odor of hay or freshly mowed grass. **Diphosgene** is similar in character to phosgene, but is able to penetrate chemical filters and has a shorter duration of onset. Once exposed to chemical choking agents, symptoms of cough, mucous membrane irritation, and changes in phonation can occur within minutes; pulmonary edema develops from 4 to 24 hours after exposure. Cutaneous and ocular burns are also expected after exposure to these agents. **Treatment** of lung injury from choking agents is primarily supportive; in addition to humidified oxygen, bronchodilators, nebulized sodium bicarbonate and systemic N-acetylcysteine may be useful. Ventilatory support and mechanical ventilation may be required.

 2. **Vesicant agents** cause blistering of exposed surfaces and include the mustard and arsenic gases.

    a. **Mustard gases** are sulfur- or nitrogen-based compounds that derive their name from the characteristic odor and color of mustard. At room temperature, mustard agents are oily, amber liquids. They can be vaporized, and at high concentration can also be inhaled. Once skin is exposed to mustard agents, filaments at the junction of the dermis and epidermis are destroyed; blisters and chemical burns begin to form at approximately 72 hours. Notably, street clothing does not confer any protection from these agents. After exposure, corneal edema occurs and results in eye pain, photophobia, and visual impairment. If inhaled at high concentrations, mustard gases can also cause epithelial sloughing and respiratory distress. Secondary to DNA disruption, mustard gases are mutagenic and carcinogenic as well. Though mortality from traditional mustard gases is approximately 5%, significant morbidity can occur from mustard gas burns and from potential superinfection and sepsis. Prolonged exposure to mustard gases cause global hematopoietic depression, which is a poor prognostic sign. Leukopenia will develop after 5 to 7 days, followed by anemia and thrombocytopenia.

b. **Lewisite** is an arsenic-based vesicant agent with properties similar to mustard gases. Upon contact with skin, lewisite hydrolyzes to **hydrochloric acid** and **chlorovinylarsenious** acid, the vesicant agents. More potent and lipophilic than its sulfur- and nitrogen-based counterparts, skin penetration occurs in 15 minutes, and blisters and chemical burns develop thereafter. The arsenic compound of lewisite binds pyruvate dehydrogenase and prevents the synthesis of acetyl CoA, resulting in cell death and systemic arsenic toxicity. This is manifest predominantly by GI symptoms of abdominal pain, nausea, and vomiting. GI mucosal sloughing and hematochezia can occur.

c. **Treatment** of vesicant agents is essentially focused on initial **decontamination,** followed by supportive management. Clothing should be removed, and patients should undergo decontamination. Notably, mustard gas is inactivated by chlorine, and water alone is insufficient for decontamination. Instead, a 1:10 diluted solution of 5% bleach can be used to decontaminate patients. Dry decontamination can also be performed by applying any absorbent powder to the skin, and removing it with a moist cloth. In addition, fluid from skin blisters does not contain vesicant and is not toxic to health care personnel. Treatment is otherwise largely supportive. Every patient exposed to a vesicant merits a careful eye examination and ophthalmology consult. Irrigation of the eye with saline is the preferred method of decontamination. Cycloplegics and topical pain medication should also be used. Systemic symptoms may respond to N-acetylcysteine, thiosulfate, steroids, and nitric oxide synthase (NOS) inhibitors. Granulocyte colony-stimulating factor (GCSF) may be useful for bone marrow suppression. British anti-lewisite (BAL) is an arsenic chelator used as an antidote for lewisite exposure; compounds related to BAL are commercially known as Succimer or Chemet, and can be given orally or IV.

3. **Nerve agents** are colorless, odorless liquids at room temperature that induce paralysis in exposed victims. They can be inhaled as vapor or absorbed through the skin. Inhalational toxicity of nerve agents is measured by LCt_{50}, the concentration of vapor necessary to kill 50% of an unprotected population. Like organophosphate pesticides, toxicity results from direct inactivation of acetylcholinesterase (AChE). Symptoms result from excess acetylcholine throughout the nervous system, initially stimulating and ultimately paralyzing neurotransmission. Initial clinical manifestations are similar to **anticholinergic toxicity** and include miosis, bronchorrhea, urination, salivation, and lacrimation.

After exposure to high concentrations of gas, loss of consciousness and seizure occur. Status epilepticus and cardiac conduction problems are common. Death occurs in minutes, usually as a result of central apnea rather than diaphragmatic paralysis. There are two major classes of nerve agents.

a. **The "G" agents.** There are four known G agents: tabun (GA), sarin (GB), soman (GD), and cyclosarin (GF). Tabun was the first known nerve gas and is the least potent of the G agents (LCt_{50} of 400 mg min/m^3). Sarin, soman, and cyclosarin were developed sequentially thereafter, each more potent than the prior. Cyclosarin is approximately 13 times more potent than tabun (LCt_{50} of 30 mg min/m^3). G agents are volatile and evaporate quickly.

b. **The "V" agents** are far more potent than the G agents and include the most toxic known nerve gas, VX (LCt_{50} of 10 mg min/m^3). V agents are more difficult to vaporize and can also be absorbed through skin, though clothing is protective.

c. **Treatment** of nerve gas exposure is centered on reactivating AChE and must be done as early as possible. **IV pralidoxime** will reactive the enzyme, but only for limited time after gas exposure. The length of time prior to this permanent inactivation is referred to as "aging" and is an intrinsic property of the nerve gas. Soman (GD) will age in 2 minutes, sarin (GB) after 5 to 8 hours. Tabun (GA) and VX will age after approximately 40 hours. Approach to treatment is immediate decontamination followed by ventilatory support and administration of atropine and pralidoxime. Succinylcholine should be avoided if muscle relaxants are used for intubation, as decreased levels of AChE will significantly prolong its duration of action. **Atropine** is targeted at relieving anticholinergic symptoms and should be administered 2 mg IV every 2 to 3 minutes until ventilation is normal. **Pralidoxime** is recommended for all exposures and must be given as soon as possible to be effective. The dose is 1 to 2 g over 10 minutes followed by a continuous infusion of 500 mg/h; treatment continues until patient is improving. Notably, soman (GD) ages too quickly for pralidoxime to be effective. In this case, physostigmine may be used as a competitive blocking agent.

d. **Systemic asphyxiants, or "blood agents"** act by creating intracellular hypoxia.

(1) **Cyanide** forces anaerobic metabolism within the cell by blocking the electron transport system. This results in impaired oxygen utilization as well as increased lactate production. Symptoms are based on level of hypoxemia and can result in loss of consciousness, arrhythmias, and hypotension. Cyanosis is a late sign. Elevated venous oxygen saturation, as well as anion-gap metabolic acidosis and elevated serum lactic acid may be clues to the diagnosis. The antidote for cyanide toxicity is **sodium nitrite.** Sodium nitrite (300 mg of a 3% solution) reverses cyanide blockade of the electron transport system, and should be followed by sodium thiosulfate (12.5 g of 25% solution). **Sodium thiosulfate** acts as purely as a sulfur donor, scavenging cyanide and allowing it to be excreted as thiocyanate in urine. Sodium nitrite can cause profound hypotension on administration, and can also induce methemoglobinemia. Methemoglobin levels should be followed. Hydroxocobalamin can be used as an alternative antidote (4–5 g over 30 minutes).

(2) Hydrogen sulfide also blocks electron transport; it is a more potent inhibitor than cyanide but because it has less binding affinity, it is more easily reversible. Unlike cyanide toxicity, early signs of exposure are absent. Hydrogen sulfide is rapidly absorbed in the white matter of the brain and results in sudden loss of consciousness. It has a characteristic sulfur odor, which may be recognizable to rescue workers. It cannot be dermally absorbed, and no special protection is required. Patients with toxicity from hydrogen sulfide may require limited support, and systemic toxicity is limited; 90% of hydrogen sulfide is metabolized in the body within 20 minutes. Given its rapid metabolism, specific data regarding an antidote are limited.

E. **Radiation injury** occurs as a consequence of transfer of energy from radioactive materials to body tissues. Radiation exposure can result from the intentional placement of a device that releases a sustained dose of radiation over time, or via a "dirty bomb" that spreads radioactive material during a blast or explosion. In the event of explosion, recognition of radiation exposure may be delayed as attention is focused on burns and concomitant traumatic injuries. Suspicion for radioactive threats must remain high until its absence can be confirmed with a detection device. As with chemical weapons, **decontamination** is crucial in limiting the spread of hazardous material and protecting rescue workers.

1. **Ionizing radiation** comes from the decay of intrinsically unstable radionuclides, ^{137}Cs and ^{60}Co among the highest risk. Radiation is emitted as α-particles, β-particles, γ-rays, x-rays, and neutrons. All of these components transfer energy to tissues in varying degrees. In addition to energy transfer, neutrons make the target substance radioactive, and therefore a persistent source of ionizing radiation. As tissues are energized, free radicals are generated and cellular death occurs, primarily via disruption of DNA. Cells with high turnover, particularly the GI and hematopoietic systems, are the most at risk of injury from radiation exposure.

2. **Principles to triage.** In-house radiation safety specialist should be notified of any potential exposure, and adequate **decontamination** must be rapidly achieved. This begins with removal of clothing, followed by a shower with soap and warm water. Hot water should be avoided as it can increase vasodilation and subsequent radionuclide absorption. Decontamination can be monitored with serial measurements of emitted radiation. Personnel protection should aim to minimize the radiation exposure to as low as reasonably achievable. This can be done in several ways:

   a. Minimize the amount of time each worker needs to be exposed to radioactive material.

   b. Maximize distance from the radioactive source; the dose of radiation absorbed decreases based on square of distance.

   c. Shielding from radiation; standard personal protective equipment will block α- and β-particles, but usually not γ-rays. Lead and other high-density materials provide increased protection.

   d. Real-time monitoring of radiation should be available to all staff in close contact with the patient and should be no greater than 0.1 mGy/h.

3. **Clinical presentation** of disease from whole-body radiation exposure is referred to as **acute radiation sickness (ARS)**. In general, manifestation of radiologic injury is delayed, and most asymptomatic patients

require only baseline laboratory studies and outpatient follow-up; inpatient admission is not mandated. Initial prodromal symptoms of acute radiation sickness are nausea, vomiting, and diarrhea, and time to onset of prodromal symptoms is predictive of total body radiation dose. Symptoms at less that 30 minutes indicate >600 rad of exposure, whereas symptoms >24 hours after presentation indicates exposure <70 rads. Without medical support, total body exposure of 600 rad carries 100% mortality. In contrast, doses of less than 70 rad may only result in modest decreases in lymphocytes. Ultimately, patients with high levels of radiation exposure will develop illness from hematopoietic derangement, including immunosuppression, bleeding diatheses, and sepsis. Prognosis is directly correlated with a 48-hour lymphocyte count: >1,200 or <300 confer good and poor prognoses respectively. Treatment for ARS is completely supportive.

IV. Organizational planning

A. An effective response to mass casualty within the ICU involves coordination of hospital personnel with federal, state, and local officials. The *National Response Framework* presents the guiding principles that enable all response partners to prepare for and provide a unified national response to disasters and emergencies and establishes a comprehensive, national, all-hazards approach to domestic incident response. This framework is administered by the Federal Emergency Management Agency (FEMA), and describes how communities, the private sector, and nongovernmental partners are integrated in an effective national response. It can be reviewed at www.fema.gov/emergency/nrf/.

B. Training and disaster drills. Proficiency in work assignments is crucial to effective response in time of disaster. The key to successful disaster preparedness is preparation for such events, and accurate anticipation of potential scenarios may aid in planning. The main component to managing disaster begins with analysis of hazards to which an area is susceptible, and consideration of potential consequences of these events. Geographic locations, including potential for weather-related incidents, natural disasters, or likelihood of terrorist attacks should be considered. Disaster drills should be developed and implemented yearly; several professional medical organizations offer courses in disaster planning and emergency preparedness that may serve as foundations for the development of institutional protocols:

- http://www.facs.org/trauma/disaster/dmep_course.html
- http://training.fema.gov/IS/crslist.asp
- http://www.aapsus.org/academies/disaster-medicine/index.html
- http://www.hhs.gov/aspr/opeo/ndms/index.html
- www.ifrc.org

Selected References

Flynn DF, Goans RE. Nuclear terrorism: triage and medical management of radiation and combined-injury casualties. *Surg Clin North Am* 2006;86:601–636.

Hotchkin DL, Rubinson L. Modified critical care and treatment space considerations for mass casualty critical illness and injury. *Respir Care* 2008;53:67–74.

http://sis.nlm.nih.gov/enviro/biologicalwarfare.html

http://www.cdc.gov/nceh/demil/guidelines.htm

Kman NE, Nelson RN. Agents of bioterrorism: a review for emergency physicians. *Emerg Med Clin North Am* 2008;26:2.

Mahoney EJ, Biffl WL, Cioffi WG. Mass-casualty incidents: how does an ICU prepare? *J Intensive Care Med* 2008;23:219–235.

Muskat PC. Mass casualty chemical exposure and implications for respiratory failure. *Respir Care* 2008;53:58–63.

Parker MM. Critical care and disaster management. *Crit Care Med* 2006;34(suppl):S52–S55.

Rubinson L, Hick JL, et al. Definitive care for the critically ill during a disaster: a framework for optimizing critical care surge capacity: from a Task Force for Mass Critical Care summit meeting. *Chest* 2008;133(5 suppl):18S–31S.

Harwood-Nuss' clinical practice of emergency medicine. 4th ed. Lippincott, 2005.

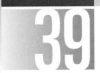

ICU Care After Vascular Surgery

Ross Blank and Rae Allain

I. **General considerations.** The vascular surgical patient presents many perioperative challenges. In addition to the inherent risks of major vascular surgery, these patients often have advanced age and significant comorbidities. Common coexisting diseases include hypertension, coronary artery disease, congestive heart failure, chronic obstructive pulmonary disease (COPD), chronic renal insufficiency, and diabetes mellitus. The presence or absence of these conditions may influence the decision to proceed with elective vascular procedures. The reader is referred to the corresponding chapters for a more detailed discussion of these comorbidities.

II. **Carotid artery stenosis.** Atherosclerotic disease at or near the carotid bifurcation represents a major risk factor for ischemic stroke. In several large, randomized controlled trials, surgical repair has led to a clear reduction in 5-year stroke rates for patients with symptomatic disease and high-grade ($\geq$ 70%) stenosis. Benefit in symptomatic patients with < 70% stenosis is more modest. The decision to operate on asymptomatic patients depends on three main factors: (1) degree of stenosis, (2) plaque density, and (3) progression of disease over time.

A. **Carotid endarterectomy (CEA)**
  1. CEA is the standard operative intervention for carotid stenosis. It involves cross-clamping the carotid artery with subsequent incision and removal of the occlusive plaque.
  2. The surgery may be performed under general or regional anesthesia.
  3. Most patients do not require postoperative critical care unless they encounter complications or have significant comorbidities.
  4. Complications
    a. **Neurologic**
      (1) **Stroke** within 30 days of surgery occurs in approximately 3% of patients. Causes include thromboembolism, hemorrhage, and ischemia secondary to carotid cross-clamping. A new deficit in the immediate postoperative period is an emergency that may necessitate angiographic studies or re-exploration.
      (2) **Cerebral hyperperfusion syndrome** (incidence, 0%–3%) occurs secondary to a profound increase in ipsilateral perfusion following revascularization in the setting of hypertension and impaired regional cerebral autoregulation. It can manifest as headache, seizures, and focal neurologic deficits, and may progress to cerebral edema, hemorrhage, and death. The mainstay of therapy is blood pressure control with agents (e.g., β-blockers) that do not cause cerebral vasodilatation.
    b. **Cardiac**
      (1) There is a high correlation between cerebrovascular and coronary artery disease, and postoperative **myocardial infarction**

occurs in 2.2% of CEA patients. Myocardial ischemia without infarction is presumably even more common.

(2) **Bradyarrhythmias** and **hypotension** can be seen after manipulation of the carotid sinus and exposure of baroreceptors to higher arterial pressures with removal of the plaque.

(3) **Hypertension** is also common and is likely multifactorial (exacerbation of baseline hypertension, carotid sinus dysfunction, pain, hypercarbia, etc.). Whatever the cause, high blood pressures should be treated to reduce shear stress on a fresh vascular anastomosis and to minimize cerebral hyperperfusion.

c. **Airway and pulmonary**

(1) **Airway obstruction** may be the result of an **expanding wound hematoma** compressing the trachea or impaired lymphatic drainage leading to laryngeal edema. Vocal cord dysfunction from recurrent laryngeal nerve injury may also contribute. Bedside hematoma evacuation may be performed by opening the surgical incision under local anesthesia, but this may not fully relieve airway obstruction if airway edema is the predominant mechanism. Imminent airway loss, regardless of the etiology, demands immediate **endotracheal intubation** with subsequent therapy dictated by specific circumstances.

(2) **Hypoxia** and **hypercarbia** may result from dysfunction of the carotid body chemoreceptors. These risks are higher in patients who have previously undergone contralateral CEA.

B. **Carotid artery stenting**

1. Endovascular stenting of the carotid artery is a less invasive alternative to CEA.

2. The fundamental rationale is relief of obstruction as opposed to removal of a disease process as with CEA.

3. Early use was limited by postprocedure compression of the stent as well as embolization of atheromatous debris. Crush-resistant stents and embolic protection devices have been developed to address these problems.

4. Meta-analysis of clinical trials of carotid artery stenting versus CEA for symptomatic stenosis has revealed no significant differences in 30-day mortality, stroke, and disabling stroke rates. Data on longer-term outcomes and newer devices will continue to evolve.

5. Stenting may be the preferred option for patients for whom open surgery poses a particularly high risk due to age, comorbidities, or prior surgery.

III. **Aortic aneurysmal disease**

A. **Ascending aortic aneurysm**

1. Aneurysms of the ascending thoracic aorta and aortic arch most commonly result from cystic medial degeneration leading to loss of smooth muscle and elastic fibers in the arterial wall and subsequent dilatation. Advanced age and hypertension are common risk factors for cystic medial degeneration. It is also seen in patients with Marfan's syndrome, familial thoracic aortic aneurysm syndrome, and bicuspid aortic valve.

2. Other causes of ascending aortic aneurysm include syphilis, large-vessel vasculitis, chronic aortic dissection (AD), and aortic trauma.

3. Repair of the ascending aorta and arch have traditionally been the domain of cardiac surgeons.

B. Descending thoracic and thoracoabdominal aortic aneurysms (DTA and **TAA)** are the primary indications for procedures on the thoracic aorta. Estimated incidence is 6 to 10 per 100,000 person-years and is likely increasing due to an aging population.

  1. Etiology and classification

    a. Unlike those of the ascending aorta and arch, aneurysms of the descending thoracic (i.e., distal to the left subclavian artery) and abdominal aorta are most commonly characterized by atherosclerotic changes in the vessel wall. Less common etiologies include chronic dissection, connective tissue disease, infection, and vasculitis.

    b. Common risk factors for atherosclerotic aneurysms include smoking, age, hypertension, hyperlipidemia, and family history.

    c. Such aneurysms may be limited to the descending thoracic aorta or, if simultaneously involving the thoracic and abdominal aorta, they may be described by the Crawford classification system (**Fig. 39-1**).

      (1) Type I originates in the proximal descending thoracic aorta and extends to the abdominal aorta proximal to the renal arteries.

      (2) Type II, the most extensive, originates in the proximal descending thoracic aorta and extends to the abdominal aorta distal to the renal arteries.

      (3) Type III originates in the middescending thoracic aorta (sixth intercostal space) and extends to the abdominal aorta distal to the renal arteries.

      (4) Type IV is a total abdominal aneurysm, originating below the diaphragm proximal to the celiac artery and extending to the abdominal aorta distal to the renal arteries.

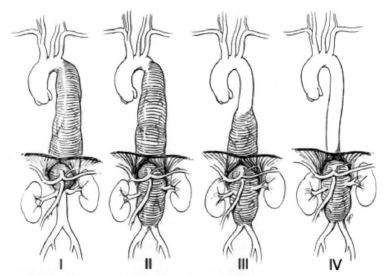

FIGURE 39-1 The Crawford classification of thoracoabdominal aortic aneurysms. From Conrad MF, Cambria RP. Contemporary management of descending thoracic and thoracoabdominal aortic aneurysms: endovascular versus open. *Circulation* 2008;117:841–852. With permission.

2. Elective repair of DTA/TAA is undertaken when the risk of rupture is judged to exceed the risk of repair. Aneurysm diameter >6 cm is a generally accepted threshold for surgical intervention. Other aneurysm risk factors for rupture include rate of expansion (>10 mm/y) and presence of dissection. Patient risk factors for rupture include age, hypertension, smoking, COPD, renal insufficiency, pain symptoms, female gender, Marfan's syndrome, and possibly preoperative steroid treatment.

3. Open repair and complications

   a. After exposure via left thoracotomy or thoracoabdominal incision, the operation entails (1) cross-clamping of the thoracic aorta proximal to the aneurysm, (2) incision of the aorta distal to the clamp to allow creation of the proximal anastomosis between native aorta and synthetic graft, (3) reconstruction of critical intercostal arteries with attachment directly to the graft, (4) reconstruction of the visceral aortic segment, often accomplished by including the adjacent ostia of the celiac, superior mesenteric, and right renal arteries in a button sutured to the graft, (5) reconstruction of the left renal artery via reimplantation or, more commonly, via a separate sidearm graft from the primary aortic graft, and (6) creation of the distal anastomosis. These steps may be modified or excluded due to variations in vascular and aneurysm anatomy.

   b. Despite improvements in surgical and organ preservation techniques, operative **mortality** remains high, in the 2% to 16% range in published series from academic centers. Retrospective studies of "real-world" conditions reveal in-hospital mortality rates of approximately 22% in elective settings. Moreover, 30-day or in-hospital mortality rates likely underestimate significantly 1-year mortality rates. Emergent repair of a ruptured or leaking aneurysm is associated with large increases in operative mortality. Preoperative renal insufficiency, intraoperative hypotension, intraoperative transfusion requirement, postoperative spinal cord ischemia, and postoperative renal failure all increase postoperative mortality in retrospective analysis.

   c. A particularly devastating complication of surgery on the thoracic aorta is **spinal cord ischemia (SCI)** leading to lower extremity weakness or paralysis. The anterior spinal cord receives its blood supply through the anterior spinal artery, which itself is supplied largely by intercostal arteries (primary branches of the thoracic aorta) including the artery of Adamkiewicz at the critical T8-L1 levels. However, there is a rich collateral network of vessels, which include intercostal vessels above and lumbar vessels below the critical zone as well as branches of the subclavian and iliac arteries. Prevention of SCI (details below) is a major focus of perioperative care with contemporary rates of paraplegia/paraparesis in the 2% to 10% range. Factors that increase SCI risk include types I and II TAAs, intraoperative sacrifice of critical intercostal vessels, prolonged intraoperative cross-clamp, preoperative aneurysm rupture, and prolonged intraoperative or postoperative hypotension. Neurologic deficits may be observed immediately postoperatively or may be delayed for days to weeks. During the immediate postoperative period, sedation should be lightened frequently to allow neurologic exam of the lower extremities.

      (1) Analogous to the concept of cerebral perfusion pressure, **spinal cord perfusion pressure** is determined by the difference between

mean arterial pressure and cerebrospinal fluid (CSF) pressure. Accordingly, relative **hypertension** (typical SBP goal, 120– 160 mm Hg) is the goal to maintain adequate spinal cord perfusion in the face of a surgically interrupted blood supply. Higher goals are generally avoided to prevent excessive shear stress on the aortic anastomosis and workload on the left ventricle. Perioperative blood pressure goals may need to be increased in the setting of new-onset lower extremity weakness or paralysis. Anecdotal literature and experience at the Massachusetts General Hospital support that induced hypertension may lead to resolution of neurologic symptoms.

(2) In order to decrease CSF pressure, it has become standard to institute **CSF drainage** intraoperatively and to continue drainage 48 to 72 hours postoperatively. Drains are placed in the lumbar subarachnoid space and allowed to passively drain to approximately 10 mm Hg (13 cm H$_2$O). Cases of delayed neurologic deficit have responded favorably to reinstitution of CSF drainage.

(3) **Epidural cooling** is a method of spinal cord protection that was developed at the MGH in the 1990s. The principle of the technique was to decrease spinal cord metabolism and the risk of SCI by actively cooling the spinal cord via an iced saline solution infused into the epidural space throughout the period of aortic cross-clamping. Although initial promising results were published from the MGH experience, similar success was not observed in other centers and the technique is no longer practiced routinely. Some centers advocate **systemic cooling** with DTA/TAA repairs performed with cardiopulmonary bypass with deep hypothermic circulatory arrest.

(4) **Left heart bypass** (**Fig. 39-2**) is an intraoperative maneuver designed to maintain blood supply to the anterior spinal artery, visceral organs, and kidneys during cross-clamping. Most commonly, a bypass circuit from the left atrium (accessed via the pulmonary veins) to the femoral artery is created. This allows for retrograde perfusion of the descending thoracic and abdominal aorta during proximal reconstruction.

(5) **Intercostal artery reimplantation,** particularly in the critical T8-L1 zone, is commonly employed in an attempt to preserve spinal cord perfusion. The benefit of reimplantation must be weighed against the risk of prolonging cross-clamp time. Often, several intercostal vessels are included together as a button to expedite the process.

(6) Intraoperative **motor evoked potentials** allow for a real-time assessment of anterior cord function and may guide blood pressure management and extent of intercostal revascularization in the OR. Recent literature suggests a diminished SCI rate (4.2% early, 2.9% delayed in 70 type II TAA patients) with this technique combined with CSF drainage and left heart bypass.

(7) It should be recognized that postoperative paraplegia may be due to **spinal or epidural hematoma** compressing the spinal cord. Clinicians must have a high index of suspicion for these entities, especially in cases where neuraxial catheters have been placed with subsequent coagulopathy related to the surgical procedure. When suspicion is high, immediate diagnostic imaging (preferably

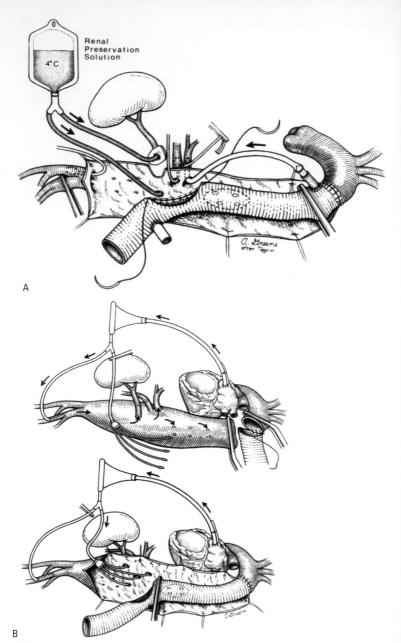

FIGURE 39-2 Operative techniques for TAA repair. Image A depicts renal cold perfusion, in-line mesenteric shunting, and intercostal button. Image B depicts left heart bypass in which perfusion distal to the cross-clamp initially is maintained via the femoral artery and then by multiple perfusion catheters once reconstruction proceeds distally. From Conrad MF, Cambria RP. Contemporary management of descending thoracic and thoracoabdominal aortic aneurysms: endovascular versus open. *Circulation* 2008;117:841–852. With permission.

MRI) should be obtained followed by surgical decompression if indicated.

d. **Cardiac complications,** including dysrhythmia, myocardial infarction, and congestive heart failure, are common ($\sim$15%) in this high-risk population.

   (1) Mobilization of "third-space" fluids on postoperative days 2 to 3 may precipitate intravascular volume overload.

   (2) Postoperative hemodynamic management is commonly facilitated by monitoring cardiac output with pulmonary artery catheterization, transpulmonary thermodilution with pulse contour analysis, or echocardiography. Baseline values from the operating room are useful benchmarks.

e. **Pulmonary complications,** specifically prolonged postoperative ventilation, pneumonia, reintubation, and tracheostomy, are exceedingly common and may approach 50%. The causes are multifactorial and likely include preoperative COPD, surgical division of the diaphragm to facilitate exposure, phrenic nerve injury, left lung trauma during surgical dissection, left lung collapse and reexpansion to facilitate exposure, and right lung ventilator–induced lung injury during prolonged one-lung ventilation.

   (1) It is standard to place a left-sided chest tube upon conclusion of the procedure.

   (2) Patients with intraoperative left lung trauma may require vigorous suctioning of blood and clots from the endotracheal tube postoperatively.

   (3) If a right-sided double-lumen endotracheal tube is used intraoperatively, right upper lobe collapse due to obstruction of the right upper lobe bronchus may be seen.

f. **Postoperative renal failure,** generally defined as a doubling of the baseline creatinine or an absolute value >3 mg/dL, has an incidence close to 20% with approximately 5% of all patients requiring dialysis, and is an independent risk factor for death. Intraoperative measures for renal protection include minimization of cross-clamp time and direct installation of cold renal preservation solution (lactated Ringer's $\pm$ mannitol and methylprednisolone) into the renal artery ostia during cross-clamping, and left heart bypass (**Fig. 39-2**). Renal artery endarterectomy/stenting or bypass grafting may also be performed if significant stenoses are found. The etiologies of postoperative renal failure may be multifactorial (see **Table 39-1** and **Chapter 24**). Depending on clinical circumstances, diagnostic workup may involve urine studies (urinalysis, urine sediment, urine eosinophils, and urine electrolytes to calculate fractional excretion of sodium) and vascular imaging studies (Doppler ultrasound or CT).

g. **Gut ischemia** has an incidence of approximately 2%. Hepatic and bowel ischemia may precipitate coagulopathy. In addition, ischemic colitis may result from sacrifice/ligation of the inferior mesenteric artery in the absence of adequate collateral flow.

   (1) Intraoperatively, left heart bypass may be employed to perfuse visceral organs during construction of the proximal anastomosis. Once reconstruction proceeds distally with the aorta open, the bypass circuit can be redirected from the femoral artery to multiple perfusion catheters placed directly into vessel ostia (**Fig. 39-2**).

   (2) In the absence of left heart bypass, in-line mesenteric shunting may be employed. This technique involves suturing a side arm to

TABLE 39-1	Etiology of Renal Failure After Aortic Surgery

Type	Cause
Contrast nephropathy	Pre- or intraoperative studies using iodinated contrast
Ischemic acute tubular necrosis (ATN)	Aortic cross-clamp above renal arteries Failure (occlusion, kinking) of renal artery bypass grafts Perioperative hypotension and/or hypovolemia Atheromatous (cholesterol) embolization
Nephrotoxic ATN	Myoglobin deposition due to rhabdomyolysis (limb ischemia, compartment syndrome)
Allergic interstitial nephritis (AIN)	Perioperative medications including antibiotics

the primary aortic graft just distal to the proximal anastomosis. After completion of the anastomosis, the clamp is moved distal to the sidearm and a perfusion catheter is extended from the side arm to either the celiac or the superior mesenteric artery ostium (**Fig. 39-2**). This allows pulsatile perfusion throughout the period of distal aortic reconstruction.

h. **Hematologic complications**
   (1) From 2% to 5% of DTA/TAA patients experience **postoperative bleeding.**
   (2) The intraoperative transfusion requirement has been shown to correlate with perioperative mortality.
   (3) Massive resuscitation from intraoperative hemorrhage may result in a wide variety of complications including **dilution of clotting factors** and platelets, hypothermia, hypocalcemia, abdominal compartment syndrome, and **disseminated intravascular coagulation (DIC**, see also **Chapter 26).**
   (4) Postoperative care to treat hypothermia and coagulopathic bleeding may include the use of fluid-warming devices, forced hot air systems, and increased ambient temperature.
   (5) The use of an **autotransfusion** or a "cell saver" system may significantly decrease the need for transfusion of banked packed red blood cells (pRBCs), because up to 50% of blood turnover during DTA/TAA resection may be returned to the patient via these methods.
   (6) Minimizing mesenteric ischemia is also critical to avoiding coagulopathic bleeding.
   (7) **Postoperative thrombocytopenia** is a common finding that may result from dilution following resuscitation or consumption in the case of ongoing bleeding. Thrombocytopenia may also be explained by platelet adhesion to or activation by the synthetic aortic graft, especially in the case of extensive aortic replacement. Less commonly, heparin-induced thrombocytopenia (**HIT**) may be the etiology (**Chapter 26**).

4. Endovascular repair and complications
   a. In recent years, **thoracic endovascular aneurysm repair (TEVAR, Fig. 39-3)** has emerged as an attractive alternative for DTA. This

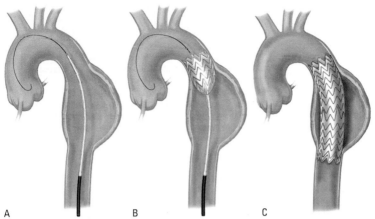

A   B   C

FIGURE 39-3 Diagram of thoracic endovascular aneurysm repair (TEVAR). From Conrad MF, Cambria RP. Contemporary management of descending thoracic and thoracoabdominal aortic aneurysms: endovascular versus open. *Circulation* 2008;117:841–852. With permission.

procedure typically involves percutaneous access to the aorta via the femoral artery, with delivery and deployment of an expandable aortic graft under fluoroscopic guidance. Patients are spared the risks of thoracotomy and aortic cross-clamping.

   b. With current technology, TAAs are generally not amenable to this technique since the aneurysm involves major branch vessels that would become excluded from circulation after placement of the stent. Branched and/or fenestrated stents may make endovascular treatment of TAAs more feasible in the future.

   c. TEVAR patients at risk for SCI often require postoperative critical care for close neurologic monitoring and CSF drainage. In addition, those who suffer procedural complications may require critical care.

   d. **Malpositioning of the stent** may occlude flow to major vessels with resultant visceral, renal, or lower extremity ischemia requiring open surgical intervention.

   e. **Rare operative hemorrhage** may result from aneurysm rupture or injury to access vessels necessitating conversion to open surgical repair.

   f. Major neurologic complications include **stroke** and **SCI**. Although the risk of embolic stroke may be affected by wire manipulation of the aortic arch, perioperative stroke rates of approximately 2% to 4% in multicenter studies compare favorably to those seen with open repair. Paraplegia incidence is reduced (~1%–3%) but not eliminated due to stent coverage of critical intercostal arteries. CSF drainage is often advocated when aneurysm anatomy or prior aortic replacement surgery (e.g., infrarenal abdominal aortic aneurysm [AAA]) suggests heightened risk for SCI.

   g. **Endoleak** is the term used to describe continued entry of blood into the aneurysm sac following stent placement and is classified into five types (**Table 39-2**). Types I and III specifically are considered ongoing risk factors for aneurysm rupture and often indicate additional procedures for repair.

TABLE 39-2	Classification of Endoleak
Classification	**Description**
Type I	Leak at proximal or distal stent attachment sites to arterial wall
Type II	Filling of aneurysm sac by collateral vessel
Type III	Leak due to stent component failure
Type IV	Leak through porous graft material
Type V	"Endotension"; continued aneurysm expansion despite no visible angiographic leak

5. **Hybrid techniques** are creative combinations of open and endovascular interventions with a goal of achieving aneurysm repair with less morbidity. **Open left carotid-to-subclavian bypass** may create a safe proximal landing zone for a thoracic stent when the aneurysm location would otherwise lead to subclavian exclusion (with possible resultant cerebral and upper extremity ischemia) after stent deployment. Analogously, **visceral rerouting** procedures involve construction of bypass grafts from the infrarenal abdominal aorta or iliac arteries to the celiac, superior mesenteric and renal arteries to create a safe distal landing zone for stent repair of a TAA (**Fig. 39-4**).

C. **Abdominal aortic aneurysm (AAA)** is far more common than thoracic aortic aneurysm with a prevalence of approximately 5% in men >65 years.
   1. Atherosclerosis is the most common underlying pathology.
   2. Balancing the risks of aneurysm rupture with **operative mortality,** large prospective studies have established aneurysm diameter >5.5 cm as the most common indication for repair. This threshold may be reduced in patients with rapidly growing or symptomatic aneurysms, and for female gender.
   3. Open repair carries a mortality rate of 4% to 6%, which increases in low-volume settings. Preoperative risk factors for death include advanced age, renal insufficiency, and prior myocardial infarction.
   4. Complications associated with open AAA repair are similar to those of TAA repair although they occur at a lower rate for specific entities (i.e., SCI, pulmonary complications). The majority of deaths are from cardiac complications. Aneurysm anatomy dictates the level of aortic cross-clamping and influences the likelihood of gut and renal ischemia.
   5. **Endovascular aneurysm repair (EVAR)** is now more commonly employed than open repair for infrarenal AAAs with suitable anatomy. Short-term perioperative morbidity and mortality are decreased compared to open surgery.
   6. Complications of EVAR that may require ICU admission are similar to those of TEVAR (see **Section III.B.4**), although both stroke and SCI are rare.

IV. **Aortic dissection (AD)**
   A. AD refers to a tear in the aortic intima allowing blood to flow in a false lumen separating the intima from the media or adventitia. Dissection spreads anterograde and/or retrograde from the entry tear.
   B. The common pathophysiologic pathway appears to be weakening of the aortic media by acquired or congenital conditions. Risk factors include

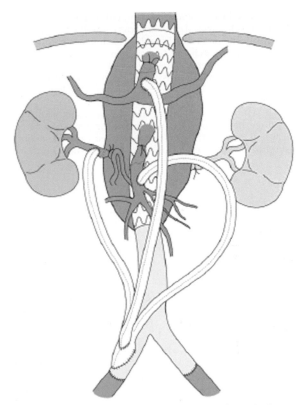

FIGURE 39-4 Diagram of hybrid repair of type IV TAA with visceral rerouting (bypass grafts from right iliac artery to celiac, superior mesenteric and right renal arteries) and endovascular aortic stent. From Peterson BG, Pearce WH, Resnick SA, Eskandari MK. Stent-graft treatment of thoracoabdominal aortic aneurysms after complete visceral debranching. *J Vasc Interv Radiol* 2006;17: 1522, with permission.

hypertension (seen in 72% of cases and by far the most common factor), advanced age, atherosclerosis, cocaine use, prior aneurysm or dissection, connective tissue disease (Marfan's or Ehlers-Danlos syndrome), vasculitis, bicuspid aortic valve, and iatrogenic injury from cardiac/aortic surgery or interventional cardiology procedures.

C. AD is an acute aortic syndrome, a classification that also includes intramural hematoma and atherosclerotic ulcer.

D. Incidence, estimated at 3 cases per 100,000 person-years, is far lower than that of aortic aneurysm.

E. The classic symptom is acute onset of tearing chest pain radiating to the back. However, a large international database has revealed that sharp chest pain alone is more common.

F. Additional symptoms depend on the location and extent of the dissection. Presentations may include cardiac tamponade (extension into pericardial space), aortic insufficiency (involvement of aortic valve), myocardial ischemia (involvement of coronary arteries), ischemic stroke and/or syncope (involvement of aortic arch branch vessels), and spinal cord/visceral/renal/limb ischemia (involvement of corresponding branches of descending thoracic and abdominal aorta).

G. The **Stanford** and **DeBakey** classification systems are depicted in **Fig. 39-5**. The Stanford system is most commonly used in the literature, and largely determines contemporary therapeutic strategy.

H. Because AD is uncommon and shares symptoms with other entities (myocardial infarction, pulmonary embolism, pericarditis, etc), it is notoriously difficult to diagnose. The classic chest x-ray findings of a widened mediastinum and abnormal aortic contour may both be absent in >20%

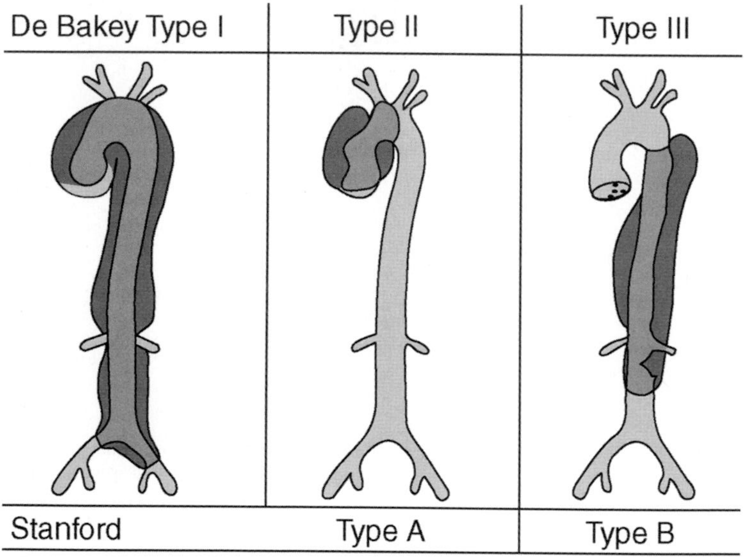

De Bakey Type I	Type II	Type III
Stanford	Type A	Type B

De Bakey

Type I	Originates in the ascending aorta, propagates at least to the aortic arch and often beyond it distally
Type II	Originates in and is confined to the ascending aorta
Type III	Originates in the descending aorta and extends distally down the aorta or, rarely, retrograde into the aortic arch and ascending aorta

Stanford

Type A	All dissection involving the ascending aorta regardless of the site of origin
Type B	All dissection not involving the ascending aorta

FIGURE 39-5 DeBakey and Stanford classifications of aortic dissection. From Nienaber CA, Eagle KA. Aortic dissection: new frontiers in diagnosis and management. Part I: from etiology to diagnostic strategies. *Circulation* 2003;108:628–635. With permission.

of cases. CT angiography has become the most common confirmatory study although transesophageal echocardiography, MRI, and conventional angiography may all be utilized.

I. **Initial medical therapy** upon diagnosis is aimed at preventing dissection extension and rupture. Control of both heart rate and systemic blood pressure likely minimizes these risks by reducing the force of left ventricular contraction (dP/dt). β-Blockers are typically first-line treatment with a goal systolic blood pressure of 100 to 120 mmHg and heart rate <60 bpm. Calcium channel blockers that affect the AV node (i.e., diltiazem and verapamil) may be used in patients with documented intolerance to β-blockers. Agents that lower blood pressure through vasodilatation may be added to β-blockers but are not useful initial therapy as they may cause a reflex tachycardia.

J. **Definitive treatment**

1. **Stanford type A** (i.e., involving the ascending aorta) AD is a surgical emergency because mortality approaches 20% by 24 hours and 30% by 48 hours. Such repairs are performed by cardiac surgeons under cardiopulmonary bypass. Concurrent injuries that preclude systemic anticoagulation may contraindicate immediate surgical repair.

2. **Stanford type B** (i.e., not involving the ascending aorta) AD is generally managed conservatively with medical therapy alone as worse short-term outcomes have been observed in patients taken to surgery. Indications for surgery are complications of dissection including aortic rupture, malperfusion of visceral organs/kidneys/limbs, dissection progression, and intractable pain.

3. Increasingly, **endovascular techniques** are being employed to augment or replace traditional surgical/medical therapy. Primary **stenting** of the true lumen with coverage of the entry tear in patients with type B dissection is currently being compared with medical management in a prospective multicenter trial. In addition, for patients with type A or B dissections suffering from malperfusion syndromes of the descending thoracic or abdominal aorta, interventional therapy may include stent placement in the aortic lumen and/or compromised branch vessels as well as **fenestration** of the intimal flap between true and false lumen to promote adequate flow between both lumens.

V. **Aortic trauma** typically results from a high-speed deceleration mechanism and presents as a tear injury between the fixed aortic arch and more mobile descending aorta. Traditionally, diagnosis was challenging, and treatment was open surgical repair, often in high-risk patients with multiple injuries. Currently, the diagnosis is most often made by CT scan, and treatment has evolved to favor **endovascular stenting**; see **Chapter 9**.

VI. **Peripheral vascular disease**

A. Patients who are admitted to the ICU following peripheral revascularization procedures (e.g., femoral to popliteal bypass graft) generally are suffering from complications of comorbid conditions, commonly cardiac disease and diabetes.

B. Severe peripheral vascular disease with ischemia, ulceration, and infection may rarely result in development of a **"septic limb"** with all the associated sequelae of sepsis. These patients are best managed by emergent amputation of the affected extremity and treatment with antibiotics, initially broad-spectrum, until they can be tailored according to operative cultures.

C. Occlusion of peripheral vascular grafts due to thrombosis or kinking may lead to limb ischemia causing severe pain. Prolonged ischemia may lead to elevated creatine phosphokinase levels, rhabdomyolysis, and even compartment syndrome. Treatment options include surgical exploration, pharmacologic thrombolysis with intra-arterial catheters directed at the site of thrombosis, and amputation.

D. Repeated or unexplained graft thromboses merit an investigation for a possible acquired or inherited hypercoagulable state.

Selected References

Cina CS, Abouzahr L, Arena GO, et al. Cerebrospinal fluid drainage to prevent paraplegia during thoracic and thoracoabdominal aortic aneurysm surgery: a systematic review and meta-analysis. *J Vasc Surg* 2004;40:36–44.

Conrad MF, Cambria RP. Contemporary management of descending thoracic and thoracoabdominal aortic aneurysms: endovascular versus open. *Circulation* 2008;117:841–852.

Conrad MF, Crawford RS, Davison JK, et al. Thoracoabdominal aneurysm repair: a 20-year perspective. *Ann Thorac Surg* 2007;83:S856–S861.

Demetriades D, Velmahos GC, Scalea TM, et al. Diagnosis and treatment of blunt thoracic aortic injuries: changing perspectives. *J Trauma* 2008;64:1415–1419.

Golledge J, Eagle KA. Acute aortic dissection. *Lancet* 2008;372:55–66.

Greenhalgh RM, Powell JT. Endovascular repair of abdominal aortic aneurysm. *NEJM* 2008;358:494–501.

Griepp RB, Griepp EB. Spinal cord perfusion and protection during descending thoracic and thoracoabdominal aortic surgery: the collateral network concept. *Ann Thorac Surg* 2007;83:S865–S869.

Gurm HS, Nallamothu BK, Yadav J. Safety of carotid artery stenting for symptomatic carotid artery disease: a meta-analysis. *Eur Heart J* 2008;29:113–119.

Hagan PG, Nienaber CA, Isselbacher EM, et al. The international registry of acute aortic dissection (IRAD): new insights into an old disease. *JAMA* 2000;283:897–903.

Hallett Jr JW, Mills JL, Earnshaw JJ, Reekers JA. *Comprehensive vascular and endovascular surgery*. Edinburgh: Mosby, 2004.

Howell SJ. Carotid endarterectomy. *Br J Anaesth* 2007;99:119–131.

Isselbacher EM. Thoracic and abdominal aortic aneurysms. *Circulation* 2005;111:816–828.

Jacobs MJ, Mess W, Mochtar B, et al. The value of motor evoked potentials in reducing paraplegia during thoracoabdominal aneurysm repair. *J Vasc Surg* 2006;43:239–246.

Meschia JF, Brott TG, Hobson RW. Diagnosis and invasive management of carotid atherosclerotic stenosis. *Mayo Clin Proc* 2007;82:851–858.

van Mook WNKA, Rennenberg RJMW, Schurink GW, et al. Cerebral hyperperfusion syndrome. *Lancet Neurol* 2005;4:877–888.

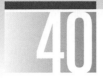

ICU Care After Thoracic Surgery

Kathrin Allen, Henning Gaissert, and Luca Bigatello

INTRODUCTION

Patients undergoing thoracic operations often need close postoperative supervision, either in an ICU or a stepdown level of care. Thoracic procedures may be associated with considerable cardiopulmonary dysfunction, resulting in significant patient morbidity that requires early recognition and appropriate management. In institutions with a high thoracic volume, ICU care is best selected in patients with important comorbid conditions, after long operations, and for mechanical ventilation. Recommendations regarding the level of postoperative care are made with the high-volume center in mind and may need adjustment where thoracic procedures are performed infrequently.

I. Thoracic surgical procedures

A. Pulmonary resection. ICU admission is determined by factors related either to patient (severe preoperative cardiopulmonary dysfunction, intraoperative myocardial ischemia) or procedure (pneumonectomy, large blood loss, associated chest wall resection). Many admissions are for temporary vasoactive support and therefore of short duration. Intra-arterial blood pressure monitoring is useful during and early after lung resection.

1. **Partial lung resections** are lobectomy, segmentectomy, and wedge resection. Commonly, these procedures incur limited blood loss and minimal third spacing of fluids, and require no postoperative mechanical ventilation, resulting in low perioperative risk and short hospital recovery. Pulmonary complications related to aspiration, pulmonary edema, arrhythmia, and impaired clearance of secretions are rare, but an important potential concern. The recent shift to thoracoscopic techniques has reduced pain and narcotic-related complications.

   a. **Wedge resection** refers to the nonanatomic excision of a part of a pulmonary lobe by either video-assisted thoracic surgery (**VATS**) or thoracotomy. Except for patient-related factors, ICU care is rarely required.

   b. **Lobectomy,** the anatomic removal of a pulmonary lobe, is performed either through a standard thoracotomy or by VATS, the severity of incisional pain being the main difference. The selection of approach is based on surgeon preference and tumor extent; thoracotomy, for example, is often chosen for larger tumors and known lymph node metastases.

   c. **Sleeve lobectomy** is a parenchyma-sparing operation for central lung tumors invading the main stem bronchus. The affected lobe is removed along with a bronchial segment, reimplanting the airway of the remaining lobe into the main stem bronchus. Sleeve lobectomy is applied to patients with compromised lung function and those who could not tolerate a more radical pneumonectomy. Mucociliary function in the reimplanted bronchus is temporarily impaired. Retained secretions and atelectasis are treated with early use of bronchoscopy. In experienced hands, breakdown of the bronchial anastomosis with formation of a bronchopleural or vascular fistula are unusual events occurring in less than 5% of procedures.

2. **Pneumonectomy,** the removal of an entire lung, raises the operative mortality and morbidity of lung resection. Careful preoperative testing is obligatory to identify appropriate candidates for pneumonectomy (see **Chapter 21** of the *Anesthesia Procedures of the Massachusetts General Hospital,* 7th edition). During the operation, a strategy of fluid restriction, hemodynamic support, and "lung-protective ventilation" has reduced the incidence of **postpneumonectomy acute lung injury (ALI, Section III.A.1).** Closure of the bronchus and its reinforcement with vascularized tissue are important details to prevent bronchial stump leak, a highly lethal complication. Attention in the early postoperative period is directed to any increase in the requirement for supplemental oxygen. Hypoxia should prompt evaluation of the remaining lung. A slow rise of the pleural air–fluid level in the pneumonectomy space is expected, while hemodynamic instability associated with rapid opacification of the hemithorax should arouse the suspicion of hemorrhage. **Atrial fibrillation**, while common after pneumonectomy, may not be tolerated well and often indicates associated, potentially lethal, complications (**Section III.B**).

3. **Extrapleural pneumonectomy** refers to pneumonectomy with added resection of parietal pleura, ipsilateral pericardium, and diaphragm; both pericardium and diaphragm are replaced with prosthetic membrane. The operative indications are malignant pleural mesothelioma and selected thymic carcinomas. Careful patient selection should establish excellent lung function and the absence of right- or left-heart dysfunction. Because of the large wound surface, intra- and postoperative blood loss and fluid shift may be substantial compared to standard pneumonectomy. Fluid resuscitation in turn is a challenge because these patients are at risk of developing **postpneumonectomy ALI** (**Section III.A**). However, their fluid losses may be significant, due to diffuse bleeding from the chest wall, often requiring substantially more fluid replacement than a standard pneumonectomy. Postoperative hypotension may also be caused by a tight pericardial patch, cardiac tamponade, or cardiac herniation through the patch. Central venous pressure monitoring, hematologic parameters, and echocardiography are important for evaluation.

4. **Lung volume reduction surgery (LVRS)**. Patients with advanced nonbullous emphysema and severe dyspnea on maximal medical management may be candidates for LVRS. The procedure aims to resect nonfunctioning, destroyed lung in heterogeneous emphysema via VATS or sternotomy. Selection criteria obligatory for reimbursement through Medicare and other payers have been published. The management of even carefully selected patients is challenging because clinical improvement after LVRS is not immediate. The development of **intrinsic positive end-expiratory pressure (auto-PEEP)** is common in these patients due to the severe airflow limitation related to their underlying disease Understanding the physiologic effects of auto-PEEP on the circulation and the work of breathing is important to properly diagnose and treat this phenomenon (see **Chapters 4** and **21**). Immediate extubation and the avoidance of mechanical ventilation are paramount to success, as is a careful balance between epidural pain control and the prevention of excessive sedation. Pleural air leaks are common because

of the extensive architectural destruction of emphysema. Multiple well-placed chest tubes and the least amount of applied negative pleural pressure to achieve expansion of the lung have been found useful.

B. **Tracheal resection and reconstruction** are indicated for postintubation tracheal stenosis, tracheal tumors, and tracheoesophageal fistula. Surgical reconstruction restores the airway in almost all patients without a need for tracheal tubes. Consequently, the postoperative airway requires utmost attention—the sole reason why these patients are observed in the intensive care unit. Airway complications include partial separation or dehiscence of the anastomosis; these occur as a function of anastomotic tension. While unusual, airway obstruction is life threatening and requires immediate attention. Intravenous steroids are rarely of help because they threaten healing at the anastomosis, while temporary administration of a helium–oxygen gas mixture ("heliox") may reduce stridor (see **Chapter 21**). The early recovery is characterized by a fine balance between analgesia, anxiolysis, and the need to promote effective cough and airway clearance. A tracheostomy must be considered when airway obstruction develops.

C. The indications for **esophageal resection** are carcinoma and functional impairment due to stricture or motility disorder. There are four common surgical approaches to the esophagus: the left thoracoabdominal approach, the laparotomy and right thoracotomy approach according to Ivor Lewis, the transhiatal approach with abdominal and left neck incision, and the minimally invasive combination of laparoscopy and thoracoscopy. Additional variations of less invasive approaches are used, all aimed at avoiding or reducing the size of the thoracotomy. The first two approaches, which allow for excellent intraoperative exposure and lymph node dissection, are disruptive in terms of intraoperative tissue dissection and trauma, the need for one-lung ventilation, and postoperative fluid management, respiratory insufficiency, and pain.

   1. Since these operations involve two body cavities, **fluid management** is similar to major abdominal gastrointestinal surgery. These patients tend to have a large intravenous fluid requirement in the first 24 hours and begin to diurese in the subsequent days.

   2. **Airway management.** Esophageal resection may have a long operative duration. The lateral decubitus position and fluid administration may lead to oropharyngeal swelling. The surgical dissection to separate trachea and esophagus may impair membranous portion function. While these factors may result in obstruction of the upper airway and impair cough, the need for postoperative intubation has consistently decreased over the last 10 years. **Aspiration of saliva or gastric contents** is very common early after esophageal surgery. The patient's head should be elevated more than 30°, and gastric acid suppressive agents should be used. A nasogastric Levine tube is inserted at the time of surgery as a continuous sump on 30 mm Hg suction, and must be carefully kept patent with repeated aspiration and irrigation using a syringe to decompress the intrathoracic stomach.

D. **Mediastinal surgery.** Certain large and central mediastinal masses may compress the airway, the right or left ventricle, or the superior vena cava. Preoperative recognition and airway management in the ICU may improve the planning of diagnostic or therapeutic interventions.

   1. **Evaluation and risk assessment** includes the assessment of postural changes, the location and degree of airway and/or cardiovascular compression with computed tomography (CT), and the use of rigid or fiberoptic bronchoscopy.

2. **Acute airway obstruction or cardiovascular collapse** may be precipitated by postural change or loss of spontaneous ventilation. Supine positioning can increase the pressure on the airway and/or increase central blood flow increasing the size of the mass. Spontaneous respiration and normal diaphragmatic movement maintain normal transpulmonary pressures and minimize the collapsibility of the airway. Therefore, patients should be maintained in their optimal position (usually upright), and sedation, if needed, should be administered with great caution. If **respiratory distress** develops, spontaneous respiration should be maintained and, if time allows, intubation occur in an operating room with an experienced thoracic anesthesiologist and surgeon. Awake fiberoptic intubation may allow direct visualization of the compressed tracheal area and ensure passage of an endotracheal tube beyond while the patient maintains normal transpulmonary pressures. Venous access in the saphenous vein or a femoral vein is advised if the superior vena cava is obstructed.

3. **The need for postoperative ICU care** is based on intraoperative findings, the severity of preoperative airway compromise, and any signs of early postoperative compromise such as stridor and dyspnea with or without position change.

4. **The need for central monitoring** should be carefully considered before emergence from general anesthesia and tracheal extubation, because placement of a central line in respiratory distress from upper airway obstruction is difficult. In addition, careful consideration must be given to possible anatomic abnormalities of the central veins due to the underlying pathology. Ultrasound guidance may be very helpful under these circumstances.

E. **Lung transplantation:** see **Chapter 41**

II. **General considerations of postoperative care**

A. **Airway management.** The care team, nurses, residents, fellows, and attendings must be aware of the potential for postoperative airway compromise and prepare options for airway support at the bedside. This may consist of placing a set of small (4–6 mm) endotracheal tubes next to the patient after tracheal resection or a fiberoptic bronchoscope after sleeve lobectomy. A plan of action should be conceived before the emergency arises, if at all possible.

B. **Pulmonary care.** Chest wall pain, interstitial edema and inflammation after prolonged lung collapse during one-lung ventilation, and retained bronchial secretions in the down lung, all impair gas exchange and oxygenation. Vigorous pulmonary toilet with chest wall percussion, incentive spirometry, and early mobilization are important to prevent and reverse these changes.

C. **Drainage of the pleural space.** After thoracotomy, one or more chest tubes drain air and fluid from the thoracic cavity and maintain lung expansion. Pleural drainage is a seemingly simple mechanical system, but failure of any component can result in significant complications. **Figure 40-1** shows a diagram of the function of a **three-chamber drainage thoracostomy system.** Proper function of the chest tube and drainage system may be monitored by asking a few basic questions: Is the chest tube in the patient's chest? Is the drainage system securely connected to the tube and can its fluid chambers accommodate the drainage? Is suction being applied to the pleural cavity?

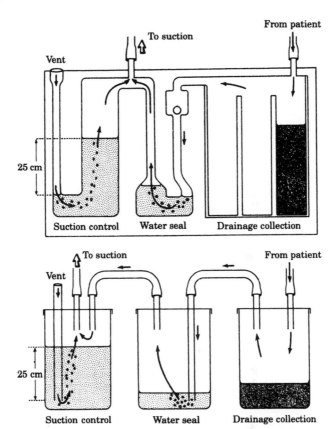

FIGURE 40-1 Chest tube drainage system. Panel A shows a commercial apparatus. The proximal chamber (on the right) is for pleural drainage, the middle is the water seal chamber, which prevents air or fluid from being driven into the thorax, and the distal (on the left) is the chamber that regulates the level of negative pressure applied. Panel B shows a traditional "three-bottle system" show for comparison.

D. **Fluid management.** Aside from esophageal resection and extrapleural pneumonectomy, a strategy of conservative fluid administration is generally employed to minimize pulmonary edema of traumatized lung tissue and suture lines. Low urine output is common after lung resection and requires careful evaluation. In the absence of neurologic compromise, severe anemia, metabolic acidosis, or arterial hypotension, a low urine output (≥ 20 mL/h) may be observed. A limited number (2–3) of small (250 mL) **intravenous fluid boluses** are often safe to administer. Prolonged blood pressure support after seemingly adequate fluid resuscitation mandates **central venous access**. Patients on angiotensin-converting enzyme inhibitors for chronic hypertension receiving postoperative epidural analgesia require occasionally prolonged vasoactive support.

E. **Postoperative analgesia** is paramount not only for proper patient comfort, but also to facilitate pulmonary toilet, deep breathing and coughing, and early ambulation. Occasionally, however, hypotension associated with epidural analgesia may require its temporary reduction and the consideration of alternative means of providing analgesia.

1. **Epidural analgesia** is the preferred method of pain management for the thoracotomy patient. Epidural analgesia may be provided with a local anesthetic, a narcotic, or, most commonly, a combination of both. A low concentration of local anesthetic (0.1% **bupivacaine**) with a low-dose narcotic (2 μg/mL **fentanyl** or 20 μg/mL **hydromorphone**) is commonly used. Choice of epidural narcotic is often based on lipophilicity. The more lipophilic the narcotic, the less it spreads along the epidural space. This results in less sedation, but also less analgesia at dermatomes far from the tip of the epidural catheter.

2. **Nonsteroidal anti-inflammatory agents (NSAIDS)** may be used alone or as adjuncts to epidural and parenteral narcotics. **Ketorolac** offers high-grade analgesia without respiratory depression or sedation. All NSAIDs (see **Appendix**) should be used cautiously in patients with renal dysfunction, patients with gastritis, and those who are prone to bleeding.

3. **Parenteral opiates** are effective analgesics but must be used cautiously because of their respiratory depressant effect. **Patient-controlled analgesia (PCA)** has been shown to be superior to prn administration of analgesia and safe following thoracic surgery.

F. **Chest radiography**

1. Daily chest x-rays should be followed while chest tubes are in place and as clinically indicated to follow resolution of atelectasis, pneumothorax, and pneumonia.

III. **Complications of thoracic surgery.** The following paragraphs detail many of the common complications observed during the routine care of patients with thoracic surgical problems. Experience teaches that, while complications may occur in isolation, often a combination of abnormalities converges on individual patients. The diagnosis of one complication should therefore initiate a search for other, associated abnormalities.

A. **Acute respiratory failure**

1. **Early postoperative failure**

a. **Mechanical problems.** Upper airway edema, vocal cord paralysis, laryngospasm, and upper airway obstruction from the soft tissue and tongue may temporarily preclude tracheal extubation. Retained bronchial secretions may require careful blind suctioning; a fiberoptic bronchoscopy, usually in the awake patient under local anesthesia, is the preferred method to assess and treat secretions.

b. **Acute pulmonary edema** leading to hypoxia requires prompt diuresis, and may benefit from continuous positive airway pressure (**CPAP**) or **noninvasive positive-pressure ventilation (NPPV)** delivered through a facemask (see **Section III.A**). With disciplined administration of intravenous fluid, pulmonary edema is uncommon.

c. **Narcotic overdose** from intraoperative or postoperative opiate administration requires prompt recognition to avoid increasing CO_2 retention and hypoxia. Elderly patients are particularly susceptible to narcotic side effects. If the patient has some degree of upper-airway obstruction but adequate minute ventilation, NPPV may serve as a temporizing measure while the narcotic wears off. **NPPV should not be given to patients after esophagectomy** to prevent thoracic gastric distension. Small doses of naloxone (0.04 mg every 2–5 minutes) may also be administered incrementally. However, if the patient is unarousable and becoming hypoxic, tracheal intubation provides the most reliable airway control.

2. **Post-lung resection ALI,** also described as **postpneumonectomy pulmonary edema,** is a syndrome of acute respiratory failure after lung resection, accompanied by radiographic pulmonary infiltrates without a clearly identifiable cause (**Fig. 40-2**). This complication has most commonly been described after pneumonectomy, but can occasionally occur after smaller resections.

   a. **Epidemiology.** Reported incidences range from 4% to 8% after pneumonectomy and 1% to 7% after lobectomy. Mortality is very high, in particular after right pneumonectomy.

   b. **Pathogenesis.** The sequence of events leading to this syndrome is still poorly understood. Although in the past much emphasis was put on the excessive administration of intravenous fluids, this view is simplistic. The absence of left ventricular failure, the delayed time of onset of the syndrome, and the ineffectiveness of diuretic administration, all point to a more complex pathogenesis. Very likely, this is an inflammatory reaction in response to perioperative lung injury. Such injury may include surgical trauma, mechanical ventilation with high inspiratory pressures and volumes, increased pulmonary artery and capillary pressure, and compromised pulmonary blood flow leading to ischemia-reperfusion of the remaining lung. Pre-existing risk factors have also been identified, including the severity of COPD, age over 60 years, male gender, and ETOH abuse.

   c. **Treatment.** No specific therapeutic measures have been shown to improve outcome. However, as this is felt to be a form of acute lung injury/acute respiratory distress syndrome (ALI/ARDS, **Chapter 20**), we employ a strategy of fluid restriction and lung-protective mechanical ventilation.

   (1) Limitation of fluid administration

      i. Excessive fluid administration in the perioperative period has been identified as a risk factor for developing ALI/ARDS after thoracic surgery. Furthermore, a recent controlled trial showed improved lung function and a shorter duration of mechanical ventilation when a **conservative fluid administration** strategy was used.

      ii. **Colloids versus crystalloids.** The type of fluid administered has not been shown to affect either the incidence or the duration of ALI after lung resection.

      iii. **Blood products,** whether red cells or plasma components, have never been shown to improve the course of any type of ALI/ARDS. In fact, all blood products can trigger an inflammatory reaction in the lung (transfusion-related acute lung injury [**TRALI**]) and should not be administered unless for specific hematologic indications.

   (2) Vigilance for infections. Pneumonia is a devastating complication in the setting of ALI, and a high index of suspicion must be maintained throughout the course of postlung resection ALI. The prophylactic use of antibiotics has not been shown to be effective.

   (3) β-Adrenergic agonists. In addition to their bronchodilator effect, there is some evidence that β-adrenergic agonists may

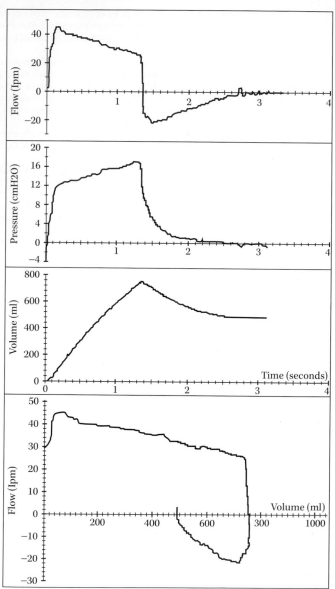

FIGURE 40-2 Semiquantification of the volume loss occurring in the presence of an air-leak due to a bronchopleural fistula. Note that in the flow trace (*top*), the area under the curve (i.e., the tidal volume) is smaller during exhalation, indicating a loss of volume. The flow-volume loop (*bottom*) fails to close at the end of exhalation, also indicating a loss of volume. *Reprinted with permission* from Lucangelo U, Bernabe F, Blanch L. Respiratory mechanics derived from signals in the ventilator circuit. *Resp. Care* 2005;50:55–65.

attenuate lung vascular injury and accelerate the resolution of alveolar edema.

   i. **Noninvasive positive pressure ventilation (NPPV)** has been demonstrated to be effective in treating acute respiratory failure following lung resections, acute pulmonary edema, and acute exacerbation of COPD. However, prolonged use of NPPV increases the risk of aspiration and fatigue; after 24 to 48 hours of NPPV, its benefits and risks as an alternative to tracheal intubation must be reconsidered.

3. **Postpneumonectomy syndrome** is characterized by extreme shift and rotation of the mediastinum late after a pneumonectomy. The syndrome results in obstruction of a main stem or lobar bronchus and air trapping leading to dyspnea, additional work of breathing, and ultimately hemodynamic instability. Diagnosis is usually made by a combination of chest radiograph, chest CT, echocardiogram, and flexible bronchoscopy. Treatment is surgical and consists of repositioning of the mediastinum in midline by implantation of saline-filled prosthesis (such as breast implants) into the vacant pleural cavity.

4. **Bronchopleural fistula (BPF)** is any communication between the airways and the pleural space. BPF may occur after lung resection, trauma, airway laceration, and alveolar rupture secondary to alveolar overdistension. Early in the postoperative course, BPFs manifest first with a **persistent air leak from the thoracostomy tube.** Small air leaks are relatively common after lobectomy or lesser resections and result from the visceral pleura or the fissure. In these cases, air leaks are generally self-limited and do not require intervention. In contrast, any **air leak after pneumonectomy** and a **large, persistent air leak following lobectomy** raise the suspicion of a disrupted bronchial suture line. The patient is threatened by pleural sepsis, pulmonary sepsis, and by respiratory insufficiency.

   a. **Evaluation.** The bronchial stump may be inspected by bronchoscopy, either in the operating room or in the ICU at the bedside in a critically ill patient. A small leak in a stable patient may also be identified on ventilation scintigraphy.

   b. **Treatment** depends on the time of diagnosis and patient condition. Surgical closure may be attempted early after resection in a stable patient without sepsis. Conversely, if closure is delayed, adequate pleural drainage with appropriately placed chest tubes is important. In patients with large bronchial disruptions complicated by pulmonary or pleural sepsis who require mechanical ventilation, exclusion of the lobar or main stem bronchus with selective intubation or balloon occlusion limits the pressure applied across the disrupted airway. However, management of selective pulmonary ventilation is complex, due to the inherent instability of the systems used to provide lung isolation, such as double-lumen endotracheal tubes and bronchial blockers (see **Section IV**). Effective approaches to limit airflow through the BPF during mechanical ventilation include limiting positive inspiratory and expiratory pressures, preventing the development of auto-PEEP, and reducing the tidal volume. It is important to note that the pressure that keeps the fistula open is the **transmural alveolar pressure** rather then just the pressure applied at the airway. Hence, during assisted ventilation (**Chapter 5**), the pressure that keeps the BPF open at end inspiration is equal to the positive pressure applied by the machine plus the negative pressure applied by the patient (which is not routinely measured).

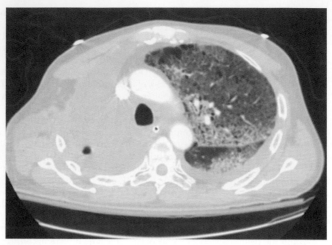

FIGURE 40-3 Postpneumonectomy acute lung injury (ALI). MGH Surgical ICU, November 2004.

   c. **Quantifying the size of the BPF,** and thus amount of wasted ventilation per breath, may assist in following the progress of the disease and guiding the ventilator settings. With modern ventilators, the ability to display flow and volume traces may provide helpful information, as illustrated in **Fig. 40-3.**

   d. **Specific ventilatory techniques** and modes of ventilation, such as **high-frequency ventilation** and **airway pressure release ventilation** (**Chapter 5**), have been used successfully to support patients with large BPFs. However, no controlled trial has showed the superiority of these modes over traditional approaches. It is likely that the success of each technique depends more on individual experience rather than the actual superiority of one mode or another. It is important to note that CO_2 is often sufficiently cleared with flow through the fistula without actual tidal ventilation.

B. **Atrial dysrhythmias** are common following thoracotomy. While often self-limited, resulting primarily from surgical manipulation of the heart and pulmonary veins, supraventricular tachycardia is the first presentation of many patients who succumb after thoracic surgical procedures. Specific causes should therefore be considered including myocardial ischemia, pulmonary embolism, electrolyte imbalances, fluid overload, and pneumothorax. The evaluation of a first atrial arrhythmia should include a chest radiograph, an electrocardiogram, and the determination of serum electrolytes. If an underlying cause cannot be found and corrected, or if the exact electrocardiographic diagnosis is unclear, the consultation of a cardiologist may be helpful. β-**Blockers** and **calcium channel blockers** are first-line drugs for rate control. **Amiodarone** is effective for rate control and possibly conversion, but isolated reports of acute pulmonary fibrosis limit the use of this effective drug after lung resections.

IV. Selected postoperative thoracic emergencies

   A. Pulmonary arterial hemorrhage with or without hemoptysis. Most episodes of hemoptysis after intrathoracic operations are self-limited. Bleeding from a pulmonary artery due to erosion of a tumor, abscess, or suture line may cause massive, immediate blood loss. Perforation by the tip of a pulmonary artery catheter is a well-recognized complication. Death from exsanguination can occur within seconds, and surgical evaluation with consideration of exploration should proceed.

      1. Expeditious airway suctioning and **intubation** may be extremely difficult due to large amounts of blood in the airway. A **double-lumen tube** may isolate and protect the nonbleeding lung. The side of bleeding is determined by review of radiographs.

      2. **Rigid bronchoscopy** to identify the source may be performed in the absence of active bleeding.

      3. **Surgical repair or resection** or **angiographic embolization** constitute ultimate therapeutic options.

   B. Tension pneumothorax can occur with or without an existing chest tube, and should be sought in any patient developing unexplained hypoxia, hypotension, or sudden increased airway pressures. The diagnosis may be established clinically by the absence of breath sounds on the affected side. **Needle decompression** with a 14-g cannula in the second intercostal space along the midclavicular line may be performed until a chest tube is placed. However, the insertion of a needle obligates chest tube placement because the lung may be injured during this maneuver. When the life of the patient is threatened, lateral open thoracostomies accomplish the same goal with a lower risk of injury.

   C. Cardiac herniation and **torsion** may occur after traumatic rupture of the pericardium or through a surgical defect in the pericardium. Because the heart is fixed on the right side by the vena cava and the aorta, herniation into the right pleural space after right extrapleural pneumonectomy is more common. Caval obstruction diminishes inflow to the right heart. Signs include cardiovascular collapse, superior vena cava syndrome and myocardial ischemia, characteristically occurring after changes in position, or coughing. Patients should then be hemodynamically supported and prepared for emergent surgery.

V. Common thoracic ICU procedures

   A. Tube thoracostomy allows drainage of the pleural space in the setting of pneumothorax or pleural effusion. Chest tubes may also be used to introduce sclerosing agents for persistent pleural effusion. Commercially available closed drainage systems derived from the original **three-bottle systems** are used to drain the pleural space (**Fig. 40-1B**). Chest tubes are initially placed to 10 to 20 cm H_2O suction. When no air leak is detected, the suction can be discontinued and the chest tube left only on water seal. Once the drainage is minimal (usually <150 mL over 24 hours) and there is no pneumothorax and no air leak, the chest tube should be removed. Prophylactic antimicrobial coverage is not required.

      1. **Ultrasound guidance** is often used to perform tube thoracostomy and thoracentesis (see **Chapter 3**).

      2. **Complications** of tube thoracostomy include intraparenchymal placement of the tube, with consequent possible lung contusion, hemorrhage, and BPF, hemothorax from injury to intercostals vessels, and subcutaneous emphysema.

B. **Fiberoptic bronchoscopy** is used liberally to clear secretions (especially large mucous plugs causing atelectasis) and to obtain a sputum culture in the diagnosis of pneumonia (see **Chapter 29**).
   1. **In the intubated patient**, bronchoscopy is a safe procedure in the hands of an experienced operator. Precise description of the bronchial anatomy and the use of sterile technique to culture secretions enhance the yield of the procedure.
   2. **In the nonintubated patient**, bronchoscopy requires a high level of skill because of the risks of limiting ventilation and causing hypercarbia and hypoxemia.
      a. The use of **topical anesthesia** (2%–4% lidocaine via a nebulizer or atomizer) is effective at anesthetizing the upper airway, but we caution that spraying the vocal cords may temporarily facilitate aspiration of oral contents into the airway.
      b. A light sedation with **remifentanil** (0.05–0.1 μg/kg/min) or **dexmedetomidine** (0.1–0.5 μg/kg/h) titrated by an experienced operator may be effective. The avoidance of sedation eliminates potential side effects; an experienced bronchoscopist will carefully explain the procedure and administer effective pharyngolaryngeal mucosal anesthesia.

Selected References

Alam N, Park BJ, Wilton A, et al. Incidence and risk factors for lung injury after lung cancer resection. *Ann Thorac Surg* 2007;84:1085–1091.
Auriant I, Jallot A, Herve P, et al. Noninvasive ventilation reduces mortality in acute respiratory failure following lung resection. *Am J Respir Crit Care Med* 2001;164:1231–1235.
Fernandez-Perez ER, Keegan MT, Brown DR, et al. Intraoperative tidal volume as a risk factor for respiratory failure after pneumonectomy. Anesthesiology 2006;105:14–18.
Grillo HC, Shepard JO, Mathisen DJ, et al. Postpneumonectomy syndromes: diagnosis, management, and results. *Ann Thorac Surg* 1992;54:638–651.
Hulscher JBF, Van Sandick JW, de Boer AG, et al. Extended transthoracic resection compared with limited transhiatal resection for adenocarcinoma of the esophagus. *N Engl J Med* 2002;347:1662–1669.
Licker M, Tschop JM, Roberts J, et al. Aerosolized salbutamol accelerates the resolution of pulmonary edema after lung resection. *Chest* 2008;133:845–852.
Martin GS, Mangialardi RJ, Wheeler AP, et al. Albumin and furosemide therapy in hypoproteinemic patients with acute lung injury. *Crit Care Med* 2002;30:2175–2182.
Slinger PD. Perioperative fluid management for thoracic surgery: the puzzle of postpneumonectomy pulmonary edema. *J Cardiothorac Vasc Anesth* 1998;9:442–451.
Spira A, Ettinger DS. Multidisciplinary management of lung cancer. *N Engl J Med* 2004; 350:379–392.
www.cms.hhs.gov/transmittals/downloads/R3NCD.pdf

41

ICU Care Following Liver, Kidney, and Lung Transplantation

Jason Wertheim and William Benedetto

I. Principles of care for transplant patients

A. Time course. The complex clinical picture of transplant patients may be simplified by considering time periods that emphasize different issues.

1. **First 7 days: donor and recipient surgery.** As a rule, the allograft is the organ most affected by hemodynamic changes. Proper allograft function will usually lead to swift overall clinical improvement. Allograft dysfunction, on the other hand, requires investigating the contribution of the recipient's preoperative status, intraoperative course, the quality of the donor organ, and the possibility of technical complications.

2. **After 1 week: acute rejection.** Because there are numerous steps in the complex cascade leading to full T-cell differentiation and activation, clinically detectable acute rejection does not usually occur until several days to weeks after transplantation. As long as technical complications have been ruled out (e.g., vascular thrombosis, biliary leak, and preservation injury), organ dysfunction at this time is usually attributed to rejection and can be treated with increased immunosuppression. At times, a liver biopsy in hepatitis C patients may be helpful to distinguish acute rejection from disease recurrence. In renal transplantation, an early rejection episode may herald an antibody- or cellular-mediated mechanism, and the result of a biopsy may dictate different lines of therapy.

3. **After 6 months: chronic issues.** The risk of opportunistic infections increases with the degree of recipient immunosuppression. Thus, infections are more typical in the late postoperative period, especially if repeated bouts of rejection have required multiple courses of heightened immunosuppression. Late allograft dysfunction raises the possibility of disease recurrence or chronic rejection, both of which may lead to steadily worsening allograft failure and will be unresponsive to increased immunosuppression.

B. Immunosuppression. Administration of any immunosuppressive agent is limited by side effects. By combining different agents, it is possible to increase immunosuppression while limiting troublesome, unwanted effects. For this reason, most whole-organ transplant patients receive either double- or triple-drug immunosuppression (**Table 41-1**).

1. **Calcineurin inhibitors: Cyclosporine** and **tacrolimus** specifically target the activation of T lymphocytes (the immune cells principally responsible for rejection). **Calcineurin** inhibitors are the core of most current immunosuppressive protocols. Either one may be started perioperatively and taken orally as long-term maintenance. Both are nephrotoxic and require careful adjustment based on blood levels. Other side effects include hypertension, hyperkalemia, hyperglycemia (especially in patients on high-dose steroids), neurotoxicity (seizures and tremors), and hyperuricemia (gout).

41-1	Immunosuppressive Medications

Medication Name	Class/Function
Cyclosporine (Neoral, Gengraf, Prograf)	Calcineurin inhibitor
Sirolimus (Rapamune)	Antiproliferative (mTOR inhibitor)
Mycophenolate mofetil (Cellcept)	Antiproliferative (IMPDH inhibitor)
Azathioprine (Imuran)	Antiproliferative (purine antimetabolite)
Methyl prednisone, prednisone	Corticosteroids
Basiliximab (Simulect), daclizumab (Zenapax)	IL-2 receptor antagonists
Muromonab-CD3 (Orthoclone OKT3)	CD3-specific monoclonal antibody
Antithymocyte globulin (Atgam, thymoglobulin)	Nonspecific polyclonal antibody

2. **Antilymphocyte-depleting antibodies and IL-2 blocking antibodies: OKT3, antithymocyte globulin, basiliximab,** and **daclizumab** also target T cells, but can only be given intravenously. The antibody-based agents are used for induction of immunosuppression, for treating steroid-resistant acute rejection, and as part of newer "tolerance"-inducing protocols. Multiple courses may have a decreased efficacy and can lead to infection and malignancy in the long term. In patients with postoperative renal failure, cyclosporine or tacrolimus may be discontinued, with OKT3 or thymoglobulin being substituted as equivalent, but nonnephrotoxic immunosuppression. This simplifies the early postoperative management, but expends an important therapeutic option, which may then be unavailable to treat subsequent resistant rejection later in the postoperative course.

3. **Antimetabolite agents: Mycophenolate** and **azathioprine** inhibit DNA or RNA synthesis and therefore block active lymphocyte proliferation. Dose reduction may be required if leukopenia, thrombocytopenia, or anemia occurs. Mycophenolate is also limited by gastrointestinal side effects that include mild ileus, gastritis, nausea, and vomiting.

4. **Corticosteroids** provide relatively nonspecific immunosuppression. High-dose intravenous **methylprednisolone** typically is initiated on the day of transplantation and tapered over the next 4 to 5 days to a maintenance level. **Prednisone** is substituted for methylprednisolone when feeding resumes. If rejection occurs, high-dose methylprednisolone boluses (500 mg intravenously every day for 2 days) are given as initial treatment. Patients may require stress dose supplementation for major procedures while receiving steroids. Intravenous **hydrocortisone** (100 mg IV every 8 hours) is given on the day of surgery and tapered over 3 days. During this time, maintenance immunosuppression is continued with either oral prednisone or intravenous methylprednisolone. Patients on high-dose steroids are at risk for developing hyperglycemia and gastrointestinal bleeding, which may be mitigated by prophylactic histamine-2 (H_2) blockers.

5. **Efforts to wean immunosuppressive agents.** There is ongoing research directed at the generation of true "transplantation tolerance" (specific immunologic nonreactivity toward the donor organ) and the development of clinical protocols for the reduction of traditional triple-drug immunosuppression down to monotherapy.

6. **Drug interactions.** The transplant patient's complex drug regimen should constantly be reevaluated and simplified. This approach will

improve compliance and avoid potentially catastrophic and sometimes unpredictable drug interactions. In particular, the addition of new medications to an immunosuppressive regimen should be carefully considered. For example, **allopurinol,** if administered in combination with azathioprine, may precipitate life-threatening leukopenia. Numerous medications (e.g., **sucralfate, verapamil,** and **erythromycin**) may alter cyclosporine absorption and thus precipitate rejection or toxicity.

C. **Infections**

1. **Prophylactic strategies.** Between 60% and 80% of liver transplant patients will develop some form of infection occurring days, weeks, or years after transplantation. However, different opportunistic infections occur within predictable time periods in the postoperative course, and prophylactic antibiotic regimens have been established (**Chapter 12**). Long-term, low-dose **trimethoprim-sulfamethoxazole** effectively prevents *Pneumocystis* infections and may prevent urinary tract infections as well. During periods of heightened immunosuppression, **ganciclovir** or **acyclovir** (or their derivatives **valganciclovir** or **valacyclovir**) is added to lower the incidence of cytomegalovirus (CMV) and Epstein-Barr virus (EBV) infections. Because invasive procedures increase the risk of bacterial infections, systemic antibiotics are administered during the perioperative period and prior to cholangiograms or percutaneous biopsies.

2. **Preventative measures** include minimizing immunosuppression, avoiding endotracheal intubation and intravascular catheters, correcting malnutrition, and tight glycemic control. Evaluation of possible hematomas, abscesses, or fluid collections should be pursued by serial ultrasound or computed tomography (CT), and appropriate drainage should be expeditiously undertaken if there is a suspicion of active infection. Because immunosuppression blunts the usual signs of inflammation, an aggressive surveillance and diagnostic approach is crucial, with routine cultures (e.g., biweekly cultures of sputum, urine, bile, and wound drainage) and daily chest radiographs while the recipient is receiving mechanical ventilation.

II. **Liver transplantation**

A. **Indications**

1. **Decompensated cirrhotic liver failure, acute fulminant hepatic failure, metabolic disorders, and liver failure with preserved hepatocyte function** are all indications for liver transplantation and are discussed in detail in **Chapter 25**.

B. **Donor allograft**

1. **Donor.** The likelihood of early allograft failure is correlated with donor characteristics (obesity, prolonged ICU stay, malnutrition, terminal hypotension, and fatty liver changes). Although the characteristics of the "ideal donor" are well described, there has been increasing use of "marginal" or suboptimal donor grafts in the United States. This practice is a response to the insufficient supply of needed donor organs and has had a proportionate impact on recipient performance in the postoperative period. In many cases, recipients who are unlikely to receive organs because of severe illness may receive marginal grafts as an alternative to dying without a transplant.

2. **Efforts to increase organ availability.** In addition to the use of marginal donors, other efforts to increase the number of available organs include the use of **donors after cardiac death** (DCD), splitting cadaveric

grafts for two recipients, and the use of living donors. DCD liver grafts probably give inferior overall graft and patient survival, whereas grafts from living donors function well but place additional risk on a healthy donor. Quantitative algorithms using donor characteristics have been developed to better pair donor and recipient organ allocation to maximize utilization of donor organs. Splitting of well-chosen cadaveric organs for an adult–child recipient pair with one member critically ill has shown promising results.

3. **Preservation.** Prolonged ischemia time is also correlated with allograft dysfunction. Cold ischemia time usually is ideally limited to less than 12 hours for livers, and is less in marginal donor livers. During procurement, the donor allograft is flushed with University of Wisconsin (UW) solution, which has been the gold standard in preservation solutions, and stored in ice until transplantation. Other preservation solutions such as Histidine-tryptophan-ketoglutarate and Celsior, which both lack starch, are currently being investigated as alternatives to UW Solution.

C. Recipient operation

1. **Native hepatectomy.** The coagulopathy of end-stage liver disease and the multiple venous collaterals of portal hypertension can lead to **massive blood loss,** which is directly correlated with postoperative morbidity and mortality. Therefore, this phase of the transplant procedure is often the most technically difficult. Once the liver is removed, patients frequently develop a **metabolic acidosis,** requiring correction prior to reperfusion. Overcorrection with sodium bicarbonate, however, may lead to severe postoperative **metabolic alkalosis.** This phenomenon results from the metabolism of the **citrate** administered with transfused blood products to bicarbonate by the functioning allograft.

2. **Donor liver implantation** may be accomplished by different techniques with regard to the vena cava anastomosis. The traditional method utilizes anastomosis between the donor and recipient vena cava at the supra- and infrahepatic locations. Blood flow through the vena cava is typically disrupted, and a venovenous bypass circuit allows blood to shunt from the femoral and portal veins into the internal jugular or axillary vein. Alternately, the "piggyback" technique creates an end to side anastomosis between the donor suprahepatic vena cava and recipient vena cava, allowing for a continuous return of blood to the heart if a side-biting clamp is used while sewing the anastomosis. This is followed by portal vein, hepatic artery, and bile duct anastomosis (either a choledochocholedochostomy or Roux-en-Y choledochojejunostomy). A biliary stent or T-tube may be placed across the anastomosis and allowed to drain percutaneously. Peritoneal drains are also placed in the supra- and infrahepatic spaces.

3. **Reperfusion of the allograft,** usually within 60 minutes of warm ischemia time, returns a sudden bolus of cold, hyperkalemic, acidotic blood from the lower body and liver and may cause severe **pulmonary artery (PA) vasoconstriction** with resultant hypotension and possible dysrhythmia ("reperfusion phenomenon"). Reperfusion of the ischemic liver may also precipitate accelerated **fibrinolysis.** Aggressive replacement of coagulation factors and antifibrinolytic agent administration (see **Chapter 10**) may be required to achieve hemostasis.

D. Posttransplant management

1. **General care.** In addition to routine physical examination (checking mental status, abdomen, wound, and peritoneal and biliary drains) and

invasive monitoring, evaluation includes serial laboratory studies, chest x-ray, and Doppler ultrasound examination in the first 48 hours to screen for hepatic artery thrombosis (HAT) (see later discussion). Neurologic complications are frequently attributable to encephalopathy, neurotoxicity due to immunosuppressants, cerebral hemorrhage, and stroke. Hypothermia must be avoided in the immediate postoperative setting and can be corrected by prewarming the ICU room, application of warm blankets, and the use of forced–air warming machines. Maintenance intravenous fluids should always contain dextrose to avoid depletion of glycogen stores in the liver. Patients often tolerate sips by 24 to 48 hours after surgery, although feeding is resumed cautiously in patients with a Roux-en-Y choledochojejunostomy. On the fifth postoperative day, a cholangiogram is obtained if a biliary tube was placed. If no obstruction or leak is evident, the biliary stent or T-tube is clamped with removal planned for 3 to 6 months post transplant.

2. **Cardiovascular**
   a. **Hemodynamics.** The high cardiac output and low peripheral vascular resistance typical of end-stage liver disease commonly persist into the early postoperative period, so that inotropic agents are rarely required in liver transplant recipients.
   b. **Hypotension.** The usual first therapeutic response is volume administration. Excessively high central venous pressures should be avoided because transmission back to the hepatic sinusoids may exacerbate allograft edema already present from reperfusion injury. If hypotension persists without detectable hypovolemia or cardiac dysfunction, sepsis should be suspected, blood cultures obtained, and empiric antibiotic therapy initiated. The use of prostaglandin E infusion to counter reperfusion injury may contribute iatrogenically to postoperative hypotension.
   c. **Hypertension.** Postoperative hypertension may be precipitated by pain, anxiety, fluid overload, and pre-existing hypertension. Because of the increased risks of cerebral edema, hemorrhage, and seizures, sustained hypertension requires aggressive treatment.
3. **Respiratory.** In the presence of good graft function, successful endotracheal extubation usually can be accomplished within 12 to 48 hours, but may be delayed by hepatic hydrothorax or right diaphragmatic paralysis from intraoperative placement of the suprahepatic vascular clamp and by metabolic alkalosis. "Fast-track" extubation after an uneventful orthotopic liver transplantation is becoming the norm at high-volume centers. Occasionally, diuresis is needed prior to extubation to reverse the effects of high-volume resuscitation. Judicious use of narcotics that are relatively unaffected by hepatic dysfunction (e.g., fentanyl) may facilitate early extubation.
4. **Renal.** Many liver allograft recipients develop mild postoperative renal dysfunction because of pre-existing renal insufficiency, intraoperative caval occlusion, bleeding, hypotension, postimplantation hepatic allograft dysfunction, and nephrotoxic drugs such as cyclosporine and tacrolimus. Other nephrotoxic drugs, such as aminoglycosides, may cause intrinsic renal dysfunction and should be avoided. **Prostaglandin E_1** may have a beneficial effect on the liver recipient's renal function during the early postoperative period. Some patients whose preoperative renal dysfunction is a result of their liver failure (i.e., those with the hepatorenal syndrome) will show posttransplant improvement. If postoperative oliguria persists despite optimized hemodynamics, a

nonnephrotoxic antibody immunosuppressant is substituted for tacrolimus or cyclosporine. With this approach, dialysis usually can be avoided. **Continuous venovenous hemofiltration** (see **Chapter 24**) has less fluid shifts and electrolyte disturbances than intermittent hemodialysis, and is preferred if renal replacement therapy is indicated. Dialysis should be used with extreme caution because rapid osmotic shifts may worsen brain swelling already present in patients with hepatic failure. Mortality is high in patients whose renal dysfunction progresses to the need for dialysis.

5. **Hematology.** Leukopenia and thrombocytopenia secondary to hypersplenism typically persist into the early postoperative period, sometimes requiring a dose reduction of azathioprine. Should the white blood cell count fall below 1,500/mm^3, **granulocyte colony-stimulating factor** (see also **Chapter 35**) can be administered to decrease the incidence of postoperative infections. The postoperative hematocrit is maintained in the range of 25% to 30%. In the absence of ongoing hemorrhage, an international normalized ratio between 1.5 and 2, a platelet count greater than $50 \times 100/L$ and a fibrinogen level >100 mg/dL is generally permissible, yet specific benchmarks vary among institutions. The likelihood of significant postoperative bleeding is related directly to the degree of intraoperative bleeding and the quality of immediate allograft function. If major blood loss persists despite reversal of coagulopathy, surgical reexploration is indicated. Even in patients whose early bleeding stops, reexploration may be indicated to evacuate clot. This may improve ventilation by reducing abdominal distension and prevent the development if secondarily infected hematomas if coagulated blood is left in the abdomen.

E. **Allograft dysfunction**

1. **Primary graft nonfunction (PGNF),** defined as initial poor hepatic allograft function, occurs in approximately 2% to 10% of recipients, and is a common cause of early retransplantation.

   a. PGNF must be differentiated from the reversible preservation injury that is frequently noted in the first 2 postoperative days. Preservation injury is typically associated with a serum glutamic-oxaloacetic transaminase (SGOT) peak less than 2,000 U/L and rapid clinical improvement. Technical problems with any of the vascular anastomoses must be ruled out as well and is typically done with abdominal ultrasonography (later discussion). In contrast, PGNF is associated with a marked elevation of bilirubin and transaminases (e.g., SGOT >2,000 U/L), persistent hepatic encephalopathy, minimal bile output (<30–60 mL/d, often colorless or white), uncorrectable coagulopathy, acidosis, hyperkalemia, worsening renal function, and profound hypoglycemia.

   b. **Treatment** consists of early prostaglandin E$_1$ infusion, intensive support, and retransplantation.

2. **Acute rejection.** Both acute rejection and acute viral hepatitis (B, C) or CMV may be heralded by a bilirubin and transaminase elevation. Acute rejection is uncommon following liver transplantation, but can occur during the first or second postoperative weeks, whereas recurrent hepatitis commonly occurs later. A percutaneous biopsy may be necessary to establish the correct diagnosis. Nearly half of recipients suffer some degree of acute rejection; of these, nearly 90% typically respond to steroid boluses. Retransplantation is rarely required due to uncontrolled rejection.

3. **Technical complications**
   a. **Hepatic artery thrombosis (HAT)** is more common in pediatric recipients, especially those with small or multiple allograft arteries. Presentation varies: Approximately one-third demonstrate acute hepatic failure, with marked elevation of transaminases (SGOT 2,000–10,000 U/L), or bile duct leak because the hepatic artery is the sole blood supply to the bile ducts; one-third have recurrent septic episodes with or without hepatic abscess; and one-third are asymptomatic with the diagnosis found as an incidental finding. The late sequelae of HAT may include biliary dysfunction or ductal stricture. Doppler ultrasound is used liberally to screen for HAT, whereas an arteriogram may be required to confirm the diagnosis. Treatment options depend on the presentation, and include retransplantation, reoperation, selective urokinase injection, and observation.
   b. **Bile duct complications** may be detected by the appearance of bile in a drain or abdominal pain and an unexplained rise in serum bilirubin. Endoscopic retrograde cholangiopancreatography (see **Chapter 26**) or reexploration may be required.
   c. **Other complications,** such as portal vein or vena cava thrombosis (manifested by ascites, variceal bleeding or detected by radiographic studies), are exceedingly rare. Treatment options usually include medical support, radiologic intervention, and operative thrombectomy. Postoperative infections are the primary cause of death after liver transplantation, and are a frequent cause of readmission to the ICU. Common sites of infection are the lungs and abdominal cavity.

III. **Renal transplantation**
   A. **Indications.** The most common indications for renal transplantation include **chronic glomerulonephritis, diabetic nephropathy, chronic pyelonephritis, malignant nephrosclerosis,** and **polycystic kidney disease.**
   B. **Renal transplant recipients** are at significant risk for cardiovascular complications. Diabetes is a leading indication for renal transplantation, and hypertension and hypercholesterolemia often complicate renal failure. Cardiovascular complications are nevertheless relatively rare in the immediate postoperative period, because aggressive pretransplant screening and preoperative treatment of occult coronary artery disease is the rule.
   C. **Donor allograft.** Adverse donor characteristics, such as advanced age, terminal or prolonged hypotension, and the need for vasopressors, are highly correlated with posttransplant acute tubular necrosis (ATN). Nevertheless, as long as the allograft has reasonable underlying parenchyma (established by biopsy), recovery may be expected. Prolonged cold ischemia time, associated with shipping renal grafts long distances and the use of DCD donors, can also contribute to poor intra- and postoperative graft function. Delayed allograft function is much easier to manage in kidney recipients than in liver recipients because of the availability of dialysis. ATN is extremely rare in living donor recipients. Though efforts at HLA matching have proven successful in lengthening the half-life of well-matched renal allografts, no difference in perioperative immunosuppression or performance is expected.
   D. **Recipient operation.** The allograft is implanted in the pelvis, with the renal artery and vein sewn into the corresponding iliac vessels. If the ureter is

implanted into the bladder, a Foley catheter should be left in place for 5 days to prevent bladder distention and strain on the ureter–bladder anastomosis. On the other hand, if an ureteroureterostomy is constructed (after a native nephrectomy), prolonged bladder catheter drainage is not required. In either case, a Jackson-Pratt drain is left in place at the site of the ureteral anastomoses.

E. **Immediate postoperative course**
   1. Immediate allograft function is heralded by a massive diuresis necessitating aggressive fluid replacement (e.g., per hour rate equal to the previous hour's urine output in milliliter plus 30 mL, limited to 400 mL/h) and diligent electrolyte monitoring.
   2. Oliguria in the early postoperative course is usually due to reversible ATN, but technical complications must be excluded.
F. **Late course.** Elevated creatinine in the postoperative period leads to a decision about whether to reduce the dose of a nephrotoxic immunosuppressant (cyclosporine or tacrolimus) or to increase immunosuppression in an attempt to treat rejection. A biopsy often is required to determine the cause of graft dysfunction.
G. **Complications.** The most common vascular complication following kidney transplant is renal artery stenosis, which often manifests as severe hypertension. Treatment may be surgical or via percutaneous balloon-based techniques. Urologic complications include leak from the bladder closure or ureteral anastomosis, and ureteral obstruction. Lymphocele of the transplant bed can be avoided with careful ligation of the surrounding lymphatics during recipient preparation.

IV. **Lung transplantation**
   A. **Indications** include end-stage chronic obstructive pulmonary disease (COPD), cystic fibrosis, pulmonary fibrosis, α-1-antitrypsin deficiency, sarcoidosis, bronchiectasis, lymphangioleiomyomatosis, occupational lung diseases, and pulmonary hypertension. Candidates have end-stage pulmonary disease with an estimated survival of 2 to 3 years without transplantation.
   B. **Donor organs.** Improved organ preservation and perioperative management have expanded the pool of potential donor organs, but **the lung remains more susceptible to ischemic injury than any other transplanted organ.** Ischemic time for lung transplantation should be limited to 6 to 8 hours; lungs from older donors are less tolerant of long ischemic times than those from younger donors. **Living related lung donation** (with two donors each donating a lung lobe) is an option, which is exercised with increasing frequency in experienced centers. DCD has also been performed for lung transplantation.
   C. **Recipient characteristics** affect the postoperative course. For example, patients with systemic disease such as cystic fibrosis may suffer from other organ involvement. Similarly, years of tobacco use may be associated with peripheral vascular disease and pulmonary disease in single-lung recipients, postoperatively.
   D. **Recipient operation**
      1. **Monitoring.** Patients undergoing single- or double-lung transplantation are usually monitored with pulmonary and systemic arterial catheters and possibly with transesophageal echocardiography. The procedure necessitates endotracheal intubation with a technique that allows for selective lung ventilation, usually with double-lumen tracheal tube.
      2. **The recipient surgical operation** consists of a posterior lateral thoracotomy for single-lung transplantation or a bilateral antero-thoracosternotomy

for bilateral-lobe transplantation. Double-lung transplantation with a single tracheal anastomosis is rarely performed due to anastomotic complications.

E. Postoperative management

    1. General. Postoperative issues in the lung transplant patient generally involve management of respiratory status, hemodynamics, prevention and treatment of infection, continuation of immunosuppressive regimen, and pain control.

    2. Respiratory management. The goal of postoperative respiratory management in the lung transplant patient is to achieve adequate oxygenation and ventilation while avoiding oxygen toxicity and barotrauma. PEEP is generally added to a level of 5 to 10 cm H_2O. Limiting tidal volume and peak airway pressures to less than 40 cm H_2O is thought to decrease barotrauma and bronchial anastomotic complication. Pulmonary reimplantation response is a phenomenon of noncardiogenic pulmonary edema lasting up to 3 weeks and requiring ventilatory support, but is generally associated with a good prognosis. Following extubation, lung transplant patients demonstrate a hypoventilatory response to hypercapnia, though the etiology is not fully delineated.

    3. Hemodynamic management. Postoperative hemodynamic management of the lung transplant patient is a fine balance between adequate volume for vital organ function and prevention of pulmonary edema, and, thus, monitoring with a PA catheter may facilitate management. Hemorrhage is more common following transplantation in which cardiopulmonary bypass (CPB) has been utilized. CPB may also increase postoperative transfusion requirement, intubation duration, and overall hospital stay. Pulmonary hypertension is common in the immediate postoperative period; patients may benefit from treatment with inhaled nitric oxide to decrease PA pressures without systemic hypotension.

    4. Pain management generally involves either systemic opioids or epidural analgesia. Those with chronic respiratory failure due to either COPD or cystic fibrosis may be particularly susceptible to the development of hypercapnia when treated with systemic opioids. Although epidural opioids may also cause hypercapnia, equivalent analgesia may generally be achieved with a significantly lower opioid dose. Epidural analgesia may decrease times to extubation and discharge from the ICU. However, their use is institution dependent and may be contraindicated in the setting of anticoagulation when CPB is used.

    5. Immunosuppression. Most centers initiate immunosuppression in the operating room. Almost all protocols include a nonspecific antiinflammatory corticosteroid. Side effects of corticosteroids such as hyperglycemia and myopathy must be considered. A calcineurin inhibitor such as **cyclosporine** is generally initiated as well. Side effects include nephrotoxicity, hypertension, and neurotoxicity. **Tacrolimus** has essentially the same mechanism of action as cyclosporine but is more effective in preventing acute rejection. Tacrolimus does have higher rates of neurotoxicity, nephrotoxicity, and new-onset diabetes. **Azathioprine** or **mycophenolate,** both of which inhibit lymphocyte proliferation, may be adjunct immunosuppressant agents. Toxicities include leukopenia, hepatitis, and cholestasis. Finally, antilymphocyte preparations such as polyclonal **antilymphocyte globulin, ATG,** and **OKT3** may be initiated.

6. **Infections.** Immunosuppression increases the transplant recipient's incidence of both bacterial and viral infection. Early infections tend to be bacterial, with gram-negative organisms predominating. **CMV** is the most common early viral infection and may be due to reactivation of an infection in a seropositive recipient (secondary) or, more commonly, new infection in a seronegative recipient from the seropositive donor organ (primary). The most serious manifestation of CMV is pneumonitis or pneumonia; treatment is with **ganciclovir**, which, when given prophylactically, may decrease the incidence. *Aspergillus fumigatus* is the most common fungal infection, with a peak incidence within the first 2 months. Manifestations include ulcerations, pseudomembranes, and tracheobronchitis.

7. **Rejection.** Hyperacute, acute, and chronic rejection may be encountered in the intensive care unit. Hyperacute rejection is extremely uncommon, occurring within the first minutes to hours after transplantation, and is almost universally fatal. It is due to preformed antibodies against HLA and ABO antigens and may be confused with ischemia–reperfusion injury. Acute rejection occurs within the first 3 to 6 months. Symptoms of acute rejection include fever, cough, dyspnea, and anorexia. Decreases in pulmonary spirometry or diffusion capacity may aid the diagnosis, which requires biopsy for confirmation. Treatment of acute rejection consists of a course of high-dose steroids and elimination of other causes of symptoms. Chronic rejection occurs generally between 6 and 12 months and is typically manifested as bronchiolitis obliterans (BO). The pathophysiology of BO is poorly understood, but the syndrome is typically characterized by airflow limitation due to fibroproliferation in the small airways. Treatment includes corticosteroids and immunosuppressants, but mortality remains high despite treatment.

Selected References

Abt PL, Desai NM, Crawford MD, et al. Survival following liver transplantation from non-heart-beating donors. *Ann Surg* 2004;239:87–92.

Allan JS. Immunosuppression for lung transplantation. *Semin Thorac Cardiovasc Surg* 2004;16:333–341.

Arcasoy SM, Kotloff RM. Lung transplantation. *N Engl J Med* 1999;340:1081–1091.

Busuttil RW, Klintmaim GB. *Transplantation of the liver*. 2nd ed. Philadelphia: Elsevier Saunders, 2005.

Busuttil RW, Shaked A, Millis JM, et al. One thousand liver transplants. The lessons learned. *Ann Surg* 1994;219:490–497.

Consensus conference on standardized listing criteria for renal transplant candidates. *Transplantation* 1998;66:962.

DeMeo DL, Ginns LC. Clinical status of lung transplantation. *Transplantation* 2001;72:1713–1724.

Feng S, Goodrich NP, Bragg-Gresham JL, et al. Characteristics associated with liver graft failure: the concept of a donor risk index. *Am J Transplant* 2006;6:783–790.

Findlay JY, Jankowski CJ, Vasdeve GM, et al. Fast track anesthesia for liver transplantation reduces postoperative ventilation time but not intensive care unit stay. *Liver Transpl* 2002;8:670–675.

Ghobrial RM, Busuttil RW. Future of adult living donor liver transplantation. *Liver Transpl* 2003;9:S73–S79.

Kawai T, Cosimi AB, Spitzer TR, et al. HLA-mismatched renal transplantation without maintenance immunosuppression. *N Engl J Med* 2008;358:353–361.

Ng CY, Madsen JC, Rosengard BR, Allan JS. Immunosuppression for lung transplantation. *Front Biosci* 2009;14:1627–1641.

Organ Procurement and Transplantation Network Web site. Available at www.optn.org.

Ploeg RJ, D'Alessandro AM, Knechtle SJ, et al. Risk factors for primary dysfunction after liver transplantation—a multivariate analysis. *Transplantation* 1993;55:807–813.

Renz JF, Emond JC, Yersiz H, et al. Split-liver transplantation in the United States: outcomes of a national survey. *Ann Surg* 2004;239:172–181.

Singh H, Bossard FR. Perioperative anaesthetic considerations for patients undergoing lung transplantation. *Can J Anaesth* 1997;44:284–299.

Sleiman C, Mal H, Fournier M, et al. Pulmonary reimplantation response in single-lung transplantation. *Eur Respir J* 1995;8:5–9.

Sollinger HW, Knechtl SJ, Reed A, et al. Experience with 100 consecutive simultaneous kidney-pancreas transplants with bladder drainage. *Ann Surg* 1991;214:703–711.

Starzl TE, Murase N, Abu-Elmagd K, et al. Tolerogenic immunosuppression for organ transplantation. *Lancet* 2003;361:1502–1510.

Tolkoff RN, Rubin RH. The infectious disease problems of the diabetic renal transplant recipient. *Infect Dis Clin North Am* 1995;9:117–130.

Tzakis AG, Gordon RD, Shaw BW Jr, et al. Clinical presentation of hepatic artery thrombosis after liver transplantation in the cyclosporin era. *Transplantation* 1985;40:667–671.

42

ICU Care of the Obese Patient

Jeremy Goldfarb and Jean Kwo

I. **Introduction.** Obesity has reached epidemic proportions in the United States with an age-adjusted prevalence of 30% in adults. Up to 26% of patients in a medical–surgical intensive care unit are obese, and the prevalence of *morbid* obesity in the ICU is up to 7%. Not only do obese patients often present with multiple comorbidities, which complicate their perioperative course, but also obesity is an independent risk factor for many postoperative complications. Hence, special consideration must be given to this population.

II. **Morbid obesity** is defined as **body mass index (BMI)** $\geq$**40 (Table 42-1).**
   BMI = Weight(kg)/Height(m)^2

III. **Physiologic changes** associated with obesity (**Table 42-2**).
   A. **Cardiovascular**
   1. **Hypertension** is the most common overweight- and obesity-related health condition. The etiology is multifactorial. Blood pressure values closely correlate with BMI.
   2. **Heart failure**
      a. Excess adipose tissue and increased loading of supporting muscle and bone **elevate metabolic demand.**
      b. Circulating blood volume and cardiac output increase to meet this demand. The increased blood volume results in increased ventricular wall stress, which can eventually lead to left ventricular enlargement and, coupled with hypertension, **left ventricular hypertrophy.**
      c. The resulting systolic and diastolic dysfunction, often in association with ischemic heart disease, can lead to **left ventricular failure.**
      d. Left ventricular failure, combined with chronic hypoxemia and hypercapnia, leads to pulmonary arterial hypertension and **right ventricular failure.**
   3. **Coronary artery disease.** Hypertension, hypercholesterolemia, and type II diabetes mellitus are all significantly correlated with obesity and are all risk factors for the development of atherosclerosis. Obesity is an independent risk factor for coronary artery disease.
   4. **Dysrhythmias.** Hypoxemia, hypercapnia, electrolyte abnormalities, coronary artery disease, increased circulating catecholamines, and heart failure predispose the obese patient cardiac dysrhythmias and sudden cardiac death.
   B. **Respiratory**
   1. **Altered respiratory mechanics**
      a. Obesity is associated with a **decreased compliance of the respiratory system** (see **Chapter 3**). Adipose tissue within the thoracic cage, diaphragm, and abdomen coupled with an exaggerated thoracic kyphosis and lumbar lordosis **decrease the compliance of the chest wall.** Decreased lung volumes, particularly the functional residual capacity (**FRC**), contribute to **decreasing** the **compliance of the lung.**

BMI and Weight Classification

BMI	Classification
18.5–24.9	Healthy weight
25–29.9	Overweight
30–34.9	Class I (moderate) obesity
35–39.9	Class II (severe) obesity
≥40 or 35 with comorbidities	Class III (morbid) obesity

BMI, body mass index.

    b. The obese abdomen restricts diaphragm descent, especially in the supine position. In the supine position, the FRC will decrease further, and may fall within the closing capacity resulting in airway closure, ventilation–perfusion mismatch, and hypoxemia during normal tidal volume ventilation.

2. Gas exchange

    a. Oxygen consumption and carbon dioxide production are increased due to the elevated metabolic demand.

    b. Maintaining eucapnia requires increased minute ventilation and **increased work of breathing.**

    c. Hypoxemia due to ventilation perfusion mismatch, intrapulmonary shunt, and coexisting respiratory disease results in respiratory insufficiency.

3. Obstructive sleep apnea (OSA) and **obesity hypoventilation syndrome (OHS)**

    a. OSA is characterized by frequent episodes of apnea or hypopnea, snoring, excessive daytime somnolence, and psychological changes.

    b. OSA causes hypoxemia and an increase in circulating catecholamines, which lead to **pulmonary** and **systemic hypertension.** The presence of **polycythemia** suggests long-standing hypoxemia.

    c. Patients with suspected OSA should be referred to a sleep specialist for evaluation and polysomnography before elective surgery.

    d. OHS is characterized by *central* (nonobstructive) apneic/hypopneic episodes resulting in sustained hypercarbia and hypoxemia.

    e. Long-standing hypoxemia and hypercarbia from **OSA** and **OHS** can lead to **pulmonary hypertension** and **right ventricular failure.**

C. Other pathophysiologic changes

    1. Gastrointestinal. Obesity is associated with increased gastric volume, diaphragmatic hernia, and gastroesophageal reflux.

    2. Hepatobiliary

        a. Abnormalities in lipid and cholesterol metabolism lead to fatty infiltration of the liver. In some cases, this can lead to cirrhosis, liver failure, or hepatocellular carcinoma.

        b. Cholelithiasis is common and found in up to 27% preoperatively. Up to 41% of gastric bypass patients will need cholecystectomy.

    3. Renal. Increased circulating blood volume and cardiac output results in an increased glomerular filtration rate. This, in addition to other comorbidities such as hypertension and type II diabetes mellitus can lead to chronic renal insufficiency and failure.

    4. Hematologic

        a. Obesity is associated with a **hypercoagulable state** and impaired fibrinolysis.

TABLE 42-2	Major Organ-System Derangements in Obesity
Organ System	**Pathology**
Respiratory	↓ FRC, TLC, VC, IC, ERV ↑ FEV$_1$/FVC Obstructive sleep apnea
Cardiovascular	↑ Blood volume ↑ Vascular tone ↓ Ventricular contractility
Renal	↑ Clearance of renally excreted drugs Hypertensive, diabetic nephropathy
Hematologic	↑ Fibrinogen ↑ PAI-1 ↓ AT-III Venous stasis
Gastrointestinal	Hiatal hernia ↑ Gastric secretion volume ↓ Gastric pH
Metabolic/endocrine	↑ Resting energy expenditure Insulin resistance ↑ Proteolysis
Immunologic	↑ IL-6 Impaired neutrophil function

↑, increased; ↓, decreased; AT-III, antithrombin III; ERV, expiratory reserve volume; FEV$_1$/FVC, ratio of forced expiratory volume in 1 second to forced vital capacity; FRC, functional residual capacity; IC, inspiratory capacity; IL-6, interleukin-6; PAI-1, plasminogen activator inhibitor; TLC, total lung capacity; VC, vital capacity.
From Pieracci FFM, Barie PS, Pomp A. Critical care of the bariatric patient. *Crit Care Med* 2006;34(6)1796–1804.

  b. Vena caval compression and immobility lead to venous engorgement and stasis.
  c. These changes increase the risk of **deep venous thrombosis (DVT)** and **thromboembolism** in the obese.
 5. Endocrine. Obesity is associated with hyperglycemia, insulin resistance, and hyperinsulinemia resulting in **type II diabetes** mellitus.
 6. Metabolic syndrome
  a. The metabolic syndrome is defined by the presence of three or more of abdominal obesity, high triglyceride level, low HDL cholesterol level, hypertension, and/or high fasting plasma glucose level. The incidence increases with waist circumference and BMI.
  b. This cluster of coronary artery disease risk factors has in common insulin resistance and is likely due to obesity and/or an inherited genetic defect.
 7. Immunologic. Adipose tissue is metabolically active and secretes cytokines and hormones. **Inflammatory cytokines** such as tumor necrosis factor-α and interleukin-6 and markers of inflammation such as C-reactive protein are produced by adipose tissue.
 8. Integument. Intertriginous dermatitis is common.
 9. Psychobehavioral. Depression and poor self-esteem.

IV. **Management of the obese patient** in the critical care setting can be challenging due to technical difficulties encountered, pre-existing comorbidities, as well as biases of clinicians and other providers who care for these patients.
   A. **Airway management**
      1. **High Mallampati** score and **large neck circumference** predict difficulty with laryngoscopy and intubation. Obesity and BMI per se are not predictive of a difficult intubation.
      2. Redundant soft tissue can compromise **mask ventilation**.
      3. Proper positioning is critical to securing an airway.
         a. Placing a person in sniff position by using bolsters to "ramp" the patient's head, neck, and shoulders can improve the view of the glottic opening during intubation.
         b. Using a short handle can minimize contact with the patient's chest.
         c. **Preoxygenation** with the patient in a 25° head-up position increases FRC and allows a longer time to desaturation.
      4. Because of the above challenges, many anesthesiologists may choose a **rapid sequence** or even an awake intubation.
   B. **Respiratory failure**
      1. Hospitalized obese patients are at increased risk of developing respiratory complications. Postoperative pulmonary complications are twice as likely in the obese patients.
      2. **Mechanical ventilation**
         a. To avoid lung injury during mechanical ventilation, initial **tidal volumes** should be based on ideal body weight instead of actual body weight. Tidal volumes can then be adjusted aiming for a reasonable inspiratory pressure limit (keeping in mind decreased chest wall compliance) and $Paco_2$.
         b. **Positive end-expiratory pressure** (**PEEP**) should be used to prevent airway closure, atelectasis, and shunt.
         c. In patients with OHS and pulmonary hypertension with RV dysfunction, the increased intrathoracic pressure and pulmonary vascular resistance from intubation and mechanical ventilation can lead to **systemic hypotension**.
         d. Anesthesia can blunt the response to chronic hypoxic vasoconstriction, which can increase the intrapulmonary shunt fraction and worsen hypoxemia.
      3. **Noninvasive ventilation** (NIV) can be considered for patients with potentially reversible causes of respiratory failure (e.g., cardiogenic pulmonary edema or narcotic overdose). NIV has been shown to be safe in the postoperative gastric bypass patient.
         a. Patients must be observed closely for failure of NIV. Intubation should be planned for patients who do not demonstrate early improvements in respiratory rate, pH, Pao_2, and $Paco_2$.
         b. Patients with OSA/OHS are encouraged to bring their CPAP or BiPAP machine from home for increased comfort, decreased anxiety, and improved ventilation.
      4. **Weaning from mechanical ventilation** (**Chapter 23**) may be difficult due to lack of pulmonary reserve and respiratory drive. **Tracheostomy** should be considered early, to enhance comfort and possibly decrease the level of support.
         a. Tracheostomy may be technically difficult due to the increased amount of pretracheal tissue and anatomical distortions. **Custom-made tracheostomy tubes** may be necessary in patients with particularly pronounced excess tissue in the neck. A tracheostomy tube with an adjustable flange (e.g., Rusch, Bivona) may be used temporarily.

     b. Morbid obesity is associated with an increased risk of tracheostomy-related **complications** including tube obstruction and malposition.

C. Hemodynamic monitoring. Due to pre-existing cardiovascular comorbidities, the critically ill obese patient is often a candidate for invasive hemodynamic monitoring.

    1. An **arterial catheter** provides more reliable blood pressure measurement due to the difficulty in obtaining an optimal fit with the noninvasive blood pressure cuff.

    2. Central venous and **pulmonary artery catheterization** may aid in evaluation of volume status and cardiac function in the setting of pre-existing cardiovascular abnormalities (increased intravascular volume, hypertension, heart failure, ischemic heart disease, etc) and renal insufficiency.

D. Vascular access

    1. Excessive subcutaneous tissue may obscure landmarks and make access technically difficult. **Ultrasound guidance** may be helpful in identifying blood vessels.

    2. Intertriginous dermatitis in the femoral crease may preclude placement of femoral venous and arterial catheters.

E. Sedation and analgesia

    1. Respiratory depression is an important concern in the obese, especially in those with pre-existing OSA or OHS whose respiratory drive may already be compromised.

    2. Opiates should be given **intravenously** and not intramuscularly or subcutaneously, as these routes may result in unreliable plasma levels. **Patient-controlled analgesia** with initial doses based on ideal body weight and carefully titrated thereafter should be chosen.

    3. Epidural infusion of an opiate and local anesthetic may provide effective analgesia.

        a. Epidural placement may be technically challenging due to obscurity of the usual bony landmarks as well as difficulty in placing the patient in the optimal position.

        b. Catheter maintenance in the epidural space may also prove difficult due to the thick layer of subcutaneous tissue between the point of surface and ligament contact.

        c. Local anesthetic volume should be reduced by 20% to 25% as the volume of the epidural space is reduced by fatty infiltration and venous engorgement from increased intra-abdominal pressure.

        d. Analgesic adjuncts such as **nonsteroidal anti-inflammatory** agents, **ketamine,** or α-2 adrenergic agonists such as **clonidine** and **dexmedetomidine** should be utilized unless contraindicated.

F. Pharmacology (also see **Appendix**)

    1. Little information exists regarding the **pharmacokinetics** and **pharmacodynamics** of drugs in obese individuals. Alteration in distribution, binding, and elimination necessitates titration of dose based on clinical endpoints and serum concentrations as opposed to weight.

    2. Obesity decreases the enzymatic activity of **cytochrome P-450.** Steatosis and/or biliary dysfunction may decrease hepatic metabolism and clearance.

    3. Increased circulating blood volume increases the initial **volume of distribution** for a given drug.

    4. Renal clearance may be decreased by chronic renal insufficiency in the presence of congestive heart failure or atherosclerotic vascular disease.

    5. Plasma protein binding is affected by increased concentrations of α-1 acid glycoprotein and hyperlipidemia.

6. **Drug dosing** is complicated. Some suggest dosing drugs based on ideal body weight or ideal body weight plus some fraction of the difference between total body weight and ideal body weight.

7. A **sensible approach** is to use short-acting, readily titratable drugs such as propofol and fentanyl and muscle relaxants with predictable kinetics such as cisatracurium.

8. **Specific drugs**
   a. **Succinylcholine** dosing should be based on total body weight when used for rapid sequence induction.
   b. The volume of distribution of certain **antibiotics,** such as **vancomycin,** correlates with total body weight and thus should be dosed accordingly. **Fluoroquinolones** and **aminoglycosides** should be based on adjusted body weight.
   c. **Sedatives** may have a prolonged effect in the obese patient.
      (1) **Midazolam** has a prolonged effect due to accumulation in adipose tissue and inhibition of cytochrome P-450 by other drugs and/or obesity.
      (2) **Fentanyl,** but not morphine, shows a cumulative effect after prolonged use in the obese.
   d. Drugs with narrow **therapeutic indices** such as **aminophylline, aminoglycosides,** and **digoxin** may become toxic if dosed based on weight.

G. **Wound infection** is twice as common in the obese due to several factors. The thick, hypovascular adipose layer provides a rich **substrate for bacterial growth.** Hyperglycemia as well as chronic inflammation lead to impaired neutrophil migration and activation.

H. **Integument**
   1. **Thorough assessment and monitoring** of skin integrity is a must in the obese.
   2. Multiple deep skin folds harbor moisture and bacteria, and are commonly infected with fungus. Frequent washing with thorough drying and application of an antifungal powder may prevent skin-related complications.
   3. Large, open wounds are effectively treated with **vacuum-assisted closure.**
   4. **Mobilization** of the patient is critical to prevent skin breakdown and decrease risk of DVT. Special equipment may be required, including beds, lifts, and a dedicated "lift team."

I. **DVT prophylaxis** should be started preoperatively and continued until the patient is ambulatory with **low-molecular-weight heparin** and serial compression devices. The use of subcutaneous **enoxaparin** 40 mg twice daily is most extensively studied in the bariatric surgical population and is preferred. Placement of an inferior vena cava filter should be considered when anticoagulation is contraindicated, but its value as an adjunct to standard prophylaxis is not proven at this time.

J. **Nutrition**
   1. During periods of metabolic stress, the obese are unable to mobilize their fat stores. Reliance on carbohydrates to fuel gluconeogenesis accelerates protein catabolism and increases the risk of **protein malnutrition.**
   2. **Nutritional support** in the form of enteral or parenteral nutrition in the critically ill obese is a necessity.
   3. Nitrogen balance should be maintained by providing 1.5 to 2.0 g/kg of ideal body weight of protein.
   4. **Indirect calorimetry** is the only validated method to measure the energy expenditures in the obese patient and should be used if possible.
   5. Most enteral feeding regimens recommend patients receive 20 to 30 kcal/kg of ideal body weight per day; however, the use of weight-based

protocols may lead to overfeeding the obese patient. Recent studies employing **hypocaloric, high-protein** feeds suggest improved outcomes in the critically ill obese and may become more prevalent in the future.

6. The Roux-en-Y gastric bypass procedure typically does not lead to malnutrition. However, other malabsorptive procedures may lead to bacterial overgrowth and protein calorie malnutrition.

7. Steatorrhea may cause a **fat-soluble vitamin deficiency.**

8. Gastrectomy may lead to an **acquired intrinsic factor/B$_{12}$ deficiency** and iron deficiency anemia.

K. **Elimination**

1. A **Foley catheter** should be placed until the patient can control micturition.

2. **Fecal incontinence** appliances often fail to fit properly, which may lead to soiling and infection. Rectal tubes are an option but may cause rectal necrosis. When used, the balloon should be deflated every 2 hours for 15 minutes.

L. **Equipment.** The standard ICU bed may not be adequate for the obese patient. **Special bariatric beds** are available with an 850-lb weight limit, a low air loss treatment surface, built-in scale, chair egress, rotational therapy, and percussion option.

M. **Outcomes.** The influence of obesity on outcomes among critically ill patients remains controversial, with some studies suggesting increased mortality and other studies showing either a decrease or no association. The most likely reason for the conflicting data is that these studies represent a heterogeneous patient population with multiple different etiologies of critical illness.

1. The **relationship between BMI** and **mortality** is best described with a U-shaped curve (**Fig. 42-1**). The highest odds of mortality occur at the lowest BMIs and decline to a minimum between BMIs of 35 to 40. Mortality increases thereafter with higher BMIs.

2. Obese patients undergo a longer **duration of mechanical ventilation** when compared to nonobese patients.

3. Obese patients have longer ICU **length of stay** when compared to nonobese patients.

4. **Complications** such as respiratory failure, pneumonia, urinary tract infections, and decubitus ulcers are more common in obese patients. Patients with BMI >40 have twice the number of complications when compared to patients with BMI <25.

V. **Bariatric surgery.** Surgical treatment for obesity is the most effective treatment for weight loss.

A. **Indications** include BMI ≥40 or >35 with serious coexisting conditions, failure of nonsurgical attempts at weight loss, absence of endocrine disorders that cause obesity, and psychological stability.

B. **Surgical approach.** Several types of bariatric surgery exist including gastric restrictive (stapled gastroplasty, gastric banding, and Roux-en-Y gastric bypass) and malabsorptive (biliopancreatic bypass) operations (**Fig. 42-2**).

1. **Gastric bypass** is associated with 60% to 70% of extra body weigh loss and >70% of control of comorbidities. Thus, it is currently the most commonly performed type of bariatric surgery in the United States, accounting for 80% to 90% of all weight loss procedures. Currently, 70% of the Roux-en-Y gastric bypass procedures are done laparoscopically.

2. The **complication rate** associated with laparoscopic gastric bypass (LGB) is lower than open gastric bypass (OGB). LGB is associated with

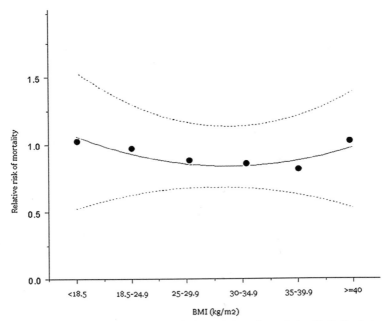

FIGURE 42-1 U-shaped correlation between body mass index and mortality in critically ill patients. From Akinnusi MA et al. *Crit Care Med* 2008; *reproduced with permission.*

lower rates of pulmonary complications, pulmonary embolus, wound infection, incisional hernia, and perioperative mortality. However, LGB is associated with higher rates of bowel obstruction, intestinal hemorrhage, and stomal stenosis when compared to OGB.

   3. Laparoscopic **adjustable gastric banding** is more popular outside the United States because its use in the United States was not approved until 2001. It is associated with less weight loss and less improvement of comorbidities when compared with gastric bypass procedures. However, it is also associated with a lower mortality and complication rate when compared to gastric bypass.

   C. The **benefits** of bariatric surgery include improved quality of life as well as reduction in obesity-related comorbidities.

   1. Diabetes resolves in 77% of patients and improves in up to 86% of patients.

   2. Hyperlipidemia resolves or improves in up to 70% of patients.

   3. Hypertension resolves in 66% and improves in up to 79% of patients.

   4. OSA resolves in up to 86% of patients.

   D. Complications

   1. The risk of **DVT** and **PE** in the obese patient having nonmalignant abdominal surgery is twice that of the lean patient.

   2. Obese patients are at risk of postoperative **respiratory failure** due to underlying OSA, and OHS, as well as postoperative respiratory muscle insufficiency, splinting, and atelectasis.

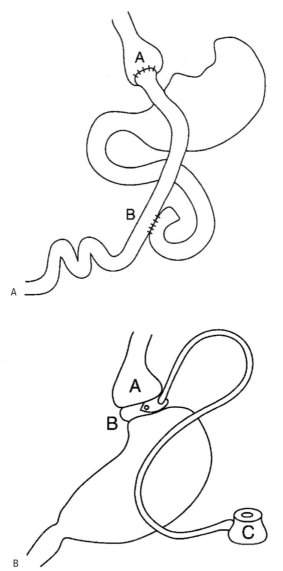

FIGURE 42-2 A: Types of bariatric surgery. Roux-en-Y gastric bypass. A 15- to 30-mL gastric pouch is formed and anastomosed to the proximal jejunum (A). A jejunojejunostomy is formed distally (B). **B:** Adjustable gastric banding. An adjustable, inflatable band (B) is placed around the proximal stomach (A) to limit oral intake. Saline is injected or removed through a needle port (C) to vary the size of the band. From Ogunnaike BO, Jones SB, Jones DB, Provost D, Whitten CW. Anesthetic considerations for bariatric surgery. *Anesth Analg* 2002;95:1793–1805.

3. Poor **wound healing** in the obese leads to anastomotic breakdown and gastrointestinal leaks, stomal stenosis and/or obstruction, and bleeding.
   a. **Anastomotic leak** complicates approximately 1% to 2% of cases of bariatric surgery.
   b. The most frequent **perioperative complication** associated with both laparoscopic and OGB is **wound infection**.
   c. The most frequent **late complication** after LGB is anastomotic stomal stenosis and after OGB is incisional hernia.
4. Perioperative **mortality** associated with bariatric surgery is approximately 0.5%.
5. **Risk factors**
   a. The patient's age, degree of obesity, coexisting medical conditions, and type of surgery affect risk of perioperative complications.
   b. Patients with respiratory insufficiency, venous stasis, higher BMI, male sex, diabetes, cardiovascular disease, age >50, or those experiencing intraoperative complications are at higher risk for postoperative complications and should be considered for triage to an ICU.

Selected References

Akinnusi ME, Pineda LA, El Solh AA. Effect of obesity on intensive care morbidity and mortality: a meta analysis. *Crit Care Med* 2008;36:151–158.

Buchwald H, Avidor Y, Braunwald E, et al. Bariatric surgery: a systematic review and meta-analysis. *JAMA* 2004;292(14):1724–1737.

Dixon BJ, Dixon, JB, Carden JR, et al. Preoxygenation is more effective in the 25° head-up position than in the supine position in severely obese patients. *Anesthesiology* 2005;102 (6):1110–1115.

Hall JE, Crook ED, Jones DW, et al. Mechanisms of obesity-associated cardiovascular and renal disease. *Am J Med Sci* 2002;324:127–137.

Koenig SM. Pulmonary complications of obesity. *Am J Med Sci* 2001;321:249–279.

Goodman LD, Patel M, et al. Critical care of the obese and bariatric surgical patient. *Crit Care Clin* 2003;19:11–32.

Maggard MA, Shugarman LR, Suttorp M, et al. Meta-analysis: surgical treatment of obesity. *Ann Intern Med* 2005;142(7):547–559.

Nasraway SA Jr, Hudson-Jinks TM, Kelleher RM. Multidisciplinary care of the obese patient with chronic critical illness after surgery. *Crit Care Clin* 2002;18:643–657.

Newell MA et al. Body mass index and outcomes in critically injured blunt trauma patients: weighing the impact. *J Am Coll Surg* 2007;204:1056–1064.

O'Brien JM, Phillips GS, Ali NA, et al. Body mass index is independently associated with hospital mortality in mechanically ventilated adults with acute lung injury. *Crit Care Med* 2006;34:738–744.

Pieracci FFM, Barie PS, Pomp A. Critical care of the bariatric patient. *Crit Care Med* 2006; 34(6):1796–1804.

Stelfox HT et al. Hemodynamic monitoring in obese patients: the impact of body mass index on cardiac output and stroke volume. *Crit Care Med* 2006;34(4):1243–1246.

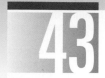

The Intensivist Outside the ICU

Edward George and Edward Bittner

The role of intensivists is increasing outside of the ICU. This is related to an increasing number and acuity of patients, and the unique skills that intensivists possess. There is increasing interest in identifying patients prior to clinical deterioration requiring ICU care, optimizing utilization of critical care resources through appropriate triage, and following up of patients after ICU discharge to reduce ICU readmission.

I. **Overview.** Critically ill patients routinely receive care in the setting of an ICU, where specialized equipment and staff facilitate high-intensity monitoring and implement a complex plan of care. However, critically ill patients may also be encountered in several settings outside of the traditional ICU.

A. **The emergency department (ED)** is a common site where critically ill patients can be encountered. While it is common for critically ill patients to be transferred between institutions directly to an ICU, it is not uncommon for patients to present to the ED in distress and experience a rapid clinical deterioration requiring the initiation of critical care. Most commonly requiring ventilatory and/or hemodynamic support, these patients may require more specialized care (e.g., neurologic ICU for stroke intervention). EDs are generally staffed and equipped to provide short-term critical care while preparing transfer to an ICU setting. However there are often delays in transferring these patients from the ED to an appropriate ICU. Delays may be due to bed unavailability, the need for additional studies (x-ray, CT, vascular studies, etc), or clinical instability. Many institutions benefit from a close relationship between ED and ICU staff. An intensivist can be engaged, either remotely (phone, computer, etc) or at the bedside, to assist in the care of the patient while awaiting transfer to an ICU.

B. **Specialized assets as a function of institution.** While utilization of the specialized skills and training of an intensivist outside of the ICU offers many advantages, several issues may impact the scope and range of this capability. A large academic medical center may have a sufficient cadre of intensivists to provide round-the-clock in-house coverage; however, smaller or more specialized hospitals may only have a single ICU and a limited number of intensivists, or may staff the ICU with physicians without specific training in critical care medicine. Thus, the ability to provide the benefit of an intensivist's expertise may be limited by time of day or on-site versus remote access.

C. **Benefit of intensivist-directed care.** Literature suggests that an intensivist-led multidisciplinary care team managing or comanaging patient care in an ICU results in optimal care of the critically ill. The intensivist model appears to be beneficial over a wide range of institution types and sizes. The ability to provide intensivist-directed care to the critically ill has been shown to reduce morbidity and mortality.

D. **Joint Commission guidelines.** The Joint Commission in 2007 has suggested that institutions develop the capability to immediately respond to key indicators suggestive of deterioration in a patient's clinical condition, with the expectation that earlier intervention may prevent further deterioration. This concept, already established in a wide range of institutions, is most commonly referred to as a **rapid response team (RRT)**. The composition of such a team is variable and may be limited by available assets. Involvement by critical care physicians in RRTs offers the ability to apply key expertise to patient care outside of the ICU in a more timely and efficacious manner.

II. Roles of the intensivist outside of the ICU
A. Clinical
1. **Management of patients in the postanesthesia care unit (PACU) and step-down units.** Institutions are increasingly utilizing PACU facilities as short-term ICUs for postoperative patients. In such settings, a surgical intensivist provides immediate oversight of such patients. Additionally, with the advent of dedicated step-down units for patients with chronic respiratory issues, the intensivist is able to offer the insight of a clinician accustomed to the requirements of the ventilator-dependent patient.

    The nature of procedures admitted to overnight coverage in the PACU is variable. Virtually, all surgical services have patients requiring a predictably brief course of critical care. In the PACU these patients remain closely monitored and are routinely transferred to a general care surgical service on the first postoperative day.

2. **Triage.** Ideally, patients would be admitted or discharged strictly on their potential to benefit from ICU care. However, the number of potential ICU patients can exceed the available beds, and a method of prioritizing or triaging is necessary. The need for triage is minimized when ICU admissions are rigorously screened, and evaluation for discharge is ongoing.

    a. **Admission.** A variety of models have been proposed for facilitating triage decisions for the ICU (**Figure 43-1**).

        (1) A **prioritization** model defines those patients that will most benefit from ICU care (Priority 1) to those that will not benefit at all (Priority 4).

        (2) A **diagnosis** model uses specific conditions or diseases to determine appropriateness of ICU admission.

        (3) An **objective parameters** model uses objective parameters such as vital signs, laboratory values, radiological and other testing results that are consistent with severity of illness for assessing the necessity of ICU resources.

    b. **Discharge.** The status of patients admitted to the ICU should be examined regularly to identify patients who may no longer require ICU level of care. Discharge is appropriate when

        (1) Patient's physiologic status has stabilized, and the need for ICU monitoring and care is no longer necessary.

        (2) When a patient's physiologic status has deteriorated and active interventions are no longer planned.

3. **Rapid response team (RRT)**

    a. **An RRT** is a group of clinicians who bring critical care expertise to the patient's bedside (or wherever is needed). The team assists in assessing and stabilizing the patient's condition and organizing information to be communicated to the patient's physician. The RRT can also serve as an educational asset for the institution.

  b. **Goal/function/benefit.** Studies suggest that patients frequently display clinical signs of deterioration as much as 8 to 12 hours before a cardiac arrest or other critical event requiring some form of urgent/emergent intervention. Early recognition of these indicators followed by prompt treatment may reduce morbidity and mortality and also decrease hospital resource utilization. Other potential benefits of an RRT include improved relationships between staff, increased staff satisfaction, and decreased health care costs.

  c. **Criteria/mechanism for activation.** Each organization should determine which criteria are used to call the RTT. Triggers for activation are typically based on physiologic parameters (**Table 43-1**).

  d. **Situation-Background-Assessment-Recommendation (SBAR).** The SBAR format provides a reliable framework for communication between members of the health care team about a patient's condition. A standardized approach to information sharing is important to ensure that patient information is consistently and accurately imparted. This is essential during critical events, handoffs, or patient transfers.

  (1) **(S) Situation:** What is happening at the present time?
    Identify self, the patient, patient location, briefly state the problem, when it happened or started, and the severity.

  (2) **(B) Background:** What are the circumstances leading up to this situation? Admitting diagnosis and date of admission, list of current medications, allergies, IV fluids, most recent vital signs, laboratory results, and other clinical information including code status.

  (3) **(A) Assessment:** What do I think the problem is?

  (4) **(R) Recommendation:** What should we do to correct the problem?

  e. **Roles of the RRT**

  (1) **Assess.** Initial assessment may often be at the level of the "ABCs" of basic life support. The RRT may be summoned to assist in the care of a patient experiencing a gradual clinical deterioration over hours (or days) or may be urgently called to care for a patient experiencing an acute change (i.e., shortness of breath, mental status change, etc). The ability to quickly assess the situation and plan/initiate corrective action(s) offers the potential to avoid further decline in clinical status. Members of the RRT may offer expertise gained from special training, such as the Society for

TABLE 43-1	Example of Rapid Response Team Calling Criteria
Physiologic Measure	**Parameter**
Heart rate	<40 or >130 bpm
Systolic blood pressure	<90 mm Hg
Respiratory rate	<8 or >28/min or threatened airway
Oxygen saturation	<90% despite oxygen administration
Conscious state	Any deterioration
Urine output	<50 mL in 4 h
Staff concern	Any concern about the patient

Critical Care Medicine's **Fundamentals of Critical Care Support Course (FCCS)**.

(2) **Stabilize.** In the setting of a patient experiencing a clinical deterioration, the RRT offers the capability of a coordinated resource, providing additional expertise in the care of the unstable/ critically ill patient.

(3) **Communicate.** The RRT can facilitate the communication of key clinical information to coordinate with personnel not present at the bedside.

(4) **Educate and support.** Given their specialized education and training, RRT personnel and support structures can be utilized as a training resource. In their role as educators, the RRT members have the unique opportunity to educate the non-ICU staff at the time of the call, in patient assessment and stabilization strategies. In addition, the RRT can serve as educators for other acute care courses, such as BLS and ACLS.

(5) **Transfer.** The goal of the RRT is to provide additional expertise and resources to the care of a clinically deteriorating patient, with the goal of preventing further decompensation. However, additional care for the patient may necessitate transfer to a different facility within the institution (intensive care unit, step-down unit, operating room, etc) or transfer to an outside facility.

f. **Structure of the RRT.** Multiple models have been implemented successfully. Key characteristics of team members should include

(1) Availability to respond immediately without being constrained by competing responsibilities.

(2) Be on-site and accessible.

(3) Must have critical care skills necessary to appropriately assess and initiate therapy as required.

(4) Established clinical role(s) in the institution to facilitate collaboration.

g. **Documentation.** A structured documentation form should be completed for each call to the RRT (**Fig. 43-1**). The form captures information on reasons for the RRT request and types of interventions required. In addition, the form can be used to organize information about the patient's condition prior to calling the primary physician, and is a record of therapeutic interventions performed.

h. **Feedback mechanism.** A mechanism for incident debriefing is critical to the function of any team charged with response to an urgent/ emergent clinical situation. The debriefing must be conducted in a nonattributable manner and must be as proximal to the event as possible. All personnel must be engaged and leadership must identify and critique in a nonpunitive manner any perceived areas of compromise (as well as demonstrated strengths). Suggested guidelines for critical incident debriefing are shown in **Table 43-2**.

i. **Effectiveness.** Three key metrics are suggested to evaluate the effectiveness of the RRT:

(1) Codes per 1000 discharges.

(2) Codes outside of the ICU.

(3) Utilization of the RRT.

   i. Secondary measures can involve assessment of staff satisfaction with the RRT, survival to discharge, and safety culture survey data.

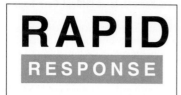

DATA COLLECTION

Your Name: _____ o Senior Resident o Clinical Supervisor o Respiratory

Date: ___/___/___ Time Paged: _____ Time Arrived: _____ Time Ended: _____

Who activated the Rapid Response Team? _____

o Medical o Surgical o Neuro o Other: _____

Urgency: o urgent (intervention within hours to prevent adverse event)
o Life-threatening (immediate intervention to avoid death)
Clinicians present:
 Intern/Junior Resident o yes o no Bedside Nurse o yes o no
 Critical care: o yes o no Other Staff (specify) _____

Trigger: (check all that apply)

Cardiac:
❑ Bradycardia
❑ Tachycardia
❑ Hypotension
❑ Hypertension
❑ Chest pain unresponsive to NTG

Respiratory:
❑ Respiratory Depression
❑ Tachypnea
❑ New onset of difficulty breathing
❑ BiPAP/CPAP with no improvement
❑ Bleeding into airway
❑ Oxygen saturation <90%

Medical:
❑ Urine output <50 mL for 4 hours

❑ Uncontrolled bleeding

Neurological:
❑ Mental status change
❑ Acute Loss of Consciousness
❑ Seizure
❑ Suspected acute stroke
❑ Unexplained agitation or delirium

Other:
❑ Pain
❑ "I am very concerned"
❑ > 1 stat page
❑ Other: _____

Response to this call:
 o Code called
 o Physician called (specify): _____
 o Other person called (specify): _____
 o Follow-up needed: _____

Disposition:
 o Remained on unit
 o Expired
 o Transfer to: _____
 o Other: _____

Brief description of call:

FIGURE 43-1 Structured documentation form used by the MGH rapid response team.

4. **Emergency department (including trauma team).** In the setting of a critically ill patient arriving in the ED, the intensivist may be called upon to assist in guiding initial therapy and performance of invasive procedures such as central line placement and airway management (**Table 43-3**). With participation in the implementation of goal-directed therapies, the intensivist can provide continuity of care as the patient is transferred to an ICU. In the context of a trauma team, the intensivist may assist with initial management, coordination of transport, and act as an additional resource in multiple trauma situations.

5. **Code team.** Oversight of the code team is often the responsibility of an intensivist. Whether providing team training, overseeing team design and coordination, or directly participating as the code team leader,

TABLE 43-2	Guidelines for critical incident debriefing	
Action	**Goal**	**Result**
Orientation	Introduce the concept of debriefing	Personnel appreciate the needs and benefits of debriefing
Situation	Description of events	Opportunity for a brief incident review to include solicitation of differing perceptions
Execution	How the event was conducted	Qualitative and quantitative description of activities
Analysis	Describe strengths and weaknesses of team	Opportunity for open critique without fear of retribution
Closure	Summation of events to include any needed follow- up	Empowers the team in a manner to promote efficiency, growth, and satisfaction of service

intensivists are involved in code teams. Code situations can be chaotic and often suffer from either an absence of clear leadership or competing perspectives from the responders. In this setting, the intensivist can establish appropriate control and either serve as the team leader or facilitate the function of the team leader.

6. **Invasive procedures outside of the ICU.** The capability to perform invasive procedures at the bedside is often a function of physician experience and support capabilities. Many physicians do not perform a sufficient number of specialized procedures, such as central line placement, to maintain competency. The involvement of an intensivist to perform or supervise such procedures at the bedside provides an added measure of safety and the enrichment of a training program.

7. **ICU patients follow-up.** Patients are at increased risk of deterioration after discharge from the ICU. This can be the result of premature discharge and/or residual organ dysfunction. Both can lead to readmission, which is associated with higher in-hospital mortality. The introduction of a follow-up service has been shown to reduce post-ICU deaths and may reduce the number of readmissions to the ICU. In addition, follow-up of patients discharged from the ICU has been recommended as a means of service evaluation. Without benefit of follow-up data, ICU staff can only

TABLE 43-3	Most Common Interventions Performed by Critical Care Outreach Team

Guiding tracheostomy management
Performing tracheal suction and chest physiotherapy
Guiding management of CPAP
Optimizing patient position
Administration of nebulizer treatment
Requesting repeat blood tests
Increasing the frequency of CVS/respiratory observations
Starting hourly fluid balance monitoring
Requesting samples be sent for microculture and sensitivity

CPAP, continuous positive airway pressure; CVS, cardiovascular system.

utilize mortality or hospital discharge information as clinical outcomes on which to judge practice performance. Knowledge of common physical and psychological problems that patients experience after ICU discharge and implementation of treatment to address these issues may play a role in preventing ICU readmission, decreasing mortality, and increasing quality of life (**Table 43-4**).

8. **ICU telemedicine.** Telemedicine involves the use of electronic information and communications technologies to provide and support health care workers when distance separates the participants (**Fig. 43-2**). Rationale for the use of telemedicine technologies in the ICU include
   a. Achieving "**24 hour/7 days a week**" ICU physician coverage for providing optimal care. Most hospitals have been unable to implement this level of service because of a national shortage of intensivists and the high cost of providing full-time coverage.
   b. Improving the effectiveness of patient care by automating the collection, evaluation, and presentation of large volumes of clinical data generated in modern ICUs.
   c. Potentially increasing the efficiency of critical care delivery, and partially compensating for the shortage of intensivists.
   d. Staffing with a single intensivist capable of directing and coordinating patient management with on-site health care providers.

B. **Administrative**
   1. **Departmental.** Intensivists are commonly engaged in variety of departmental support and oversight roles. Through in participation on committees within an anesthesia department, such as quality assurance, as well as in oversight of assets within the department, such as specialized intraoperative care teams for complex patients and/or those requiring specialized invasive monitoring requiring

	Common Physical and Psychological Problems of Patients after Discharge from the ICU
TABLE 43-4	

Physical Disorders

Muscle wasting, fatigue, and weakness including reduced cough and pharyngeal weakness
Joint stiffness
Numbness, paresthesia (peripheral neuropathy)
Taste changes, poor appetite
Sleep disturbances
Cardiac decompensation: postural hypotension
Reduced pulmonary reserve: breathlessness on mild exertion
Recovering organ failure (lung, kidney, liver, etc)
Iatrogenic: tracheal stenosis (from intubation), nerve palsies, scarring

Psychological Disorders

Depression
Impaired memory, concentration
Anxiety, panic attacks
Recurrent nightmares
Posttraumatic stress disorder

Adapted from Broomhead LR, Brett SJ. Clinical review: intensive care follow-up, what has it told us? *Critical Care* 2002;6:411–417 and Griffiths RD, Jones C. ABC of intensive care: recovery from intensive care. *BMJ* 1999;319:427–429.

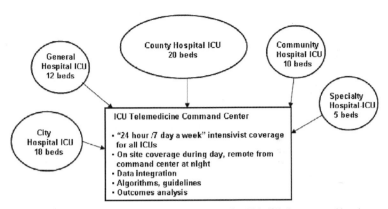

FIGURE 43-2 Example of ICU telemedicine: management of multiple ICUs from a central location.

specialized invasive monitoring, intensivists are called upon to provide guidance for intraoperative care and coordination between the operating room and the ICU.

2. **Institutional.** Assignments for intensivists may vary, in part as a function of the size of the institution. However, in addition to the typical role(s) as a member of a critical care oversight committee for the institution, assignments can include oversight of the institution's emergency response teams, patient safety groups, and institutional review boards.

3. **National.** Opportunities to serve at the national level (e.g., American Society of Critical Care Anesthesiologists, Society of Critical Care Medicine) offer the opportunity to influence the growth of the discipline. Additional service can include involvement at the federal level, such as serving in the National Disaster Medical Teams of the Department of Health and Human Services. Providing advice to the public health sector can influence planning and allocation of resources for critically ill patients in the setting of disasters, epidemics.

APPENDIX 43-1
Models for Facilitating Triage to the ICU

Prioritization Model

Priority 1. Critically ill, unstable patients in need of intensive treatment and monitoring that cannot be provided outside of the ICU. These treatments include ventilator support, vasoactive drug administration, etc. These patients generally have no limits placed on the extent of therapy they are to receive.

Priority 2. The patients require intensive monitoring and may potentially need immediate intervention. No therapeutic limits are generally stipulated for these patients.

Priority 3. These unstable patients are critically ill, but have a reduced likelihood of recovery because of underlying disease or nature of their acute illness. These patients may receive intensive treatment to relieve acute illness, but limits on therapeutic efforts may be set.

Priority 4. These are patients who are generally not appropriate for ICU admission. Admission of these patients should be made on an individual basis at the discretion of the ICU director.

Diagnosis Model

1. **Cardiac disorders.** Acute MI with complications, cardiogenic shock, complex arrhythmias, acute CHF with respiratory failure and/or requiring hemodynamic support, hypertensive emergencies, unstable angina, post-cardiac arrest, cardiac tamponade with instability, dissecting aortic aneurysms.

2. **Pulmonary disorders.** Acute respiratory failure requiring ventilatory support, pulmonary embolism with hemodynamic instability, patients in an intermediate care unit with respiratory deterioration, massive hemoptysis, respiratory failure with imminent intubation.

3. **Neurologic disorders.** Acute stroke with altered mental status, coma, intracranial hemorrhage, acute SAH, meningitis with altered mental status or respiratory compromise, CNS or neuromuscular disorders with deteriorating neurologic or pulmonary function, status epilepticus, brain dead or potentially brain dead patients who are being aggressively managed for organ donation.

4. **Drug ingestion and overdose.** Hemodynamically unstable drug ingestion, significantly altered mental status, inadequate airway protection, seizures following drug ingestion.

5. **Gastrointestinal disorders.** Life-threatening GI bleeding, acute hepatic failure, severe pancreatitis.

6. **Endocrine.** Complicated DKA, thyroid storm or myxedema coma, hyperosmolar state with coma, adrenal crisis, severe hypercalcemia with altered mental status, hypo-/hypernatremia with seizures or altered mental status, hypomagnesemia with hemodynamic compromise/arrhythmias, hypophosphatemia with muscular weakness.

7. **Surgical.** Postoperative patients requiring hemodynamic monitoring/ventilatory support or extensive nursing care.

8. **Miscellaneous.** Septic shock, clinical conditions requiring ICU level nursing care, environmental injuries (lightning, near drowning, hypo-/hyperthermia), new/experimental therapies with potential for complications.

Objective Parameters Model

1. **Vital signs.** HR <40 or >50, SBP <80 or 20% below baseline, MAP <60 mm Hg, DBP >120 mm Hg, RR >35.

2. **Laboratory values.** Serum Na <110 or >170 mEq/L, serum K <2.0 or >7.0, Pao_2 <50, pH <7.1 or >7.7, serum glucose > 800 mg/dL, serum Ca >15 mg/dL, toxic level of drug or substance in a hemodynamically or neurologically compromised patient.

3. **Radiology.** Cerebral hemorrhage, contusion, or SAH with neurologic deficit; ruptured viscera, esophageal varices with hemodynamic instability, dissecting aortic aneurysm.
4. **Electrocardiogram.** MI with complex arrhythmias, hypotension or CHF, sustained ventricular arrhythmia, complete heart block.
5. **Physical findings.** Acute obtundation, anuria, airway obstruction, continuous seizures, cardiac tamponade.

CHF, congestive heart failure; CNS, central nervous system; DBP, diastolic blood pressure; GI, gastrointestinal; HR, heart rate; MAP, mean arterial pressure; MI, myocardial infarction; RR, respiratory rate; SAH, subarachnoid hemorrhage; SBP, systolic blood pressure.
This document is adapted from: Task Force of the American College of Critical Care Medicine, Society of Critical Care Medicine. Guidelines for intensive care unit admission discharge and triage. *Crit Care Med* 1999;27:633–638, Lippincott.

Selected References

Breslow MJ, Rosenfeld BA, Doerfler M, et al. Effect of a multiple-site intensive care unit telemedicine program on clinical and economic outcomes: an alternative paradigm for intensivist staffing. *Crit Care Med* 2004;32:31–38.

Broomhead LR, Brett SJ. Clinical review: intensive care follow-up, what has it told us? *Crit Care* 2002;6:411–417.

Griffiths RD, Jones C. ABC of intensive care: recovery from intensive care. *BMJ* 1999; 319:427–429.

Task Force of the American College of Critical Care Medicine, Society of Critical Care Medicine. Guidelines for intensive care unit admission discharge and triage. *Crit Care Med* 1999;27:633–638.

Joint Commission Practice Guidelines for establishment of a rapid response team. http://jointcommission.org Accessed March 16, 2009.

Leapfrog recommendations for intensivist-managed ICUs. http://www.leapfroggroup.org. Accessed March 16, 2009.

Institute for Healthcare Improvement. Sample Rapid Response Team Education and Training Packet. http://www.ihi.org/IHI/Topics/CriticalCare/IntensiveCare/Tools/SampleRapidResponseTeamEducationandTrainingPacket.htm. Accessed July 17, 2008.

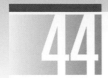

Obstetric Critical Care

Amy Ortman and Richard Pino

I. **Introduction.** The obstetric patient population is in general healthy, but pre-existing comorbid conditions and several pregnancy-related disorders may be associated with significant morbidity and mortality.

II. **Preeclampsia** is part of a spectrum of hypertensive disorders specific to pregnancy. Although the precise etiology of preeclampsia remains unknown, it is a disease which occurs only in the presence of placental tissue. The maternal manifestations are consistent with a process of vasospasm, ischemia, and changes in the normal balance of humoral and autocoid mediators. Preeclampsia is diagnosed in 3% to 5% of all pregnancies in the United States and is most common in nulliparous women. A patient meets the criteria for a diagnosis of preeclampsia if she has persistently elevated blood pressure after 20 weeks' gestation in the setting of previously normal blood pressure, and proteinuria of greater than 300 mg in 24 hours. The diagnosis of preeclampsia is divided into mild and severe based upon the presence or absence of specific signs, symptoms, and abnormal laboratory values (**Table 44-1**).

   A. Two additional diagnoses, **HELLP syndrome** and **eclampsia,** are a part of this spectrum of disease.

      1. **HELLP syndrome** (**H**emolysis, **E**levated **L**iver enzymes, and **L**ow **P**latelets) involves a constellation of laboratory abnormalities, and is generally regarded as a subset of severe preeclampsia. The diagnosis of HELLP syndrome is also associated with an increased risk of adverse outcomes including abruption, renal failure, hepatic subcapsular hematoma formation, liver rupture, and fetal and maternal death.

      2. **Eclampsia** is defined as the occurrence of **seizures** in a woman with preeclampsia that cannot be attributed to other causes. Eclamptic seizures may occur antepartum, intrapartum, or postpartum. Eclampsia is a cause of significant maternal and fetal morbidity, and is present in approximately 50% of maternal deaths associated with preeclampsia.

   B. **Management**

      1. **Delivery.** The only definitive treatment for preeclampsia is delivery of the fetus and placenta. The decision of when to deliver is made based on the gestational age and the severity of the disease. Each patient and clinical situation should be individualized with a management strategy that seeks to balance and minimize both maternal and fetal morbidity.

      2. **Pharmacologic therapy**

         a. **Seizure prophylaxis.** Although the mechanism of action is unknown, **magnesium sulfate** is the medication of choice for prophylactic prevention and treatment of eclamptic seizures. Dosage of magnesium is 4 g intravenous (IV) bolus over 30 minutes followed by 2 g/h IV. The drug is administered during labor, delivery, and for 24 to 48 hours post-delivery. Because of its relaxant effect on vascular and visceral smooth muscle, magnesium may decrease maternal blood pressure and predispose to postpartum atony and hemorrhage.

Diagnostic Criteria for Mild and Severe Preeclampsia

	Mild Preeclampsia	Severe Preeclampsia
Blood pressure	>140/90 but <160/110 mm Hg	>160/110 mm Hg
Proteinuria	0.3–5 g in 24-h urine collection	>5 g in 24-h urine collection
	OR	OR
	1–2+ on urine dip	3–4+ on urine dip
Additional signs or symptoms	None	Persistent headache
		Cerebral or visual disturbances
		Impaired liver function
		Epigastric or RUQ pain
		Thrombocytopenia
		Pulmonary edema or cyanosis
		Fetal growth restriction (IUGR)
		Oliguria <500 mL in 24 h

    b. **Antihypertensive medications** such as **labetalol, hydralazine,** and **calcium channel blockers** are frequently administered for control of blood pressure. The goal is not to normalize blood pressure, but to keep patients from progressing to a hypertensive crisis, encephalopathy, or stroke. When administering antihypertensive medications, it is important to remember that the placenta has no ability to autoregulate flow. Thus, a sudden drop in maternal blood pressure may decrease placental perfusion and result in significant compromise to the fetus.

III. **Acute fatty liver of pregnancy (AFLP)** is a rare but potentially fatal complication of pregnancy involving microvesicular fat deposition in the liver and characterized by liver dysfunction, DIC, hypoglycemia, encephalopathy, and renal insufficiency. Patients usually present in the third trimester although the disease has been described as early as 23 weeks' gestation.
    A. **Pathophysiology.** The precise pathogenesis of AFLP remains unknown, but the disease has been associated with long-chain 3-hydroxyacyl-CoA dehydrogenase (LCHAD) deficiency in the fetus. It is thought that abnormal fatty acid metabolites from a fetus with LCHAD deficiency enter the maternal circulation and overwhelm the maternal mitochondrial oxidation pathway resulting in fatty infiltration and profound liver dysfunction.
    B. **Clinical manifestations.** Patients frequently present with nonspecific symptoms such as malaise, nausea and emesis, jaundice, epigastric or right upper quadrant pain, headache, and anorexia.
    C. **Diagnosis and laboratory findings.** The hallmark laboratory finding of acute fatty liver of pregnancy is **hyperbilirubinemia** with serum levels of 3 to 40 mg/dL reported. Patients also have elevated serum ammonia levels, mild to moderate transaminase elevations, prolonged prothrombin time, profoundly decreased antithrombin III, and hypoglycemia. Proteinuria and hypertension are common findings in AFLP. Less consistent findings include an elevated serum creatinine due to renal insufficiency, and hyponatremia from diabetes insipidus which is present in up to 10% of patients. Liver biopsy is rarely required and should be performed only when absolutely necessary because of the concomitant coagulopathy.

D. Management. The liver dysfunction and failure associated with AFLP is reversible in virtually all patients, and **supportive care** and **delivery** are the mainstays of treatment. AFLP is a medical emergency which requires immediate evaluation. The most important component of treatment is the delivery of the fetus. Supportive measures include careful assessment of fluid status and regular evaluation of electrolytes. **Serum glucose levels** should be checked every 1 to 2 hours and hypoglycemia aggressively treated; all patients should receive an infusion of at least 5% dextrose, and many will require higher concentrations with intermittent boluses to maintain normoglycemia. **Coagulation studies** should be followed at regular intervals and postpartum hemorrhage anticipated. Regardless of the mode of delivery, patients should have adequate IV access and cross-matched blood products available. If the patient requires a cesarean section, attempts should be made to improve or correct the coagulopathy prior to incision.

IV. Neurologic disease
A. Stroke. In pregnancy, the incidence of stroke is estimated at 5 to 15 per 100,000 deliveries with cerebrovascular events accounting for 5% of maternal deaths. A significant proportion of strokes occur late in pregnancy, with the highest incidence in the peripartum period. **Ischemic events** account for one-half to two-thirds of cerebrovascular events in pregnancy, whereas **hemorrhagic strokes** are slightly less common.
   1. **Clinical manifestations.** **Headache** is the most common presenting symptom. Other symptoms include focal neurologic deficits and seizures.
   2. **Diagnosis.** In addition to physical examination, neurologic imaging is critical for establishing the diagnosis and etiology. Attempts should be made to minimize fetal exposure to radiation, but appropriate diagnostic imaging should not be avoided entirely.
   3. **Etiologies.** Cerebral infarctions may be divided into arterial or venous etiologies. **Arterial etiologies** include vasculopathies, dissections, and embolic events; **venous infarctions** may result from hypercoagulable states, dehydration, or infections. **Hemorrhagic events** are largely a result of aneurysms, vascular malformations, preeclampsia, or trauma.
   4. **Management** in the pregnant patient is similar to the treatment of non-pregnant patients. Care is supportive and directed at the underlying etiology. For preservation of fetal well-being, oxygenation, intravascular volume, and normal blood pressure should be maintained, and extreme hypocarbia and maternal seizures avoided. Delivery of the fetus may be complicated by the risk of aneurysm or arteriovenous malformation (AVM) rupture, thrombolytic therapy, or anticoagulation; both the route of delivery and anesthetic management should be tailored to each individual patient.
B. Seizure disorders. Approximately 0.5% of all parturients have a chronic, pre-existing seizure disorder. Half of women with epilepsy will experience little or no change in the frequency of their seizures during pregnancy; of the remaining 50%, most will notice an increase, and the remainder will have a decrease in their seizure frequency. Despite the potential for teratogenic effects, patients should remain on antiseizure medications throughout pregnancy to minimize the risk of uncontrolled seizure activity.
   1. **Status epilepticus** (see also **Chapter 31**). Although the frequency of seizure activity is increased in a significant portion of parturients, pregnancy itself does not increase the likelihood of status epilepticus.

    a. Should status epilepticus occur in a pregnant patient, **treatment goals** include (a) maintaining an adequate airway, (b) ensuring adequate oxygenation, (c) determining the cause of the seizure, and (d) stopping the seizure. The patient should be placed in the lateral position and supplemental oxygen administered.

    b. **Pharmacologic therapy** should be initiated after 2 to 5 minutes of prolonged seizure activity and consists of the same medications used in the nonpregnant population.

    c. For **intractable seizure activity,** electroencephalographic monitoring, suppression of seizure activity with medications, tracheal intubation, and mechanical ventilation may be necessary.

2. **Eclampsia.** The diagnosis of eclampsia should be entertained and ruled out in any pregnant woman who presents with a new-onset seizure disorder after 20 weeks' gestation. Management of eclamptic seizures includes magnesium sulfate and prompt delivery.

V. **Acute respiratory distress syndrome (ARDS,** see **Chapter 20)** is a rare but serious complication in pregnancy and when present, may result in significant maternal and fetal mortality. No large studies are available, but data from the last several decades place maternal mortality rates in the range of 30% to 40% and fetal mortality over 20%.

A. **Risk factors specific to pregnancy** include gastric aspiration, medications used for tocolysis, preeclampsia, amniotic fluid or trophoblastic embolism, and abruption.

B. **Management.** As in the nonpregnant population, the mainstay of treatment is supportive care. However, the following should be considered when managing a pregnant patient with ARDS.

1. **Ventilation.** In animal experiments, permissive hypercapnia with a $Paco_2$ up to 60 mm Hg has not significantly impacted uterine blood flow, but human data are lacking. Maternal oxygen consumption increases in pregnancy by 20% to 30% at term—largely because of increased consumption by the fetus and placenta. To minimize fetal effects, the maternal Pao_2 should be maintained at more than 60 mm Hg.

2. **Maintenance of maternal cardiac output** is critical for placental perfusion and fetal oxygenation. Thus, standard treatments in ARDS therapy such as high levels of PEEP, diuretics, and vasopressors must be weighed against the risk of decreased venous return, decreased cardiac output, and changes in maternal blood flow distribution—all of which may decrease placental perfusion and fetal oxygenation. Additionally, after 20 weeks' gestation, patients should be positioned with uterine displacement or in the lateral position to minimize aortocaval compression.

C. **Obstetric considerations.** Fetal assessment should be performed at regular intervals to evaluate fetal well-being. Patients with ARDS in pregnancy are at increased risk of preterm labor and delivery and should be monitored appropriately. Lastly, some authors suggest that delivery of the preterm fetus after 28 weeks' gestation in patients with ARDS may improve maternal outcome.

VI. **Cardiovascular disorders**

A. **Valvular heart disease** (see also **Chapter 18)**

1. Chronic **regurgitant lesions** are well-tolerated with the normal physiologic changes of pregnancy. A decrease in systemic vascular resistance, reduced left ventricular afterload, and a modest increase in heart rate all lead to a reduction in regurgitation. However, in the immediate postpartum period, the sudden increase in venous return and vascular resistance may lead to decompensation, and patients should be carefully monitored for the first 24 to 48 hours. **Endocarditis prophylaxis** is not recommended in this patient population.

   a. **Aortic regurgitation (AR)** with preserved LV function is well-tolerated in pregnancy. In symptomatic, severe AR, the treatment is **salt restriction, diuretics,** and **digoxin.** Vasodilators such as **hydralazine** and **nitrates** may be used as substitutes to ACE inhibitors, which are contraindicated in pregnancy.

   b. **Mitral regurgitation (MR)** during pregnancy is usually due to rheumatic valvular disease or the myxomatous degeneration of mitral valve prolapse. Patients with MR in pregnancy will rarely become symptomatic, but if decompensation occurs, medical management with **vasodilators** and **diuretics** may be helpful.

   c. As in the nonpregnant population, **acute regurgitant lesions** are poorly tolerated and constitute a medical and surgical emergency.

2. In contrast to regurgitant lesions, **stenotic lesions** are not as well-tolerated in pregnancy. Increased intravascular volume, increased heart rate, and the decreased systemic vascular resistance of pregnancy adversely affect these patients. Known predictors of poor maternal–fetal outcome include prior cardiac event or arrhythmia, impaired left ventricular function, pulmonary hypertension, severe stenotic lesions, and impaired New York Heart Association functional class at the initiation of prenatal care. The autotransfusion and increased venous return associated with delivery may lead to further decompensation, and patients should be closely monitored for the first 24 to 48 hours postpartum. **Endocarditis prophylaxis** is not recommended in patients with stenotic lesions.

   a. **Aortic stenosis (AS)** in pregnant women is usually congenital. Women with mild to moderate disease will tolerate pregnancy provided they are followed closely and managed appropriately. In contrast, women with severe AS are at risk of deterioration with development of heart failure and preterm delivery.

      (1) **Medical management** consists of **diuretics** and **maintenance of sinus rhythm.**

      (2) If possible, patients with severe disease should undergo preconceptual valve replacement or valvuloplasty. In the setting of an established pregnancy, valvuloplasty is the procedure of choice to minimize the risk of fetal loss.

      (3) For delivery, hemodynamic monitoring, early epidural placement, and an assisted second stage are recommended.

   b. **Mitral stenosis (MS)** is the most common acquired valvular lesion in pregnancy. The increased stroke volume and heart rate in the setting of a significantly narrowed valve lead to increased left atrial pressure, arrhythmias, and worsened symptoms.

      (1) Patients contemplating pregnancy with severe stenosis should be offered valvuloplasty or replacement; in patients who are already pregnant, valvuloplasty is preferred.

      (2) Optimal **medical management** of the pregnant patient involves administration of β-**blockers** for reducing heart rate and left atrial pressure. **Diuretics** and **salt restriction** may also be necessary. **Anticoagulation** should be considered in patients with severe MS and an enlarged left atrium, even in the absence of atrial fibrillation.

(3) Hemodynamic monitoring, early epidural anesthesia, and an assisted second stage are recommended for delivery. Patients with MS are particularly vulnerable to failure following delivery, and diuretics may be necessary to prevent failure.

   c. Isolated **pulmonic stenosis (PS)**, even when severe, is well-tolerated in pregnancy. In symptomatic patients, balloon valvuloplasty is a treatment option.

3. Prosthetic cardiac valves are associated with additional risks during pregnancy. Despite the replacement of a malfunctioning valve, some degree of myocardial, valvular, or pulmonary dysfunction usually persists.

   a. Anticoagulation. Thromboembolic events are of particular concern in pregnancy, and all obstetric patients with mechanical valves or bioprosthetic valves in atrial fibrillation should receive anticoagulation. Women with bioprosthetic valves and no risk factors do not require anticoagulation. Anticoagulation in pregnancy is usually accomplished with **unfractionated heparin** or **low-molecular-weight heparin (LMWH)**, although warfarin may be used in particularly high-risk patients prior to 35 weeks' gestation. **Endocarditis prophylaxis** is recommended in this patient population.

B. Congenital heart disease. Pregnant women with a history of repaired congenital disease are becoming increasingly common as more survive to childbearing age, and congenital heart lesions are now the most common cause of cardiac disease in the pregnant population. Many will be **asymptomatic** with relatively normal pressures and flow patterns, and such patients will not require special treatment during pregnancy. However, others will **present with a partially repaired or completely uncorrected lesion,** making management considerably more complex. Known predictors of poor maternal–fetal outcome include the following preconceptual markers: elevated pulmonary artery pressure, depressed right or left ventricular function, cyanosis, and impaired New York Heart Association functional class. **Endocarditis prophylaxis** should be given to patients with unrepaired cyanotic heart disease, repaired disease with residual defects adjacent to prosthetic material, or a repair involving placement of prosthetic material within the previous 6 months.

   1. Left-to-right intracardiac shunting may occur via several common congenital lesions: **atrial septal defect (ASD), ventricular septal defect (VSD),** or a **patent ductus arteriosis.** De-airing of IV lines and injections must be performed in all patients with a shunt as shunt reversal and paradoxical embolism may occur in association with straining at delivery or with the reduction in SVR following regional blockade. Mild degrees of shunting are usually well-tolerated and mortality is rare.

   2. Tetralogy of Fallot is characterized by (1) a VSD, (2) right ventricular hypertrophy, (3) right ventricular outflow tract (RVOT) obstruction, and (4) an aorta that overrides the right and left ventricles. Very few women will survive to childbearing age without surgical correction. Correction typically involves closure of the VSD and widening of the RVOT, and if successful will result in an asymptomatic patient. Even after successful repair, patients remain at risk for development of arrhythmias in pregnancy, and physiologic changes of pregnancy may unmask a small residual VSD. Patients with uncorrected or palliated lesions may develop increased right-to-left shunting, cyanosis, biventricular failure, arrhythmias, and paradoxical emboli. Fetal outcome is closely associated with the development of cyanosis.

3. **Uncorrected coarctation of the aorta** puts patients at risk for left ventricular failure, aortic rupture or dissection, and endocarditis. The coarctation is usually located just distal to the left subclavian artery, and patients will have a gradient between blood pressures measured in the upper and lower limbs. The pathophysiologic manifestations include a fixed obstructive lesion with distal hypoperfusion, and commonly associated comorbidities include a bicuspid aortic valve and cerebral aneurysms. There may be an increased risk of fetal mortality because of decreased uterine perfusion, although the data are mixed. During delivery, intravascular volume should be maintained and blood pressure measurements distal to the constriction should be used to estimate uterine perfusion pressure.

4. **Eisenmenger syndrome** is the result of a chronic, uncorrected left-to-right shunt, which leads to elevated right-sided pressures, ventricular hypertrophy, and eventually a right-to-left shunt. Hemodynamic changes of pregnancy are poorly tolerated, and the maternal mortality rate approaches 50% with an estimated fetal mortality rate of 40%. Pregnancy is thought to be contraindicated and termination is recommended. In patients who elect to continue the pregnancy, limited activity, supplemental oxygen, and prophylactic anticoagulation are recommended. Vaginal delivery is preferred, but few will tolerate labor and cesarean section is common. Arterial pressure and intravascular volume status should be carefully followed. Because increased complications have been reported with the use of pulmonary artery pressure catheters, they are not recommended.

C. **Myocardial infarction** is uncommon in pregnancy with an estimated incidence of 3 to 10 per 100,000 deliveries, and a case fatality rate of 5% to 20%. Possible etiologies include atherosclerotic disease and coronary dissection, vasospasm, or thrombus. Risk factors for MI in pregnancy include advanced maternal age, hypertension, diabetes, thrombophilia, smoking, cocaine abuse, transfusion, and postpartum hemorrhage.

1. The balance between **myocardial oxygen supply and demand** is affected by the physiologic changes of pregnancy leading to an increase in heart rate, contractility, and wall tension. Additionally, labor and delivery are associated with a significant increase in cardiac output, myocardial oxygen consumption, and elevated levels of circulating catecholamines. While pregnancy itself is not thought to be a risk factor for MI, the changes of pregnancy may place high-risk individuals at even greater risk; compared to nonpregnant individuals of the same age, the incidence of MI may be three- to fourfold higher in pregnancy.

2. **Diagnosis.** As in nonpregnant individuals, the diagnosis of MI is made by history, examination, and appropriate diagnostic tests. **Troponins** remain sensitive and specific in the pregnant population. However, in pregnancy, minor electrocardiographic (ECG) changes such as T-wave inversions and ST-segment depressions are common, diminishing specificity of ECG interpretation for ischemia. **Cardiac catheterization** should be considered despite the small risk of ionizing radiation to the fetus; with shielding and limited fluoroscopy, the total radiation dose may be limited to approximately 1 rad, well below the 5 rad teratogenic threshold. Lastly, an echocardiogram may be useful for evaluating ventricular function.

3. **Management** of an acute MI in pregnancy is guided by the same principles as in the nonpregnant population with several important considerations.

a. **Medical management.** β-Blockers and nitrates may be used safely in pregnancy, although hypotension should be avoided. **Low-dose aspirin** has been shown to be safe even with chronic use. Conversely, ACE inhibitors and statins are contraindicated in pregnancy, and both should be avoided.

b. **Anticoagulation** may be safely achieved with **unfractionated heparin** or **LMWH.** There is very limited information about the safety and efficacy of **thrombolytic therapy** in pregnancy; although successful use has been reported, there is an increased risk of puerperal hemorrhage and placental abruption.

c. **Revascularization.** Both **PCI** and **CABG** have been successfully used to treat pregnancy-associated acute MI, and the choice of treatment modality should be individualized to the patient. Pregnancy is not a contraindication to cardiopulmonary bypass and good maternal and fetal outcomes are possible, although fetal loss is estimated to be between 20% and 40%.

d. **Obstetrical management.** The fetus should be carefully monitored and a plan for delivery established in the event of sudden maternal or fetal decompensation.

D. **Peripartum cardiomyopathy (PPCM)** is a rare dilated cardiomyopathy which has an estimated incidence of 1 in 4,000 to 15,000 live births. The etiology remains unclear, although risk factors include multiple gestation, advanced maternal age, obesity, and preeclampsia.

1. **Clinical presentation and diagnosis.** Patients present with symptoms of heart failure such as dyspnea, fatigue, and edema, which may be difficult to distinguish from normal changes in pregnancy. The diagnosis requires echocardiographic evidence of cardiomyopathy and three criteria: (1) onset within a 6-month period, from the last month of pregnancy to 5 months postpartum; (2) no prior history of cardiomyopathy or pre-existing heart failure; and (3) exclusion of all other identifiable causes of cardiomyopathy.

2. **Medical management** is supportive and similar to the treatment of other forms of heart failure. Patients may benefit from **inotropic support, sodium restriction, diuretics,** and **ventricular afterload reduction.** Patients with PPCM are at high risk of thromboembolism, and **anticoagulation** should be considered. Pregnant patients should not receive ACE inhibitors, and nitroprusside should be used cautiously because of the risk of fetal cyanide toxicity with prolonged use. Finally, mechanical support with a **ventricular assist device** or **intra-aortic balloon pump** should be considered as a bridge to transplant in patients who fail to respond to medical management.

3. **Obstetrical management.** Delivery should be strongly considered in pregnant patients diagnosed with PPCM, particularly if the fetus is at risk, the patient is not responding to medical management, or if the patient also has preeclampsia.

4. **Prognosis and recurrence.** Fifty percent of patients diagnosed with PPCM will have a significant improvement in cardiac function. The remainder will have progression of their disease requiring heart transplant, or resulting in an early death. The overall estimated mortality of patients who acquire PPCM ranges from 15% to 50%. There is no clear consensus on the recurrence of PPCM in subsequent pregnancies, but the data would suggest patients with residual left ventricular impairment at the time of conception have an increased risk of recurrence and mortality.

E. **Pulmonary hypertension** is defined as a systolic pulmonary artery pressure (PAP) >35 mm Hg or a mean PAP >25 mm Hg at rest, and is commonly classified as either primary or secondary. Right ventricular failure can rapidly ensue when pregnancy-induced increases of blood volume and cardiac output are superimposed on pre-existing pulmonary hypertension.

   1. **Primary pulmonary hypertension (PPH)** is a progressively fatal disease of unknown etiology. The pathophysiology involves pulmonary vasoconstriction, vascular wall remodeling, and thrombosis, leading to right ventricular failure and death. In contrast to secondary pulmonary hypertension, patients with PPH respond to vasodilator therapy.

      a. **Medical management** should be individualized in each case, and a multidisciplinary team approach adopted. **Oxygen,** either continuous or for several hours each day, reduces PAP and improves cardiac output. **Anticoagulation** with unfractionated heparin or LMWH is recommended to prevent pulmonary emboli, which may be fatal. **Specific pulmonary vasodilator therapy** includes **inhaled nitric oxide;** inhaled, subcutaneous, or IV **prostacyclin;** and **sildenafil.** Use of **bosentan and iloprost** are contraindicated in pregnancy due to teratogenicity.

      b. Throughout pregnancy and delivery, the hemodynamic goals should be (1) to prevent pain, hypoxemia, acidosis, and hypercarbia; (2) to maintain intravascular volume and preload, but with careful monitoring to avoid volume overload and RV failure in the peripartum period; (3) to maintain systolic blood pressure greater than PAP to ensure adequate coronary perfusion of the RV; (4) to augment cardiac output as needed; and (5) to avoid tachydysrhythmias.

   2. **Secondary pulmonary hypertension** can develop from long-standing mitral valve disease or untreated left-to-right shunts. The mortality rate in pregnancy of these patients is 25% to 50% and may be due to embolism, dysrhythmia, right ventricular failure, or myocardial infarction.

VII. **Venous thromboembolism (VTE)** is the leading cause of maternal mortality in the United States. Several normal physiologic changes of pregnancy increase the risk of VTE, including venous stasis in the lower extremities from mechanical compression of the uterus, increased production of coagulation factors, and increased platelet activation. Antepartum bedrest, cesarean delivery, and postpartum tubal ligation further increase the risk.

   A. **The incidence** of pulmonary thromboembolism (PE) in pregnancy is estimated to be 0.5%. Up to one-quarter of pregnant patients with untreated deep vein thrombosis will experience a pulmonary embolus, and of those who do, the mortality rate is 12% to 15%.

   B. **Risk factors.** In addition to the factors listed above, obesity, increased age and parity, and acquired or congenital hypercoagulable states are associated with an increased risk of VTE.

   C. **Diagnosis.** Pregnant patients present with the same signs and symptoms as the nonpregnant population. However, confirming the diagnosis may be more complex. The D-dimer is not specific for VTE in pregnancy. **Doppler ultrasonography** of the lower extremities may be used without safety concern in pregnancy. Although the imaging studies commonly used to diagnose PE (**spiral computerized tomography, perfusion scan,** and **pulmonary angiography**) do expose the fetus to radiation, the exposure is considerably less than 5 rad.

   D. **Treatment** of VTE in pregnancy is summarized in **Table 44-2**.

	The American College of Chest Physicians Guidelines for Antithrombotic Therapy During Pregnancy
Condition	**Recommendation**
Previous VTE prior to current pregnancy or thrombophilia with or without VTE	Surveillance, heparin (5,000 U SQ q12h or adjusted to an anti-Xa level of 0.1–0.3 U/mL), or prophylactic LMWH (dalteparin 5,000 U SQ q24h or enoxaparin 40 mg SQ q24 h to keep anti-Xa level 0.2–0.6 U/mL) throughout pregnancy followed by postpartum anticoagulation for 4–6 weeks. The indication for active prophylaxis is stronger in antithrombin-deficient women
VTE or PE during current pregnancy	Adjusted-dose LMWH (weight adjusted, full treatment doses [e.g., dalteparin 200 U/kg q24h or enoxaparin 1 mg/kg q12h]) or heparin in full IV doses for 5–10 d, followed by q12h SQ injections to prolong 6-h postinjection PTT into the therapeutic range and then held for delivery followed by postpartum anticoagulation for 6 weeks
Planning pregnancy in patients who are being treated with long-term oral anticoagulants	Either heparin SQ q12h to prolong 6-h postinjection PTT into the therapeutic range, or Frequent pregnancy tests and substitute heparin (as above) for warfarin when pregnancy is achieved
Mechanical heart valves	Either heparin SQ q12h to prolong 6-h postinjection PTT into therapeutic range or LMWH to keep a 4-hour postinjection anti-Xa level at approximately 1.0 U/mL, or Adjusted-dose SQ heparin or LMWH as above until week 13, warfarin (target INR 2.5–3.0) until the middle of the third trimester, then restart SQ heparin or LMWH until delivery
APLA and more than one previous pregnancy loss	Antepartum aspirin and heparin or LMWH as for previous DVT above
APLA and no or one previous pregnancy loss	Surveillance, aspirin 80–325 mg q24h, heparin 5,000 U SQ q12h, or prophylactic LMWH (dalteparin 5,000 U SQ q24h or enoxaparin 40 mg SQ q24h to keep anti-Xa level 0.2–0.6 U/mL)
APLA and previous venous thrombosis	Either heparin q12h SQ to prolong 6-h postinjection PTT into the therapeutic range or LMWH to keep 4-h postinjection anti-Xa level at approximately 1.0 U/mL. Resumption of long-term anticoagulation postpartum

APLA, antiphospholipid antibodies; INR, international normalized ratio; LMWH, low-molecular-weight heparin; PE, pulmonary embolism; PTT, activated partial thromboplastin time; q12h, every 12 hours; q24h, every 24 hours; SQ, subcutaneous; VTE, venous thromboembolism.
Adapted from Ginsberg JS, Greer I, Hirsh J. Use of antithrombotic agents during pregnancy. *Chest* 2001;119:122S–131S. With permission.

VIII. Hemorrhage. Blood volume increases 30% to 40% during pregnancy, which helps to compensate for the blood loss that may occur at the time of delivery. Even with significant bleeding, most parturients will recover quickly and completely; however, a small number require ICU care for treatment of hemorrhage. Despite improvements in resuscitation strategies, hemorrhage—both antepartum and postpartum—remains a significant source of maternal morbidity, and is the second most common cause of maternal mortality.

A. Antepartum vaginal bleeding occurs in approximately 6% of pregnancies, and is frequently a marker for abnormal placentation. The patient at greatest risk is the fetus, and premature delivery may be required. **Etiologies** include

1. **Placenta previa,** which is diagnosed when the placenta comes up to or covers the internal cervical os. **Risk factors** for previa include a uterine scar from a previous surgery or procedure, increasing multiparity, and advanced maternal age. The classic presentation is painless vaginal bleeding. Ultrasound confirms the diagnosis.

2. **Placental abruption,** which is defined as a premature separation of the placenta from the uterus. Bleeding occurs because of the exposed vessels, and fetal distress may ensue from a loss of placental surface for oxygen and nutrient exchange. Etiology remains unclear, but **risk factors** are hypertension, advanced maternal age, increasing multiparity, trauma, prior history of abruption, tobacco and cocaine use, and preterm premature rupture of membranes. The classic presentation is vaginal bleeding, uterine tenderness, and painful, frequent contractions. The diagnosis is largely clinical, although ultrasound and laboratory tests such as a Kleihauer-Betke, a blood test which measures the amount of fetal hemoglobin transferred into maternal circulation, may be helpful.

3. **Uterine rupture** is an uncommon complication of pregnancy with potential for significant maternal and fetal morbidity. The major **risk factor** is a previous uterine scar; in patients with a previous lower uterine segment incision, the incidence is less than 1%. However, in patients with a history of a classical uterine incision, the incidence is higher; in these patients rupture is associated with greater morbidity because of the vascularity of the anterior uterine wall and the possible disruption of the placental bed.

4. **Management.** In all cases of antepartum bleeding, the first steps are maternal stabilization and assurance of fetal well-being. Adequate IV access should be obtained and preliminary laboratory tests sent. Placental abruption and previa may be expectantly managed, depending upon the degree of bleeding and gestational age. For significant bleeding, prompt delivery and aggressive volume resuscitation is critical. Previa and abruption place patients at increased risk for atony and development of coagulopathy, which should be anticipated and aggressively treated. Uterine rupture requires immediate delivery of the fetus. The uterus may be repaired, but hysterectomy is sometimes required.

B. Postpartum hemorrhage. The average blood loss for a vaginal delivery and cesarean delivery is <500 cc and <1,000 cc, respectively. Postpartum hemorrhage may be defined as blood loss in excess of the above, or clinically as a 10% decrease in hematocrit from admission to the postpartum period. **Etiologies** include

1. **Uterine atony,** which is the most common cause of primary postpartum hemorrhage and a frequent indication for peripartum hysterectomy.

Risk factors include prolonged labor, multiple gestation, high parity, chorioamnionitis, augmented labor, precipitous labor, tocolytic agents, and use of volatile anesthetics. Once the diagnosis is made, initial treatment should include bimanual massage, placement of large-bore IV access, and **oxytocin** infusion. Further pharmacologic therapy may include administration of uterotonic medications such as **Methergine 0.2 mg IM, misoprostol 800 to 1,000 μg PR**, and **15-methyl prostaglandin $F_{2\alpha}$ 250 μg IM**. Surgical intervention may be required, including a peripartum hysterectomy as well as significant volume resuscitation.

2. **Placenta accreta,** which is defined as a placenta adherent to the uterine wall. There are two additional types of placenta accreta: **placenta increta,** defined as invasion into the myometrium, and **placenta percreta,** defined as invasion through the uterine serosa. **Risk factors** for placenta increta include a previous uterine incision or instrumentation, advanced maternal age, multiparity, and a low-lying placenta or placenta previa. The incidence of accreta rises significantly when placenta previa is present in a patient with one or more previous uterine incisions. Management includes having a high index of suspicion in patients with risk factors and preparing appropriately for a large-volume resuscitation. Although in some cases the uterus may be preserved, peripartum hysterectomy is usually necessary.

3. **Uterine inversion,** which is the turning inside out of all or part of the uterus. A rare event, it may cause significant hemorrhage. First-line treatment is the replacement of the uterus, followed by aggressive medical management (administration of uterotonic medications) to improve uterine tone and limit further blood loss.

4. **Retained placenta,** which is a frequent cause of postpartum hemorrhage. Management involves removal of the placenta manually or with curettage, and volume resuscitation as required.

IX. **Sepsis** is an uncommon, but critical, event in pregnancy. Bacteremia is estimated to occur in approximately 7.5 of every 1,000 obstetric admissions, and sepsis develops in 8% to 10% of this bacteremic population. Worldwide, sepsis is one of the five leading causes of maternal mortality with significantly higher rates of sepsis and death reported in developing nations. Obstetrical sepsis primarily arises from chorioamnionitis, endometritis, urologic infections, septic abortions, and wound infections.

A. **Pathophysiology.** Overall, obstetric patients with sepsis have a favorable outcome as compared to the general population, likely due to an absence of comorbid conditions. However, some physiologic changes of pregnancy may complicate the diagnosis and disease state.

1. **Pulmonary.** Because of a lower oncotic pressure, decreased total lung capacity, and an increased oxygen consumption, pregnant patients are susceptible to the development of pulmonary edema and rapid onset of hypoxemia.

2. **Cardiovascular.** Pregnancy is associated with an increase in heart rate, a decrease in blood pressure, and an increase in cardiac output. These changes may mask some early signs of sepsis and may further compromise organ perfusion in the septic patient.

3. **Hematologic.** Pregnancy is associated with a procoagulant state from increased production of clotting factors and decreased activity of the fibrinolytic system. In the setting of sepsis, these changes may predispose to the development of DIC.

B. **Management.** Early diagnosis with prompt and aggressive treatment is critical for minimizing morbidity and mortality. Although no studies have specifically addressed the management of sepsis in obstetric patients, most evidence-based recommendations for improving survival in sepsis may be applied to pregnancy (see **Chapter 30**). Pregnant patients who develop sepsis are at high risk for preterm delivery and fetal loss. In the setting of sepsis, fetal compromise is usually the result of maternal decompensation and thus, initial efforts toward maternal resuscitation should be the priority. Regular and frequent cardiotocographic monitoring should be performed for assessment of fetal well-being and for surveillance for preterm labor. When choosing antibiotics, attempts should be made to maximize the effectiveness for the mother and minimize fetal harm, although this may not always be possible. Finally, the physiologic changes of pregnancy may change the pharmacokinetics of antibiotics and require adjustments in dosing and monitoring.

X. **Endocrine disorders** (see **Chapter 28**)
  A. **Diabetic ketoacidosis (DKA)** is infrequent in pregnancy, with an estimated incidence between 1% and 2% in pregnancies complicated by pre-existing or gestational diabetes. In recent years, maternal mortality associated with DKA has improved, but fetal loss remains high with estimates ranging from 9% to 35% in affected pregnancies.
   1. **Clinical presentation** and **laboratory abnormalities** are identical to those in the nonpregnant population. In addition, evidence of fetal compromise is frequently present.
   2. **Risk factors** for DKA in pregnancy include emesis of any cause, use of β-sympathomimetics, infection, previously undiagnosed diabetes, and poor patient compliance.
   3. Several **physiologic changes of pregnancy** predispose patients to developing DKA. Pregnancy is a state of relative insulin resistance and increased lipolysis, with a tendency toward ketone body formation. Additionally, increases in minute ventilation cause a mild respiratory alkalosis which is compensated by increased renal excretion of bicarbonate; this compensated respiratory alkalosis leaves patients less capable of buffering serum ketone acids.
   4. **Fetal concerns.** Maternal acidosis decreases uterine blood flow and causes a leftward shift in the maternal oxyhemoglobin dissociation curve, both of which compromise fetal oxygenation. Ketoacids dissociate and cross the placenta contributing to a metabolic acidosis in the fetus. Lastly, glucose readily crosses the placenta causing fetal hyperglycemia, osmotic diuresis, and hypovolemia.
   5. **Medical management** is unchanged from the nonpregnant population. Aggressive fluid resuscitation, glucose control, treatment of the underlying etiology, and control of electrolyte abnormalities are the mainstays of treatment.
   6. **Obstetric management.** Fetal status may be measured indirectly by fetal heart rate tracings or biophysical profile. Maternal resuscitation is imperative to improving the fetal outcome, and delivery for fetal indications should be reserved for fetal compromise, which continues after appropriate maternal resuscitation.
  B. **Ovarian hyperstimulation syndrome (OHSS)** is a rare, iatrogenic complication of ovulation induction which may occur in response to almost every agent used to stimulate the ovaries. It usually occurs in the luteal phase or within the first week post-conception. The seminal event in

the genesis of OHSS is ovarian enlargement, with an acute fluid shift out of the intravascular space resulting in ascites and intravascular hypovolemia.

1. The reported **prevalence** of the most severe form is 0.5% to 5% with an estimated mortality of 1 per 450,000 to 1 per 50,000 patients.

2. **Clinical presentation.** Signs and symptoms result from increased vascular permeability and arterial dilation which leads to extravasation of intravascular fluid into the extravascular spaces. Patients may present with ascites, oliguria, renal failure, hydrothorax, or ARDS. Laboratory abnormalities include electrolyte imbalances (hyponatremia and hyperkalemia), elevated creatinine, hemoconcentration, leukocytosis, and thrombocytosis.

3. **Management.** Treatment of OHSS is supportive. Patients should be carefully monitored, administered isotonic fluids to restore intravascular volume, and treated for electrolyte disturbances. Increased intra-abdominal pressure from ascites may result in poor pulmonary function and impaired renal perfusion, and may have significant deleterious effects on maternal circulation. **Ultrasound-guided paracentesis** has been shown to improve creatinine clearance, urine output, dyspnea, and osmolarity, but care must be taken to avoid inadvertent puncture of ovarian cysts with subsequent intraperitoneal hemorrhage. These patients also are at risk of developing thromboses in either the arterial (25%) or venous (75%) circulations, and prophylactic **anticoagulation** should be initiated.

4. **Resolution.** After a period of several days, patients begin to mobilize the extravascular fluid and a natural diuresis occurs. Complete resolution typically takes 2 weeks from the onset of symptoms.

XI. Amniotic fluid embolism (AFE) is a rare but possibly catastrophic complication of pregnancy. Because AFE remains a diagnosis of exclusion, the true incidence is unknown but is estimated to be between 3 and 5 per 100,000 live births. However, the mortality rate among affected parturients is as high as 85%, and the disease accounts for up to 12% of all maternal deaths overall. Among survivors, significant and permanent neurologic sequelae are common.

A. Clinical presentation. Classically, patients present during labor or delivery, or in the immediate postpartum period, with acute hypoxia and hypotension which rapidly deteriorates to cardiovascular collapse, coagulopathy, and death.

B. Pathophysiology. The etiology is likely multifactorial and is poorly understood. It is thought that the inciting event is a breach in the barrier between the maternal and fetal compartments leading to the presence of fetal cells, amniotic fluid, and inflammatory mediators in the maternal circulation.

C. Manifestations affect multiple organ systems and presentation may vary depending upon the predominant physiologic change.

1. **Cardiovascular.** Hypotension is a hallmark feature, present in 100% of patients with severe disease. A biphasic model of shock has been proposed to explain the findings seen in patients with AFE. The initial transient response is pulmonary hypertension, likely from the release of vasoactive substances, causing hypoxia and right heart failure. Patients who survive the initial insult develop a second phase of left heart failure and pulmonary edema, although the etiology of the left-sided heart dysfunction remains unclear.

2. **Pulmonary.** Hypoxia is an early manifestation, arising from acute pulmonary hypertension with subsequent ventilation–perfusion mismatch. Later, pulmonary edema develops in association with left ventricular dysfunction. A substantial portion of patients will also manifest noncardiogenic pulmonary edema after left ventricular function improves.

3. **Coagulation.** Disruption of the normal clotting cascade occurs in up to two-thirds of patients. It remains unclear whether the coagulopathy is the result of a consumptive process, or from massive fibrinolysis. However, patients may experience significant bleeding, massive hemorrhage, and DIC.

D. **Management** involves aggressive resuscitation; supportive care is aimed at minimizing additional hypoxia and subsequent end-organ damage. Goals of therapy include maintenance of oxygenation, circulatory support, and correction of the coagulopathy. (1) Most patients will require tracheal intubation, mechanical ventilation, and supplemental oxygen. (2) Hemodynamic instability should be corrected with fluid resuscitation and pressor support as needed. (3) **Lines and monitors** should include adequate IV access, continuous pulse oximetry, invasive blood pressure monitoring and a pulmonary artery catheter, and/or transesophageal echocardiography to assess ventricular function. (4) **Laboratory studies** should be sent at regular intervals and coagulopathy aggressively treated. (5) If the event occurs before delivery, the fetus should be delivered as quickly as possible to minimize fetal hypoxia and to aid maternal resuscitation. (6) Rescue therapies such as cardiopulmonary bypass, extracorporeal membrane oxygenation, and intra-aortic balloon counterpulsation have been described in the literature as successful options for the treatment of refractory AFE.

XII. **Trauma (Chapter 9)** is the most common cause of nonobstetric mortality and morbidity in pregnancy, complicating 5% to 10% of all pregnancies. Common causes include motor vehicle accidents, assault, falls, and burns.

A. **Management.** Standard guidelines for care of trauma patients apply to pregnant patients with several important modifications. (1) Patients at 20 weeks' gestation or more who are placed on a backboard should be angled 15 degrees to the left to minimize aortocaval compression. (2) Efforts should be made to transfuse only O-negative blood in the event that transfusion is required before a type and cross can be performed. (3) Blood pressure and intravascular volume should be maintained. (4) Early evaluation for pregnancy complications and assessment of fetal well-being should be performed.

B. **Maternal complications** will vary based upon the mechanism and severity of injury. Women at more than 20 weeks' gestation should have **cardiotocographic monitoring** for the first 2 to 6 hours after injury. Early, frequent contractions are a sensitive indicator of abruption. The period of monitoring and observation should be increased in women with contractions, abdominal tenderness, or significant maternal injury. Additional testing specific to pregnancy may include a **Kleihauer-Betke test,** which may indicate the severity of uterine-placental trauma. Lastly, all patients should have a type and screen, and Rh-negative patients with a positive Kleihauer-Betke should be given **Rh-immune globulin.**

1. **Blunt trauma.** Because of increased vascularity and shifting of abdominal contents by the gravid uterus, splenic and retroperitoneal injury is more common in pregnant women, while bowel injury is less frequent.

Placental abruption may be present in up to 40% of women with severe maternal trauma.

2. **Penetrating trauma.** Because of anatomical changes, pregnant women have a fourfold decrease in death from penetrating trauma, as opposed to nonpregnant women. However, the same anatomic changes lead to an increased risk of bowel injury when penetrating trauma occurs in the upper abdomen.

C. **Fetal outcome** is dependent upon maternal outcome and the mechanism of injury. Maternal death is the most common cause of fetal death, and severe maternal injuries result in fetal death in 20% to 40% of cases. In significant penetrating abdominal trauma, fetal injuries are common with fetal mortality ranging from 40% to 70%, due to direct fetal injury or premature delivery. Fetal evaluation should include a thorough **ultrasound evaluation** of the fetus and placenta and continuous **fetal heart-rate monitoring** for the first 2 to 6 hours or longer.

XIII. **Local anesthetic toxicity.** Systemic absorption or inadvertent intravascular injection of local anesthetics may result in toxicity which is typically manifested by central nervous system (CNS) symptoms and cardiovascular compromise. Toxicity of local anesthetics is correlated to potency and their rank in order of increasing toxicity is as follows: 2-chloroprocaine, mepivacaine, lidocaine, etidocaine, tetracaine, and bupivacaine.

A. **CNS symptoms** reported by patients correlate with increased plasma concentrations of local anesthetics. At lower levels, **periorbital numbness** and **metallic taste** are reported. As the serum concentration increases, **loss of consciousness, seizures,** and **respiratory arrest** may occur.

B. **Cardiovascular manifestations** occur at much higher serum concentrations than CNS symptoms. They may progress from **increased blood pressure** to **bradycardia, ventricular dysfunction, ventricular tachycardia,** and **fibrillation.** As in nonpregnant patients, the more potent amide local anesthetics such as bupivacaine have a smaller margin of safety and may cause refractory arrhythmias. Despite this, bupivacaine remains the most common local anesthetic in obstetric anesthesia.

C. Pregnancy increases the risk of adverse outcomes from local anesthetic toxicity by several mechanisms: decreased concentrations of plasma proteins result in a higher free serum concentration, and vascular engorgement may increase the risk of epidural catheter placement into an epidural vein. Additionally, resuscitation is more difficult because of rapid development of hypoxemia, and the technical difficulty of performing effective chest compressions in pregnant patients.

D. **Management** is largely supportive. Seizures should be terminated with **benzodiazepines** or **barbiturates.** Additionally, resuscitation with **intralipid** therapy should be considered based on literature reports of success in pregnant patients. All patients should be given supplemental oxygenation, and tracheal intubation should be considered. Monitoring should include the fetal heart rate. Blood pressure should be supported with fluids, vasoactive medications, and if needed, CPR.

XIV. **Cardiopulmonary resuscitation (CPR).** Cardiac arrest complicates 1 in 30,000 pregnancies, with a higher incidence in women with underlying cardiopulmonary disease. In general, CPR algorithms are unchanged for pregnant women, since maternal resuscitation is the best therapy for the fetus. **Vasoactive medications** and **defibrillation** should be administered as in the nonpregnant population. There are some important differences:

A. **Airway.** The pregnant patient should be intubated soon after initiation of CPR to protect the airway from aspiration and facilitate oxygenation and ventilation.

B. **Circulation.** Cardiac output is significantly affected by patient positioning after approximately 20 weeks' gestation. Uterine compression of the IVC and aorta can considerably compromise preload and cardiac output. A critical component of resuscitation in the obstetric population involves left uterine displacement, accomplished with a wedge or pillow under the patient's right hip, or by manual displacement of the uterus to the left.

C. **Delivery.** If cardiac arrest occurs before 24 weeks' gestation (age of fetal viability), the rescuer's efforts should be directed exclusively toward the mother. If arrest occurs after 24 weeks, the fetus should be delivered if CPR has not been successful within 4 to 5 minutes to optimize both maternal and fetal outcomes. Prompt delivery of the fetus minimizes the risk of hypoxic insult and improves maternal cardiac output by relieving aortocaval compression, decreasing metabolic demands, and allowing for more effective chest compressions. Delivery may be considered even in a nonviable pregnancy to improve resuscitation of the mother.

D. **Venous access** should be secured in the upper extremities.

E. Both **cardiopulmonary bypass** and **open cardiac massage** have been advocated if closed-chest resuscitative efforts are unsuccessful.

Selected References

Bandi VD, Munnur U, Matthay MA. Acute lung injury and acute respiratory distress syndrome in pregnancy. *Crit Care Clin* 2004;20:577–607.

Budev MM, Arroliga AC, Falcone T. Ovarian hyperstimulation syndrome. *Crit Care Med* 2005;33:S301–S306.

Carroll MA, Yeomans ER. Diabetic ketoacidosis in pregnancy. *Crit Care Med* 2005;33: S347–S353.

Duhl AJ, Paidas MJ, Ural SH, et al. Antithrombotic therapy and pregnancy: consensus report and recommendations for prevention and treatment of venous thromboembolism and adverse pregnancy outcomes. *Am J Obstet Gynecol* 2007;197:457e1–457e21.

Elkayam U, Bitar F. Valvular heart disease and pregnancy: part I: native valves. *J Am Coll Cardiol* 2005;46:223–230.

Fernandez Perez ER, Salman S, Pendem S, Farmer JC. Sepsis during pregnancy. *Crit Care Med* 2005;33:S286–S293.

Harnett M, Mushlin PS, Camann WR. Cardiovascular disease. In: Chestnut DH, ed. *Obstetric anesthesia: principles and practice.* St. Louis, MO: Mosby, 2004:707–733.

James AH, Jamison MG, Biswas MS, Brancazio LR, Swamy GK, Meyers ER. Acute myocardial infarction in pregnancy: a United States population-based study. *Circulation* 2006;113: 1564–1571.

Muench MV, Canterino JC. Trauma in pregnancy. *Obstet Gynecol Clin N Am* 2007;34:555–583.

O'Shea A, Eappen S. Amniotic fluid embolism. *Int Anesthesiol Clin* 2007;45:17–28.

Stout KK, Otto CM. Pregnancy in women with valvular heart disease. *Heart* 2007;93:552–558.

Tidswell M. Peripartum cardiomyopathy. *Crit Care Clin* 2004;20:777–788.

Turan TT, Stern BJ. Stroke in pregnancy. *Neurol Clin* 2004;22:831–840.

Wilson W et al. Prevention of infective endocarditis: guidelines from the American Heart Association. *Circulation* 2007;116:1736–1754.

Supplemental Drug Information

Alan DiBiasio, Robert Hallisey, Jr., and Kathryn Kalafatas Davis

---

Abciximab (Reopro)

Indications	To prevent thrombus formation following percutaneous transluminal coronary angioplasty (PTCA) and following stent placement
Dosage	Bolus: 0.25 mg/kg administered 10–60 minutes prior to PTCA Maintenance dose: 0.125 µg/kg/min to maximum 10 µg/min for 12 hours postprocedure
Effect	Glycoprotein IIB/IIIA inhibitor, preventing platelet adhesion and aggregation
Onset	2 hours
Duration	2–4 hours for bleeding; up to 24 hours for platelet recovery
Comments	Anaphylaxis may occur; hypotension with bolus dose; bleeding complications and thrombocytopenia are common side effects

---

Acetazolamide (Diamox)

Indications	Metabolic alkalosis; alternative antiepileptic agent; increased intraocular and intracranial pressures, diuretic
Dosage	125–500 mg IV over 1–2 minutes or orally not to exceed 2 g in 24 hours
Effect	Carbonic anhydrase inhibitor that increases the excretion of bicarbonate ions
Onset	IV: 2 minutes
Duration	Extended-release capsule: 18–24 hours Tablet: 8–12 hours IV: 4–5 hours
Clearance	From 70% to 100% excreted unchanged in the urine within 24 hours
Comments	May increase insulin requirements in diabetic patients and cause renal calculi in patients with past history of calcium stones; may cause hypokalemia, thrombocytopenia, aplastic anemia, increased urinary excretion of uric acid, and hyperglycemia; initial dose may produce marked diuresis; tolerance to desired effects of acetazolamide occurs in 2–3 days; rare hypersensitivity reaction in patients with sulfa allergies

---

Acetylcysteine (Mucomyst, Acetadote)

Indications	1. Acetaminophen overdose 2. Contrast-induced nephropathy prophylaxis
Dosage	1. Oral: 140 mg/kg orally × 1 dose; then 70 mg/kg every 4 hours × 17 doses

IV: Load 150 mg/kg in 200 mL D_5W × 1 dose over 15 minutes; then 50 mg/kg in 500 mL D_5W × 1 dose over 4 hours; then 100 mg/kg in 1,000 mL D_5W × 1 dose over 16 hours

2. Oral: 600 or 1,200 mg orally twice daily × 4 doses; 2 doses prior to contrast and 2 doses post-contrast

Effect   The exact mechanism of action in acetaminophen toxicity is unknown; thought to act by providing substrate for conjugation with the toxic metabolite. The presumed mechanism in preventing contrast-induced nephropathy is its ability to scavenge oxygen-derived free radicals and improve endothelium-dependent vasodilation

Clearance   Renal

Comments   Acetadote (200 mg/mL) is for IV use only. Mucomyst (200 mg/mL) is for oral use and inhalation only

Acyclovir (Zovirax)

Indications   1. Treatment of initial and prophylaxis of recurrent mucosal and cutaneous herpes simplex (HSV-1 and HSV-2) infections
2. HSV encephalitis
3. Varicella zoster infections
4. Herpes zoster, genital herpes, and varicella zoster infections in immunocompromised patients

Dosage   May vary with specific indication
Adult:
1. IV: 5 mg/kg/dose every 8 hours for 7–14 days
2. IV: 10–15 mg/kg/dose every 8 hours for 10–14 days
3. IV: 10 mg/kg/dose every 8 hours for 7–10 days
Oral: 800 mg/dose 4 times/d for 5 days
4. IV: 10 mg/kg/dose or 500 mg/m^2/dose every 8 hours for 7 days
Oral: 800 mg every 4 hours (5 times/d) for 7–10 days
Pediatric:
1. IV: 750 mg/m^2/d divided every 8 hours or 15 mg/kg/d divided every 8 hours for 5–10 days
2. IV: 1,500 mg/m^2/d divided every 8 hours or 30 mg/kg/d divided every 8 hours for 10 days
3. IV: 1,500 mg/m^2/d divided every 8 hours or 30 mg/kg/d divided every 8 hours for 5–10 days
Oral: 10–20 mg/kg/dose (up to 800 mg) 4 times/d
4. IV: 7.5 mg/kg/dose every 8 hours
Oral: 250–600 mg/m^2/dose 4–5 times/d
Neonate:
HSV infection:
IV: 1,500 mg/m^2/d divided every 8 hours or 30 mg/kg/d divided every 8 hours for 10–14 days

Effect   Antiviral; inhibits herpes DNA synthesis and viral replication

Onset   Oral: within 1.5–2 hours
IV: within 1 hour

Duration   Half-life:
Neonates: 4 hours
Children 1–12 years: 2–3 hours
Adults: 3 hours

| Clearance | Primary route is the kidney (30%–90% of a dose is excreted unchanged); hemodialysis removes ~60% of the dose, whereas while removal by peritoneal dialysis is to a much lesser extent |
| Comments | Dose should be reduced in patients with renal impairment; use with caution in patients with pre-existing renal disease or in those receiving other nephrotoxic drugs concurrently; use with caution in patients with underlying neurologic abnormalities and in patients with serious renal, hepatic, or electrolyte abnormalities or substantial hypoxia |

Adenosine (Adenocard)

Indications	Paroxysmal supraventricular tachycardia, Wolff-Parkinson-White syndrome
Dosage	Adult: 6–12 mg IV bolus
	Pediatric: 50 μg/kg IV
Effect	Slow or temporary cessation of AV node conduction and conduction through reentrant pathways
Onset	Immediate
Duration	<10 seconds
Clearance	Red blood cell and endothelial cell metabolism
Comments	Its effects are antagonized by methylxanthines such as theophylline; adenosine is contraindicated in patients with high-degree heart block or sick sinus syndrome; hypotension can occur; not effective in atrial flutter or fibrillation; asystole for 3–6 seconds is common

Albuterol (Proventil, Ventolin)

Indications	Bronchospasm
Dosage	Adult:
	Aerosolized: 2.5 mg in 3 mL of saline via nebulizer, 180 or 200 μg (two puffs) via inhaler
	Oral: 2 mg
	Pediatric:
	Oral: 0.1 mg/kg (syrup 2 mg/5 mL)
Effect	β_2-Receptor agonist
Onset	Immediate
Duration	3–6 hours
Clearance	Hepatic metabolism; renal elimination
Comments	Possible β-adrenergic overload, tachydysrhythmias

Alprostadil (Prostaglandin E1)

Indications	Pulmonary vasodilator, maintenance of patent ductus arteriosus
Dosage	Starting dose: 0.05–0.1 μg/kg/min
	Standard mix: 500 μg/250 mL of D_5W or NS
Effect	Prostaglandin E1 will cause vasodilation, inhibition of platelet aggregation, vascular smooth muscle relaxation, and uterine and intestinal smooth muscle stimulation
Onset	Immediate
Duration	60 minutes
Clearance	Pulmonary metabolism; renal elimination
Comments	May cause hypotension, apnea, flushing, and bradycardia

Alteplase (recombinant tPA, tissue plasminogen activator, Activase, Cathflo)

Indications	1. Lysis of thrombi in coronary arteries in hemodynamically unstable patients with acute myocardial infarction 2. Management of acute massive pulmonary embolism in adults 3. Acute embolic stroke 4. Catheter clearance
Dosage	1. Loading dose: Patient weight >67 kg: 15-mg bolus, then 50 mg over the next 30 minutes. Institute heparin therapy with a bolus. Infuse remaining 35 mg of TPA over the next hour (total dose of TPA = 100 mg) Patient weight <67 kg: 5-mg bolus, then 0.75 mg/kg (maximum 50 mg) over 30 minutes. Initiate heparin therapy with a bolus. Then 0.5 mg/kg (maximum 35 mg) over the next hour 2. 100 mg continuous infusion over 2 hours 3. Total of 0.9 mg/kg (maximum 90 mg), administer 10% as a bolus and the remainder over 60 minutes. Do not start heparin within 24 hours 4. Patients <30 kg: 110% of the internal lumen volume of the catheter, not to exceed 2 mg/2 mLs; retain in catheter for 0.5–2 hours; may instill a second dose if catheter remains occluded Patients ≥30 kg: 2 mg (2 mL); retain in catheter for 0.5–2 hours; may instill a second dose if catheter remains occluded
Effect	Tissue plasminogen activator
Onset	Rapid
Duration	80% cleared within 10 minutes of discontinuing infusion
Clearance	Rapid hepatic clearance
Comments	After acute myocardial infarction, aspirin (325 mg) should be given at the initiation of therapy; heparin should be started (1,000 U/h) by continuous infusion 1 hour from the initiation of alteplase Doses above 150 mg have been associated with an increased incidence of intracranial hemorrhage; use within 6 hours of coronary occlusion for best results; contraindicated with active internal bleeding, history of hemorrhagic stroke, intracranial neoplasm, aneurysm, or recent (within 2 months) intracranial or intraspinal surgery or trauma; should be used with caution in patients who have received chest compressions and patients who are receiving heparin, warfarin, or antiplatelet drugs

Aminocaproic acid (Amicar)

Indications	Hemorrhage due to fibrinolysis
Dosage	Load: 4–5 g given over 1 hour Maintenance: 6–24 g given continuously over 24 hours Total 24-hour dose should not exceed 30 g Standard mix: 6 g/250 mL D_5W or NS
Effect	Stabilizes clot formation by inhibiting plasminogen activators and plasmin
Clearance	Primarily renal elimination
Comments	Contraindicated in disseminated intravascular coagulation

Amiodarone (Cordarone)

Indications	Refractory or recurrent ventricular tachycardia or ventricular fibrillation; rapid supraventricular arrhythmias, particularly atrial fibrillation
Dosage	Oral loading dose: 800–1,600 mg/d in divided doses orally $\times$ 1–3 weeks; then 600–800 mg/d in divided doses orally $\times$ 4 weeks Oral maintenance dose: PO: 100–400 mg/d IV loading dose: 150 mg in 100 mL D_5W over 10 minutes (15 mg/min) IV maintenance dose: 360 mg over the next 6 hours (1 mg/min); then 540 mg over the next 18 hours (0.5 mg/min) Arrest, pulseless VF or VT: 300 mg IV bolus; may repeat 150 mg IV bolus in 3–5 minutes
Effect	Depresses the sinoatrial node; prolongs the PR, QRS, and QT intervals; and produces α- and β-adrenergic blockade
Onset	Oral: days to months
Duration	Weeks to months
Clearance	Biliary elimination
Comments	May cause severe sinus bradycardia, ventricular dysrhythmias, AV block, liver and thyroid function test abnormalities, hepatitis, and cirrhosis; pulmonary fibrosis may follow long-term use; increases serum levels of digoxin, oral anticoagulants, diltiazem, quinidine, procainamide, and phenytoin **Black- Box warning from the Food and Drug Administration (FDA)** 'Amiodarone is not indicated for patients with life-threatening arrhythmias, because of risk of exacerbation of arrhythmias. Such risk may be increased with concomitant use of other antiarrhythmic agents and of drugs that prolong the QTc interval. Patients should be monitored over time for liver toxicity and lung damage

Argatroban

Indications	Therapeutic anticoagulation in patients with strongly suspected or confirmed heparin-induced thrombocytopenia (HIT type II)
Dosage	0.5–2 μg/kg/min titrated to 1.5–3 times activated partial thromboplastin time (aPTT) control; do not exceed 10 μg/kg/min
Effect	Inhibitor of bound and soluble thrombin
Clearance	Hepatic (primary), renal (2%–10%)
Comments	Discontinue and remove all heparin products, obtain a baseline aPTT prior to initiating therapy (except in cath lab); once a stable dose is achieved, draw aPTT every 24 hours; obtain order for each change in dose; there is no antidote or reversal agent for argatroban; the INR and aPTT may also be elevated, but should not be considered monitoring parameters; administer via a dedicated line, argatroban is not compatible with other drugs

Atenolol (Tenormin)

Indications	Hypertension, angina, following myocardial infarction
Dosage	PO: 50–100 mg/d
Effect	β_1-Selective adrenergic receptor blockade
Onset	Orally: 30–60 minutes

Duration	Orally: >24 hours
Clearance	Renal, intestinal elimination unchanged
Comments	High doses block β_2-adrenergic receptors; relatively contraindicated in congestive heart failure, asthma, and heart block; caution in patients on calcium channel blockers; rebound angina may occur with abrupt cessation

Atropine

Indications	1. Antisialagogue
	2. Bradycardia
Dosage	Adult:
	1. 0.2–0.4 mg IV
	2. 0.4–1.0 mg IV
	Pediatric:
	1. 0.01 mg/kg/dose IV/IM (<0.4 mg)
	2. 0.02 mg/kg/dose IV (<0.4 mg)
Effect	Competitive blockade of acetylcholine at muscarinic receptors
Onset	Rapid
Duration	Variable
Clearance	50%–70% hepatic metabolism, renal elimination
Comments	May cause tachydysrhythmias, AV dissociation, premature ventricular contractions, dry mouth, or urinary retention; CNS effects occur at high doses

Azathioprine (Imuran)

Indications	1. Adjunct for prevention of rejection in allotransplantation
	2. Rheumatoid arthritis
Dosage	May vary with specific indication
	Adult:
	1. Renal transplantation:
	Urally, IV: 200–300 mg/d to start
	Maintenance dose: 50–200 mg/d
	2. Rheumatoid arthritis:
	PO: 50–100 mg/d for 6–8 weeks; increase by 0.5 mg/kg every 4 weeks until response or up to 200 mg/d
	Maintenance therapy: the lowest effective dose
	Pediatric:
	1. Renal transplantation:
	PO, IV: 3–5 mg/kg/d to start
	Maintenance dose: 1–3 mg/kg/d
Effect	Antimetabolite, immunosuppressant
Clearance	Extensively metabolized by hepatic xanthenes oxidase to 6-mercaptopurine (active)
Comments	Dose should be reduced for white blood cell count (WBC) <4,000 cells/mm^3 and/or held for WBC <3,000 cells/mm^3; azathioprine metabolism is competitively inhibited by allopurinol, and dose reduction is required; use with caution in patients with liver disease, renal impairment; chronic immunosuppression increases the risk of neoplasia; has mutagenic potential to both men and women and with possible hematologic toxicities

Bicarbonate, sodium

Indications	1. Metabolic acidosis
	2. Prophylaxis of adult contrast-induced nephropathy
Dosage	1. IV dose in mEq $NaHCO_3$ = Base deficit $\times$ weight (kg) $\times$ 0.3 (subsequent doses titrated against patient's pH)
	2. Sodium bicarbonate 150 mEq in 1,000 mL D_5W infuse 3 mL/kg/h $\times$ 1 hour pre-procedure, then 1 mL/kg/h $\times$ 6 hours post-procedure
Effect	Metabolic acid neutralization
Onset	Rapid
Duration	Variable
Clearance	Plasma metabolism; pulmonary, renal elimination
Comments	May cause metabolic alkalosis, hypercarbia, hyperosmolality; may decrease cardiac output, systemic vascular resistance, and myocardial contractility; in neonates, may cause intraventricular hemorrhage; crosses placenta; an 8.4% solution is approximately 1 mEq/mL; a 4.2% solution is approximately 0.5 mEq/mL

Bumetanide (Bumex)

Indications	Edema, hypertension, intracranial hypertension
Dosage	0.5–1 mg IV, repeated to a maximum of 10 mg/d
Effect	Loop diuretic with principal effect on the ascending limb of the loop of Henle; causes increased excretion of Na^+, K^+, Cl^-, and H_2O
Onset	Immediate, peak 15–30 minutes
Duration	2–4 hours
Clearance	Hepatic metabolism, 81% renal excretion (45% unchanged)
Comments	May cause electrolyte imbalance, dehydration, and deafness; patients who are allergic to sulfonamides may show hypersensitivity to bumetanide; effective in renal insufficiency

Calcium chloride, calcium gluconate

Indications	Hypocalcemia, hyperkalemia, hypermagnesemia, severe hypotension
Dosage	Calcium chloride (CaCl): 5–10 mg/kg IV prn
	(10% $CaCl_2$ = 13.6 mEq Ca^{2+}/10 mL and 273 mg Ca^{2+})
	Calcium gluconate: 15–30 mg/kg IV prn
	(10% calcium gluconate = 4.5 mEq Ca^{2+}/10 mL and 93 mg Ca^{2+})
Effect	Maintenance of cell membrane integrity, muscular excitation–contraction coupling, glandular stimulation–secretion coupling, and enzyme function. It increases blood pressure
Onset	Rapid
Duration	Variable
Clearance	Incorporated into muscle, bone, and other tissues; rapid onset; variable duration
Comments	May cause tachycardia, bradycardia, and dysrhythmia (especially with digitalis); CaCl should not be administered peripherally undiluted except in emergency situations; CaCl has three times more available elemental calcium

Captopril (Capoten)

Indications	Hypertension, congestive heart failure
Dosage	Loading dose: 12.5–25 mg orally 2–3 times/d
	Maintenance dose: 25–150 mg orally 2–3 times/d
Effect	Angiotensin I-converting enzyme inhibition decreases angiotensin II and aldosterone levels; reduces both preload and afterload in patients with congestive heart failure
Onset	15–60 minutes, peak 60–90 minutes
Duration	4–6 hours
Clearance	Hepatic metabolism; 95% renal elimination (40%–50% unchanged)
Comments	Can be used in hypertensive emergency; may cause neutropenia, agranulocytosis, hypotension, or bronchospasm; avoid in pregnant patients; exaggerated response in renal artery stenosis and with diuretics

Chlorothiazide (Diuril)

Indications	Edema, heart failure, acute/chronic renal failure, hypertension
Dosage	Adult: 250–500 mg IV push at 50–100 mg/min
	Maximum: 2,000 mg over 24 hours
	Pediatric: 20 mg/kg/d orally in two divided doses every 12 hours
Effect	Thiazide diuretic
Onset	2 hours
Duration	Oral: 6–12 hours
	IV: ~2 hours
Clearance	Renal elimination
Comments	Enhances activity of antihypertensives, digoxin; may enhance activity of loop diuretics in renal failure; may increase insulin requirements in diabetic patients

Clonidine (Catapres)

Indications	Hypertension; adrenergic overload due to narcotic withdrawal
Dosage	0.1–1.2 mg/d orally in divided doses (2.4 mg/d maximum dose); also available as a transdermal patch delivering 0.1, 0.2, or 0.3 mg/d for 7 days
Effect	Central α_2-adrenergic agonist, resulting in decrease in systemic vascular resistance and heart rate
Onset	Oral: 30–60 minutes, peak 2–4 hours
	Transdermal: 48 hours
Duration	8 hours
Clearance	50% hepatic metabolism; elimination 20% biliary, 80% renal
Comments	Abrupt withdrawal may cause rebound hypertension or dysrhythmias; may cause drowsiness, nightmares, restlessness, anxiety, or depression; IV injection may cause transient peripheral α-adrenergic stimulation

Dalteparin (Fragmin)

Indications	1. Prophylaxis of deep venous thrombosis and pulmonary embolism (DVT/PE)

2. Therapeutic anticoagulation for treatment or prevention of thrombosis

3. Acute coronary syndrome

Dosage
1. 2,500–5,000 U SQ daily
2. 100 U/kg SQ every 12 hours
3. 120 U/kg SQ every 12 hours

Effect
Binds with antithrombin III, and accelerates inactivation of factors IIa (thrombin), Xa, IXa, XIa, and XIIa

Onset
2 hours

Duration
10–24 hours

Clearance
Renal

Comments
Therapeutic doses should be used with caution in patients with renal impairment; factor Xa levels are of little value in determining therapeutic response; incompletely and unpredictably reversed by protamine; do not use in patients with heparin-induced thrombocytopenia

---

Dantrolene (Dantrium)

Indications
Malignant hyperthermia, skeletal muscle spasticity, neuroleptic malignant syndrome

Dosage
Prophylactic treatment is generally not recommended
Malignant hyperthermia: 2.5 mg/kg IV bolus; if syndrome persists after 30 minutes, repeat dose, up to 10 mg/kg
Neuroleptic malignant syndrome: 1 mg/kg; may repeat dose up to maximum cumulative dose of 10 mg/kg, then switch to oral dosage form. Therapy should be in conjunction with bromocriptine

Effect
Reduction of Ca^{2+} release from sarcoplasmic reticulum

Onset
30 minutes

Duration
8 hours

Clearance
Hepatic metabolism; renal elimination

Comments
Mix 20 mg in 60 mL of sterile water; dissolves slowly into solution; may cause muscle weakness, gastrointestinal upset, drowsiness, sedation, or abnormal liver function (chronically); additive effect with neuromuscular blocking agents; tissue irritant. **Black- Box warning from the Food and Drug Administration (FDA)** 'Dantrolene Sodium can cause hepatotoxicity from hepatitis, idiosyncratic or hypersensitivity. The lowest possible effective dose for the individual patient should be prescribed.

Desmopressin acetate (DDAVP)

Indications
1. Coagulation improvement in von Willebrand's disease, hemophilia A, uremic bleeding
2. Antidiuretic

Dosage
Adult:
1. 0.3 μg/kg IV (diluted 50 mL NS), infused over 15–30 minutes preoperatively and/or every 12–24 hours to a maximum of 3 days
2. Diabetes insipidus: 2–4 μg/d usually in 2 divided doses
Pediatric:
<10 kg: Dilute adult dose in 10 mL of NS
>10 kg: See adult dose

Effect	Increases plasma levels of factor VIII activity by causing release of von Willebrand's factor from endothelial cells; increases renal water reabsorption
Onset	Minutes; peak 15–30 minutes
Duration	3 hours for von Willebrand's disease, 4–24 hours for hemophilia A
Clearance	Renal elimination
Comments	Chlorpropamide, carbamazepine, and clofibrate potentiate the antidiuretic effect; for bleeding diathesis, repeated doses will have diminished effect compared to initial dose

Dexamethasone (Decadron)

Indications	Cerebral edema from CNS tumors; airway edema
Dosage	Loading dose: 10 mg IV
	Maintenance dose: 4 mg IV every 16 hours (tapered over 6 days)
Effect	Anti-inflammatory and antiallergic effect; mineralocorticoid effect; stimulation of gluconeogenesis; inhibition of peripheral protein synthesis; membrane-stabilizing effect; has 25 times the glucocorticoid potency of hydrocortisone; minimal mineralocorticoid effect
Onset	IV: immediate
Duration	IV: 4–6 hours up to 24 hours
Clearance	Primarily hepatic metabolism; renal elimination
Comments	May cause adrenocortical insufficiency (Addison's crisis) with abrupt withdrawal, delayed wound healing, CNS disturbances, osteoporosis, or electrolyte disturbances

Dexmedetomidine (Precedex)

Indications	Short-term use as a sedative for patients undergoing mechanical ventilation in the intensive care setting
Dosage	Loading infusion: 1 μg/kg over 10 minutes
	Maintenance dose: 0.2–0.7 μg/kg/h
Effect	Selective α-2 adrenoreceptor agonist used for short-term therapy as a sedative for patients undergoing mechanical ventilation in the intensive care setting
Onset	30 minutes
Duration	Up to 4 hours
Clearance	Hepatic
Comments	Hypotension can occur in approximately 30% of patients; transient hypertension may be associated with bolus dosing; hypoxia can occur in nonventilated patients

Dextran 40 (Rheomacrodex)

Indications	Inhibition of platelet aggregation; improvement of blood flow in low-flow states (e.g., vascular surgery); intravascular volume expander
Dosage	Adult:
	Loading dose: 30–50 mL IV over 30 minutes
	Maintenance dose: 15–30 mL/h IV (10% solution)
	Pediatric:
	<20 mL/kg/24 hours of 10% dextran

Effect	Immediate, short-lived plasma volume expansion; adsorption to red blood cells (RBC) surface preventing aggregation, decreasing blood viscosity and platelet adhesiveness
Onset	Rapid
Duration	4–8 hours
Clearance	100% renal elimination
Comments	*Promit* (dextran monomer) is no longer available in the United States. May cause volume overload, anaphylaxis, bleeding tendency, interference with blood cross-matching, or false elevation of blood sugar; can cause renal failure

Digoxin (Lanoxin)

Indications	Heart failure, tachydysrhythmias, atrial fibrillation, atrial flutter
Dosage	Adult: Loading dose: 0.5–1 mg/d IV or orally in divided doses Maintenance dose: 0.125–0.5 mg IV or orally daily, reduce dose in renal failure
Effect	Increase in myocardial contractility; decrease in conduction in AV node and Purkinje fibers
Onset	15–30 minutes
Duration	2–6 days
Clearance	Renal elimination (50%–70% unchanged)
Comments	May cause gastrointestinal intolerance, blurred vision, ECG changes, or dysrhythmias; toxicity potentiated by hypokalemia, hypomagnesemia, hypercalcemia; cautious use in Wolff-Parkinson-White syndrome and with defibrillation; heart block potentiated by β-blockade and calcium channel blockade

Diltiazem (Cardizem)

Indications	Angina pectoris, variant angina from coronary artery spasm, atrial fibrillation/flutter, paroxysmal supraventricular tachycardia, hypertension
Dosage	IV loading dose: 0.25 mg/kg (~15–20 mg; maximum dose 25 mg) direct IV bolus over 2 minutes; for inadequate response an additional 0.35 mg/kg IV over 2 minutes (~25–30 mg) may be given 15 minutes after initial dose IV Maintenance dose: 10 mg/h (5 mg/h if hemodynamically unstable); titrate by 2.5 mg/h every 0.5–2 hours to achieve desired heart rate; recommended maximum 30 mg/h Oral maintenance dose: 30–60 mg every 6 hours Maximum: 540 mg/d for hypertension, 480 mg/d for angina
Effect	Calcium channel antagonist that slows conduction through sinoatrial and AV nodes, dilates coronary and peripheral arterioles, and reduces myocardial contractility
Onset	IV: 1–3 minutes Oral: 1–3 hours
Duration	IV: 1–3 hours Oral: 4–24 hours
Clearance	Primarily hepatic metabolism; renal elimination

| Comments | May cause hypotension, bradycardia, and heart block; may interact with β-blockers and digoxin to impair contractility; causes transiently elevated liver function tests; avoid use in patients with accessory tracts, AV block, IV β-blockers, or ventricular tachycardia |

Diphenhydramine (Benadryl)

Indications	Allergic reactions, drug-induced extrapyramidal reactions, sedation
Dosage	Adult: 10–50 mg IV every 6–8 hours
	Pediatric: 5 mg/kg/d IV in 4 divided doses (maximum 300 mg)
Effect	Antagonism of histamine action on H_1 receptors; anticholinergic; CNS depression
Onset	Rapid
Duration	4–6 hours
Clearance	Hepatic metabolism; renal excretion
Comments	May cause hypotension, tachycardia, dizziness, urinary retention, seizures; it should be administered IV or IM; do NOT administer subcutaneously

Dobutamine (Dobutrex)

Indications	Heart failure, hypotension
Dosage	Standard mix: 250 mg in 250 mL of D_5W or NS
	Adult: Start infusion at 2 μg/kg/min and titrate to effect
	Pediatric: 5–20 μg/kg/min
Effect	$β_1$-adrenergic agonist
Onset	1–2 minutes
Duration	<5 minutes
Clearance	Hepatic metabolism; renal elimination
Comments	May cause hypertension, hypotension, dysrhythmias, or myocardial ischemia; can increase ventricular rate in atrial fibrillation; doses >20 μg/kg have a high rate of cardiac dysrhythmia

Dopamine (Intropin)

Indications	1. Hypotension, heart failure
	2. Oliguria
Dosage	Standard mixes: 200, 400, or 800 mg in 250 mL D_5W or NS
	1. Infusion at 5–20 μg/kg/min IV, titrate to effect
	2. Infusion at 1–3 μg/kg/min IV
Effect	Dopaminergic, α- and β-adrenergic agonist
Onset	5 minutes
Duration	<10 minutes
Clearance	75% metabolized in the liver, kidneys, and plasma by monoamine oxidase and catechol O-methyltransferase to inactive homovanillic acid
Comments	May cause hypertension, dysrhythmias, or myocardial ischemia; primarily dopaminergic effects (increased renal blood flow) at 1–5 μg/kg/min; primarily α- and β-adrenergic effects at ≥10 μg/kg/min; run via central line

Droperidol (Inapsine)

Indications	1. Nausea, vomiting
	2. Agitation, sedation, adjunct to anesthesia
Dosage	Adult:
	1. 0.625–2.5 mg IV prn
	2. 2.5–10 mg IV prn
	Pediatric:
	1. 0.05–0.06 mg/kg every 4–6 hours
Effect	Dopamine (δ_2)-receptor antagonist; apparent psychic indifference to environment, catatonia, antipsychotic, antiemetic
Onset	3–10 minutes
Duration	3–6 hours
Clearance	Hepatic metabolism; renal excretion
Comments	May cause anxiety, extrapyramidal reactions, or hypotension (from moderate α-adrenergic and dopaminergic antagonism); residual effects may persist $\geq$24 hours. Potentiates other CNS depressants; and may cause fatal ventricular arrhythmia. **A Black- Box warning from the Food and Drug Administration (FDA)** reports that QT prolongation, ventricular arrhythmia such as *torsade de pointes,* and even death have been reported. Droperidol should not be administered in men with QTc intervals >440 ms or in women with QTc intervals >450 ms. ECG monitoring should continue for 2–3 hours after completion of droperidol treatment; at-risk patients, according to the manufacturer, include those with congestive heart failure, bradycardia, cardiac hypertrophy, hypokalemia, or hypomagnesemia; also those using diuretics or other drugs known to cause QT-interval prolongation

1. Intramuscular (Solution)
a) Cases of QT prolongation and/or torsade de pointes have been reported in patients receiving droperidol at doses at or below recommended doses. Some cases have occurred in patients with no known risk factors for QT prolongation and some cases have been fatal. b) Due to its potential for serious proarrhythmic effects and death, droperidol should be reserved for use in the treatment of patients who fail to show an acceptable response to other adequate treatments, either because of insufficient effectiveness or the inability to achieve an effective dose due to intolerable adverse effects from those drugs. c) Cases of QT prolongation and serious arrhythmias (e.g., torsade de pointes) have been reported in patients treated with droperidol. Based on these reports, all patients should undergo a 12-lead ECG prior to administration of droperidol to determine if a prolonged QT interval (i.e., QTc greater than 440 msec for males or 450 msec for females) is present. If there is a prolonged QT interval, droperidol should not be administered. For patients in whom the potential benefit of droperidol treatment is felt to outweigh the risks of potentially serious arrhythmias, ECG monitoring should be performed prior to treatment and continued for 2–3 hours after completing treatment to monitor for arrhythmias. d) Droperidol is contraindicated in patients with known or suspected QT prolongation, including patients with congenital long QT syndrome. e) Droperidol should

be administered with extreme caution to patients who may be at risk for development of prolonged QT syndrome (e.g., congestive heart failure, bradycardia, use of a diuretic, cardiac hypertrophy, hypokalemia, hypomagnesemia, or administration of other drugs known to increase the QT interval). Other risk factors may include age over 65 years, alcohol abuse, and use of agents such as benzodiazepines, volatile anesthetics, and IV opiates. Droperidol should be initiated at a low dose and adjusted upward, with caution, as needed to achieve the desired effect (Prod Info Droperidol intravenous solution, intramuscular solution, USP, 2002).

Enalapril/enalaprilat (Vasotec)

Indications	Hypertension, congestive heart failure
Dosage	Oral loading dose: 2.5–5 mg daily
	Oral maintenance dose: 10–40 mg daily
	IV: 0.125–5 mg every 6 hours (as enalaprilat)
Effect	Angiotensin-converting enzyme inhibitor; synergistic with diuretics
Onset	1 hour
Duration	6–24 hours
Clearance	Renal/fecal elimination; hepatic metabolism of enalapril to active metabolite (enalaprilat)
Comments	Hyperkalemia, increased renal blood flow, volume-responsive hypotension; subsequent doses are additive in effect; may cause angioedema, blood dyscrasia, cough, lithium toxicity, or worsening of renal impairment

Enoxaparin (Lovenox)

Indications	1. DVT/PE prophylaxis
	2. Therapeutic anticoagulation for treatment or prevention of thrombosis, acute coronary syndrome
Dosage	1. 30 mg SQ twice daily or 40 mg SQ daily
	2. 1 mg/kg SQ every 12 hours
Effect	Binds with antithrombin III and accelerates inactivation of factors IIa (thrombin), Xa, IXa, XIa, and XIIa
Onset	2 hours
Duration	10–24 hours
Clearance	Renal
Comments	Therapeutic doses should be used with caution in patients with renal impairment; factor Xa levels are of little value in determining therapeutic response; incompletely and unpredictable reversed by protamine; do not use in patients with heparin-induced thrombocytopenia

Ephedrine

Indication	Hypotension
Dosage	5–50 mg IV prn
Effect	α- and β-adrenergic stimulation; norepinephrine release at sympathetic nerve endings
Onset	Rapid

Duration	1 hour
Clearance	Mostly renal elimination, unchanged
Comments	May cause hypertension, dysrhythmias, myocardial ischemia, CNS stimulation, decreased uterine activity, or mild bronchodilation; avoid giving to patients taking monoamine oxidase inhibitors; minimal effect on uterine blood flow; tachyphylaxis with repeated dosing

Epinephrine (Adrenaline)

Indications	1. Heart failure, hypotension, cardiac arrest
	2. Bronchospasm, anaphylaxis
	3. Airway edema, bronchospasm
Dosage	Standard mix: 2 mg in 250 mL of D_5W or NS
	Adult:
	1. 0.1–1 mg IV or (intracardiac) every 5 minutes prn: 1–3 mg intratracheal during CPR
	2. 0.1–0.5 mg SQ, 0. 1–0.25 mg IV, or 0.25–1.5 μg/min IV infusion
	3. 2.5–5 mg inhaled via nebulizer every 1–4 hours prn
	Pediatric:
	1. Neonates: 0.01–0.03 mg/kg every 3–5 minutes
	Children: 0.01 mg/kg IV or intratracheal every 3–5 hours (up to 5 mL 1:10,000)
	2. 0.01 mg/kg IV up to 0.5 mg; 0.01 mg/kg SQ every 15 minutes by 2 doses up to 1 mg/dose
	3. 0.25–0.5 mL/kg (maximum: 5 mLs) in 3 mL NS nebulized *prn*
Effect	α- and β-adrenergic agonist
Onset	Rapid
Duration	1–2 minutes
Clearance	Monoamine oxidase/catechol *O*-methyltransferase metabolism
Comments	May cause hypertension, dysrhythmias, or myocardial ischemia; dysrhythmias potentiated by halothane; topical or local injection 1:80,000–1:500,000 causes vasoconstriction; crosses placenta

Ergonovine (Ergotrate)

Indication	Postpartum hemorrhage due to uterine atony
Dosage	For postpartum hemorrhage: IV (emergency only): 0.2 mg in 5 mL of NS over ≥1 minute
	IM: 0.2 mg every 2–4 hours prn for up to 5 doses; then oral: 0.2–0.4 mg every 6–12 hours for 2 days or prn
Effect	Constriction of uterine and vascular smooth muscle
Onset	IV: 1 minute
	IM: 2–3 minutes
	Oral: 6–15 minutes
Duration	IV: 45 minutes
	Oral / IM: 3 hours
Clearance	Hepatic metabolism; renal elimination
Comments	May cause hypertension from systemic vasoconstriction (especially in eclampsia and hypertension), dysrhythmias, coronary spasm, uterine tetany, or gastrointestinal upset; IV route is only used in emergencies; overdose may cause convulsions or stroke

Esmolol (Brevibloc)

Indications	Supraventricular tachydysrhythmias, myocardial ischemia
Dosage	Start with 5–10 mg IV bolus and increase every 3 minutes prn to total 100–300 mg; infusion 1–15 mg/min
Effect	Selective β_1-adrenergic blockade
Onset	Rapid
Duration	10–20 minutes following discontinuation
Clearance	Degraded by RBC esterases; renal elimination
Comments	May cause bradycardia, AV conduction delay, hypotension, congestive heart failure; β_2 activity at high doses

Esomeprazole (Nexium)

Indications	Gastric acid hypersecretion or gastritis, gastroesophageal reflux
Dosage	IV: 20 mg or 40 mg once daily; change to oral therapy as soon as appropriate
Effect	Inhibition of H^+ secretion by irreversibly binding H^+/K^+-ATPase
Onset	1 hour
Duration	>24 hours
Clearance	Extensive hepatic metabolism; 72%–80% renal elimination, 18%–23% fecal elimination
Comments	Increases secretion of gastrin; more rapid healing of gastric ulcer than with histamine-2 blockers; effective in ulcers resistant to histamine-2 blocker therapy; inhibits some cytochrome P-450 enzymes

Ethacrynic acid (Edecrin)

Indications	Edema, congestive heart failure, acute/chronic renal failure
Dosage	Adult: IV: 25–100 mg IV over 5–10 minutes; 24-hour cumulative dose: 400 mg Oral: 50–200 mg/d in 1–2 divided doses Pediatric: IV: 1 mg/kg/dose; repeat doses with caution due to potential for ototoxicity Oral: 25 mg/d to start, increase by 25 mg/d until response is obtained; maximum 3 mg/kg/d
Effect	Diuretic
Onset	IV: 5 minutes Oral: within 30 minutes
Duration	IV: 2 hours Oral: 12 hours
Clearance	Hepatically metabolized to active cysteine conjugate (35%–40%); 30%–60% excreted unchanged in bile and urine
Comments	May potentiate the activity of antihypertensives, neuromuscular blocking agents, and digoxin and increase insulin requirement in diabetic patients; oral preparations are not readily available; long-term therapy is generally not feasible

Fenoldopam (Corlopam)

Indications	1. Hypertension 2. Oliguria

Dosage	Adult:
	1. Hypertension: initial, 0.03–0.1 μg/kg/min IV; increase every 15 minutes by 0.05–0.1 μg/kg/min based on response, maximum 1.6 μg/kg/min
	2. Oliguria: 0.03 μg/kg/min with no dose adjustments
	Pediatric:
	1. Hypertension: initial, 0.2 μg/kg/min IV; increase in increments of up to 0.3–0.5 μg/kg/min every 20–30 minutes; doses >0.8 μg/kg/ min have resulted in tachycardia with no observation of additional benefit
Effect	Selective δ-1 receptor agonist
Onset	15–30 minutes
Duration	Up to 4 hours
Clearance	Hepatic (insignificant)
Comments	Hypotension, increases in heart rate, and asymptomatic T-wave flattening on the electrocardiogram have been reported; other adverse effects include headache, dizziness, flushing, nausea and vomiting, and increases in portal pressure in cirrhotic patients

Filgrastim (G-CSF, granulocyte-colony stimulating factor, Neupogen)

Indications	Neutropenia secondary to immunosuppressive drug therapy
Dosage	Adult and pediatric:
	Initial dosing recommendation: 5 μg/kg/d administered SQ. May be given IV for neutropenic patients.
	Doses may be increased in increments of 5 μg/kg as titrated to patient response, according to the duration and severity of the absolute neutrophil count nadir
Effect	Promotes neutrophil production
Onset	Rapid elevation in neutrophil counts within the first 24 hours, reaching a plateau in 3–5 days
Duration	Absolute neutrophil count decreases by 50% within 2 days after discontinuing G-CSF; white counts return to the normal range in 4–7 days
Clearance	Systemically metabolized
Comments	Filgrastim dose should be adjusted to coincide with available single-use containers (300 μg, 480 μg) whenever possible

Flumazenil (Romazicon)

Indication	1. Reversal of benzodiazepine sedation
	2. Benzodiazepine overdose
Dosage	1. 0.2–1 mg IV every 20 minutes at 0.2 mg/min
	2. 3–5 mg IV at 0.5 mg/min
Effect	Competitive antagonism of CNS benzodiazepine receptor
Onset	1–2 minutes
Duration	1–2 hours (dose dependent)
Clearance	100% hepatic metabolism; 90%–95% renal elimination of metabolite
Comments	Duration of action depends on dose and duration of action of benzodiazepine; flumazenil will reverse CNS sedation, but has little effect on respiratory (CO_2 dependent) drive; may induce CNS excitation including seizures, acute withdrawal, nausea, dizziness, agitation; does not reverse non–benzodiazepine-induced CNS depression

Folic acid (Folacin, Folate)

Indications	Megaloblastic and macrocytic anemias
Dosage	Adult:
	Oral, IM, IV, SQ:
	Initial dose: 1 mg/d
	Maintenance dose: 0.5 mg/d; pregnant and lactating women: 0.8 mg/d
	Pediatric:
	Oral, IM, IV, SQ:
	Initial dose: 1 mg/d
	Maintenance dose:
	1–10 years: 0.1–0.3 mg/d
	Infants: 15 μg/kg/d or 50 μg/d
Effect	Vitamin B complex substrate
Onset	Within 0.5–1 hour
Comments	Folic acid may alleviate the hematologic complications of pernicious anemia while allowing neurologic sequelae to occur; therefore, it should be administered with extreme caution to patients with undiagnosed anemia; may produce allergic reactions

Fondaparinux (Arixtra)

Indications	1. Prophylaxis of DVT and PE in orthopedic surgery and hip fractures
	2. Treatment of DVT and PE
Dosage	1. 2.5 mg SQ daily
	2. <50 kg: 5 mg SQ daily
	50–100 kg: 7.5 mg SQ daily
	>100 kg: 10 mg SQ daily
Effect	Anti-Xa pentasaccharide
Onset	60–90 minutes
Duration	17–21 hours
Clearance	Renal (avoid in patients with creatinine clearance <30 mLs)
Comments	Renally excreted; does not cross-react with PF4 heparin antibodies

Fosphenytoin (Cerebyx)

(See Chapter 29 for treatment of seizures.)

Indications	1. Seizures, seizure prophylaxis
	2. Digoxin-induced dysrhythmias
	3. Refractory ventricular tachycardia
Dosage	1. Seizures
	IV loading dose:
	Neonates: 15–20 mg **phenytoin equivalents (PE)**/kg IV
	Infants, children, and adults: 15–18 mg PE/kg in a single or divided dose
	IV maintenance dose:
	Neonate: 2.5 mg PE/kg/dose every 12 hours
	Infants and children: Initial: 5 mg PE/kg/d in 2–3 divided doses;
	Usual doses: (dosing based on recommended IV phenytoin doses)
	0.5–3 years: 8–10 mg PE/kg/d

4–6 years: 7.5–9 mg PE/kg/d
7–9 years: 7–8 mg PE/kg/d
10–16 years: 6–7 mgPE/kg/d
Adults: Usual: 300 mg PE/d or 4–6 mg PE/kg/d in 2–3 divided doses
2, 3. Arrhythmias:
Children and adults: dosing based on recommended IV phenytoin doses
IV loading dose: 1.25 mg PE/kg every 5 minutes, may repeat up to
total loading dose 15 mg PE/kg.
IV maintenance dose:
Children: 5–10 mg PE/kg/d in 2–3 divided doses

Effect	Anticonvulsant effect via membrane stabilization; antidysrhythmic effects similar to those of quinidine or procainamide
Onset	3–5 minutes
Duration	Dose dependent; half-life is dose dependent in therapeutic range
Clearance	Hepatic metabolism; renal elimination (enhanced by alkaline urine)
Comments	**PE = phenytoin equivalents.** Fosphenytoin is a prodrug of phenytoin, and its anticonvulsant effects are attributed to phenytoin. May cause nystagmus, diplopia, ataxia, drowsiness, gingival hyperplasia, gastrointestinal upset, hyperglycemia, or hepatic microsomal enzyme induction; IV bolus may cause bradycardia, hypotension, respiratory arrest, cardiac arrest, CNS depression; tissue irritant; crosses placenta; significant interpatient variation, from 7.5 to 20.0 μg/mL, in the dose needed to achieve therapeutic concentration; determination of unbound phenytoin levels may help in patients with renal failure or hypoalbuminemia

Furosemide (Lasix)

Indications	Edema, hypertension, renal failure, hypercalcemia
Dosage	Adult: 10–40 mg IV (initial dose, dose individualized) at a rate not to exceed 10 mg/min Pediatric: 1–2 mg/kg/dose
Effect	Increase in excretion of Na^+, Cl^-, K^+, PO_4^{3-}, Ca^{2+}, and H_2O by inhibiting reabsorption in loop of Henle
Onset	5 minutes
Duration	6 hours
Clearance	Hepatic metabolism; 88% renal elimination
Comments	May cause electrolyte imbalance, dehydration, transient hypotension, deafness, hyperglycemia, or hyperuricemia; sulfa-allergic patients may exhibit hypersensitivity to furosemide. May be given as a continuous infusion in the ICU setting

Ganciclovir (Cytovene)

Indications	Treatment of cytomegalovirus (CMV) retinitis in immunocompromised individuals; treatment of CMV colitis and pneumonitis
Dosage	Adult and pediatric: Initial IV: 5 mg/kg every 12 hours for 14–21 days Followed by 5 mg/kg IV as a single dose for the duration of patient's immunosuppression; adjust dose for renal impairment
Effect	Antiviral
Onset	Oral absorption increased with food

Duration	Half-life: 1.7–5.8 hours; increases with impaired renal function
Clearance	Majority (94%–99%) excreted unchanged drug in the urine
Comments	Dose adjustment or interruption of ganciclovir therapy may be necessary in patients with neutropenia and/or thrombocytopenia and patients with impaired renal function

Glucagon

Indications	1. Duodenal or choledochal relaxation
	2. Hypoglycemia
	3. β-Blocker overdose
Dosage	1. 0.25–0.5 mg IV every 20 minutes prn
	2. 0.5–1 mg, may repeat in 20 minutes as needed
	3. 5-mg bolus followed by an infusion of 1–5 mg/h up to 10 mg/h as titrated to patient response
Effect	Catecholamine release
Onset	45 seconds
Duration	9–25 minutes (dose dependent)
Clearance	Hepatic and renal proteolysis
Comments	May cause anaphylaxis, nausea, vomiting, hyperglycemia, or positive inotropic and chronotropic effects; high doses potentiate oral anticoagulants

Glycopyrrolate (Robinul)

Indications	1. Decrease gastrointestinal motility, antisialagogue
	2. Bradycardia
Dosage	Adult:
	1. IV/IM/SQ: 0.1–0.2 mg; oral: 1–2 mg
	2. 0.1–0.2 mg/dose IV
	Children:
	1. Oral: 40–100 mcg/kg/dose 3–4 times/d
	IM, IV: 4–10 mcg/kg/dose every 3–4 hours
Effect	See atropine
Onset	IV: 1–4 minutes
	IM: 30–45 minutes
Duration	IV: 2–4 hours
	IM: 2–7 hours
Clearance	Renal elimination
Comments	See atropine; doses do not cross blood–brain barrier or placenta; with less chronotropy than atropine; erratic oral absorption

Haloperidol (Haldol)

Indications	1. Psychosis, agitation, delirium
	2. Delirium in the ICU
Dosage	1. 0.5–5 mg IV prn 2–3 times/d (dose individualized)
	2. IV 2–5 mg; may repeat bolus doses every 20–30 minutes until calm achieved then administer 25% of the maximum dose every 6 hours; monitor ECG and QT_c interval

Effect	Antipsychotic effects due to dopamine (D_2)-receptor antagonism; CNS depression
Onset	IV peak effect <20 minutes
Duration	IV half-life 14 hours
Clearance	Hepatic metabolism; renal/biliary elimination
Comments	Monitor ECG and QT_c interval. May cause extrapyramidal reactions or very mild α-adrenergic antagonism; may precipitate neuroleptic malignant syndrome; contraindicated in Parkinson's disease, toxic CNS depression, coma

Heparin

Indications	1. Anticoagulation for thrombosis, thromboembolism 2. Cardiopulmonary bypass 3. Disseminated intravascular coagulation

Dosage	Adult:
	1. Loading dose: 50–150 U/kg IV
	   Maintenance dose: 15–25 U/kg/h IV; titrate dosage with partial thromboplastin time or activated clotting time
	2. Loading dose: 300 U/kg IV
	   Maintenance dose: 100 U/kg/h IV; titrate with coagulation tests
	3. Loading dose: 50–100 U/kg IV
	Pediatric:
	Loading dose: 50 U/kg IV
	Maintenance dose: 15–25 U/kg/h IV; titrate with coagulation tests

Effect	Potentiates action of antithrombin III; blockade of conversion of prothrombin and activation of other coagulation factors
Onset	IV: immediate SQ: 1–2 hours
Duration	Half-life: 1–6 hours; increases with dose
Clearance	Primarily by reticuloendothelial uptake, hepatic biotransformation
Comments	May cause bleeding, **heparin-induced thrombocytopenia (HIT)**, allergic reactions, or diuresis (36–48 hours after a large dose); half-life increased in renal failure and decreased in thromboembolism and liver disease; does not cross placenta; reversed by protamine

Hydralazine (Apresoline)

Indication	Hypertension
Dosage	2.5–20 mg IV every 4 hours or prn (dose individualized)
Effect	Relaxation of vascular smooth muscle (arteriole > venule)
Onset	5–20 minutes, peak effect 10–80 minutes
Duration	2–6 hours
Clearance	Extensive hepatic metabolism; renal elimination
Comments	May cause hypotension (diastolic > systolic), reflex tachycardia, systemic lupus erythematosis syndrome, or Coombs'-positive hemolytic anemia; increases coronary, splanchnic, cerebral, and renal blood flows

Hydrocortisone (SoluCortef—see also Chapter 27 for comparison of various corticosteroids.)

Indications	1. Adrenal insufficiency
	2. Inflammation and allergy
	3. Status asthmaticus
Dosage	1. 100 mg IV bolus, then 300 mg/d in divided doses every 8 hours
	2. Oral, IM, IV: 15–240 mg every 12 hours
	3. IV: 1–2 mg/kg/dose every 6 hours for 24 hours, then maintenance of 0.5–1 mg/kg every 6 hours
Effect	Anti-inflammatory and antiallergic effect; mineralocorticoid effect; stimulation of gluconeogenesis; inhibition of peripheral protein synthesis; membrane-stabilizing effect
Onset	1 hour
Duration	6–8 hours (dose/route dependent)
Clearance	Hepatic metabolism; renal elimination
Comments	May cause adrenocortical insufficiency (Addison's crisis) with abrupt withdrawal, delayed wound healing, CNS disturbances, osteoporosis, or electrolyte disturbances

Hydroxyzine (Vistaril, Atarax)

Indications	Anxiety, nausea and vomiting, allergies, sedation
Dosage	Oral: 25 = 200 mg every 6–8 hours
	IM: 25–100 mg every 4–6 hours
	Not an IV drug. Injection for IM use only
Effect	Antagonism of histamine action on histamine-1 receptors, CNS depression, antiemetic
Onset	15–60 minutes
Duration	4–6 hours
Clearance	Hepatic (P-450) metabolism; renal elimination
Comments	May cause dry mouth; minimal cardiorespiratory depression; IV injection may cause thrombosis; crosses placenta

Insulin

Indications	1. Hyperglycemia
	2. Diabetic ketoacidosis
Dosage	1. Individualized: usually 5–10 U IV/SQ prn (regular insulin)
	2. Loading dose: 10–20 U IV (regular insulin)
	Maintenance dose: 0.05–0.1 U/kg/h IV (regular insulin), titrated against plasma glucose level
Effect	Facilitation of glucose transport intracellularly; shift of K^+ and Mg^{2+} intracellular
Onset	SQ: insulin aspart, lispro: rapid acting: 10–20 minutes
	Regular: 30 minutes
	NPH: 1–2 hours
	Glargine: 3–4 hours
Duration	SQ: insulin aspart: rapid acting: 3–5 hours
	Lispro: 60–90 minutes
	Regular: 5–7 hours
	NPH: 18–24 hours

Glargine: 24 hours

Clearance   Hepatic and renal metabolism; 30%–80% renal elimination;
                      unchanged insulin is reabsorbed

Comments   May cause allergic reactions, synthesis of insulin antibodies; may
                      be absorbed by plastic in IV tubing; when initiating insulin therapy,
                      use human rather than beef or pork insulin to minimize the develop-
                      ment of antibodies (see also **Chapter 28**)

Isosorbide dinitrate (Isordil)

Indications	Angina, hypertension, myocardial infarction, congestive heart failure
Dosage	5–20 mg orally every 6 hours
Effect	See nitroglycerin
Onset	15–40 minutes
Duration	4–6 hours
Clearance	Nearly 100% hepatic metabolism; renal elimination
Comments	See nitroglycerin; tolerance develops

Ketorolac (Toradol)

Indications	Nonsteroidal anti-inflammatory analgesic drug (NSAIDs) for moder-ate pain; useful adjunct for severe pain when used with parenteral or epidural opioids
Dosage	IM/IV: 30 mg, then 15–30 mg every 6 hours For patients older than 65 years, maximum suggested dose is 15 mg every 6 hours
Effect	Limits prostaglandin synthesis by cyclooxygenase inhibition
Onset	30–60 minutes
Duration	4–6 hours
Clearance	<50% hepatic metabolism, renal metabolism; 91% renal elimination
Comments	Adverse effects are similar to those with other NSAIDs: peptic ulceration, bleeding, decreased renal blood flow; duration of treat-ment not to exceed 5 days

Labetalol (Normodyne, Trandate)

Indications	Hypertension, angina
Dosage	IV: 5- to 10-mg increments at 5-minutes intervals, to 40–80 mg/dose Standard mix: 500 mg in 250 mL D_5W or NS (5 mg/mL); start at 0.05 µg/kg/min
Effect	Selective α1-adrenergic blockade with nonselective β-adrenergic blockade; ratio of α/β blockade is 1:7
Onset	Minutes
Duration	2–12 hours
Clearance	Hepatic metabolism; renal elimination
Comments	May cause bradycardia, AV conduction delays, bronchospasm in patients with asthma, and postural hypotension; crosses placenta

Levothyroxine (Synthroid)

Indications	Hypothyroidism
Dosage	Adjust according to individual requirements and response Adults:

Oral: 0.1–0.2 mg/d up to a maximum of 0.5 mg/d
IV: 75% of oral dose
Pediatric:
Oral:
0–6 months: 25–50 µg/d or 8–10 µg/kg/d
6–12 months: 50–75 µg/d or 6–8 µg/kg/d
1–5 years: 75–100 µg/d or 5–6 µg/kg/d
6–12 years: 100–150 µg/d or 4–5 µg/kg/d
>12 years: >150 µg/d or 2–3 µg/kg/d
IV: 75% of oral dose

Effect	Exogenous thyroxine
Onset	Oral: 3–5 days
	IV: within 6–8 hours
Duration	Peak effect at approximately 24 hours
Clearance	Metabolized in the liver to triiodothyronine (active); eliminated in feces and urine
Comments	Contraindicated with recent myocardial infarction or thyrotoxicosis, or uncorrected adrenal insufficiency; phenytoin may decrease levothyroxine levels; increases effects of oral anticoagulants; tricyclic antidepressants may increase toxic potential of both drugs; intravenous therapy can be given at three-fourths of the oral dose

Lidocaine (Xylocaine)

Indications	1. Ventricular dysrhythmias
	2. Local anesthesia
Dosage	Adult:
	1. **Loading dose: 1 mg/kg IV over 1 minute.** Additional loading doses: 0.5 mg/kg at 10-minute intervals up to 3 mg/kg
	Maintenance dose: 15–50 µg/kg/min IV (1–4 mg/min)
	2. 5 mg/kg maximum dose for infiltration or conduction block
	Pediatric:
	1. Loading: 0.5–1 mg/kg IV (second dose 20–30 minutes after first dose)
	Maintenance dose: 15–50 µg/kg/min IV
Effect	Antiarrhythmic effect; sedation; neural blockade; decreased conductance of sodium channels
Onset	Rapid
Duration	5–20 minutes
Clearance	Hepatic metabolism to active/toxic metabolites; renal elimination (10% unchanged)
Comments	May cause dizziness, seizures, disorientation, heart block (with myocardial conduction defect), or hypotension; crosses placenta; therapeutic concentration is 1–5 mg/L; avoid in patients with Wolff-Parkinson-White syndrome

Magnesium sulfate

Indications	1. Preeclampsia/eclampsia
	2. Hypomagnesemia
	3. Polymorphic ventricular tachycardia (torsades de pointes)
Dosage	Adult:
	1. Loading dose: 2–6 g over 20–30 minutes IV (2 g/100 mL or 40 g/1,000 mL)

Maintenance dose: 1–4 g/h infusion (2 g/100 mL or 40 g/1,000 mL)

2. 1 g (8 mEq) every 6 hours × 4 doses

3. 1–2 g in 10 mL of D_5W over 1–2 minutes; 5–10 g may be administered for refractory dysrhythmias

Effect	To replete serum magnesium; for the prevention and treatment of seizures or hyperreflexia associated with preeclampsia/eclampsia
Onset	Rapid
Duration	4–6 hours
Clearance	100% renal elimination for IV route
Comments	Potentiates neuromuscular blockade (both depolarizing and nondepolarizing agents); potentiates CNS effects of anesthetics, hypnotics, and opioids; toxicity occurs with serum concentration ≥10 mEq/L; avoid in patients with heart block; may alter cardiac conduction in digitalized patients; caution in patients with renal failure

Mannitol (Osmitrol)

Indications	1. Increased intracranial pressure 2. Oliguria, or anuria associated with acute renal injury
Dosage	Adult: 1. 0.25–1 g/kg IV as 20% solution over 30–60 minutes (in an acute situation, can give a bolus of 1.25–25 g over 5–10 minutes 2. 0.2 g/kg test dose over 3–5 minutes then 50–100 g IV over 30 minutes if adequate response Pediatric: 1. 0.2 g/kg test dose, with maintenance of 2 g/kg over 30–60 minutes
Effect	Increase in serum osmolality, which reduces cerebral edema and lowers intracranial and intraocular pressure; also causes osmotic diuresis and transient expansion of intravascular volume
Onset	15 minutes
Duration	2–3 hours
Clearance	Renal elimination; onset 15 minutes, duration 2–3 hours
Comments	Rapid administration may cause vasodilation and hypotension; may worsen or cause pulmonary edema, intracranial hemorrhage, systemic hypertension, or rebound intracranial hypertension; hyponatremia common. Administer using in-line 5-μm filter set

Methylene blue

Indications	1. Surgical marker for genitourinary surgery 2. Methemoglobinemia
Dosage	1. 100 mg (10 mL of 1% solution) IV 2. 1–2 mg/kg IV of 1% solution over 10 minutes; repeat every 1 hour prn
Effect	Low dose promotes conversion of methemoglobin to hemoglobin; high dose promotes conversion of hemoglobin to methemoglobin
Onset	Immediate
Clearance	Tissue reduction; urinary and biliary elimination
Comments	May cause RBC destruction (prolonged use), hypertension, bladder irritation, nausea, diaphoresis; may inhibit nitrate-induced coronary artery relaxation; interferes with pulse oximetry for 1–2 minutes; may cause hemolysis in patients with glucose-6-phosphate dehydrogenase deficiency

Methylergonovine (Methergine)

Indication	Postpartum hemorrhage
Dosage	IV (EMERGENCY ONLY, after delivery of placenta): 0.2 mg in 5 mL of NS/dose over ≥1 minute
	IM: 0.2 mg every 2–4 hours (<5 doses)
	Oral: (after IM or IV doses): 0.2–0.4 mg every 6–12 hours × 2–7 days
Onset	IV: immediate
	IM: 2–5 minutes (maximum response after 30 minutes)
	PO: 5–10 minutes
Duration	1–3 hours
Clearance	Hepatic metabolism; renal elimination
Comments	See ergonovine; hypertensive response is less marked than with ergonovine

Methylprednisolone (Solu–Medrol)

Indications	Adrenal insufficiency, chronic obstructive pulmonary disease, cerebral edema, inflammatory diseases, immunosuppression
	Spinal cord injury
	Transplant rejection
	Reduction of allergenic drug response
	Asthma exacerbations
Dosage	Adult:
	1. For non–life-threatening conditions: 10–250 mg IV every 4–24 hours (IV given over 1 minute)
	For life-threatening conditions: 100–250 mg IV every 2–6 hours, or 30 mg/kg IV (given over 15 minutes) every 4–6 hours
	2. IV loading dose: 30 mg/kg in 50 ml over 15 minutes
	IV maintenance: 5.4 mg/kg/h × 23 hours. Start 45 minutes after the loading dose is finished
	3. 500 mg IV × 1 dose. 1,000 g IV × 1 dose for cardiac transplant patients
	4. Oral: 32 mg. Given 12 hours and 2 hours before administration of offending drug
	5. Load 2 mg/kg/dose then 0.5–1 mg/kg/dose every 6 hours for up to 5 days
	Pediatric:
	1. For life-threatening conditions: no more than 0.5 mg/kg in a 24-hour period
	2. See adult dosing above
	3. 250–500 mg IV × 1 dose
	5. See adult dosing above
Effect	See hydrocortisone; has five times the glucocorticoid potency of hydrocortisone; almost no mineralocorticoid activity
Onset	Minutes
Duration	6 hours
Clearance	Hepatic metabolism; renal elimination (dose/route dependent)
Comments	See hydrocortisone

Metoclopramide (Reglan)

Indications	Gastroesophageal reflux, diabetic gastroparesis, premedication for patients needing pulmonary aspiration prophylaxis, antiemetic

Dosage	Adult:
	IV: 10 mg 4 times/d
	Oral: 10 mg 4 times/d
	Pediatric: IV, oral: 0.1–0.2 mg/kg/dose 4 times/d. Not to exceed
	0.5 mg/kg/d
Effect	Facilitates gastric emptying by increasing gastrointestinal motility and lower esophageal sphincter tone; antiemetic effects are secondary to antagonism of central and peripheral dopamine receptors
Onset	IV: 1–3 minutes
	Oral: 30–60 minutes to peak effect
Duration	IV, oral: 1–2 hours
Kinetics	Hepatic metabolism; renal elimination
Comments	Avoid in patients with gastrointestinal obstruction, pheochromocytoma, and Parkinson's disease; extrapyramidal reactions in 0.2%–1% of patients; may exacerbate depression. Reduce dose in renal dysfunction

Metoprolol (Lopressor)

Indications	Hypertension, angina pectoris, dysrhythmia, hypertrophic cardiomyopathy, myocardial infarction, pheochromocytoma
Dosage	IV: 2.5–10 mg every 6 hours
	Oral: 50–100 mg orally every 6–8 hours
Effect	β_1-adrenergic blockade (β_2-adrenergic antagonism at high doses)
Onset	15 minutes
Duration	6 hours
Clearance	Hepatic metabolism, renal elimination
Comments	May cause bradycardia, bronchoconstriction (with doses >100 mg), dizziness, fatigue, insomnia; may increase risk of heart block; crosses placenta and blood–brain barrier

Milrinone (Primacor)

Indications	Congestive heart failure
Dosage	Loading dose: 50 μg/kg IV over 10 minutes
	Maintenance dose: titrate 0.375–0.750 μg/kg/min to effect
Effect	Phosphodiesterase inhibition causing positive inotropy, vasodilation
Onset	Immediate
Duration	2–3 hours
Clearance	Renal elimination
Comments	Short-term therapy; may increase ventricular ectopy

Nadolol (Corgard)

Indications	Angina pectoris, hypertension
Dosage	40–240 mg/d orally
Effect	Nonselective β-adrenergic blockade
Onset	1–2 hours
Duration	>24 hours
Clearance	No hepatic metabolism; renal elimination
Comments	May cause severe bronchospasm in susceptible patients (see propranolol)

Naloxone (Narcan)

Indications	Reversal of systemic opioid effects
Dosage	Adult: 0.04–2 mg/dose IV, may repeat every 2–20 minutes
	Pediatric:
	For total reversal of narcotic effect:
	Infants and children ≤5 years or ≤20 kg: 0.1 mg/kg
	Children >5 years or >20 kg: 2 mg/dose
	Pediatric postanalgesic narcotic reversal: 0.01 mg/kg, may repeat 2–3 minutes as needed
Effect	Antagonism of opioid effects by competitive inhibition
Onset	Rapid
Duration	Dose dependent; lasting 20–60 minutes
Clearance	95% hepatic metabolism; primarily renal elimination
Comments	May cause reversal of analgesia, hypertension, dysrhythmias, rare pulmonary edema, delirium, or withdrawal syndrome (in opioid-dependent patients); renarcotization may occur because antagonist has short duration; caution in hepatic failure

Nifedipine (Procardia)

Indications	Coronary artery spasm, hypertension, myocardial ischemia
Dosage	Oral:
	Immediate release: 10–40 mg 3 times/d
	Sustained release: 30–60 mg twice a day
Effect	Blockade of slow calcium channels in heart; systemic and coronary vasodilation and increase in myocardial perfusion
Onset	Oral: 20 minutes
Duration	4–24 hours
Clearance	Hepatic metabolism
Comments	May cause reflex tachycardia, gastrointestinal upset, or mild negative inotropic effects; little effect on automaticity and atrial conduction; may be useful in asymmetric septal hypertrophy; drug solution is light sensitive

Nitric oxide (Inomax)

Indications	Hypoxemic acute respiratory failure in term and near-term neonates
Dosage	1–40 ppm by continuous inhalation
Effect	Cyclic GMP-mediated pulmonary vasodilation of ventilated lung regions
Onset	5–10 minutes
Duration	Variable
Clearance	Bound to hemoglobin; metabolized to nitrates/nitrites
Comments	Off-label uses may include acute respiratory distress syndrome, cardiogenic shock, acute right ventricular failure, post–lung or heart transplant ischemia–reperfusion injury, and post–cardiopulmonary bypass pulmonary hypertension

Nitroglycerin

Indications	Angina pectoris, myocardial ischemia/infarction, hypertension, congestive heart failure, esophageal spasm

Dosage	IV infusion initially at 10 μg/min; titrate to effect;
	Standard mix: 200 mg/500 mL (0.4 mg/mL = 400 μg/mL)
	SL: 0.15–0.6 mg/dose every 5 minutes $\times$ 3 doses
	Topical: 2% ointment, 0.5–2.5 in every 6–8 hours
Effect	Smooth muscle relaxation by enzymatic release of nitric oxide, causing systemic, coronary, and pulmonary vasodilation (veins > arteries); bronchodilatation; biliary, gastrointestinal, and genitourinary tract relaxation
Onset	IV: 1–2 minutes
	SL: 1–3 minutes
	Oral: 1 hour
	Topical: 30 minutes
Duration	IV: 10 minutes
	SL: 30–60 minutes
	Oral: 8–12 hours
	Topical: 8–24 hours
Clearance	Nearly complete hepatic metabolism; renal elimination
Comments	May cause reflex tachycardia, hypotension, headache; tolerance with chronic use may be avoided with a 10- to 12-hour nitrate-free period; may be absorbed by plastic in IV tubing; may cause methemoglobinemia at very high doses

Nitroprusside (Nipride, Nitropress)

Indications	Hypertension, controlled hypotension, congestive heart failure
Dosage	IV: infusion initially at 0.1 μg/kg/min, then titrated against patient response to maximum 10 μg/kg/min (total dose <1–1.5 mg/kg over 2–3 hours)
	Standard mix: 50 mg in 250 mL of D_5W or NS
Effect	Direct nitric oxide donor causing smooth muscle relaxation (arterial > venous)
Onset	1–2 minutes
Duration	1–10 minutes after stopping of infusion
Clearance	RBC and tissue metabolism; renal elimination
Comments	May cause excessive hypotension, reflex tachycardia, accumulation of cyanide with liver dysfunction; thiocyanate with kidney disfunction; cyanide/thiocyanate buildup with prolonged infusion; avoid with Leber's hereditary optic atrophy, tobacco amblyopia, hypothyroidism, or vitamin B_{12} deficiency; solution and powder are light sensitive and must be wrapped in opaque material

Norepinephrine (Levarterenol, Levophed)

Indication	Hypotension
Dosage	Start at 1–8 μg/min, then titrate to desired effect
	Standard mix: 4 mg in 250 mL of D_5W or NS
Effect	α- > β-adrenergic agonist
Onset	Rapid
Duration	1–2 minutes following discontinuation
Clearance	Monoamine oxidase/catechol O-methyltransferase metabolism
Comments	May cause hypertension, dysrhythmias, myocardial ischemia, increased uterine contractility, constricted microcirculation, or CNS stimulation

Octreotide (Sandostatin)

Indication	1. Upper GI tract bleeding, acute variceal hemorrhage
	2. Control of symptoms in patients with metastatic carcinoid and vasoactive intestinal peptide–secreting tumors; pancreatic tumors, gastrinoma, secretory diarrhea
	3. Off-label uses include AIDS-associated secretory diarrhea, cryptosporidiosis, Cushing's syndrome, insulinomas, small-bowel fistulas, postgastrectomy dumping syndrome, chemotherapy-induced diarrhea, graft-versus-host disease–induced diarrhea, Zollinger-Ellison syndrome
Dosage	1. Adults:
	IV bolus: 25–50 μg followed by continuous IV infusion of 25–50 μg/h
	2, 3. Adults:
	SQ: initial 50 μg 1–3 times/d, and titrate dose based on patient tolerance and response
	Carcinoid: 100–600 μg/d in 2–4 divided doses
	VIPomas: 200–300 μg/d in 2–4 divided doses
	Diarrhea: IV, initial 50–100 μg every 8 hours; increase by 100 μg/dose at 48-hour intervals; maximum dose 500 μg every 8 hours
	Pediatric: SQ: 1–10 μg/kg every 12 hours beginning at the low end of the range and increasing by 0.3 μg/kg/dose at 3-day intervals
Effect	Somatostatin analogue that suppresses release of serotonin, gastrin, vasoactive intestinal peptide, insulin, glucagon, and secretin
Onset	IV: minutes
Duration	6–12 hours
Clearance	Hepatic and renal (32% eliminated unchanged); decreased in renal failure
Comments	May cause nausea, decreased gastrointestinal motility, transient hyperglycemia; duration of therapy should be no longer than 72 hours due to lack of efficacy beyond this time

Omeprazole (Prilosec)

Indications	Gastric acid hypersecretion or gastritis, gastroesophageal reflux
Dosage	20–40 mg orally 1–2 times/d
Effect	Inhibition of H^+ secretion by irreversibly binding H^+/K^+-ATPase
Onset	1 hour
Duration	>24 hours
Clearance	Extensive hepatic metabolism; 72%–80% renal elimination, 18%–23% fecal elimination
Comments	Increases secretion of gastrin; more rapid healing of gastric ulcer than with histamine-2 blockers; effective in ulcers resistant to histamine-2 blocker therapy; inhibits some cytochrome P-450 enzymes

Ondansetron hydrochloride (Zofran)

Indications	Prevention and treatment of perioperative nausea, vomiting
Dosage	Adult:

	IV: Perioperative 4 mg undiluted over > 30 seconds
	Oral: 2–8 mg
	Pediatric:
	$<$40 kg: 0.1 mg/kg IV $\times$ 1
	$>$40 kg: 4 mg IV $\times$ 1
Effect	Selective serotonin 5-HT$_3$ receptor antagonist
Onset	30 minutes
Duration	4–8 hours
Clearance	95% hepatic, 5% renal excretion
Comments	Used in much higher doses for chemotherapy-induced nausea; mild side effects: headache, reversible transaminase elevation

Oxytocin (Pitocin)

Indications	1. Postpartum hemorrhage, uterine atony
	2. Augmentation of labor
Dosage	1. IV infusion at rate necessary to control atony (e.g., 0.02–0.04 U/min)
	2. Labor induction: 0.0005–0.002 U/min
	Standard mix: 30 U in 500 mL of NS
Effect	Reduced postpartum blood loss by contraction of uterine smooth muscle; renal, coronary, and cerebral vasodilation
Onset	Immediate
Duration	1 hour
Clearance	Tissue metabolism; renal elimination
Comments	May cause uterine tetany and rupture, fetal distress, or anaphylaxis; IV bolus can cause hypotension, tachycardia, dysrhythmia

Pentamidine (Pentam)

Indications	Prevention and treatment of pneumonia caused by *Pneumocystis carinii*
Dosage	IV adult and pediatric: 4 mg/kg/d IV for 14 days. Maximum dose 300 mg
	Inhalation pediatric: 300 mg every 3–4 weeks via nebulizer
	Inhalation adult: 300 mg every 4 weeks via nebulizer
Effect	Antiprotozoal
Duration	Terminal half-life is 6–9 hours; may be prolonged in patients with severe renal impairment
Clearance	33%–66% excreted unchanged in urine
Comments	Concomitant use of nephrotoxic drugs may increase risk of nephro-toxicity

Phenobarbital

Indications	1. Sedative/hypnotic
	2. Anticonvulsant
Dosage	1. Adult and pediatric: 1–3 mg/kg orally
	2. Adult, infant, and pediatric:
	Loading dose: 10–20 mg/kg, additional 5 mg/kg doses every 15–30 minutes for control of status epilepticus, maximum 30 mg/kg

	Maintenance dose:
	Infants: 5–6 mg/kg/d in 1–2 divided doses
	Children 1–5 years: 6–8 mg/kg/d in 1–2 divided doses
	Children 5–12 years: 4–6 mg/kg/d in 1–2 divided doses
	Children >12 years and adults: 1–3 mg/kg/d in 1–2 divided doses
Onset	5 minutes, allow 60–90 minutes for full sedative effect
Duration	10–12 hours; half-life may be >100 hours
Clearance	Hepatic metabolism: 25%–50% renal elimination unchanged
Comments	May cause hypotension; multiple-drug interactions through induction of hepatic enzyme systems; therapeutic anticonvulsant concentration 15–40 μg/mL at trough (just before next dose)

Phenoxybenzamine (Dibenzyline)

Indication	Preoperative preparation for pheochromocytoma resection
Dosage	10–40 mg/d divided 2–3 times/d orally titrated (start at 10 mg/d and increase dose by 10 mg/d every 4 days prn)
Effect	Nonselective noncompetitive α-adrenergic antagonist
Onset	Hours
Duration	3–4 days
Clearance	Hepatic metabolism; renal/biliary excretion
Comments	May cause orthostatic hypotension (which may be refractory to norepinephrine), reflex tachycardia; nasal congestion expected

Phentolamine (Regitine)

Indications	1. Hypertension from catecholamine excess as in pheochromocytoma
	2. Extravasation of α-agonist
Dosage	1. 1–5 mg IV prn for hypertension
	2. Infiltrate area with a small amount (e.g., 1 mL) of solution (made by diluting 5–10 mg in 10 mL of NS) within 12 hours of extravasation
Effect	Nonselective, competitive α-adrenergic antagonist
Onset	Minutes
Duration	Half-life: 19 minutes
Clearance	Unknown metabolism; 10% renal elimination unmetabolized
Comments	May cause hypotension, reflex tachycardia, cerebrovascular spasm, dysrhythmias, stimulation of gastrointestinal tract, or hypoglycemia

Phenylephrine (Neo-Synephrine)

Indication	Hypotension
Dosage	IV: infusion initially at 10 μg/min, then titrated to response
	IV bolus: 40–100 μg/dose
	Standard mix: 20 mg in 250 mL D_5W or NS
Effect	α-Adrenergic agonist
Onset	Rapid
Duration	5–20 minutes
Clearance	Hepatic metabolism; renal elimination
Comments	May cause hypertension, reflex bradycardia, constricted microcirculation, uterine contraction, or uterine vasoconstriction

Phenytoin (Diphenylhydantoin, Dilantin)

Indications	1. Seizures, seizure prophylaxis
	2. Digoxin-induced dysrhythmias
	3. Refractory ventricular tachycardia
Dosage	1. Seizures
	IV: see Fosphenytoin
	Oral loading dose: 15–20 mg/kg; based on phenytoin serum concentrations and recent dosing history; administer oral loading dose in 3 divided doses given every 2–4 hours
	Maintenance dose: 300 mg/d or 5–6 mg/kg/d in 3 divided doses or 1–2 divided doses using extended release formulation
	2, 3. Arrhythmias:
	Children and adults:
	IV loading dose: **see Fosphenytoin**
	Children:
	Oral maintenance dose: 5–10 mg/kg/d in 2–3 divided doses
	Adults:
	Oral loading dose: 250 mg 4 times/d for 1 day, then 250 mg twice daily for 2 days
	Oral maintenance dose: 300–400 mg/d in divided doses 1–4 times/d
Effect	Anticonvulsant effect via membrane stabilization; antidysrhythmic effects similar to those of quinidine or procainamide
Onset	3–5 minutes
Duration	Dose dependent; half-life is dose dependent in therapeutic range
Clearance	Hepatic metabolism; renal elimination (enhanced by alkaline urine)
Comments	May cause nystagmus, diplopia, ataxia, drowsiness, gingival hyperplasia, gastrointestinal upset, hyperglycemia, or hepatic microsomal enzyme induction; IV bolus may cause bradycardia, hypotension, respiratory arrest, cardiac arrest, CNS depression; tissue irritant; crosses placenta; significant interpatient variation, from 7.5 to 20 μg/mL, in the dose needed to achieve therapeutic concentration; determination of unbound phenytoin levels may help in patients with renal failure or hypoalbuminemia; divide daily dose into 3 doses when using suspension, chewable tablets, or immediate release preparations; extended-release preparations may be dosed in adults every 12 or 24 hours if patient is not receiving concomitant enzyme-inducing drugs and apparent half-life is sufficiently long

Phosphorus (Phospho-Soda; Neutra-Phos; potassium phosphate; sodium phosphate)

Indications	1. Treatment and prevention of hypophosphatemia
	2. Short-term treatment of constipation
	3. Evacuation of the colon for rectal and bowel examinations
Dosage	1. Mild to moderate hypophosphatemia:
	Children <4 years:
	PO: 2–3 mmol/kg/d in divided doses
	Children >4 years and adults:
	PO: 250–500 mg 3 times/d for 3 days
	IV: 0.08–0.15 mmol/kg over 6 hours

Moderate to severe hypophosphatemia:
IV:
Children <4 years: 0.15–0.3 mmol/kg over 6 hours
Children >4 years and adults: 0.15–0.25 mmol/kg over 6–12 hours
2. Laxative [Fleet(R) Phospho(R)-Soda]:
Oral:
Children 5–9 years: 5 mL as a single dose
Children 10–12 years: 10 mL as a single dose
Children >12 years and adults: 20–30 mL as a single dose
3. Colonoscopy prep regimen [Fleet(R) Phospho(R)-Soda]:
Oral:
Adults: 45 mL diluted to 90 mL with water the evening prior to the
examination and repeat the dose again the following morning

Effect Electrolyte replacement
Onset Cathartic: 3–6 hours
Clearance 80% of dose reabsorbed by the kidneys
Comments Infuse doses of IV phosphate over a 4- to 6-hour period; risks of
rapid IV infusion include hypocalcemia, hypotension, muscular irritability, calcium deposits, renal function deterioration, and
hyperkalemia; orders for IV phosphate preparations should be written in mmol (1 mmol = 31 mg); use with caution in patients with cardiac disease and renal insufficiency; do not give with magnesium-
and aluminum-containing antacids or sucralfate, which can bind
with phosphate

Physostigmine (Antilirium)

Indications Postoperative delirium, tricyclic antidepressant overdose, reversal
of CNS effects of anticholinergic drugs
Dosage 0.5–2 mg IV every 15 minutes prn
Effect Inhibition of cholinesterase, central and peripheral cholinergic effects
Onset Rapid
Duration 30–60 minutes
Clearance Cholinesterase metabolism
Comments May cause bradycardia, tremor, convulsions, hallucinations, psychi-
atric, or CNS depression, mild ganglionic blockade, or cholinergic
crisis; crosses blood–brain barrier; antagonized by atropine; con-
tains sulfite

Potassium Chloride (KCl)

Indication Hypokalemia, digoxin toxicity
Dosage Adult:
20 mEq of KCl administered IV over 60–120 minutes
Usual maximum rate of infusion: 10 mEq/h
Pediatric:
0.5–1 mEq/kg/dose. Usual rate: 0.3–0.5 mEq/kg/h, up to a maximum
rate of 1 mEq/kg/h
Standard mix: 20 mEq in 250 mL of D_5W or NS
Effect To correct severe hypokalemia
Onset Immediate
Duration Variable

Clearance	Renal
Comments	Bolus administration may cause cardiac arrest; not to exceed a maximum single dose of 40 mEq in adults; serum potassium levels should be checked prior to repeat administration; a central venous line is preferable for administration

Procainamide (Pronestyl)

Indications	Atrial and ventricular dysrhythmias
Dosage	Loading dose: 10–50 mg/min IV until toxicity or desired effect occurs, up to 12 mg/kg; stop if $\geq$50% QRS widening, or if PR-interval lengthening occurs Maintenance dose: 2 mg/kg/h
Effect	Class IA antiarrhythmic; blocks sodium channels
Onset	Immediate
Duration	Half-life 2.5–4.5 hours, depending on acetylator phenotype
Clearance	25% hepatic conversion to active metabolite N-acetylprocainamide, a class III antiarrhythmic; renal elimination (50%–60% unchanged)
Comments	May cause increased ventricular response in atrial tachydysrhythmias unless predigitalized, asystole (with AV block), myocardial depression, CNS excitement, blood dyscrasia, lupus syndrome with positive antinuclear antibody test, or liver damage; IV administration can cause hypotension from vasodilation, decrease load by one-third in congestive heart failure or shock; therapeutic concentration is 4–8 mg/L

Prochlorperazine (Compazine)

Indications	Nausea and vomiting
Dosage	IV: 5–10 mg/dose IV ($\leq$40 mg/d) IM: 5–10 mg IM every 2–4 hours prn PR: 25 mg per rectum every 12 hours prn
Effect	Central (δ_2) antagonist with neuroleptic and antiemetic effects; also antimuscarinic and antihistaminic effects
Onset	Rapid
Duration	3–4 hours
Clearance	Hepatic metabolism; renal/biliary elimination
Comments	May cause hypotension, extrapyramidal reactions, neuroleptic malignant syndrome, leukopenia, or cholestatic jaundice; contains sulfites; caution in liver disease; less sedating than chlorpromazine

Promethazine (Phenergan)

Indications	Allergies, anaphylaxis, nausea and vomiting, sedation
Dosage	IM, IV: 12.5–50 mg IV every 4–6 hours prn
Effect	Antagonist of H-1, δ-1, and muscarinic receptors; antiemetic, and sedative
Onset	IV: 3–5 minutes IM: 20 minutes
Duration	2–4 hours
Clearance	Hepatic metabolism; renal elimination

Comments	May cause mild hypotension or mild anticholinergic effects; crosses placenta; may interfere with blood grouping; extrapyramidal effects rare; contains sulfite; intra-arterial injection can cause limb gangrene ("purple glove")

Propofol (Diprivan)

Indications	Sedation during mechanical ventilation
Dosage	Starting dose: 25–75 mg/h
	Maintenance dose: titrate by 25-mg increments every 15 minutes until desired response is achieved up to a maximum of 200–250 mg/h
	Bolus dose: 10–50 mg
Effect	General anesthetic and sedation in patients with mechanical ventilation
Onset	Rapid
Duration	10 minutes
Clearance	Cytochrome P-4502B6 (CYP2B6) with a high metabolic clearance that ranges from 1.6 to 3.4 L/min in healthy 70-kg adults, suggesting extrahepatic metabolism
Comments	Side effects include hypotension vomiting, rash, pain at the site of injection; IV bolus doses are associated with histamine release; use with caution in patients with documented egg allergy
	Sulfite warnings: Baxter propofol injectable emulsion contains sodium metabisulfite; the overall prevalence of sulfite sensitivity in the general population is unknown, is probably low, and is seen more frequently in patients with asthma
	There are no preservatives in either brand of propofol; vials and ampoules are for single use only; propofol is diluted in 10% fat emulsion; propofol should not be administered in the same IV line as other medications; admixed containers and tubing must be changed every 6 hours and unused drug discarded; infusion directly from bottles should be changed every 12 hours

Propranolol (Inderal)

Indications	Hypertension, atrial and ventricular dysrhythmias, myocardial ischemia/infarction, hypertension, thyrotoxicosis, hypertrophic cardiomyopathy, migraine headache
Dosage	Adult:
	Test dose of 0.25–0.5 mg IV, then titrate ≤1 mg/min to effect
	Oral: 10–40 mg every 6–8 hours, increase prn
	Pediatric: 0.01–0.1 mg/kg IV over 10 minutes
Effect	Nonspecific β-adrenergic blockade
Onset	IV: 2 minutes
	Oral: 30 minutes
Duration	IV: 1–6 hours
	Oral: 6 hours
Clearance	Hepatic metabolism; renal elimination
Comments	May cause bradycardia, AV dissociation, and hypoglycemia; bronchospasm, congestive heart failure, and drowsiness can occur with low doses; crosses placenta and blood–brain barrier; abrupt withdrawal can precipitate rebound angina

Protamine

Indication	Reversal of the effects of heparin
Dosage	1 mg/100 U of heparin activity IV at ≤5 mg/min
Effect	Polybasic compound forms complex with polyacidic heparin
Onset	30–60 seconds
Duration	2 hours (dependent on body temperature)
Clearance	Fate of heparin/protamine complex is unknown
Comments	May cause myocardial depression and peripheral vasodilation with sudden hypotension or bradycardia; may cause severe pulmonary hypertension, particularly in the setting of cardiopulmonary bypass; the protamine/heparin complex is antigenically active; transient reversal of heparin may be followed by rebound heparinization; can cause anticoagulation if given in excess relative to amount of circulating heparin (controversial); monitor response with partial thromboplastin time or activated clotting time

Ranitidine (Zantac)

Indications	Duodonal and gastric ulcers, reduction of gastric volume, raising gastric pH, esophageal reflux
Dosage	IV: 50–100 mg every 6–8 hours Continuous infusion for GI bleed: 12.5 mg/h Oral: 150–300 mg every 12 hours
Effect	Histamine H_2-receptor antagonist; inhibits basal, nocturnal, and stimulated gastric acid secretion
Onset	IV: rapid Oral: 1–3 hours
Duration	IV: 6–8 hours Oral: 12 hours
Clearance	70% renal elimination unchanged
Comments	Doses should be reduced by 50% with renal failure

Scopolamine (Hyoscine)

Indications	Antisialagogue; amnesia, sedation, antiemetic, anti–motion sickness
Dosage	IV, IM: 0.3–0.6 mg Transdermal: 1.5 mg patch every 72 hours
Effect	Peripheral and central cholinergic (muscarinic) antagonism
Onset	IV, IM: rapid Transdermal: 4 hours
Duration	Variable
Clearance	Hepatic metabolism; renal elimination
Comments	Excessive CNS depression can be reversed by physostigmine; may cause excitement or delirium, transient tachycardia, hyperthermia, urinary retention; crosses blood–brain barrier and placenta

Terbutaline (Brethine, Bricanyl)

Indications	1. Bronchospasm 2. Tocolysis (inhibition of premature labor)

Dosage	1. Adult:
	SQ: 0.25 mg SQ; repeat in 15 minutes prn (maximum: 0.5 mg in a 4-hour period);
	PO: 2.5–5 mg orally every 6 hours prn (maximum: 15 mg/d)
	Pediatric SQ: 0.005–0.01 mg/kg/dose to a maximum of 0.4 mg/dose every 15–20 minutes for 3 doses; may repeat every 2–6 hours prn
	2. Acute IV: 2.5–10 μg/min IV infusion; increase gradually every 10–20 minutes; Effective maximum doses from 17–30 μg/min have been used with caution. Duration of infusion is at least 12 hours
	Maintenance oral: 2.5–10 mg every 4–6 hours
Effect	β_2-Selective adrenergic agonist
Onset	SQ: <15 minutes
	PO: <30 minutes
Duration	SQ: 1.5–4 hours
	Oral: 4–8 hours
Clearance	Hepatic metabolism; renal elimination
Comments	May cause dysrhythmias, pulmonary edema, hypertension, hypokalemia, or CNS excitement

Theophylline

Indications	Bronchospasm
Dosage	Adult:
	Loading dose: 200–400 mg IV bolus
	Rate not to exceed 20 mg/min
	Maintenance dose: 8–64 mg/h
	Use lower doses in elderly, congestive heart failure, hepatic disease
Effect	Inhibition of phosphodiesterase and adenosine antagonism, resulting in bronchodilation with positive inotropic and chronotropic effects
Onset	Rapid
Duration	6–12 hours
Clearance	Hepatic metabolism, renal elimination (10% unchanged)
Comments	May cause tachydysrhythmias; therapeutic concentration, 10–20 μg/mL; each mg/kg raises concentration approximately 2 μg/mL; aminophylline 100 mg = theophylline 80 mg

Thiamine (vitamin B$_1$; Betalin)

Indications	Treatment of thiamine deficiency including beriberi, Wernicke's encephalopathy syndrome, peripheral neuritis associated with pellagra, and pregnancy
Dosage	Adult:
	Non–critical thiamine deficiency: 5–50 mg/d orally for 1 month
	Beriberi: 5–50 mg IM 3 times/d for 2 weeks, then switch to 5–50 mg orally every day for 1 month
	Severe deficiency: 50–100 mg IM or slow IV over 5 minutes repeated daily until oral therapy can be substituted; Maximum dose: 300 mg/24 hours
	Recommended daily allowance: 1.4 mg (males); 1 mg (females)
	Pediatric:

Noncritical thiamine deficiency: 10–50 mg/d orally in divided doses
for 2 weeks followed by 5–10 mg/d for 1 month
Beriberi: 10–25 mg/d IM for 2 weeks, then 5–10 mg orally every day
for 1 month
Recommended daily allowance for infants and children: 0.2–1.2 mg

Effect   Vitamin supplement
Clearance   Eliminated unchanged in urine, and as pyrimidine after body storage
sites become saturated
Comments   Single vitamin B_1 deficiency is rare, suspect multiple vitamin deficiencies; the IV route of administration is not recommended
because of the risk of anaphylaxis

Thiosulfate, sodium

Indication	1. Cyanide and nitroprusside antidote, cyanide poisoning
	2. Cisplatin rescue
Dosage	Adult:
	1. 12.5 g over 10 minutes after 300 mg of sodium nitrite; may repeat with 50% of initial dose if signs of cyanide toxicity recur
	2. 12 g/m^2 over 6 hours or 9 g/m^2 IV bolus followed by 1.2 g/m^2 continuous infusion for 6 hours
	Pediatric:
	1. 412.5 mg/kg of body weight or 7 g/m^2; administered IV at a rate 0.625–1.25 g/min (2.5–5 mL/min)
	2. 12 g/m^2 over 6 hours or 9 g/m^2 IV bolus followed by 1.2 g/m^2 continuous infusion for 6 hours
Effect	Facilitates conversion of cyanide to less toxic thiocyanate by rhodanese
Clearance	Renal elimination
Comments	Give after amyl nitrite and sodium nitrite

Tromethamine (Tris buffer; Tham)

Indications	Metabolic acidosis
Dosage	Adult and pediatric: dose depends on buffer base deficit; tromethamine mL of 0.3 M solution = body weight (kg) $\times$ base deficit (mEq/L) $\times$ 1.1
	Pediatric: maximum recommended pediatric dose is 33–40 mL/kg/d or 500 mg/kg/dose
Effect	Organic proton acceptor (buffer)
Onset	Rapid
Duration	Hours
Clearance	Rapidly eliminated by kidneys (>75% in 3 hours)
Comments	Use with caution in patients with renal impairment or chronic respiratory acidosis

---

Vasopressin (Antidiuretic hormone, Pitressin)

Indications	1. Diabetes insipidus
	2. Gastrointestinal bleeding
	3. Vasopressor augmentation in hypotension

4. Shock-refractory ventricular fibrillation/pulseless ventricular tachycardia

Dosage	1. IM/SQ: 5–10 U every 8–12 hours; IV: 2.4–10 Units/h as required based on serum electrolytes, osmolality, and urine specific gravity
	2. IV continuous infusion: 0.1–0.4 Units/min
	3. IV continuous infusion: 0.01–0.04 Units/min
	4. 40 Units IV push × 1
Effect	Synthetic posterior pituitary hormone that increases urine osmolality and decreases urine volume; smooth muscle contraction; constriction in splanchnic, coronary, muscle, and skin vasculature
Onset	Immediate
Duration	2–8 hours
Clearance	Hepatic and renal metabolism; renal elimination
Comments	May cause oliguria, water intoxication, pulmonary edema; hypertension, dysrhythmias, myocardial ischemia; abdominal cramps (from increased peristalsis); anaphylaxis; contraction of gallbladder, urinary bladder, or uterus; vertigo, or nausea; patients with coronary artery disease are often treated with concurrent nitroglycerin

Verapamil (Isoptin, Calan)

Indications	Supraventricular tachycardia, atrial fibrillation or flutter, Lown-Ganong-Levine syndrome
Dosage	Adult:
	Loading dose: 2.5–10 mg (75–150 μg/kg) IV at a rate of 1 mg/min; may repeat 2.5–5 mg every 10 minutes, not to exceed 20 mg
	Maintenance dose: 5–20 mg/h as titrated to patient response
	Pediatric:
	0–1 years: 0.1–0.2 mg/kg IV
	1–15 years: 0.1–0.3 mg/kg IV; repeat once if no response in 30 minutes
Effect	Blockade of slow calcium channels in heart; prolongation of PR interval with negative inotropy and chronotropy; systemic and coronary vasodilation
Onset	Oral: 1–2 hours
	IV: 1–5 minutes
Duration	Oral: 8–24 hours
	IV: 10 minutes–2 hours
Clearance	Hepatic metabolism; renal elimination
Comments	May cause severe bradycardia, AV block (especially with concomitant β-blockade), excessive hypotension, or congestive heart failure; may increase ventricular response to atrial fibrillation or flutter in patients with accessory tracts; active metabolite has 20% antihypertensive effect

Vitamin K/Phytonadione (AquaMEPHYTON)

Indications	Deficiency of vitamin K–dependent clotting factors; reversal of warfarin effect
Dosage	IV: 1–5 mg diluted; infuse over 20 minutes
	SQ/Oral: 2.5–5 mg
	If 8 hours after IV/SQ dose, PTT is not improved, repeat dose prn
Effect	Promotion of synthesis of clotting factors II, VII, IX, and X
Onset	PO: 6–12 hours

	IV: 1–2 hours
Duration	Variable
Clearance	Hepatic metabolism
Comments	If the international normalized ratio (INR) is above the therapeutic range but below five and rapid reversal is not indicated, omit the next dose or two of warfarin sodium and resume therapy at a lower maintenance dose when the INR returns to the therapeutic range
	If the INR is >5 and <9 **or** rapid reversal is required, vitamin K 0.5–1 mg IV or vitamin K 1–2.5 mg SQ or orally may be administered; if there is a high thrombotic risk, the option to withhold warfarin for 2 or more doses may be preferred
	If the INR is >9 and <20, vitamin K 2.5 mg IV or 5 mg SQ may be administered
	If the INR is >20, administration of fresh-frozen plasma is indicated along with vitamin K 2.5 mg IV or 5 mg SQ
	IV vitamin K is associated with a small risk of severe allergic reaction; when administered IV, doses infused over 20 minutes at a rate not to exceed 1 mg/min; reversal of anticoagulation by any means (vitamin K or fresh frozen plasma) is associated with a risk of thrombosis depending on the patient's underlying need for anticoagulation

Warfarin (Coumadin, Panwarfin)

Indication	Anticoagulation
Dosage	For patients restarting warfarin, resume warfarin therapy at the patient's maintenance dose
	Initiation:
	Patients ≥80 years old, or patients <80 years old who are <60 kg in weight: 2.5 mg
	Patients <80 years old and >60 kg in weight: 5 mg
	Large loading doses (≥10 mg/d) should not be used
	Monitor the international normalized ratio (INR) frequently during the first week of warfarin therapy to assure safe and efficient anticoagulation to target INR 2.5 (range 2–3)
Effect	Interferes with utilization of vitamin K by the liver and inhibits synthesis of factors II, VII, IX, and X
Onset	12–72 hours
Duration	2–5 days
Clearance	Hepatic metabolism; renal elimination
Comments	May be potentiated by ethanol, antibiotics, chloral hydrate, cimetidine, dextran, D-thyroxine, diazoxide, ethacrynic acid, glucagon, methyldopa, monoamine oxidase inhibitors, phenytoin, prolonged use of narcotics, quinidine, sulfonamides, congestive heart failure, hyperthermia, liver disease, malabsorption, and so on; may be antagonized by barbiturates, chlordiazepoxide, haloperidol, oral contraceptives, hypothyroidism, hyperlipidemia; crosses the placenta

Key to pharmacopeia symbols

D_5W, dextrose 5% water; IM, intramuscularly; IV, intravenously; NS, normal saline; SL, sublingually; SQ, subcutaneously.

TABLE A-1 Common Intravenous Antimicrobial Agents

Drug	Usual Adult IV Dose[a]	Usual Dose Interval[b]	Comments
Amikacin	300 mg	Every 8 hours	Aminoglycoside. Dose adjustment required for renal impairment
Amphotericin B	Initial dose: 0.25 mg/kg administered over 6 hours; dose should be gradually increased, ranging up to 1 mg/kg/day or 1.5 mg/kg on alternate days	Every 24–48 hours	Broad-spectrum antifungal. Initial test dose: 1 mg infused over 30 min–hour. Do not exceed 1.5 mg/kg/d concomitant nephrotoxic drugs should be avoided if at all possible
Amphotericin liposomal	3–5 mg/kg/day over 6 hours	Every 24 hours	Broad-spectrum antifungal reserved for: Nephrotoxicity to amphotericin with a serum creatinine increase by ≥1.5 mg/dL over baseline despite adequate hydration Initial therapy of fungal infection in patients with preexisting renal disease: baseline serum creatinine ≥2.5 mg/dL Systemic reactions to amphotericin persisting for >3–5 days despite acetaminophen, meperidine, diphenhydramine, and/or corticosteroids Progression of documented fungal disease (by clinical, radiographic, or histopathologic assessment) despite a minimum total course of standard amphotericin B of 500 mg or 7 mg/kg
Ampicillin	1 g	Every 4 hours	Penicillin. Combined with sulbactam is Unasyn[1]
Ampicillin–sulbactam (2:1)	3 g	Every 6 hours	Not effective against *Pseudomonas aeruginosa*
Azithromycin	500–1,000 mg	Every 24 hours	Macrolide for atypical pneumonia and in with a third-generation cephalosporin for community-acquired pneumonia. Effective against *Legionella*
Aztreonam	1 g	Every 8 hours	Can be used for patients allergic to penicillins or cephalosporins

Drug	Dose	Interval	Comments
Cefazolin	1 g	Every 8 hours	First-generation cephalosporin. Adjust dose in renal disease.[c] Use caution in patients allergic to penicillin[d]
Cefepime	1–2 g	Every 12 hours	Fourth-generation cephalosporin. Preferred for *P. aeruginosa* and neutropenic patients with fever[c,d]
Ceftazidime	1 g	Every 8 hours	Third-generation cephalosporin[c,d]
Ceftriaxone	1 g	Every 24 hours	Second-generation cephalosporin. Preferred for empiric coverage of bacterial meningitis in higher doses[c,d]
Ciprofloxacin	400 mg	Every 12 hours	Quinolone. Good absorption via oral route (500 mg q12 h). Effective against *P aeruginosa*
Clindamycin	600 mg	Every 8 hours	Highly associated with *Clostridium difficile* colitis
Daptomycin	4 mg/kg IV	Every 24 hours	Adjust dose for renal insufficiency: Cr. clearance <30 mL/min: 4 mg/kg IV every 48 hours. Hemodialysis: 4 mg/kg IV once every 48 hours after hemodialysis
Doxycycline	100 mg	Every 12 hours	Rare hepatotoxicity, pseudotumor cerebri, and benign intracranial hypertension have been reported
Erythromycin	0.5–1 g	Every 6 hours	Macrolide. Bacteriostatic. Gastritis with orally route. Venous irritation
Fluconazole	200–400 mg	Every 24 hours	Broad-spectrum antifungal. Well absorbed orally. Dose adjustments required in renal and hepatic insufficiency
Gentamicin	60–120 mg (3–5 mg/kg/d)	Every 8–12 hours over 30 minutes	Aminoglycoside. Decrease dose in renal failure. Renal and ototoxicity. Precipitates with heparin. May prolong neuromuscular blockade
Imipenem–cilastatin	500 mg	Every 6 hours	Carbapenem. Preferred for multiple-drug resistant gram-negative bacterial infections[c,d]
Levofloxacin	500 mg	Every 24 hours	Quinolone. L-isomer of ofloxacin. Well absorbed orally. Dose adjustments required in moderate to severe renal insufficiency

(continued)

	TABLE A-1 Common Intravenous Antimicrobial Agents (continued)		
Drug	**Usual Adult IV Dose[a]**	**Usual Dose Interval[b]**	**Comments**
Linezolid	600 mg	Every 12 hours	Also available orally with equal efficacy. Anemia, thrombocytopenia, and leukopenia can occur. Will resolve with discontinuation of the drug
Meropenem	0.5–1 g	Every 8 hours	Carbapenem.[c,d] See Imipenem
Metronidazole	500 mg	Every 8 hours	Possible acute toxic psychosis; disulfiram-like reaction with convulsions, leukopenia
Micafungin	50–100 mg	Every 24 hours	Echinocandin. Broad-spectrum antifungal. Monitor liver function tests
Nafcillin	1.5 g	Every 4 hours	Preferred for antistaphylococcal coverage.[c,d] May induce interstitial nephritis
Penicillin G[1]	500,000–2,000,000 Units	Every 4 hours	Hypersensitivity is common[c,d]
Piperacillin	4 g	Every 6 hours	Usually combined with aminoglycoside for treatment of Pseudomonas[c,d]
Piperacillin–tazobactam (8:1)	3.375 g	Every 6 hours	Tazobactam expands activity to include β-lactamase–producing strains of Staphylococcus aureus, Haemophilus influenzae, Enterobacteriaceae, Pseudomonas, Klebsiella, Citrobacter, Serratia, Bacteroides, and other gram-negative anaerobes[c,d]
	4.5 g	Every 8 hours	
Ticarcillin-clavulanic acid (30:1)	3.1 g	Every 4 hours	Clavulanic acid expands activity to include β-lactamase–producing strains of S. aureus, H. influenzae, Enterobacteriaceae, P. aeruginosa, Klebsiella, Citrobacter, and Serratia[c,d]
Trimethoprim/sulfame thoxazole	8–10 mg/kg/day (based on trimethoprim component)	Every 6–12 hours	Allergic reactions common. Interferes with secretion of creatinine and potassium; values may increase
Tobramycin	60–120 mg (3–5 mg/kg/day over 15–20 minutes)	Every 8 hours	Aminoglycoside. See gentamicin

Vancomycin	500 mg–1 g over 60 minutes	Every 12 hours	Preferred for oxacillin-resistant staphylococcal infections and patients with penicillin allergy. Decrease dose in renal disease. Histamine release ("red man"), renal damage, deafness. May precipitate with other medications
Voriconazole	Load: 6 mg/kg IV q12 h for two doses Maintenance: 4 mg/kg IV q12 h	Every 12 hours	Broad-spectrum antifungal. Monitor liver function tests. May increase the concentrations of other drugs metabolized by the CYP3A4 pathway. Coadministration with phenytoin, carbamazepine, and long-acting barbiturates will decrease plasma voriconazole concentrations. Voriconazole increases the plasma concentrations of sirolimus, efavirenz, rifabutin, and ergot alkaloids

See also Chapter 12.

[a]Adult doses are those usually given to healthy 70-kg patients and may vary with the patient's condition or concomitant drug intake. Older or debilitated patients may require smaller doses.

[b]Dose adjustments may be required in patients with renal impairment, hepatic dysfunction, and altered volume status.

[c]All β-lactams in high concentrations will cause seizures and should be dosed based on the creatinine clearance.

[d]From 5% to 10% of penicillin-allergic patients will react to cephalosporins and carbapenems.

TABLE A-2 Opioids Comparison Chart

Drug	Adult Dose[a] (mg)	Pediatric Dose[a] (mg/kg)	Duration of Action (h)	Conversion Factor	Metabolism	Comments
Codeine			4		Hepatic to morphine	Avoid IV route due to large histamine release and cardiovascular effects
Parenteral	15–60	0.5–1		0.08		
Oral	15–60	0.5–1		0.05		
Fentanyl			0.5–2		Hepatic	Rapid IV injection can result in skeletal muscle and chest wall rigidity 25, 50, 75, or 100 μg/h
Parenteral	0.05–0.1	0.001–0.002		100		
Transdermal				100		Pediatric use not well established
Hydromorphone			4		Hepatic; eliminated in urine, principally as glucuronide conjugates	
Parenteral	1–2	0.015–0.05		0.67		
Oral	2–4	0.03–0.08		1.33		
Meperidine			3–4		Hepatic; normeperidine (metabolite) is dependent on renal function and can accumulate with high doses or in patients with decreased renal function	Use with caution in patients with hepatic or renal failure, seizure disorders, or receiving high doses of serotonin-uptake inhibitors. Normeperidine (CNS stimulant) may accumulate and precipitate twitching, tremor, or seizures; **contraindicated with concurrent use of MAO inhibitors**
Parenteral	50–150	1–1.5		0.1		

					Metabolism	
Methadone						
Parenteral	2–10	0.1	6–8, increases to 22–48 with repeated doses	1.3		Phenytoin, pentazocine, and rifampin may increase the metabolism of methadone and may precipitate withdrawal; increased toxicity: CNS depressants, phenothiazines, tricyclic antidepressants, and MAO inhibitors may potentiate the adverse effects of methadone
Oral	2–10	0.1–0.2		0.7	Metabolism is four times greater after oral administration than after parenteral administration	
Morphine						
Parenteral	5–10	0.1–0.2	3–5	1	In the liver via glucuronide conjugation; excreted unchanged in urine	Histamine release; may cause hypotension in patients with acute myocardial infarction
Oral[b]	10–30	0.2–0.5	4	0.33	Hepatic	
Oxycodone						
Oral	5	0.05–0.15		0.33		

See also **Chapter 7.**

CNS, central nervous system; IV, intravenous; MAO, monoamine oxidase.

[a] These doses (oral, intramuscular) are recommended starting doses for acute pain. Optimal doses for each patient are determined by titration, and the maximal dose is limited by adverse effects. For single starting intravenous doses, use *half* the intramuscular dose listed. Any oral or parenteral analgesic may be converted into its intramuscular morphine equivalent by multiplying the dose by the conversion factor.

[b] Controversy exists concerning the actual conversion factor (3:1 ratio).

TABLE
A-3

Comparison of Benzodiazepines

Drug	Adult Dose Range (mg/day)	Time to Peak Plasma Level (hours)	Half-life (hours)	Active Metabolites
Long acting				
Chlordiazepoxide (Librium)	15–100	1–4	5–30	Desmethylchlordiazepoxide Demoxepam N-Desmethyldiazepam
Clonazepam (Klonapin)	1.5–12	1–4	30–40	None
Diazepam (Valium)	6–40	0.5–2	20–80	N-Desmethyldiazepam N-Methyloxazepam (temaxepam) Oxazepam
Flurazepam (Dalmane)	15–60	2–6	40–114	N-Desalkylflurazepam
Short acting				
Alprazolam (Xanax)	0.75–4	1–2	12–15	None
Lorazepam (Ativan)	2–6	2–4	10–20	75% is converted to the glucuronide derivative (12-hour half-life), which can accumulate in prolonged dosing
Midazolam (Versed)	2.5–30	0.25–1	1–4	α-Hydroxymidazolam
Oxazepam (Serax)	30–120	2–4	5–16	None

See also Chapter 7.

Page numbers followed by f denotes figure; those followed by t denote tables